Recent Trends in Animal and Veterinary Sciences

Recent Trends in Animal and Veterinary Sciences

Editor: Hugh Patmore

Callisto Reference
www.callistoreference.com

Callisto Reference,
118-35 Queens Blvd., Suite 400,
Forest Hills, NY 11375, USA

Visit us on the World Wide Web at:
www.callistoreference.com

ISBN: 978-1-63239-961-8 (Hardback)

Printed in China.

Cataloging-in-Publication Data

Recent trends in animal and veterinary sciences / edited by Hugh Patmore.
p. cm.
Includes bibliographical references and index.
ISBN 978-1-63239-961-8
1. Veterinary medicine. 2. Animals--Diseases. 3. Animal health. I. Patmore, Hugh.
SF745 .R43 2018
636.089--dc23

Table of Contents

Preface

The branch of medicine which is concerned with the diseases and medical disorders of animals and birds is known as veterinary medicine. It helps in controlling zoonotic diseases by monitoring and treating animals. Veterinary science branches out in sub-specialties such as veterinary dentistry, veterinary ophthalmology, veterinary pharmacology, etc. This book is a valuable compilation of topics, ranging from the basic to the most complex advances in the field of veterinary science and medicine. This book, with its detailed analyses and data, will prove immensely beneficial to professionals and students involved in this area at various levels.

Significant researches are present in this book. Intensive efforts have been employed by authors to make this book an outstanding discourse. This book contains the enlightening chapters which have been written on the basis of significant researches done by the experts.

Finally, I would also like to thank all the members involved in this book for being a team and meeting all the deadlines for the submission of their respective works. I would also like to thank my friends and family for being supportive in my efforts.

Editor

1

Enrichment of bovine semen with x-bearing spermatozoa using Percoll™ and Optiprep® discontinuous gradients

Vera Hossepian de Lima[1], Mariney Flavia Di-Tanno Ramalho[2], Beatriz Costa Aguiar Alves[3], Aline Costa Lucio[1], Leticia Zoccolario Oliveira[1], Carlos Alberto Moreira Filho[3], Luísa Cunha Carneiro[1, *]

[1]Department of Preventive Veterinary Medicine and Animal Reproduction, Estadual University of Sao Paulo, UNESP, Jaboticabal, Brazil
[2]Research Center of Biotechnology, University of Sao Paulo, Sao Paulo, Brazil
[3]Department of Pediatrics, Medicine School of Estadual Universtiy of Sao Paulo, Sao Paulo, SP, Brazil

Email address:
verahossepian@gmail.com (V. H. de Lima), mramalho@fcav.unesp.br (M. F. Di-Tanno Ramalho), bcaalves@uol.com.br (B. C. A. Alves), alinelucio@hotmail.com (A. C. Lucio), leticiazoccolario@yahoo.com.br (L. Z. Oliveira), cmoreira@icb.usp.br (C. A. M. Filho), luisacunhacarneiro@hotmail.com (L. C. Carneiro)

Abstract: In cattle, sex selection has a significant economic impact when it improves herd capacity of milk or meat production. Density gradient centrifugation might be an approach to sexing spermatozoa because of the additional DNA content and volume of X-bearing sperm head. In the present work, the accuracy of sperm sexing by Percoll™ and OptiPrep® gradients centrifugation was compared. Bovine semen from three breeds (Holstein, Gir, and Red Angus) was used. The sperm viability and sexing accuracy after sperm selection by centrifugation of low and high-density discontinuous gradient composed by three layers of Percoll™ or OptiPrep® were assessed by *in vitro* embryo production (IVP) and pregnancy rate following artificial insemination (AI). After IVP, cleavage rate was higher ($P < 0.05$) for unsexed (81.3%) than for sexed (75.5%) spermatozoa. A significantly lower cleavage rate was observed for sexed (76.1%) spermatozoa when compared to sexed Red Angus (81.2%) spermatozoa. Additionally, significantly lower blastocyst rate was observed using Holstein sexed sperm by OptiPrep® gradient (23.3%) when compared with Gir (41.9%) and Red Angus (48.7%) sexed sperm by Percoll™ gradient. Nevertheless, in all breeds analyzed, a significant sex ratio deviation to females was observed. Analyzing the pregnancy rate after AI with sexed sperm by Percoll™ and OptiPrep®, semen from Gir bulls presented lower ($P <0.05$) pregnancy/AI (61.3%)when compared to Red Angus (75.9%) and Holstein (77.4%) and bulls. From the results, it was concluded that the increase in female percentage after insemination and/or IVP with bovine sexed sperm by centrifugation of high density gradient composed by three layers of Percoll™ and OptiPrep® may allow this spermatozoa sexing technique to be used in large scale which would support genetic enhancement for milk and meat production as well as for progeny tests in cattle.

Keywords: Artificial Insemination, Bovine Sexed Semen, *In Vitro* Production

1. Introduction

In cattle, sex selection has a significant economic impact. It improves the herd capacity of milk and meat production [1; 2; 3].

Since bovine X-bearing sperm cells carry 3.8% more DNA than the Y-bearing spermatozoa, these two sperm types can be separated in two sperm subpopulations by flow cytometry [4;5] according to their differences in specific sperm head volume [6,7] and differences in the intensity of specific DNA-binding fluorochrome [4]. Alternatively, density gradient centrifugation can be another approach to sperm sexing [8; 9; 10; 11; 12; 13] given that the extra DNA content and head volume of X- bearing spermatozoa is also related to a higher density of these cells, approximately 0.006% [14].

In bovines, reference [15] used two centrifugations protocols for separating X and Y sperm populations in discontinuous low density gradient of Percoll™. The gradients contained 10 layers of Percoll™ solutions (0.6 mL each layer) with density ranging from 1.034 to 1.068 g/mL at 6 °C. This method increased 75% of X-bearing and 65% of

Y-bearing sperm cells in bottom and upper fractions, respectively, which was confirmed by *in situ* hybridization. Reference [8] employing this same methodology for sperm selection, utilized the sperm cells from these two fractions for *in vitro* embryo production (IVP). The genetic sex of embryos was assessed by PCR (Polymerase Chain Reaction) and, according to the results, the use of sperm cells from upper and lower layers produced 75% and 92% of male and female embryos, respectively. A similar experiment was performed by reference [9] which observed, after *in situ* hybridization, 70% X-bearing spermatozoa in bottom fraction and 65% of Y-bearing spermatozoa in upper fraction.

In humans, reference [16] using low density gradient centrifugation at 6 °C, composed by 7 layers of Percoll™ solutions (1.050 to 1.123 g/mL) and one layer of NycoPrep™ (1.115 g/mL), detected by *in situ* hybridization 61% of X-bearing spermatozoa in the lower fraction. Recently, reference [13] were able to separate 60% of X-bearing human spermatozoa using low density gradient centrifugation at room temperature with a gradient composed by 8 layers of 38% to 84% of albumin.

However, despite those interesting results reported above, this sexing methodology has never been used as a common tool in animal reproductive procedures, mainly due to the limited success and the low repeatability of such bio technique. Hence, the aim of the present study was to evaluate if bovine sperm centrifugation on high and low discontinuos density gradients composed by three layers of Percoll™ or OptiPrep® are able to increase the X-bearing sperm population in the bottom layer of the gradient.

2. Experimental Development

All reagents used in this study were obtained from Sigma-Aldrich (St Louis, MO, USA) unless otherwise stated.

2.1. Semen Collection and Quality Control

For all trials, semen was collected from 10 bulls of three breeds (ranging from 4 to 8 years old, 2 Holstein Friesian, 4 Gir and 4 Red Angus) in a routine collection schedule using an artificial vagina. After collection, sperm concentration was determined by a hemocytometer in a 1:200 dilution.

The percentages of progressive motile sperm and vigor were determined subjectively under a bright-field microscope at 400X magnification. Only ejaculates with a concentration higher than 900x 10^6 sperm/mL, a progressive motility of at least 60% and vigor between 4 to 5 were processed. Thereafter, 3mL samples from 75 ejaculates were divided in half to produce sexed and non-sexed sperm.

Procedures for sexing, processing and freezing Percoll™ discontinuous density gradient

Percoll™ (Pharmacia Fine Chemicals, Uppsala, Sweden) stock solution (PSS; density 1.123 g/mL) was prepared adding 9 parts (v/v) of Percoll™ (density 1.130 g/mL) to 1 (v/v) of 10 X concentrated (DMEM 10 X) containing 0.01 g/L gentamicin sulfate; 6mM HEPES; pH 7.4; 280-320 mOsm/kg of H_2O. To prepare the discontinuous density gradient, PSS was diluted with DMEM 1 X (containing 0.01 g/L of gentamicin sulfate; 6 mM of HEPES; 0.3% bovine serum albumin V fraction, BSA (Calbiochem, Darmstadt, Germany; pH 7.4) to produce different densities.

Gradient 1 (G1) was prepared to be used as a control group. It was composed by 10 layers of Percoll™ solutions (1 mL each layer), with the following densities: 1.034 g/mL, 1.038 g/mL, 1.042 g/mL, 1.045 g/mL, 1.049 g/mL, 1.053 g/mL, 1.057 g/mL, 1.059 g/mL, 1.064 g/mL, 1.068 g/mL.

Gradient 2 (G2) was composed by 3 layers of 3mL each of Percoll™ solutions of densities ranging from 1.110 g/mL to 1.123 g/mL.

The Percoll™ discontinuous gradient was prepared by layering each solution of Percoll™ from the densest to the lowest in 15 mL centrifuge tubes (Corning, 430053, New York, USA), with the help of an adjustable pipette with a reservoir for automated volume dispenser (Labsystems, 4540, Helsinki, Finland).

2.2. OptiPrep® Discontinuous Density Gradient

The OptiPrep® (Axis-Shield, 1114542, New York, USA) was diluted in DMEM 1X (D1152, Sigma-Aldrich, St Louis, MO, USA) medium in different proportions to produce different densities solutions.

Gradient 3 (G3) was composed by 3 layers of OptiPrep® solution with 3 mL each, of densities ranging from 1.123 g/mL to 1.163 g/mL.

Gradient 4 (G4) was composed by 10 layers of 1 mL each of Optiprep™ solutions with densities: 1.034 g/mL, 1.038 g/mL, 1.042 g/mL, 1.045 g/mL, 1.049 g/mL, 1.053 g/mL, 1.057 g/mL, 1.059 g/mL, 1.064 g/mL, 1.068 g/mL.

The discontinuous gradient of OptiPrep® was prepared by layering each OptiPrep® solution, from the densest to the lowest, in 15 mL centrifuge tubes (Corning, 430053, New York, USA), with the help of an adjustable pipette with a reservoir for automated volume dispenser (Labsystems, 4540, Helsinki, Finland).

2.3. Spermatozoa Centrifugation in Discontinuous Density Gradients

Aliquots of 1.0 mL of semen containing 90 x 10^6 spermatozoa were layered gently on each discontinuous density gradient that was then centrifuged in a bench-top centrifuge at 500 x *g* for 15 minutes, at 22°C. Next, the supernatant was discarded using a Pasteur pipette. Pellets were resuspended with 200 µL of Tris-egg yolk extender containing 1.4 M glycerol. Sperm concentration was adjusted to 12 x 10^6 spermatozoa/straw.

2.4. Further Processing and Freezing

Sexed or non-sexed sperm of each ejaculate was cooled at 5°C for 1-2 hours and packaged in 0.25 mL French straws (IMV, Aigle, France), each containing 12 x 10^6 spermatozoa. After packaging, straws were kept in freezing racks and frozen in an automatic freezer (IMV, Aigle, France) and stored in liquid nitrogen at -196 °C. Three days after freezing, one straw of each batch was thawed at 35°C for 20 sec and quality parameters were established. The minimum values obtained immediately after thawing (0 hours) were 30% progressive motility and vigor 4; and after the resistance test (3 hours) were 20% spermatozoids with progressive motility and vigor 3.

2.5. Experiment 1 - In vitro Embryo Production Using Spermatozoa Sexed by Density Gradient Centrifugation

Ovaries collected at slaughterhouse were transported to laboratory in saline solution at 33°C. Immature cumulus oocyte complexes (COCs) were aspirated from follicles with a diameter of 3 and 6 mm.The COCs were washed in TCM-199, supplemented with 0.2 mM of sodium pyruvate, 20 mM of HEPES, 5 mM of sodium bicarbonate, and 16.67 µg/mL of amikacin. The oocytes were matured in TCM-199 with 0.2 mM of sodium pyruvate, 25 mM Na_2HCO_3, 16.67 µg/mL amikacin, 1 µg/mL 17-β estradiol, 0.5 µg/mL follicle stimulating hormone (FSH; Folltropin™, Bioniche Animal Health, Belleville, USA), 5.0 µg luteinizing hormone (LH; Lutropin-V, Vetefarm, London, UK), and 10% (v/v) fetal calf serum (FCS; Gibco-BRL, Grand Island, NY, USA). The COCs were matured in 100 µL droplets (20 oocytes per droplet) under mineral oil at 38.5 °C in 5% CO_2 humid atmosphere for 22 hours.

For IVP of bovine embryos, matured oocytes were inseminated with frozen-thawed non-sexed or sexed semen. In each group, the straws were thawed at 35 °C for 30 sec and layered on top of a gradient composed by 1 mL fraction each of 45% and 90% isotonic Percoll™. After 30 min centrifugation at 900 x *g* the supernatant was discarded and the pellet adjusted with fertilization medium to obtain a final concentration of 100 x 10^3 spermatozoa in each fertilization droplet. The oocytes and sperm were incubated for 20 h in 5% CO_2, in humidified air at 38.5 °C, in TALP-IVF medium. Presumptive zygotes were denuded and co-cultured with synthetic oviduct fluid (SOF) medium. They were then transferred to four-well dishes, and the embryo culture was done at 38.5°C in a humid atmosphere containing 5% CO_2, 5% O_2, and 90% N_2 [17]. The cleavage was assessed 48 h after IVF and the blastocyst at 7 to 8 days of culture. Fetal calf serum (FCS) was not added during *in vitro* culture, as previously recommended [18]. Embryos in blastocyst stage were frozen individually into microtubes containing 10µL of double distilled water and stored at -20 °C for further determination of the genetic sex by PCR.

2.6. Determination of Embryo Genetic Sex by PCR

Before amplification reactions, a Proteinase K (Gibco-BRL, CA, USA) digestion of each embryo was performed. Each embryo received 5µg of Proteinase K and was kept at 37 °C for 1 hour; the Proteinase K was then denatured at 98°C for 10 min.

Each sample was amplified by two distinct and independent reactions, named A and B. Reaction A consisted in the simultaneous amplification of two Y-chromosome specific segments using primer pairs 1 (forward 5'-CCTCCCCTTGTTCAAACGCCCGGAATCATT-3' and reverse 5'-TGCTTGACTGCAGGGACCGAGAGGTTTGGG-3') and 2 (forward 5'-ATCAGTGCAGGGACCGAGATG-3' and reverse 5'-AAGCAGCCGATAAACACTCCTT-3'). Primer pairs 1 and 2 amplified a 210 bp [19]and a 250 bp [20] product in bovine males, respectively; reaction B, by its turn, amplified a 280 bp product from a repetitive sequence of the bovine genome used as internal control (primer pair 3: 5'-AGGTCGCGAGATTGGTCGCTAGGTCATGCA- 3' and 5'-AAGACCTCGAGAGACCCTCTTCAACACGT-3';) [21]. Thus, female samples produced only one band of 280 bp resulted from the amplification reaction B while male samples produced 3 bands of 280 bp and 250 bp (reaction A) and of 210 bp (reaction B).

Amplification reactions were performed in 10mM Tris-HCl buffer with 1mM of EDTA, pH 8; 2mM $MgCl_2$, 1U of Taq DNA Polimerase (AmpliTaq Gold, Applied Biosystem, Forrest City, CA, USA) and 10 pmol of each primer. Reactions A were submitted to 40 cycles of 94°C for 60 sec, 58°C for 30 sec, and 72°C for 60 sec, followed by 7 min at 72°C. Reactions B were submitted to 38 cycles of 94°C for 60 sec, 58°C for 60 sec, and 72°C for 60 sec, followed by 7 min at 72°C.

Amplified products were visualized in a 5% agarose gel and analyzed with Stratagene software (Eaglesight® Software).

2.7. Experiment 2 - Artificial Insemination Using Spermatozoa Sexed by Percoll™ or OptiPrep® Discontinuous Density Gradient Centrifugation

A total of 390 extensively pasture raised heifers (*Bosindicus* X *Bos Taurus*), with age ranging from 24 and 36 months, were inseminated for the present experiment. The heifers presented body condition score higher than 4.5 in a scale from 1(emaciated) to 9 (extremely fat). Estrus detection and AI were performed by two experienced technicians. Heifers were inseminated following natural estrus [22] with semen sexed by gradients G1 or G2, or with non-sexed semen from the same ejaculate.

2.8. Fetal Sexing by Ultrasound

Transrectal ultrasonography was performed 60 to 70 days after AI to evaluate pregnancy rates (pregnancy per AI) and to identify fetal gender using a Pie Medical Scanner (200 apparatus with linear transductor of 5 MHz), according to the criteria described by reference [23].

2.9. Statistical Analysis

The effect of sexing or breed on cleavage and blastocyst rates (Experiment 1) was analyzed with multiple comparison Analyses of Variance (ANOVA) followed by the Tukey test of Multiple Comparisons. Data were expressed as percentages on mean ± SD. Pregnancy rate and fetal sex (Experiment 2) were analyzed by Chi-square (X^2).

3. Results

Regarding the proportion of sperm recovered from the bottom of density gradients after centrifugation in Percoll™ and Optiprep® gradients, no difference was observed among the groups (P > 0.05; a total of 13% in Percoll™ and 10% in Optiprep® gradients; n= 75 ejaculates from 10 bulls). The recovered sperm was used to produce 439, 406, and 368 doses of sexed sperm of Gir, Holstein, and Red Angus breeds, respectively (total of 1213 sexed doses).

Regarding semen quality after thawing, it was observed that the sexing procedure reduced (P <0.05) sperm viability. In non-sexed semen, 100% of 75 ejaculates presented a minimum sperm motility of 50% and vigor 4. In sexed semen, 66.7% (50 of 75) of the batches presented a minimum sperm motility of 50% and vigor 4. After sperm thermal resistance test (TTR), in non-sexed semen, 84% (63/75) of the batches presented a minimum sperm motility of 20% and vigor 3. In sexed semen, after TTR, 20.6% of the batches presented a minimum sperm motility of 20% and vigor.

3.1. Experiment 1 - In Vitro Embryo Production Using Sexed Spermatozoa by Density Gradient Centrifugation

Cleavage and blastocyst rates were calculated considering the total number of oocytes used for each gradient used, per breed.

No difference on cleavage rate was observed between high and low density gradients of Percoll™ and Optiprep®. For all breeds, sexed spermatozoa had an effect (P <0.01) on cleavage rate of IVP. Using non-sexed sperm, cleavage rate (81.3%) was higher (P <0.05) than using sexed sperm (75.5%) (Table 1).

Table 1. *Means of cleavage and blastocyst rates of in vitro produced bovine embryos using 75 batches of spermatozoa either non-sexed or sexed by Percoll™ (G1 and G2)[a] or OptiPrep® (G3 and G4)[b] discontinuous density gradient centrifugation from semen of Gir, Holstein, and Red Angus bulls.*

Treatment	Total number of oocytes	Cleavage rate* (% ± SD)	Blastocyst rate** (% ± SD)
Unsexed	5115	81.0 ± 7.9	38.1 ± 11.8
Sexed	5963	75.6 ± 13.1	33.4 ±13.7

*P<0.0001(Chi-square)
**P=0.0023(Chi-square)
[a]G1: densities from 1.110 g/mL to 1.123 g/mL; G2: densities from 1,034 to 1,045 g/mL
[b]G3: densities from 1.123 g/mL to 1.163 g/mL; G4: densities from 1,034 g/mL to 1,045 g/mL

Table 2. *Breed effect on cleavage rate means of in vitro produced bovine embryos using 75 baths of spermatozoa sexed by Percoll™ (G1 and G2)a or OptiPrep® (G3 and G4)b discontinuous density gradient centrifugation from semen of Gir, Holstein, and Red Angus bulls.*

Breed	Total number of oocytes	Cleavage rate (% ± SD)
Gir	3011	76.1± 13.4[c]
Holstein	4776	77.7± 8.2[cd]
Red Angus	3291	81.2±11.7[d]

[a]G1: densities from 1.110 g/mL to 1.123 g/mL; G2: densities from 1,034 to 1,045 g/mL
[b]G3: densities from 1.123 g/mL to 1.163 g/mL; G4: densities from 1,034 g/mL to 1,045 g/mL
[c-d] Means without common superscript letters differ P <0.05 (Chi-square).

Breed also had an effect on cleavage rate (P <0.05). The cleavage rate obtained from sexed semen of Red Angus (81.2%) was significantly higher when compared to cleavage rate obtained from sexed semen of Gir (76.1%) (Table 2).

Gradient centrifugation had a significant effect (P>0.01) on blastocyst rate, as shown by comparing means of blastocysts obtained from sexed (35.0%) and non-sexed (38.1%) sperm (Table 1).

Table 3. *Breed effect on blastocyst rate means of in vitro produced bovine embryos using 75 baths of spermatozoa sexed by Percoll™ (G1 and G2) or OptiPrep® (G3 and G4) discontinuous density gradient centrifugation from semen of Gir, Holstein, and Red Angus.*

Breed	Gradient[a]	Blastocyst rate (% ± SD)
Gir	G1	42.0 ± 13.3[b]
	G2	37.4 ± 11.5[b]
	G3	41.9 ± 12.5[b]
	G4	36.9 ± 12.8[b]
Holstein	G1	30.1 ± 11.8[b]
	G2	29.9 ± 9.7[b]
	G3	23.2 ± 9.8[b]
	G4	36.9 ± 12.2[b]
Red Angus	G1	36.6 ± 14.5[bc]
	G2	37.4 ± 11.4[bc]
	G3	48.6 ± 12.4[b]
	G4	30.0 ± 7.5[c]

[a]G1: densities from 1.110 g/mL to 1.123 g/mL; G2: densities from 1,034 to 1,045 g/mL; G3: densities from 1.123 g/mL to 1.163 g/mL; G4: densities from 1,034 g/mL to 1,045 g/mL.
[b-c] Means without common superscript letters differ, P<0.05 (Test Tukey)

There was an association (P<0.001) between breed and sexing for blastocyst rate. The Tukey test for sexing and breed allowed pair-wise comparison of all means, considering either breed or discontinuous density gradient (Tables 3 and 4).

Table 4. *Gradient effect on blastocyst rate means of in vitro produced bovine embryos using 75 baths of spermatozoa sexed by Percoll™ (G1 and G2) or OptiPrep® (G3 and G4) discontinuous density gradient centrifugation from semen of Gir, Holstein, and Red Angus bulls.*

Gradient[a]	Breed	Blastocyst rate (% ± SD)
G1	Gir	42.0 ± 13.3[b]
	Holstein	30.1 ± 11.8[b]
	Red Angus	36.6 ± 14.5[b]
G2	Gir	37.4 ± 11.5[b]
	Holstein	29.9 ± 9.7[b]
	Red Angus	37.4 ± 11.4[b]
G3	Gir	41.9 ± 12.5[b]
	Holstein	23.2 ± 9.8[c]
	Red Angus	48.6 ± 12.4[b]
G4	Gir	36.9 ± 12.8[b]
	Holstein	36.9 ± 12.2[b]
	Red Angus	30.0 ± 7.5[b]

[a]G1: densities from 1.110 g/mL to 1.123 g/mL; G2: densities from 1,034 to 1,045 g/mL; G3: densities from 1.123 g/mL to 1.163 g/mL; G4: densities from 1,034 g/mL to 1,045 g/mL
[b-c] Means without common superscript letters differ, P<0.05 (Test Tukey)

When breed was taken into consideration was observed that, in Red Angus, the blastocyst rate was significantly higher when the sexed semen obtained with gradient 1. No significant difference was observed with the other breeds (Table 3). When gradient was considered, was observed that sexed semen obtained from gradient 1 significantly decreased (P <0.05) blastocyst rate in Holstein (Table 4). However, for the other gradients, this effect was not significant.

Regarding the sex ratio among embryos produced in vitro, the variance analysis detected an effect of sperm sexing on sex ratio. An increased female proportion was observed after IVP with sexed semen (72.3%) compared to the female proportion after IVP with non-sexed semen (48.2%) (Table 5). No difference was observed between high and low density gradient centrifugation on female proportion.

Experiment 2 - Artificial insemination using spermatozoa sexed by density gradient centrifugation

A total of 162 crossbreed heifers were inseminated with frozen-thawed non-sexed semen of Gir, Red Angus and Holstein breeds; whereas 228 crossbreed heifers were inseminated with frozen-thawed sexed semen of Gir, Red Angus, and Holstein breeds, from either G2 or G4. Tables 6 and 7 present the pregnancy rates and sex ratios obtained 60 days following AI with non-sexed semen and with sexed semen from G2 and G4.

Table 5. *Means of female in vitro produced bovine embryos using 75 thawed batches of spermatozoa either non-sexed or sexed by Percoll™ (G1 and G2)[a] or OptiPrep® (G3 and G4)[b] discontinuous density gradient centrifugation from semen of Gir, Holstein, and Red Angus bulls.*

Treatment	Total number of embryos sexed by PCR	Female embryos*(% ± SD)
Non-sexed	3338	48.2 ± 4.4
Sexed	3605	72.3 ± 10.4

*P <0.0001

[a]G1: densities from 1.110 g/mL to 1.123 g/mL; G2: densities from 1,034 to 1,045 g/mL

[b]G3: densities from 1.123 g/mL to 1.163 g/mL; G4: densities from 1,034 g/mL to 1,045 g/mL

Table 6. *Pregnancy rates in crossbred heifers and female fetus 60 days after AI using semen either non-sexed or sexed by Percoll™ discontinuous density gradient (G1 and G2) from semen of Gir, Holstein, and Red Angus bulls.*

Breed	Treatment	Total number of heifers inseminated	Pregnancy rate (%)	Female fetus (%)
Gir	Non-sexed	31	67.7c	10 (47.6)d
	Sexed	32	61.3c	13 (68.4)e
Holstein	Non-sexed	30	86.7b	13 (50.0)d
	Sexed	31	77.4b	17 (70.8)e
Red Angus	Non-sexed	30	76.7b	12 (52.2)d
	Sexed	29	75.9b	16 (68.1)e

[a]G1: densities from 1.110 g/mL to 1.123 g/mL; G2: densities from 1,034 to 1,045 g/mL

[b-c] Means without common superscript letters differ, P<0.05 (Chi-square)

[d-e] Means without common superscript letters differ, P<0.05 (Chi-square)

Table 7. *Pregnancy rates in crossbred heifers and female fetus 60 days after AI using semen either non-sexed or sexed by OptiPrep® discontinuous density gradient (G3 and G4)[a] from semen of Gir, Holstein, and Red Angus bulls.*

Breed	Treatment	Total number of inseminated heifers	Pregnancy rate (%)	Female fetus (%)
Gir	Non-sexed	20	65.0c	7 (53.9)d
	Sexed	37	59.5c	18 (81.8)e
Holstein	Non-sexed	28	75.9b	23 (57.5)d
	Sexed	54	85.7b	17 (70.8)e
Red Angus	Non-sexed	23	73.9b	9 (52.6)d
	Sexed	45	80.0b	26 (72.2)e

[a]G3: densities from 1.123 g/mL to 1.163 g/mL; G4: densities from 1,034 g/mL to 1,045 g/mL

[b-c] Means without common superscript letters differ, P<0.05 (chi-square)

[d-e] Means without common superscript letters differ, P<0.05 (chi-square)

The sexing procedure had no significant effect on pregnancy rate when compared to non-sexed semen of the same breed 60 days following AI. However, there was a significant decrease (P <0.05) in pregnancy rate obtained with sexed and non-sexed semen of Gir breed if compared to sexed and non-sexed pregnancy rate obtained with Holstein and Red Angus breeds. Notably, AI with sexed semen of Red Angus and Holstein breeds seemed to present higher (P <0.05) pregnancy rates when compared to Gir breed. A significant sex ratio deviation (P <0.05) toward to female gender was observed when AI was performed with sexed semen obtained with all density gradients in all breeds (Table 7). The sex ratio deviation (P<0.05) of 70.7% in favor of female gender was confirmed at parturition. No occurrences of dystocia, or neonatal mortality were reported.

4. Discussion

In this work, a method for sexing bovine sperm with high and low density discontinuous gradient made with isotonic solutions from modified colloidal silica (Percoll™) or iodinated compounds (OptiPrep®) was used. The composition of these gradients allowed a lower accuracy (70%) when separating X- bearing bovine spermatozoa than that observed by reference [8] (90%), reference [9] (70%), and reference [15] (75%). After thawing, 66.7% of the straws had at least 50% of sperm with motility that produced on average 33.4% blastocysts with IVP of bovine embryos and 73% pregnancy rates after conventional artificial insemination.

Considering the samples of 75 ejaculates in one of the four gradients, on average of 16 doses of semen (12 x 10^6 sperm per straw) enriched with X-bearing sperm in each 2 mL of the ejaculate were produced every 30 minutes, using approximately 30% of each ejaculate, distributed in 36 tubes.

The discontinuous Percoll™ and OptiPrep® density gradients were employed for the selective isolation of bovine X-bearing spermatozoa. Retrieval of spermatozoa with Y chromosome in the Percoll™ and OptiPrep® discontinuous gradients was on average 5% (data not shown), as the Y chromosomes were spread out in gradients similarly to what is observed with human species [24; 25] and with bovines [8]. This low recovery of Y-bearing spermatozoa is not a relevant issue because female selection is more relevant for commercial milk and meat production from pure breed as well as for progeny tests and genetic enhancement for milk and meat production [1; 2].

The use of density gradient centrifugation to sort bovine sperm in IVP systems had been investigated in previous studies [8; 9] and provided similar results to those here presented.

The fact that was used a large number of samples (6943 embryos, 13,886 PCRs) in this study, provided great power to our statistical analysis and allowed us to observe the great deviation in sex ratio that sexing may cause. To our knowledge, the only description of embryos sexed by density gradient typed 20 embryos [8]. Interestingly, embryos sexed by reference [8] had their sex confirmed by PCR and produced 90% females, which is higher than the percentage found in this study (table 6).Besides the fact that these 20 embryos were produced with a single enriched straw of sperm and in a single procedure of IVP embryos, the greater number of embryos may have led to detect less deviation.

Cleavage and blastocyst rates in this study were higher than those described by reference [8], who found 53.4% cleavage and 20.2% blastocyts in 515 oocytes using the Percoll™ gradient centrifugation. Another noteworthy fact of their study is that the IVP did not produce over 50% male embryos, as observed in the control groups and expected to be obtained in this type of procedure. Using bovine fetal serum instead of BSA and eliminating glucose during embryo development may explain these observations. Reference [26] showed that when glucose is present, more than 75% of blastocyts produced in SOF medium were male. In SOF medium containing SFB not only was the development rate accelerated but also survival rates of male embryos increased [18].

Glucose in high concentrations not only impairs development of bovine embryos but also causes a selective block of female embryos during transition from morula to blastocyst, which leads to a higher rate of males among the expanded blastocysts [27]. This phenomenon is likely to be explained by the presence in female embryos of the two active X chromosomes, which have low tolerance for imbalances in the carbohydrate metabolism [27].

The results obtained after insemination of heifers with sperm sorted by discontinuous density gradient centrifugation suggest that the process did not affect *in vitro* fertility process nor had an effect after artificial insemination. The pregnancy rate obtained with OptiPrep® was 75.06%.

No reports of AI done in bovines using sperm centrifuged in either Percoll™ or OptiPrep® density gradient were found. The results show in this study showed that it is possible to produce pregnancies using conventional artificial insemination of semen sexed by density gradient centrifugation. In addition, it was possible to observe that this sexing method was compatible with freezing, it minimized spermatozoa loss during the process, and did not reduce pregnancy rates.

It is also important to evaluate sexing methodologies not only on their ability to precisely determine embryo sex. It is also important to evaluate the ability of sexed spermatozoa to produce pregnancies. These issues are most relevant when implementing sexing methodologies on a large scale, so that neither reproduction rates nor the genetic enhancement obtained with production of milk and meat systems are affected.

Improvements in density gradient centrifugation, especially in its precision, may allow this system of spermatozoa sexing to be used on a large scale for milk and meat production as well as for progeny tests in bovines.

Acknowledgements

This work was funded by FAPESP grant 99/11392-8. M.F.P.D-T. Ramalho was the recipient of a scholarship from FAPESP (Brazil). Semen was produced at Lagoa da Serra Ltda. Heifers were supplied by Andriju and Barreiro Farms. I.W. Santos, M.Z. Costa, and M.V. Resende diagnosed pregnancy and fetal sex using ultrasound. We would like to thank Marcia Triunfol of Publicase for writing assistance and manuscript review.

References

[1] R.K. Splan, L.V. Cundiff, L. D. Van Vleck, "Genetic parameters for sex-specific traits in beef cattle," J. Anim. Sci., v. 76, pp.2272-2278, 1998.

[2] W.D. Hohenboken, "Applications of sexed semen in cattle production", Theriogenology, v. 52, pp.14, 1999.

[3] A. De Vries, M. Overton, J. Fetrow, K. Leslie, S. Eicker, G. Rogers. "Exploring the impact of sexed semen on the structure of the dairy industry", J. Dairy Sci., v.91, pp.847–56, 2008.

[4] D. L Garner Hoechst 33342: The dye that enabled differentiation of living X-and Y-chromosome bearing mammalian sperm. Theriogenology 71, 11-21. 2009

[5] J.C. Sharpe, K.M .Evans, "Advances in flow cytometry for sexing sperm," Theriogenology, v.71, pp.4-10, 2009.

[6] E.B. Van Munster, J .Stap, R. A. Hoebe, G.J. Te Meerman, J.A Aten, " Difference in volume of X- and Y-chromosome bearing bovine sperm heads matches difference in DNA content," Citometry, v. 35,pp. 125-128. 1999a.

[7] E.B .Van Munster, J. Stap, R. A. Hoebe, G.J. Te Meerman, J.A. Aten, "Difference in sperm head volume as a theorical basis for a sorting X- and Y- bearing spermatozoa: a potencials and limitation", Theriogenology, v. 52, pp.1281-1293, 1999b.

[8] S. Blottner, M. Schwerin, M. Böttcher, C. Pitra, "Selective enrichment of bovine X- and Y-spermatozoa by Percoll™ density gradient", Arch. Tierz, v.36, pp.153-162, 1993.

[9] W. Lange, H. Pemsel, S .Blottner, R. Roselius, J. Pfeilsticker, P. Rommel, "Über de einflu des bullen auf die selective anreicherung der X-und Y- spermienmit der Percoll™-dichtegradienten-zentrifugation", Arch. Tierz. v.38, pp.155-161, 1995.

[10] V.F.M. Hossepian de Lima, M.F.P.D-T Ramalho, L.H. Rodrigues, E. B. Malheiros, C. A. Moreira-Filho, "Separation of X- and Y- bearing bovine spermatozoa by Percoll™ density gradient centrifugation", Theriogenology , v.53 pp. 280, 2000.

[11] V.F.M. Hossepian de Lima, "Methodological advances on spermatozoa sexing for using in genetic improvement and animal production." Braz. J. Anim. Sci., v. 36, pp.219-228, 2007.

[12] E. Curry, S.L. Pratt, D.R. Lapin, J.R. Gibbons,"Efficacy of a commercially available post-thaw bovine semen sexing kit in both single-ovulating and hyperstimuled cows", Anim. Reprod. Sci., v. 116, p.376-380, 2009.

[13] F. Aleahmad, H .Gourabi, B. Zeinali, S. Ashtiani,H. Baharvand., "Separation of X- and Y-bearing human spermatozoa by sperm isolation medium gradients evaluated by FISH", Reprod. Biom. OnLine, v. 18, pp.475-478, 2009.

[14] D.P. Windsor, G. Evans, I.G, "White Sex predetermination by separation of X and Y chromossome- bearing sperm: A review", Reprod. Fert. Develop. v. 5, p.155-171, 1993.

[15] H. Schwiderski, S. Blottner, M. Schwerin, "Mikroinjektion und in vitro befruchtung mit spermien aus versuchen zur anreicherung der geschlechtss pezifischen spermientypen beim rind", Reprod. Dom. Anim., v.26, pp. 143-144, 1991.

[16] C.Y. Andersen, A.G. Byskov," Enhanced separation of X and Y bearing sperm cells by a combined density gradient centrifugation evaluated by fluorescence in situ hybridization of the Y-chromosome", Acta Obstet. Gyn. Scan,v. 76, pp.131-134, 1997.

[17] G. Vajta, N. Rindom, T.T. Peura, P. Holm, T. Greve, H. Callesen , "The effect of media, serum and temperature on in vitro survival of bovine blastocysts after open pulled straw (OPS) vitrification", Theriogenologyv.52, pp.939-948, 1999.

[18] A. Gutiérrez-Adán, J. Granados, B. Pintado, J. De La Fuente, " Influence of glucose on the sex ratio of bovine IVM/IVF embryos cultured in vitro", Reprod. Fertil. Dev., v. 13, pp.1-5. 2001.

[19] K. R. Bondioli, S. B. Ellis, J. H. Pryor, M. W. Williams, M. M. Harpold, "The use of male-specific chromosomal DNA fragments to determine the sex of bovine preimplantation embryos" Theriogenology, v. 31, pp. 95-104, 1989.

[20] M. Schwerin, S.Blottner, P.D. Thomsen, D. Roschlau, G. Brockmann, "Quantification of Y chromosome bearing spermatozoa of cattle using in situ hybridization", Mol. Reprod. Dev., v. 30, pp.39-43, 1991.

[21] S. B. Ellis, K.R. Bondioli, M. E. Williams, J. H. Pryor, M. M. Harpold Sex determination of bovine embryos using male-specific DNA probes. Theriogenology 29, 242. 1988.

[22] S. Verberckmoes, A. Van Soom, I. Depauw, J. Dewulf, T. Rijsselaere, A. Kruif , "Effect of hole blood and serum on bovine sperm quality and in vitro fertilization capacity", Theriogenology, v. 61,pp. 25-33, 2004.

[23] S .Curran, J. P. Kastelic, O. J. Ginther, "Determining sex of the bovine fetus by ultrasonic assessment of the relative location of the genital tubercle", Anim. Reprod. Sci. v. 19, pp.217-227, 1989.

[24] Kaneko S, Oshio S, Kobayashi T, Mohri H, Iizuka R 1984.Selective isolation of human X- bearing sperm by differential velocity sedimentation in Percoll™ density gradients. Biomedical Research 5, 187-194.

[25] R. Iizuka, S .Kaneko, R. Aoki, T. Kobayashi, "Sexing of human sperm by discontinuos Percoll™ density gradient and its clinical application", Hum. Reprod. v. 2,pp.573-575, 1987.

[26] M. A. Larson, K. Kimura, H. M. Kubisch, R. M. Roberts, "Sexual dimorphism among bovine embryos in their ability to make the transition to expanded blastocyst and in the expression of the signaling molecule IFN-τ", Proc.Natl.Acad. Sci.v.98, pp.9677–9682, 2001.

[27] K. Kimura, H. Iwata, G. J. Thompson, "The effect of glucosamine concentration on the development and sex ratio of bovine embryos", Anim. Reprod. Sci., v.103, pp.228–238, 2008.

2

Pre and Post-natal Nutrition of Ewes on the Performances of Native Bengal Ewes and Their Lambs

Sadek Ahmed[1,*], Md. Rezaul Hai Rakib[1], Rahat Ara Karim[1], Swapon Kumar Fouzder[2], Nusrat Jahan[3], Nasrin Sultana[1], Md. Ershaduzzaman[1]

[1]Goat and Sheep Production Research Division, Bangladesh Livestock Research Institute, Savar, Dhaka, Bangladesh

[2]Department of Poultry Science, Patuakhali Science and Technology University, Patuakhali, Bangladesh

[3]Animal Biotechnology Division, National Institute of Biotechnology, Savar, Dhaka, Bangladesh

Email address:

sadek.ahmed@blri.gov.bd (S. Ahmed)

[*]Corresponding author

Abstract: The aim of the study is to determine the effects of different plane of nutrition during late pregnancy to lactation on the performances of ewes and their offspring to weaning. About 36 native Bengal ewes of last 7 weeks gestation were randomly assigned to four different groups (T_0, T_1, T_2, T_3). The T_0, T_1, T_2 and T_3 groups were supplemented a concentrate mixture at 0.0, 1.0, 1.5 and 2.0% of their body weight, respectively. Chopped German grass (*Echinochloa polystachya*) was provided as basal forages to ewes and a creep mixture (20 g/lamb/day) to the lambs from 2 weeks of age with a weakly increase of 10 g/lamb. The results shown that ewes dry matter intake ($p < 0.01$), milk yield ($p < 0.05$), days open ($p < 0.01$), live weight gain before lambing ($p < 0.01$) and at weaning ($p < 0.01$) and weight recovery from late gestation to weaning ($p < 0.05$) improved with high plane of nutrition. Higher weight recovery found in T_2 group. Litter size had an effect on ($p < 0.01$) all weight traits of lambs and ewes milk yield. Sex of lamb also affects ($p < 0.05$) the weaning weight and daily gain of lambs.

Keywords: Native Bengal Ewes, Lambs, Pre and Post-natal Nutrition

1. Introduction

Currently, the livestock sector in Bangladesh produced only 30.18% total requirement of meat and the per capita meat consumption is still very low (only 8.6 kg) compared to developing countries (42.1 kg) and world (32.2 kg) [1]. To meet this huge gap, the meat production of the country must be increased in many folds with emphasizing different non-popular species including sheep as a meat animal. Bangladesh has 3.16 million sheep which secure 3rd position in number among the ruminant species of the country [2]. Though the number of animals is satisfactory but their performance is very poor. Nutrition is one of the major limiting factors in livestock production in Bangladesh and more than 90% of the feed consumed by the ruminants in our country are rice straw [3]. During pregnancy, nutrition is one of the very important factors that determine many productive and reproductive qualities after birth. In the late gestation, the last six to eight weeks of pregnancy, 80% of fetal growth occurs, leading to a significant increase in nutrient requirements of the ewe [4]. Inadequate feed intake during late gestation might lead to a reduction in birth weight (BW), mammary development and milk production [5, 6, 7 and 8]. Besides that, when multiple bearing ewes offered additional feed in late pregnancy, lamb mortality was reduced for single and twin lambs [9]. Research also revealed that body weight (BW) of lambs were higher when the ewes were fed higher levels of protein compared to the one that fed on low levels (14.9 vs. 11.3% CP) during late gestation and early lactation [10]. Therefore, it is necessary to find out a suitable nutrition level for native Bengal ewes during late pregnancy to lactation in view of effective lamb production in Bangladesh. Thus, the research was undertaken to know the effect of different level of nutrition during late pregnancy and lactation on the performances of native ewes and their lambs until weaning.

2. Materials and Methods

2.1. Experimental Site and Duration

The experiment was carried out at the Goat and Sheep Production Research Farm, Bangladesh Livestock Research Institute (BLRI), Savar, Dhaka-1341, Bangladesh during November 2014 to April 2015.

2.2. Experimental Animals and Feeding Management

A total of thirty-six native Bengal ewes between 2 to 5 parity were randomly allocated to four different treatment groups (T_0, T_1, T_2, T_3) at the stage of last 7 weeks pregnancy. Ewes were housed in individual cage and lambs remained with their dams until weaning except for the days of milk measurement. Ewes of all the treatment groups were supplied ad libitum German grass (*Echinochloa polystachya*) by chopping into the size of 1 to 1.5 inch. The ewes of T_1, T_2 and T_3 group were supplemented with a concentrate mixture (Crushed Maize 40%, Soybean meal 26%, Wheat bran 22%, Rice polish 10%, Salt 1%, Vitamin-mineral premix 0.5% and DCP 0.5%), at the rate of 1.0, 1.5 and 2.0% of their body weight, respectively and maintaining T_0 as control. After parturition, a creep mixture (Crushed maize 68%, Soybean meal 30%, Vitamin-mineral premix 1% and Salt 1%) was supplied to lambs at the age of 2 weeks @ 20g/lamb/day and a weekly increment of 10g/lamb/week was done. Beside this, a small amount of German grass was freely offered to the lambs in *ad libitum* basis from 04 weeks and onward. The required amount of grass and concentrates were divided into two equal parts and supplied twice daily (morning and evening).

2.3. Parameter Studied

Dry matter intake (DMI), weight changes during the period of pregnancy to lactation, milk yield (MY), rectal temperature, litter size and days open (DO) of ewes with birth weight (BW), sex, daily gain (DG) and weaning weight (WW) of lambs were recorded. Weight of individual animal was measured at the onset of the trial and subsequently on weekly basis. Besides weekly weight, ewes were also weighted daily from 05 days before of their expected lambing date until lambing to identify the weight before lambing. The weights of the new natal lambs were taken immediate after parturition and before suckling milk and then weekly basis. Weight of the ewes was also taken at 06 hours after parturition i.e. after expelling placenta.

2.4. Milk Yield Measurement

Milk yield (MY) of ewes were estimated by using the Peart method [11] that is, weighing of the lambs before and after suckling and removal of residual milk by hand. Briefly, MY of ewes were measured over a total of 24 hrs period and repeated over the lactation period. On the day of measurement lambs were removed at 20.00 hrs, and weighted (M_1) at 7.00 h next morning and allowed lambs for 45 min to obtain milk, weighted again (M_2) and the differences between M_2 and M_1 assume to be amount of milk consumed. There was no residual milk after suckling of lambs. The procedure repeated on the same day at 20.00 hrs to measured MY for the other half of the day. The sums of two suckling yields measurements were assumed to be milk yield over 24 hr periods. The single weekly estimate of MY was assumed to be representing the average MY for the week in which it was measured.

2.5. Chemical Analysis of Experimental Diets

Chemical compositions of the experimental diets are presented in the Table 1. Dry matter content of the feed was determined by drying the samples at 105°C overnight, while ash was measured by burning further at 600°C for 4 hours [12]. Dried samples were ground and passed through a 1 mm sieve before analysis. The CP content was determined using the Kjeldahl method [13]. The neutral detergent fibre (NDF) and acid detergent fibre (ADF) composition were analyzed using the method described by Goering and Van Soest [14].

Table 1. Chemical composition of the experimental diets.

Diets	DM (% Fresh)	Chemical composition (%DM)					Estimated ME (MJ/kg DM)	Estimated TDN (%)
		Ash	OM	CP	ADF	NDF		
German grass	15.85	11.70	88.30	10.61	46.31	74.67	6.41	43.27
Concentrate mixture (ewe)	87.65	9.56	90.45	18.27	12.71	19.97	12.39	81.92
Creep mixture (lamb)	88.29	6.18	93.82	17.86	11.56	15.88	12.56	83.24

2.6. Experimental Design and Statistical Analysis

The experiment was arranged in a completely randomized design (CRD). The collected data were subjected to analysis of variance (ANOVA) using the general linear model (GLM) procedure of SAS 9.0 (2004). Significant differences among means were separated using the Duncan's multiple Range Test (DMRT).

3. Results and Discussion

3.1. Performances of Ewes

3.1.1. Ewes Live Weight Changes

The effect of different level of concentrate supplementation from last 06 weeks pregnancy to lactation stage on ewes live weight changes are presented in Table 2. Maternal nutrition during last stage of pregnancy plays an essential role in proper foetal and placental development that affects the health and productivity of the offspring. The results indicate that feeding concentrate had significant ($p<0.01$) effect on LWG during last 06 weeks of pregnancy. Similarly, ewes live weight recovery from last 06 weeks pregnancy stage to lamb's weaning stage also significantly increased ($p<0.05$) in supplemented groups compare to control group (T_0). Higher body weight recovery rate was found in T_2 group (96.00%). On the other hand, the type of birth had only significant effect ($p<0.05$) on weight gain of ewes during last 06 weeks of pregnancy but not in WW and WR after lambing compare to initial weight. On this regard, it is also found that during late pregnancy, ewes with high plane of feeding made significantly higher live weight gain than those on low plane [7, 8]. The higher body weight recovery of supplemented groups during lactation would be expected to improve subsequent reproductive performances in ewes [11].

Table 2. *Effect of different level of nutrition during late pregnancy to lactation and type of birth on weight (kg) changes of native Bengal ewes.*

Factors	Initial weight (kg)	LW day before lambing (kg)	LW gain before lambing (kg)	LW after lambing (kg)	LW at weaning (kg)	WR (%) from initial weight to lambing
T_0 (8)	25.84	27.42	1.58^a	23.23^a	20.95^a	81.70^a
T_1 (9)	26.42	30.81	4.39^b	26.81^{ab}	23.30^{ab}	88.55^{ab}
T_2 (9)	27.29	33.09	5.80^b	28.50^b	26.03^b	96.00^b
T_3 (7)	21.80	27.84	6.04^b	22.57^a	20.31^a	94.11^b
Overall mean	25.54	29.98	4.44	25.50	22.84	90.10
SEM	0.900	0.947	0.407	0.885	0.775	1.764
Sig. Level	NS	NS	**	*	*	*
Type of Birth	NS	NS	*	NS	NS	NS
Single (17)	25.74	29.24	3.50^a	25.55	22.94	89.98
Twin (15)	25.41	30.68	5.27^a	25.48	22.80	90.20
Triplet (1)	23.90	32.00	8.10^b	25.00	21.70	90.79
Overall mean	25.54	29.98	4.44	25.50	22.84	90.10
SEM	0.900	0.947	0.407	0.885	0.775	1.764

NS= Non significant; *$P<0.05$;** $P<0.01$; ^{ab} values within the same column with different superscripts differ significantly; LW= live weight; T_o= no concentrate supplementation, T_1= Supplementation of concentrate at 1% of LW, T_2= Supplementation of concentrate at 1.5% of LW; T_3= Supplementation of concentrate at 2% of LW.

3.1.2. Ewes Feed Intake

The effects of different amount of concentrate offered during pre and post-natal period on DM intake of native ewes are shown in Table 3. There was a significant ($p<0.01$) effect on the overall DM intake of ewes (DMI during pregnancy + lactation stage) compare to control group (T_0). Although DM intake among the groups T_1, T_2 and T_3 were not differ significantly. Likewise, DM intake during pregnancy and lactation stage also differ significantly ($p<0.01$) among the different treatment groups compare to control group (T_0). Ewes DMI from late pregnancy to lactation on their per cent body weight ware 3.05, 3.79, 3.38 and 4.06% for T_0, T_1, T_2, T_3, respectively and also differ significantly ($P<0.01$) among the groups. Other research also found a non-significant effect on total DM intake by level of concentrate from 110 days pregnancy to lambing when fed two types of hays (lucern and pasture) as basal feed [15]. They also observed intake decreased with increasing level of concentrates.

Table 3. *Effect of different level of nutrition during late pregnancy to lactation on the performances of native Bengal ewes.*

Parameters	T_0	T_1	T_2	T_3	Overall mean	SEM	Lev. Sig.
DMI of ewes (kg)	0.66^a	0.94^b	0.93^b	0.89^b	0.86	0.025	**
DMI during pregnancy (kg/day)	0.51^a	0.94^b	0.86^b	0.90^b	0.80	0.035	**
DMI during lactation (kg/day)	0.74^a	0.95^b	0.96^b	0.88^b	0.89	0.023	**
DMI on% LW of ewes	3.05^a	3.79^{bc}	3.38^{ab}	4.06^c	3.56	0.095	**
DMI on% LW of ewes during pregnancy	2.00^a	3.36^c	2.87^b	3.64^c	2.96	0.129	**
DMI on% LW of ewes during lactation	3.60^a	4.03^{ab}	3.66^a	4.31^b	3.88	0.092	*
Litter Size (no.)	1.38	1.44	1.44	1.86	1.52	0.098	NS
Daily Milk Yield (g)	339.28^a	450.87^{ab}	525.2^b	561.07^b	467.49	30.711	*
Days Open (day)	79.75^b	55.67^a	54.78^a	50.71^a	60.21	3.070	**

NS= Non significant, *$P<0.05$, ** $P<0.01$, abc values within the same raw with different superscripts differ significantly. DMI= Dry matter intake; To= no concentrate supplementation, T1= Supplementation of concentrate at 1% of LW, T2= Supplementation of concentrate at 1.5% of LW; T3= Supplementation of concentrate at 2% of LW.

Since 80% of the foetal growth takes place in the last trimester of the pregnancy [4], nutritional requirements of the ewe increase to a great extent during this period. During the last six weeks of pregnancy energy requirements of twin bearing ewe are raised by more than 80% and protein requirements by 100% [16]. At the same time, pregnancy can reduce eating capacity but increase passage rate through the digestive tract [17]. Those combined changes in late pregnancy make it difficult to fill energy requirements of the pregnant and lactating ewe without using significant amounts of concentrates along with high quality roughage [18]. However, during the last 2 weeks of pregnancy, particularly in twin- or triple-bearing ewes; voluntary feed intake declines [19] although the demand for nutrients are higher at that stage. [20]. The above discussions suggest a concentrate supplementation along with green grass to meet increasing nutrient requirement during late pregnancy to lactation in ewes. In this study, DMI of all treated groups (T_1, T_2 and T_3) significantly increased (p<0.01) compare to control group (T_0) both pregnancy and lactation stage to maintain the nutrient requirements.

3.1.3. Daily Milk Yield

The daily MY (g) of different treatment group were resulted significant differences (p<0.05) compare to control group (T_0) (Table-3). Ewes with higher level of concentrate groups (T_3) produced more milk during entire lactation period compare to control group (T_0) but not differ among the different supplemented groups (T_1, T_2 and T_3). The results showed that MY increased with increasing the level of concentrate supplement [21, 6]. MY was affected by the nutritional plane of before and after lambing.

Type of birth i.e. litter size significantly (p<0.01) affected daily MY of ewes. Highest MY found in the triplet bearing ewes (915.35 g/days) followed by twin (514.87 g/day) and single birth ewes (399.34 g /day) (Table 5). More MY also found in ewes which give birth to twins and reared twins compare to single birth ewes [6]. This may be associated with the simulation effect on the secretion cell of the udder which resulted from more frequent suckling by the lamb [22] or may be due to the sample size and genetics because in our study we got only one triplet birth.

3.1.4. Days Open

Days open (DO) also decreased significantly (p<0.01) with increasing concentrate supplementation during last 6 weeks of pregnancy to lactation (Table-3). The results indicate that supplementation improves the reproductive efficiency of ewes to reduce lambing interval. The overall DO of this study was 60.21 days however a lower value (42.73 days) reported for native Bengal ewes by other authors [23]. This variation may be due to the differences of parity of ewes, lambing season, level of nutrition, litter size and lambs sex.

Table 4. *Effect of different level of nutrition during late pregnancy to lactation on the performances of native Bengal lambs.*

Parameters	T_0	T_1	T_2	T_3	Overall mean	SEM	Lev. Sig.
Birth weight (kg)	1.92	2.13	2.31	1.70	2.04	0.091	NS
Birth weight of male (kg)	1.96	2.16	2.24	1.75	2.01	0.115	NS
Birth weight of female (kg)	1.68	2.01	2.29	1.62	1.91	0.109	NS
Weaning weight (kg)	8.96	9.31	12.31	9.44	10.07	0.536	NS
Weaning weight of male (kg)	8.77^{a}	10.91^{ab}	13.23^{b}	9.90^{a}	10.83	0.598	*
Weaning weight of female (kg)	8.43	8.78	10.57	8.26	8.96	0.511	NS
Daily live weight gain (g)	78.22	79.75	111.20	86.04	89.29	5.303	NS
Daily live weight gain of male (g)	75.68^{a}	97.18^{ab}	122.13^{b}	90.60^{a}	98.02	5.726	*
Daily live weight gain of female (g)	74.94	75.22	92.10	73.83	78.38	4.808	NS

NS= Non significant, *P<0.05,** P<0.01, ^{ab} values within the same raw with different superscripts differ significantly; T_o= no concentrate supplementation, T_1= Supplementation of concentrate at 1% of LW, T_2= Supplementation of concentrate at 1.5% of LW; T_3= Supplementation of concentrate at 2% of LW.

3.2. Performances of Lambs

The highest BW and WW were observed in T_2 supplemented group (Table 4). Similarly, the highest WW also observed in T_2 treatment group. The results showed a non-significant effect of pre-natal nutrition on post-natal weight traits of lambs. But, WW and DG of male lambs until weaning differ significantly among the treatment groups. Nevertheless, BW, WW and DG not differ significantly among the treatment groups but numerically higher values for all these traits found in T_2 treatment group that may affect lambs slaughter weight and profitability. In Hamandi ewes a non-significant effect also found on post-natal weight traits of lambs for different plane of nutrition in late pregnant ewes [6].

Table 5. *Effect of type of lamb birth and lamb's sex on the performances of native Bengal lambs and ewes providing different levels of nutrition in ewes during late pregnancy to lactation.*

Factors	Birth weight of lambs (Kg)	Weaning weight of Lambs (kg)	Daily weight gain of lambs (kg)	Daily milk yield of ewes (g)
Litter size (no.)	**	**	**	**
Single (17)	2.36^{b}	11.75^{b}	104.38^{b}	399.34^{a}
Twin (15)	1.69^{a}	8.28^{a}	73.16^{a}	514.87^{a}
Triplate (1)	1.72^{a}	8.45^{a}	74.80^{a}	915.35^{b}
Overall mean	2.04	10.07	89.29	467.49
SEM	0.091	0.537	5.303	30.711
Sex of lamb	NS	*	*	-
Male (21)	2.01	10.83^{b}	98.02^{b}	-
Female(24)	1.92	8.96^{a}	78.38^{a}	-
Overall mean	1.96	9.83	87.54	-
SEM	0.080	3.948	0.410	-

NS= Non significant, *P<0.05, ** P<0.01, ^{abc} values within the same column with different superscripts differ significantly.

It has been generally shown that BW of lambs not only depends on the nutrition of ewes during late stage of pregnancy but also correlated with litter size and sex of lambs. Similarly, growth and WW also depends on ewes' MY. So, the results of this experiment also compared according to litter size and sex of lambs (Table 5). Though lambs BW, WW and DG not differ significantly among treatment groups (Table 4) but litter size (single, twin and triplet) has significant effects ($p<0.01$) on these weight traits (Table 5). Single lambs were significantly heavier for all weight traits. This could be due to the quantities of milk available for them. With increasing litter size MY also increases, may be due to the simulation effect on the milk secretary cells of the udder which resulted from more frequent suckling by the lambs [22]. This result agrees with the findings in Hamandi ewes [6].

Although, overall BW of male lambs higher than female lambs but not differ significantly whereas, DG and WW differ significantly ($p<0.05$). Thus, the effects of ewe's nutrition during late stage of pregnancy to lactation on lamb's BW, WW and DG and ewes MY were interact with type of birth and sex of lambs.

4. Conclusions

The pre and post-natal nutrition of significantly affect all the weight traits of ewes from late pregnancy to lactation. Litter size not affect any weight traits of ewes expect weight gain before lambing. The LWR significantly increases in T_2 treatment group. DM intake also significantly improved in treatment groups compare to control group. MY significantly increases with increasing level of nutrition. Although, the BW, WW and DG of lambs not differ significantly among the treatment groups but numerically higher values observed in T_2 treatment group for all these traits that would be expected to improve subsequent weight at slaughter age and profitability. Thus, it can be concluded that ad libitum green grass and a concentrate mixture at 1.5% of their live weight containing 18% CP and 12 MJ ME/kg DM would be a suitable feeding regime during last stage of pregnancy to lactation to obtain optimum production from native Bengal ewes and their lambs.

References

[1] K. S. Huque, Changes in and challenges of Bangladesh livestock. BLRI Newsletter 3. Dhaka, Bangladesh: Bangladesh Livestock Research Institute; 2012. pp.1.

[2] DLS. Department of Livestock Services, Ministry of Fisheries and Livestock. Government of the People's Republic of Bangladesh, Dhaka, Bangladesh. 2014.

[3] M. J. Khan, K. J. Peters and M. M. Uddin, Feeding strategy for improving dairy cattle productivity in small holder farm in Bangladesh. Bang. J. Anim. Sci. 2009, 38(1&2): 67 – 85

[4] J. J. Robinson, K. D. Sinclair, R. D. Randel and A. R. Sykes, Nutritional management of the female ruminant: mechanistic approaches and predictive models. In: Proceedings of the 5th International Symposium on Nutrition of Herbivores. American Society of Animal Science, Savoy, Illinois. USA: ISNH; 1999.

[5] S. P. Ford, B. W. Hess, M. M. Schwope, M. J. Nijland, J. S. Gilbert, K. A. Vonnahme, W. J. Means, H. Han and P. W. Nathanielsz, Maternal under nutrition during early to mid-gestation in the ewe results in altered growth, adiposity and glucose tolerance in male offspring. J. Anim. Sci. 2007; 85: 1285-1294.

[6] K. O. Aziz and S. S. Al-Dabbagh, Effect of plane of nutrition during late pregnancy and early lactation on milk production and lambs growth of Hamadani ewes. Jordan J. Agr. Sci. 2008; 4 (2): 148-157.

[7] D. H. M. Hamada, G. A. R. Sameh, A. Y. H. Mohamed and A. K. A. Enas, Effect of Maternal Feeding in Late Pregnancy on Behaviour and Performance of Egyptian Goat and Sheep and Their Offspring. Global Veterinaria. 2013; 11 (2): 168-176.

[8] M. Abd-Allah, Effects of Parity and Nutrition plane during late pregnancy on metabolic responses, Colostrum production and lamb output of Rahmani ewes. Egypt. J. Anim. Prod. 2013; 50(3):132-142.

[9] G. H. Scales, R. N. Burton and R. A. Moss, Lamb mortality, birth weight and nutrition in late pregnancy. New Zeal. J. Agr. Res. 1986; 29: 75-82.

[10] P. G. Hatfield, G. D. Snowder, W. A. Head Jr, H. A. Glimp, R. H. Stobart and T. Besser, Production by ewes rearing single or twin lambs: Effects of dietary crude protein percentage and supplemental zinc methionine. J. Anim. Sci. 1995; 73: 1227-1238.

[11] J. N. Peart, Lactation of suckling ewes and does. In sheep and goat production. In: Coop IE editor. Amsterdam, Netherlands: Elsevier Scientific Publishing Company; 1982. pp. 119-134.

[12] N. Thiex, L. Novotny and A. Crawford, Determination of ash in animal feed: AOAC official method 942.05 revisited. J. AOAC Int. 2012; 95(5):1392-7.

[13] AOAC (Association of Official Agricultural Chemists). Official Methods of Analysis. 10th edition. Washington D.C. 2003.

[14] H. K. Goering and P. J. Van Soest, Forage Fiber Analysis (apparatus, reagents, procedures and some applications). Agrie. Handbook. ARS, USDA, Washington, DC. 1970. pp. 379.

[15] T. Castro, F. F. Bermúdez, C. Valdés, A. R. Mantecónb, T. Manso and I. Salzar, The voluntary intake and utilization of forage-concentrate diets by ewes in late pregnancy. J. Anim. Feed Sci. 1994; 3: 181-189.

[16] J. Sveinbjörnsson and B. L. Ólafsson, Orkuþarfir sauðfjár og nautgripa í vexti með hliðsjón af mjólkurfóðureiningakerfi [Energy requirements of sheep and growing cattle with respect to milk feed unit system]. Ráðunautafundur 1999; 127-204.

[17] J. J. Gonzalez, J. J. Robinson and C. Fraser, The effect of physiological state on digestion in the ewe and its influence on the quantity of protein reaching the abomasum. Livest. Prod. Sci. 1985; 12: 59-68.

[18] J. J. Robinson, Nutrition of the pregnant ewe. In: Haresign W editor. Sheep Production. London: Butterworths; 1983. pp. 111-131.

[19] R. J. Orr and T. T. Treacher, The effect of concentrate level on intakes of hays by ewes in late pregnancy. Anim. Prod. 1984; 39: 89-98.

[20] A. W. Bell, Regulation of organic nutrient metabolism during transition from late pregnancy to early lactation. J. Anim. Sci. 1995; 73: 2804-2819.

[21] S. Al-dain, Z. Qusay, E. A. Al-Rawi and K. A. Ayoub, Effect of using different nutrition levels on feeding pregnant Awassi ewes as affected in lamb growth, milk production and chemical composition. Tikrit J. Agric. Sci. 2003; 3(7): 48-60.

[22] J. B. Owen, Sheep Production. Bailliere and Tindall, London. 1976.

[23] M. R. Hassan and M. A. I. Talukder, Comparative performance of different regional native sheep in Bangladesh. The Bangladesh Veterinarian 2011; 28(2): 85-94.

3

Removal Cyanobacteria by Diatomite Filter from Raw Freshwater and Potential Use in Watering Domestic Animals

Belkacem Behira

University of Es-senia, Faculty of Biology, Oran, Algeria

Email address:
behira1958@yahoo.fr

Abstract: Growing harmful cyanobacteria in freshwater cause several poisoning episodes of livestock, wild and domestic animal. Conventional surface drinking water treatment utilizes coagulation; flocculation, sedimentation, filtration and disinfection are inadequate and require great financial means or application in watering domestic animals. The filtration of raw freshwater by diatomite is very simple without use of chemical products. Samples of locally diatomite were dried ant calcined and tested to verify their efficiency to removal cyanobacteria cells from raw freshwater. The results obtained shows that filtration by calcined diatomite improve high efficiency to removal cyanobacteria and decrease the level of microcystin in the filtrate solutions.

Keywords: Cyanobacteria, Diatomite, Removal, Raw Freshwater

1. Introduction

Cyanobacteria are a morphologically diverse group of photosynthetic prokaryotes that occupy a wide range of niches, from freshwater to hydrothermal vents, from desert rocks to Antarctic lakes. They most common toxic cyanobacteria in freshwater are *Microcystis spp.*, *Cylindrospermopsis raciborskii*, *Planktothrix* (*syn. Oscillatoria*) *rubescen*s, *Synechococcus spp.*, *agardhii*, *Gloeotrichia spp.*, *Anabaena spp.*, *Lyngbya spp.*, *Aphanizomenon spp.*, *Nostoc spp.*, some *Oscillatoria spp.*, *Schizothrix spp.* and *Synechocystis spp.* Toxicity cannot be excluded for further species and genera (WHO,2003).

Temperature, light, and nutrients level and composition are the main factors affecting toxin production. Variation of cellular toxin levels under different growth conditions have been studied mainly with the batch cultures of *Microcystis*, *Oscillatoria*, *Anabaena*, *Anabaena*, *Aphanizomenon,* and *Planktothrix* (Rapala 1998, Sivonen and Jones 1999). About 75% of all cyanobacteria sampled contain toxins. It is the huge conglomerations of cells that present a great concern of development of large blooms in late summer and early fall (Chorus *et al.* 2000). The production of cyanotoxins includes risks to human and animal health. Depending on the concentration in the aquatic environment, they can cause severe poisoning, produce chronic diseases such as cancer, and even lead to death. Cyanotoxins are thus an important group of chemical compounds, from the point of view of ecotoxicology, toxicology, and environmental chemistry(Bláha,2009): Several poisoning episodes of livestock, wild and domestic animals have been associated with the occurrence of cyanobacteria blooms in surface waters used for drinking (Stewart et al. 2008). Microcystins are the most frequently occurring and widespread of the cyanotoxins. Due to these adverse health effects, the World Health Organization established a provisional guideline of 1μg/L for microcystin-LR in drinking water (WHO, 1998).Conventional surface drinking water treatment utilizes coagulation, flocculation, sedimentation, filtration and disinfection as basic methods. However, conventional treatment may need to be optimized for cyanotoxin removal, relating to the form of the toxin to be removed (intra- or extracellular), the background water matrix, and possible dissolved toxin release during the treatment process (Falconer, 2005).In agreement with earlier findings that alum flocculation, filtration, and chlorination are ineffective in the removal of cyanobacteria toxins (Vuori et al. 1992). Physicochemical water treatment processes have been shown to cause cell lysis and toxin release (James and Fawell, 1991). Diatomite is a natural material formed from the remains of diatoms, which grew and were deposited in seas or lakes. The structure of diatomite is quite complex. Because there are many fine microscopic pores, cavities, and channels, it has a large specific surface area, high absorption capacity, and low density. Moreover, because of its relative low cost and abundance, it is utilized extensively as a filler, a filtering aid, an abrasive, an insulating material, a conventional catalyst support, and a membrane. Small, highly porous diatomite particles are useful in fabricating highly permeable microporous membrane filters (Vasconcelos et al., 2000). Diatomite was used in purification potable water, contaminated ground- and surface water, decontamination of sewage liquids and waste water. (Grešovnik, 2007).

The aim of this work is to test the natural and calcined diatomite as filter without chemical products use to removal cyanobacteria from raw water in watering domestic animals.

2. Materials and Methods

The raw diatomite obtained from (Sig deposit, Algeria) under investigation was subjected to treatment under various conditions. The first sample is the natural sample (S1). The second one (S2) is treated by 0.5 N Hcl, then washed by distilled water and finally dried in drying oven at 110 °C for 5 hours. The third one (S3) is calcined diatomite at 500 °C using muffle furnace. While the fourth (S4) is calcined at 700 °C. All samples milled in a ball mill machine and sieved below 200 µm to remove all particles larger than 200 µm. ideally, these fractions contain sand, rocks, clay, and other impurities. Raw water collected from eutrophic lake was used in this experiment. A pre-filtration was occurred on fine sand to removal microalgae and other large particular matters. To achieve filtration, 10 grams of diatomite were added in funnel and the pre-filtered water and one liter was filtered through the diatomite filter. The quantification and identification of cyanobacteria was determined by inverted microscopic. The morphological identification of cyanobacteria was done according to (Komárek and Zapomelova 2008). The determination of intracellular and the extracellular microcystin concentration in extracted samples was determined by HPLC following the method of Lawton et al, (1994). All chemicals used were HPLC grade. The stationary phase was a Symmetry C18 column (250 x 4.6 mm I.D., 5 µm particle size, Waters) at a flow rate of 1ml min-1 and column temperature 38 o C. The mobile phase were Milli-Q water (solvent A) and acetonitrile (solvent B) both acidified with 0.05 % v/v TFA. MC-LR stock solution was prepared by mixing MC-LR standard (Sigma) with methanol, and then it was centrifuged in 2000 RPM for 15 min. MC-LR standard solutions were prepared in different concentrations by adding desired volumes of stock solution to methanol. The prepared standard solutions were 0,01, 0.1,0.2, 0.4 ,0.6, 0.8, 1.0 , 2.0 , 4.0 , 5.0, 10.,20, 40, 80 and 100 µg/L of concentrations.

All experiments were repeated three twice.

Table 1. *cyanobacteria count in filtrate solutions (cell/ ml).*

Sample	*cyanobacteria spp.*			
	microcystis spp.	*anabaena spp.*	*Oscillatoria spp*	*Synechococcus spp*
S1	2.10^4	2.10^3	2.10^2	50
S2	$5.\ 10^3$	2.10^2	20	10
S3	80	20	10	4
S4	10	4	0	0

S1: natural diatomite, S2: Diatomite trated by 0.5 N Hcland drying at 110 °C; S3: Diaomite calcined at 500°C; S4: Diatomite calcined at 700 °C.

3. Result and Discussion

The identification and quantification in sample of raw water before filtration show that the *microcystis spp.* was the predominant genus followed respectively by *anabaena spp.*, *Oscillatory sop.,Synechococcus spp.* The colonial diameter of *microcrystals spp.* range from 300 to 400 µm. The length of filaments *anabaena spp.* range from 100 to 200 µm. *Oscillatoria spp.* The filament length range from 90 to 150 µm. The quantification of cyanobacteria was $6.\ 10^4$ cells/ml of *microcystis* spp, 4.10^3 cell/ml of *anabaena spp.*, $5.10\ ^2$ cell/ml of *Oscillatoria spp.* and 1.10^2 cells / ml of *Synechococcus spp.* The quantification of cyanobacteria in the filtrate solution flirted through the naturally diatomite (S1) shows that the number of microcystiis *spp.* decrease at 8.10^2 cell/ ml, *anabaena spp.* at 2.10^3 cell/ ml , *Oscillatoria spp.* at 2.10^2 cell/ ml and *Synechococcus spp.* at 50 cell/ ml. For the diatomite treated by 0.5 Hcl and dried at110 °C (S2), the numeration of cyanobacteria in the filtrate solution shows that the *microcystis spp.* was $6.\ 10^2$ cell/ml , following by *anabaena spp.* 2.10^2 cell/ml and 20cell/ml of *Oscillatoria spp* . The counting of the filtrate solution filtered through the calcined diatomite at 500 °C (S3) was 50 cell / ml of *microcystis* spp. , 20 cell/ml of *anabaena spp.*, 10 cell/ml of *Oscillatoria spp.*, 4 cell/ ml of. For the filtrate solution collected from the filtration by calcined diatomite at 700 °C, was detected only 10 cell/ml of *microcystis spp.* and 4 cell/ml of *anabaena spp.* The content of total microcystin LR in raw water reached 90 µg/L in the same sample the extracellular microcystin LR was 1.6 µg/L. The results of Total and extracellular microcystin in filtrate solutions were summarized in Tab. 2. the majors groups of cyanobacteria found in raw water from this eutrophic lake were *microcystis spp.* as the predominant genus. *Microcystis* genus is one of the most common bloom formers in freshwater systems on every continent except Antarctica. This genus can produce a suite of potentially harmful compounds (Fristachi and Sinclair, 2008). The Tab.1 shows that the retention of cells increases with diatomite processing method. The highest value was observed in the diatomite calcined at 700 °C. median pore size of a calcined diatomite. Lange et al. (1986) found that the grade of diatomite used affected filter performance. For the finest diatomite grade with a median particle size of 7.5

µm, turbidity reduction was close to 100%; however, for coarser grades with a median particle size of 22 µm, a 10% reduction was observed. The percent of retained cells of *microcistis spp.* increase at 33% of initial microbial charge in raw diatomite filter (SI), this value increase at 80 % in dried diatomite filter to reaching 0.01 % by calcined diatomite filter (S4). The high retention was observed at *ossilatoria spp.* 96%was removal by dried diatomite, 98% by calcined diatomite at 500 °C and 100% by calcined diatomite calcined at 700 °C. This is probably explained by the morphology of the filament that can reach 100 µm of long and the mucilage sheath. The estimation of total microcystin LR and the intracellular microcystin shows that this toxin was concentered in the cells. By subtracting, the intracellular microcystin was very high (88.4µg/L) compared to extracellular microcystin LR content (1.6 µg/L). The high rates of dissolved microcystin in filtered lake water at the end of blooming season suggest that release of cyanotoxins from cells occurs during the senescence and the decomposition periods of Microcystis cells (Park et al. 1996). The results shows that the filtration by diatomite was not contributed to increase of microcystin content in all filtrates. However the use of chemical products increases the extracellular microcystin level in the freshwater treatment by lysis of cyanobacteria cells. In similar work Zhang et al.(2011) were tested bombon-based charcoal adsorbent modified with chitosan to removal microcystin from drinking water and their conclusion was the efficiency this product depends of the pH and the organic matters dissolved in water. The diatomite filter efficiency depending of the size of the pores of the diatomite filter and the size of cyanobacterial cell, so not affected by the chemical or the physical parameters of water. Compared to sample (S4), the difference between total microcystin LR and the extracellular microcystin LR in the three samples (S1, S2, S3) is highly significant. the result of filtration shows that was conform to the guidance value for the maximal acceptable concentration of microcystin-LR in drinking water, 1 µg/L recommended by the WHO.

Table 2. *content of total microcystin LR and extracellular in filtrate solutions (µg/L).*

Sample Total	Total microcystin LR	Extracellular microcystin LR
S1	4.5	0.9
S2	10.5	0.7
S3	4.0	0.5
S4	0.6	0.5

4. Conclusion

The diatomite is a product of choice to remove toxic cyanobacteria in raw water. Filtration through natural diatomite calcined at 700 ° C exhibits a high efficiency of filtration of all the colonial and filamentous forms of cyanobacteria. This method reduces the amount of microcystins in filtered water. This simple method can be applied in the reservoirs watering domestic animals. In rural areas this method is economic and easy.

References

[1] Bláha, L.; Pavel, B.; Blahoskav, M. (2009) Toxins produced in cyanobacterial water blooms—Toxicity and risks. *Interdiscip. Toxicol.* 2009, *2*, 36–41

[2] Chorus I, Falconer I R, Salas H J and Bartram J. '(2000). Health risks caused by freshwater cyanobacteria in recreational waters. *Journal of Toxicology and Environmental Health-Part B* 3(4): 323–47.

[3] Falconer, I.R. (2005) Cyanobacterial toxins of drinking water supplies: cylindrospermopsins and microcystins. Boca Raton: CRC Press; 2005.

[4] Fristachi, A. and J.L Sinclair.(2008) Occurrence of cyanobacterial harmful algal blooms workgroup report. In: Hudnell, K.H. (Ed.), Cyanobacterial Harmful Algal Blooms: State of the Science and Research Needs. Springer, New York, pp. 45–103

[5] Grešovnik, I.(2007) The use of moving least squares for a smooth approximation of sampled data. Strojniški vestnik - Journal of Mechanical Engineering, vol. 53, no. 9, p. 582-598

[6] James, H. and Fawell, J.K. (1991) Detection and Removal of Cyanobacterial Toxins from Freshwaters. Report No. FR0211 Foundation for Water Research, Marlow, UK.

[7] Komárek, J. and Zapomělová, E. (2008) Planktic morphospecies of the cyanobacterial genus Anabaena = subg. Dolichospermum – 2. part: straight types. Fottea, Olomouc, 8(1): 1–14, 2008

[8] Lange, K.P., Bellamy, W.D., Hendriks, D.W. and Logsdon, G.S.(1986) Diatomaceous earth filtration of Giardia cysts and other substances. J. Am. Water Works Assoc., 78(1): 76–84.

[9] Lawton, L.A., Edwards, C., and Codd, G.A. (1994) Extraction and high performance liquid Microcystis and amount of microcystin in Lake Suwa, Japan. In: Yasumoto T, Oshima Y, Fukuyo

[10] Park, H.D., Iwami, C., Watanabe, M.F., Harada, K.I, Okino, T., Hayashi; H.(1996) Seasonal changesof toxic population of the toxic cyanobacterium Microcystis spp. in Lake Wannsee (Germany). Microb. Ecol. 43:107–118

[11] Rapala J and Sivonen K. 1998. Assessment of environmental conditions that favour hepatotoxic and neurotoxic *abaena* spp. strains cultured under light limitation at different temperatures. *Microbial Ecology* 36(2): 181–92

[12] Sivonen K and Jones G. 1999. Cyanobacterial toxins. *Toxic Cyanobacteria in Water: a Guide to Their Public Health Consequences, Monitoring and Management.* Pp.41–111.(Eds.) Chorus I and Bartram J E and FN Spon, London.

[13] Stewart, I., Seawright, A., Shaw, G.(2008) Cyanobacterial poisoning in livestock, wild mammals and birds - an overview. Adv Exp Med Biol 2008;619:613-37.

[14] Vasconcelos, P.V., Labrincha, J.A., and Ferreira, J.M.F.(2000) Permeability of diatomite layers processed by different colloidal techniques. J. Eur. Ceram. Soc. 20, 201

[15] Vuori. E, Himberg, K., Waris, M., Niinivaara, K.(1992) Drinking water purifiers in removal of hepato- and neurotoxins produced by cyanobacteria. In: Recent Advances in Toxinology Research. Vol 3 (Gopalakrishnakone P, Tan CK, eds). Singapore:National University of Singapore, Venom and Toxin Research Group, 1992;318-32

[16] WHO .(2003) Guidelines for safe recreational water environments Volume 1: Coastal and freshwaters. World Health Organization, Geneva, 2003.

[17] WHO.(1998) Cyanobacterial toxins: Microcystin-LR in Drinking-water. Background document for development of WHO Guidelines for Drinking-water Quality. Guidelines for drinking-water quality,. World Health Organization, Geneva,1 998.

[18] Zhang H, Zhu G, Jia X, Ding Y, Zhang M, Gao Q, Hu C, Xu (2011) Removal of microcystins-LR from drinking water using a bombon-based charcoal adsorbent modified with chitosan.. J Environ Sci (China). 2011;23(12):1983-8.

4

Purification of Staphylococcal Enterotoxin Type D and Obtaining Its Antiserum

Bidjeh Kebkiba[1, *], Ban-Bo Bebanto Antipas[2], Podkapaev Vladimir Michaelovich[3]

[1]Livestock Research Institute for Development (IRED), Ndjamena, Chad
[2]Faculty of Exact and Applied Sciences, University of Ndjamena, Ndjamena, Chad
[3]Veterinary Academy in Moscow, KI Skriyabin, Moscow, Russia

Email address:
bidjeh.kebkiba@gmail.com (B. Kebkiba), bidjehkebkiba@yahoo.fr (B. Kebkiba)

Abstract: Uncontrolled use of antibiotics in the treatment of calves suffering from gastroenteritis and dairy cows suffering from mastitis, created in pathogenic staphylococci enterotoxin producers some resistance to these drugs. These pathogens enterotoxin producers are often excreted with milk from cows with mastitis. That is why the specific and topical issue remains the isolation and identification of strains producing staphylococcal enterotoxin from cow milk and faeces of calves suffering from enteritis. Given all this, we have set a goal to get staphylococcal enterotoxin type D for use as mastitis diagnostic kit and enteritis and antigen for obtaining the antiserum. To obtain the staphylococcal enterotoxin type D we used *strain* S. *aureus No. 494 (ATSS23235)* courtesy offered by Dr. FC Fluer from Institute of Experimental Medicine, NF Gamaley, Medical Academy (USSR). Verification of the specificity of the enterotoxin) was performed using 5 *strains of S.aureus* producing different enterotoxins (enterotoxin - A; enterotoxin-B; enterotoxin C_{-1}; C_{-2} and enterotoxin - E) as well as non-enterotoxigenic staphylococcal strain (*S. aureus* Wood 46). In addition to the staphylococcal strains, five *strains of Escherichia coli*, producing thermostable and thermolabile enterotoxins were also used in the experiment. The method of purification of enterotoxin-D by precipitation twice chromatography on km - *cellulose* and gel filtration on *Sephadex* G-75 allows to obtain pure enterotoxin-D having the biological properties, immunological and antigenic characteristics. Immunization of rabbits with purified enterotoxin-D associated with incomplete Freund's adjuvant provides antiserum very active and specific.

Keywords: *Staphylococcus aureus,* Milk, *faeces*, Enterotoxin, Antiserum, Enteritis

---

1. Introduction

Some researchers VA Alikaev *et al.;* PB Barto *et al.*; MA Volovenko and BV Venskiyavitchen *[1;* 32; 40; 41] reported that a high percentage of recorded gastro enteritis in calves is mainly due to the ingested milk from cows suffering from mastitis. In the aetiology of gastro-enteritis of calves, it is important to also consider non-compliance with hygienic rearing conditions of these young animals. Many authors believe that young animals become contaminated with microorganisms such as enterotoxigenic *Staphylococcus aureus and Escherichia coli,* through the ingestion of colostrum or milk from cows suffering from mastitis [3]. The role of enterotoxigenic staphylococci in the aetiology of gastro-enteritis in calves remains to be elucidated. There are in the literature data on the purification methods of staphylococcal enterotoxin type D and its identification in the milk or colostrum and other food. However, these authors have used more complex methods for purification and for obtaining the antiserum. Also, the methods used by these authors are difficult to apply in laboratories in developing countries [4]. Milk from cows with mastitis represents a great danger to human health, particularly for infants and the elderly [18; 22].

Until the 20th century, most of authors [5; 12; 19; 20; 33; 34], used kittens for biological test to identify the staphylococcal enterotoxin, but rarely mice and pups, as they are insensitive. By cons, in the United States of America, the monkey genus *rhesus Macacca* was used for this test. Also note that the identification of staphylococcal enterotoxin by the biological test is laborious and time consuming and the results are still not satisfactory. Also, for the biological testing a significant number of animals require; In addition, this method only allows detecting the presence of enterotoxin, but does not give rise to know the serotype of the offending enterotoxin inducing Intoxication. The aim of this work is to develop a simple method of purification of staphylococcal enterotoxin type D for use as an antigen in immunization of rabbits in order to obtain the antiserum for diagnosis of enteritis due to staphylococci enterotoxin-D producing.

2. Materials and Methods

To obtain the staphylococcal enterotoxin type D we used *strain* S. *aureus No. 494 (ATSS23235)* courtesy offered by Dr. FC Fluer from Institute of Experimental Medicine, NF Gamaley, Medical Academy (USSR). To verify the specificity of the enterotoxin we used 5 *strains of S. aureus* enterotoxins producing such as: FRI 722- enterotoxin- A; FRI-243-enterotoxin- B; FRI-137-enterotoxin C_{-1}; FRI-493-enterotoxin C_{-2} and FRI-326 enterotoxin-E), and non-enterotoxigenic staphylococcal strain *(S. aureus* Wood 46). In addition to the staphylococcal strains, five *strains of Escherichia coli (E.* P16, *E.* 1012, and E.015 - H10407, thermostable enterotoxin-producing; *E.*coli-P99, producing heat-labile enterotoxin, have also been used in the experiment. The morphological, dyeing, biological and enzymatic properties of 7 *strains of S.aureus* indicated above as well as strains isolated from f*aeces* of calves with diarrhea and cow milk-producing staphylococcal enterotoxin-D were studied by the method of KI Mateveev; BA Nourmatov *et al.* and AK Akatov *et al.* [24; 23; 25]. In the experiment, 10 rabbits, genus *chinchilla* weighing 2.5-3 grams each; 180 kittens 1-3 months of age and weighing 350-700 g each, were used. Material containing the enterotoxin is obtained according to the method of. of CE Donnelly *et al.* [31] by cultivating the S. *aureus* strain No. *494* in the plastic bag under continuous stirring at a rate of 280-300 rounds / min for 24-48 hours and the ventilation method, which involves passing air through medium through the two filters using a micro compressor mark VK-1 (220V, 50Hz, 10watt). To obtain the maximum concentration of staphylococcal enterotoxin type D, 5 different culture media were tested. These are: Medium n° 1. [26], modified by VI Bougrova *et al.* [6]; Medium n°2. [29]; Medium n°3. [30], Medium n°4 [42] and Medium n°5 [46]. All of these media are prepared on the basis of casein hydrolyzat and supplemented amino acids and vitamins in different concentrations. The activity of the enterotoxin is set to kittens by the method of [33]. Purification of enterotoxin is performed according to the method of K. Bidjeh, [4], which comprises of passing (2 times) the solution containing enterotoxin on km- *cellulose* and on *sephadex* G-75 gel. The homogeneity of the enterotoxin has been defined by the disc electrophoresis method as in acid system [39] that in the basic system [28] in a gel (7.5 %) of polyacrylamyl using the reagents and the electrophoresis apparatus *(Reanal,* Hungary).Some physicochemical properties of enterotoxin-D were studied as follows: heating at 80, 90 and 100°C. for 15, 30 and 60 minutes, and by studying the action of certain enzymes such as trypsin, pepsin, renin and hemotrypsin (all at a concentration of 0. 3%).

For antisera, 8 rabbits were immunized according to the method of EP Casman *et al.* [46]. Purified enterotoxin mixed with Freund's incomplete adjuvant in equal parts, injected into rabbits intramuscularly at increasing dosis (mg protein / ml) - 0.10; 0.10; 0.15; 0.2; 0.3; 0.4; 0.6; 0.8; 0.9; 1.2; 1.6; 1.6; 1,6 at 6- 7 days interval. In the control group, two non-immunized rabbits were used. The action and specificity of the antiserum have been defined by the agar immunodiffusion reaction (AGID) in petri dishes by the method of Ouchterlony O. [38] and in tubes. For the reaction of immunoelectrophoresis (IEP) is the method of P. Graber *et al.* [48] was used. 10 days after the 13th injection, rabbits were bled. After clotting, the clot is removed and the serum is obtained by centrifuging the contents of the tubes at 3000 rpm / min for 30 minutes and stored at -20 ° C. The resulting serum of each animal is considered as a serial. A total of 4 series of serum was obtained. The sera are then distributed in tubes and kept at -20°C for further use.

3. Results

Purification of enterotoxin - D and its physicochemical properties

Purification of enterotoxin-D is carried out as follows: after passing on km-*cellulose* (twice), washing is done on the gel *Sephadex* G-75 with distilled water until obtaining the pH neutral (7.0). After lyophilization, entering the second step on km-*cellulose.* After that, it was noted that only peak 3 had biological activity and the bioassay was positive on kittens. By repeating chromatography on km-*cellulose*, it has been found that a single peak eluting had a positive biological effect on kittens. The results of the disc –electrophoresis of eluent on polyacrylamil gel obtained after the 3rd purification step, showed that enterotoxin was not homogeneous because on the gel appeared two precipitation lines, indicating the presence of the second element in the solution (eluent), which is nothing other than *α - hemolysin, which* has been shown by the action hemolytic eluent on erythrocytes of rabbits. After 4th purification step on Sephadex, only the second peak of eluting possessed a biological action on kittens. The homogeneity of the enterotoxin is demonstrated by the appearance of a single precipitation line on the gel and the absence of hemolytic activity on erythrocytes of rabbits. It has been shown that both the purified enterotoxin and unpurified were resistant to the action of proteolytic effect of enzymes (0.3%) such as pepsin, trypsin, hemotrypsin and renin. Enterotoxin both purified and non-purified is destroyed at the temperature ranged between 85 and 100°C for 25 minutes as they lose their antigenic properties.

Obtaining antiserum enterotoxin- D and its specific action by immunodiffusion tests on agar (AGID), precipitation in tubes (IPT) and the immunoelectrophoresis test (IEP)

The activity of each serum is checked by the AGID and IPT tests. Both by the AGID as other immunochemical tests, the antiserum revealed the homogeneity of enterotoxin-D to the minimum concentration of protein of 10, 62 mg/ml, which is demonstrated by the appearance of one line of precipitation between the wells containing the enterotoxin-D and those containing antiserum at different dilutions: from 1/2 to 1/32.

The specificity of the antiserum obtained was checked by various tests: Agar gel immuno diffusion (AGID), immuno-precipitation in tubes (IPT) and immunoelectrophoresis (IEP) vis-à-vis the heterogeneous enterotoxins (Table 1.). From this table, we can see that antiserum anti-enterotoxin- D has been very specific because it does not react with the filtrates of enterotoxigenic staphylococci producing enterotoxin types: A, B, C $_1$, C $_2$ and E and S. *aureus* strain producing α and β- hemolysin. As it can be seen from the said table 1, antiserum anti-enterotoxin-D does not react with any of these above mentioned antigens. Similar results were found with the supernatant of E. Coli N°1012, E; coli P16 and *E.* coli H10407 producers of thermostable enterotoxin (TS); E. *Coli* N°015-339, heat-labile enterotoxin Producer (TL). We recorded the same results with A-enterotoxin of Cl. *Perfringens.*

Table 1. *Specificity of the antiserum anti-enterotoxin-D in AGID, PT and IEP tests.*

Antigens	Protein concentration mg / ml	Results		
		IDG	IPT	IEP
S. enterotoxin-A	6000	-	-	-
S. enterotoxin-B	6000	-	-	-
S. enterotoxin C $_1$	5000	-	-	-
Enterotoxin C $_2$ S.	5000	-	-	-
S. -E enterotoxin	4000	-	-	-
A and *β-S.* hemolysins	6000	-	-	-
TS E.coli 1012	3900	-	-	-
TS P 16 E. coli	3900	-	-	-
TL E. Coli P99	3900	-	-	-
TS, TL E. coli H10407	3900	-	-	-
E.coli 015-339	3900	-	-	-
CL. perfringens-A	170	-	-	-
S. enterotoxin-D	4000	+	+	+

NB.: For staphylococcal enterotoxin types A, B, C $_1$, C $_2$, D and E, the supernatant that was used in the experiment. As for the enterotoxin-A of Cl. *Perfringens* is the purified product, which was used.

Demonstration of enterotoxin -D in the faeces of calves suffering from enteritis and in the milk or colostrum of cows suffering from mastitis.

In the study no positive reaction was found with faeces from healthy calves. By cons, among the 30 faecal samples from calves, 8 (26, 66%) reacted positively with antiserum anti-enterotoxin -D by AGID test; 2 (6.66%) yielded questionable results by the same test. The presence of enterotoxin - D has been demonstrated in 6 (75%) faecal samples from calves aged from 5 to 8 days. In 2 (25%) of cases, the results were also positive with faeces from calves aged 1 to 7 days. 2 (25%) calves, whose samples were positive with antiserum anti-enterotoxin-D, were aged between 4 and 7 days respectively. The age groups corresponding to the period when calves are often suffering from enteritis were divided as follows: 1, 3, 5 and 6 days. The study of infected pasteurilised milk with staphylococcal colonies producing enterotoxin- D at a concentration of 10^3 and 10^{5}/ ml did not reveal the presence of enterotoxin -D in any case regardless of the incubation time at 37 ° C for 3, 6, 18 and 24 hours. By cons, in the samples of pasteurellised milk infected with *S. aureus* at a concentration of 10^{6} - 10^{9} and incubated at 37°C for 18-24 h, there was secretion of enterotoxin-D, Which allows deducing that the speed of secretion of enterotoxin-D depends on the quantity of microorganisms in the medium and the incubation time. The study of 95 samples of milk with 5% dimastin solution showed that the reaction was positive in only 36 (37.8%) cases. In contrast, with the immunochemical test (AGID), no sample was positive vis-a-vis the antiserum anti-enterotoxin-D. However, of 17 samples of colostrum tested, only 2 (11.76%) reacted positively with antiserum anti-enterotoxin-D by AGID test. This is explained by the fact that among the cow milk, the concentration of enterotoxin is so low that we cannot detect with AGID test, while in cows that have given birth, the possibility of revealing the presence of enterotoxin-D is the first milking.

4. Discussion

In general, increased animal production requires industrialization in this area and the creation of large livestock complexes. However, infectious diseases such as enteritis due to staphylococci significantly reduce growth in the number of cattle in dairy farms. The information collected in different scientific journals shows the possible role of enterotoxigenic staphylococci in enteritis of calves and mastitis in dairy cows excreting enterotoxigenic staphylococci with milk and constituting potential sources of diseases such as food poisoning, gastroenteritis, etc. [1; 2; 3; 4; 9; 10; 11; 13; 14; 16; 17; 27; 35; 39; 40; 41; 45; 50]. However, the role of staphylococci producing enterotoxin- D in the aetiology of these diseases is poorly understood and the simplified method of identifying the enterotoxin in faeces of calves suffering from enteritis has not been in focus. It is the same for the milk of cow carriers of pathogenic staphylococci. EH Kato et al.[35]; MS Berdoll [43]; KN Shinagawa Kunita [49]; EP Casman *et al.*[*46*] described the methods of purification and identification of the staphylococcal enterotoxin type D in milk and colostrum from cows, but the authors used for these purposes complex methods difficult to implement in the conditions of laboratories in developing countries. These shortcomings noted have led us to use the four-step purification of staphylococcal enterotoxin-D.

Today, the most effective diagnosis of enterotoxicoses caused by staphylococci can be done with the immunochemical test that gives accurate and satisfactory results. For use, it is necessary to have the purified enterotoxin and the antiserum [4; 21; 47; 15; 44]. However, in the veterinary field, the development of such reagents requires the development of special technology for extraction, purification of enterotoxin and obtaining the homologous antiserum.

By immunizing rabbits with enterotoxin-D, it was noted that it is only at the 9th injection that was able to detect antibodies directed against enterotoxin-D (½ of dilution). Then, antibody titers increased progressively up to 1/8 according to increase in the dose of the antigen. Also note that in the immunization process, 4 rabbits (50%) died, demonstrating the toxicity of enterotoxin-D. The use of this immunization scheme of rabbits demonstrates once again that enterotoxin-D, like other staphylococcal enterotoxins have low antigenic property.

Many problems associated with the effect of colostrum from cows suffering from mastitis and carrier enterotoxigenic staphylococci. These problems have not previously found solutions, while the spread of enterotoxicoses of calves are recorded every day and this number increases rapidly [40; 3]. The antiserum obtained is one of the possible solutions to these problems. As it will detect the presence of enterotoxin-D in the milk / colostrum from cows suffering from mastitis and in the faeces of calves suffering from gastroenteritis.

5. Conclusion

The method of purification of enterotoxin-D by precipitation twice chromatography on *km- cellulose* and gel filtration on *Sephadex* G-75 allows to obtain pure enterotoxin-D having the biological properties, immunological and antigenic characteristics of staphylococcal enterotoxin.

Immunization of rabbits with purified enterotoxin-D associated with incomplete Freund's adjuvant provides antiserum very active and specific. Obtaining purified enterotoxin and the antiserum thus offering use the immunochemical method for the detection of enterotoxin-D in the supernatant of faeces of sick calves and dairy cows carrier pathogenic staphylococci.

References

[1] Alikaev VA, VV Matuchin. Fight against calves gastroenteritis. Veterinariya, 1982, 4, 51-55.

[2] Alikaev VA. Prophylaxis of cow diseases in industrial livestock complexes. Moscow kolos, 1976, 192p.

[3] Abzaloba AG. Mastitis and gastroenteritis. Uralski Nivi, 1978, 3, 52-53.

[4] Bidjeh K. Development of identification method of staphylococcal enterotoxin type D in milk /*colostrum* of cows and in the faecal samples of calves suffering from enteritis. phD *thesis,* Veterinary Academy of Moscow KI Skriyabin, Moscow, 1984, 176p.

[5] Baïliozov D. B., Panaïtova M., Visiolinov V.O. About the identification method of staphylococcal enterotoxin. JMEI, 1962, 8, 101-109.

[6] Bougrova V.I., Nikolaeva I.S. obtaining the enterotoxin- A for the diagnosis of staphylococcal intoxication. Vapros pitani, 1974.6, 47-52.

[7] Berdoll MS. The nature of staphylococcal enterotoxins. Clinical toxicol. 1972, 5, 4, 441.

[8] Berdoll MS, Huang IY, Schantz EJ. Chemistry of staphylococcal entertoxins. J. Agric. Food Chem., 1974, 22, 9-13.

[9] Winduga Bozena. Occurrence of enterotoxigenic staphylococci especially producors of entertoxin- D and E among Strains isolated from food. Acta food. Pol., 1978, 4, 2, 129-132.

[10] Kartachova V.M. Fast detection method of staphylococcal toxin in milk and dairy products. Veterinariya, 1970, 11, 105-107.

[11] Kartachova V.M. Methods for identifying staphylococci and their toxins in milk and milk products. In: Identification of pathogenic bacteries in milk and milk products, Moscow, Kolos, 1973, 108-148.

[12] Kuchko I.V., Xatmever M.L., Akatov A.K. About the possibility of the method of use of part of the intestine ligature of experimental animals for identification of enterotoxins. In: The problem of staphylococcal infections. Tch. I. Saratov, 1979, 13-15.

[13] Minor T.E., Mart E.X. Staphylocci in food products, Moscow, 1980. 231p.

[14] Niskanen A., Korainen L., Roine K. Staphylococcal enterotoxin and Thermonuclease production during the induced bovine mastitis and the clinical reaction of enterotoxin in Udders. Infection and Immunity, 1978, 19, 2, 493-498.

[15] Sabri Darvich Morgan Selim. Immunochemical Method identification of the staphylococci producing enterotoxin-A isolated from cows with mastitis. phD *thesis*, 1979 178, 178p.

[16] Santos E.C., Moreira H.A. Influence of mastitis induced by staphylococcal enterotoxin protein on the composition of bovine milk. Arg. E sc. Vet., 1976, 28, 3, 227-232.

[17] Santos E.C., Moreira H.A. Influence of staphylococcal mastitis induced by enterotoxin on production of bovine milk. Arg. E sc. Vet., 1977, 29, 1, 5-10.

[18] Slavchev G. Economic importance of sub/clinical mastitis in cows. Vet. Sb., 1982, 80, 8, 34-36.

[19] Stolmakova A.I. Food poisoning original staphylococci. University of Lvov, Lvov, 1959. 22p.

[20] Stolmakova A.I. Experimental poisoning of animals by the staphylococcal enterotoxin, 1954, 13, 5, 28-33.

[21] Fluer F.S. Some physicochemical, structural and functional properties of staphylococcal entertoxins. JMEI, 19, 80, 12, 9-17.

[22] Mutovin V.I. Fight against mastitis of cows, Moscow, 1974, 254p.

[23] Nourmatov B.A., Dvites NE. Bacteriological diagnostic of staphylococcal infections (methodological Recommendations) Tashkent, 1978, 22p.

[24] Mateveev K.I. Annals of microbiological diagnosis of infectious diseases, 2nd ed, Moscow, 1973, 624p.

[25] Akatov A.K., Zueva V.S. Staphylococci, Medicine, Moscow, 1983, 256p.

[26] Casman E.P. Serological studies of staphylococcal Enterotoxins. Public health, report, 1958, 73, 599-609.

[27] Casman E.P, Berdoll M.S., Robinson J. Designation of staphylococcal enterotoxins. J. Bacteriol., 1963, 85, 715-716.

[28] Davis B.J. Disc electrophoresis. II. Method and Application to human proteins. Ann. NY Acad. Science 1964, 121, 404-427.

[29] Jarvis A.W. and Lowrence R.C. Production of high titers of Enterotoxins for the routine testing of staphylococci. Applied Microbiology, 1970, 19, 4, 698-699.

[30] Noleto A.L. and Berdoll M.S. Staphylococcal enterotoxin Production in the non-enterotoxigenic staphylococci. Applied and Environmental Microbiology, 1980, 39, 6, 1167-1171.

[31] Donnelly C.B., leslie J.E., Black LA. Serological identification of enterotoxigenic staphylococci in cheese. Applied Microbiology, 1967, 15, 1382-1387.

[32] Barto P.B., Bush L.J., Adams G.D. Effect of sour colostrum on survival of *Staphylococcus aureus*. Animal Science Research report, 1979.104, 265-326.

[33] Dolman E.C., Wilson R G. The kitten test for staphylococcal enterotoxin. Canadian Journal of Public Health, 1940, 31, 68-71.

[34] Hammon Mcd. W. Staphylococcal enterotoxin: An Improved cat test. Chemical and immunological studies. Am. J. Public Health, 1941, 31, 1191-1198.

[35] Kato Tsuneo E. and Kume. Enterotoxigenicity of staphylococci isolated from bovine mastitis California test- positive milking. Japan. J. Vet. Res. 1980, 28, 3, 75-85.

[36] Olson J.C., Casman E.P., Berdoll M.S. Enterotoxigenicity cultures of *staphylococcus aureus* isolated from bovine mastitis of acute cases. Journal of applied microbiology, 1970, 20, 4, 605- 607.

[37] Ostachevski A.G., Obrassov V.P., Kotenko I.I. Using the precipitation reaction for the identification of enterotoxigenic staphylococci. Trudi kharkov, zoovet., Institute., 1970 (1971), 5, 29, 22-26.

[38] Ouchterlony. Antigen antibodies reactions in gels. Acta Patholol. Microbiol. Scand., 1949, 25, 507-515.

[39] Reisfeld R.A., Lewis U.J., Williams D.E. Disc electrophoresis of proteins in basic polyacrylamid gels. Nature 1962, 195, 281-283.

[40] Volovenko M.A. Effect of colostrum and milk products coming from cows with mastitis on natural resistance and morbidity of calves. *PhD Thesis*, Kharkov, 1975 173P.

[41] Venskiyavischen V.B. Effect of udder on the morbidity of calves. Bulletin of the Scientific and Technological Information, 1967.1, 46-47.

[42] Favourite G.O., Hammon W.M. Production of staphylococcal toxin, enterotoxin and alpha hemolysin in a simplified medium. Journal of bacteriology, 194,141, 305-316.

[43] Berdoll M.S. Staphylococcal poisoning. In: H. Riemann and Bryan F.L. (ed) Food borne infections and intoxications 2nd ed. Academic Press, New York, 1979, 443-494.

[44] Berdoll MS, H. Sugiyama, Dack GM. Staphylococcal enterotoxin I. Purification. Ach. Bioch. Biophys., 1959, 85, 85-89.

[45] Bozena Z.S. Enterotoxigenicity of staphylococci isolated from cow milk with mastitis. Medecin veterinariya 1980, 36, 6, 368-370.

[46] Casman E.P., Bennet R.W., Dorsey A.E. Issa J.A. Identification of staphylococcal enterotoxin D, fourth serotype. Bacteriology, 1967, 94, 6, 1875-1882.

[47] Chang H.C. and Berdoll M.S. Purification of Reduced and Some properties of staphylococcal enterotoxin-D. Biochemistry 1979, 18, 1937-1942.

[48] Graber P. Immunoelectrophoretic analysis. Methods Biochem. 1959 7, 1-38

[49] Shinagawa K., N. Kunita Simplified methods for purification of staphylococcal Enterotoxins A and C and preparation of anti – enterotoxin. Jap. Bacterial J. 1975, 30, 6, 683-692.

[50] Tingting zhang, Anning Huang, Junnian Li, Liu Xinqin, Liuli, Lu Yao, Ying Huang and Wang WinPing. Characterization of antimicrobial resistance and enterotoxin in meticillin - resistant *Staphylococcus aureus* isolated from milk and food poisoning cases. Journal of animal and veterinary advances, 201413 (7) 423-429.

5

Comparison Between Plethysmometer and Caliper Methods to Monitor Lesion-Size Induced by *Leishmania major* Infection in BALB/c Mouse Experimental Model

Hanene Attia[1, 2], Aymen Bali[1, 2], Rabiaa M. Sghaier[1, 2], Pablo A. Leon Martinez[1, 2], Ghada Mkannez[1, 2], Chiraz Atri[1, 2], Khaled Chourabi[1, 2], Fatma Z. Guerfali[1, 2], Dhafer Laouini[1, 2, *]

[1]Institut Pasteur de Tunis, LR11IPT02, Laboratory of Transmission, Control and Immunobiology of Infections (LTCII), Tunis-Belvédère, Tunisia

[2]Université Tunis El Manar, Tunis, Tunisia

Email address:

dhafer_l@yahoo.ca (D. Laouini), dhafer.laouini@pasteur.rns.tn (D. Laouini)

Abstract: In several parasitological diseases, as for leishmaniasis, measurement of the size of cutaneous lesions, which develop at the site of parasite inoculation in animal models, are the most commonly used index to assess disease progression, to compare parasites pathogenicity or virulence and to determine the effects of drug treatment and immunotherapies. The aim of this study is to compare the accuracy of two measurement tools i.e., the caliper and the plethysmometer to refine the lesion size determination. Our findings showed that the use of plethysmometer produced higher correlation with the importance of the lesion mass at experimental endpoints. These findings suggest that, for better differentiation in drug monitoring or *Leishmania* (*L.*) strains' virulence and pathogenicity, plethysmometer method is more sensitive to detect parasite-induced swelling and lesions differences at the end of experimental protocols when lesion size is important but caliper is more indicated for small lesions.

Keywords: *Leishmania major*, BALB/c Experimental Model, Lesion Size, Caliper, Plethysmometer

1. Introduction

The clinical manifestations of human cutaneous leishmaniasis caused by *Leishmania* (*L.*) *major* display a spectrum of disease severity varying from an asymptomatic infection to multiple disfiguring scars [1, 2]. This differential clinical expression is considered as the result of interaction between individual behaviour of the microorganism and the host immunologic background. Relative contribution of the host immune background and the vector components involvement are difficult to measure [1, 3, 4], especially in host-outbred individuals such as humans.

Animal models of cutaneous leishmaniasis are useful tools for dissecting mechanisms related to disease pathogenesis and vaccine or drug development [5]. Indeed, cutaneous infection of mice with *L. major* is a well-established experimental model of chronic human disease caused by an intracellular parasite. This local infection is not well controlled by the immune anti-parasite responses in susceptible BALB/c mice and the disease disseminates towards the visceral organs with fatal outcome.

Upon experimental infection with different *L. major* strains, distinct aspects of the clinical spectrum of human cutaneous leishmaniasis have been generally reflecting the spectrum of clinical manifestations in humans with reasonable success. Indeed, infection of different inbred strains of mice with *L. major* can, to certain limits, mimic the disease phenotype observed in human cutaneous leishmaniasis [6] and is routinely used for vaccine or treatment discovery [7-9].

This model is also suitable for comparing the intrinsic virulence of different isolates of *Leishmania* belonging to the same species [1, 10] and might hence reflect the pathogenicity and virulence of each isolate. It is also suitable for the determination of the effects of drug treatment, immunotherapies and vaccines.

Several previous [11, 12] as well as new [13-15] studies

used routinely the caliper to monitor the lesion development induced in the footpad of animals. This measure represents the difference between the widths and/or the thicknesses of the infected and the uninfected paws of the same mouse. Hence, caliper measurements are commonly collected along the longest two dimensions of the lesion x/y plane only, with the z-axis dimension assumed to be the same [16]. Depending on the manipulator, caliper measures may suffer errors and are not easily reproducible from an experiment to another.

Another measure tool is more and more used i. e., the plethysmometer. It is routinely used to study tumors and potential anti-inflammatory or anti-edema properties of pharmacological substances [17-20]. It is more and more routinely used to measure paw inflammation and edema in rodent models [21, 22]. Instead of measuring the lesion diameter, the size is rather determined by the difference between the volume of the infected paw and the volume of the uninfected one of the same mouse. To our knowledge, there are no studies reporting comparison between the two methods in the experimental model of *L. major* infection.

In this work, using the BALB/c experimental mice model, we aimed to compare lesion measurements obtained by both methods on the same animals infected with different *L. major* wild strains isolated from patients living in a zoonotic cutaneous leishmaniasis (ZCL) endemic area of Tunisia.

2. Materials and Methods

Eleven strains of *L. major* were isolated from fresh lesions of patients living in the Centre of Tunisia, an endemic region for ZCL. The study protocol, consent forms and procedures were reviewed and approved by the Institut Pasteur de Tunis Ethical Review Board. Patients provided written informed consent for the collection of parasites and subsequent use.

The isolates were harvested between October 2009 and March 2010, the period in which the lesions of the majority of the individuals infected during the ZCL transmission period appear.

2.1. Parasite Culture, Metacyclic form Purification

Promastigotes were cultured in NNN solid medium at 26°C, and then progressively adapted to a medium composed of RPMI 1640 and 10% of Fetal Calf Serum (FCS) and supplemented with 100 U of penicillin/ml, 100 µg of streptomycin/ml and 2 mM L-glutamine. When the stationary phase was reached, the metacyclic promastigotes were then purified by a negative selection with peanut agglutinin (PNA) (Sigma, Saint-Quentin Fallavier, France). The PNA^- and PNA^+ fractions were separated by density gradient centrifugation. The PNA-metacyclic promastigotes were washed and diluted at the desired density.

2.2. Animal Infection and Monitoring of the Disease Pattern

BALB/c female mice were obtained from the specific pathogen-free animal-breeding facility Janvier (France) and maintained in a conventional animal facility at Institut Pasteur de Tunis, Tunisia. Animal experiments were performed in compliance with the directive 86/609/EEC of the European parliament and the council on the protection of animals used for scientific purposes, in agreement with the guidelines of International Guiding Principles for Biomedical Research Involving Animals and with the approval of the Ethical Review Board of Institut Pasteur de Tunis.

For each *Leishmania* isolate (identified by an Arabic number), a group of 5 to 6 eight-week old BALB/c mice was infected with 2×10^6 metacyclic promastigotes. Isolates correspond to parasites obtained from ZCL patients with heterogeneous clinical outcomes. The parasites were suspended in 50 µl of 1X PBS and injected in the left footpad. The right footpad is considered as an uninfected control.

From the second week of infection, lesion development was assessed weekly by measuring the diameter and volume of right and left pads by the same operator and using the same devices i. e.; a vernier caliper and a plethysmometer (Model 7140; Ugo Basile, Italy). Lesion development using caliper was then assessed by measuring the thickness diameter difference between the infected and non-infected footpad of every mouse (mm). Immediately following measurements, data sets were also collected using plethysmometer device.

The water digital plethysmometer is formed by two interconnected tubes filled with a conductive solution, a platinum electrode for each chamber and a control unit. When the mouse paw is immersed in the measuring tube, the water displacement is also produced in the second tube inducing a change in the conductance between the two platinum electrodes. The control unit detects the conductance changes and generates an output signal to the digital display indicating the volume displacement measured in milliliter (0.01 ml resolution). Difference between the volume displacement of the infected and uninfected footpad indicates the lesion volume (ml). At the end of the experimental protocol, mice were sacrificed and the infected and contralateral footpads of each mouse were excised and weighed using a precision balance. Parasite load from infected mice was determined by limiting-dilution method following a protocol described elsewhere [23]. Briefly, excised pads were homogenized. A serial 10-fold dilutions were plated in duplicate in 96-well flat-bottom microtiter plates (Nunc, Roskilde, Denmark) containing Schneider's *Drosophila* medium (both from Gibco-BRL, Paisley, Scotland) supplemented with 100 U of penicillin/ml, 100 µg of streptomycin/ml, 2 mM L-glutamine, and 10% heat-inactivated fetal calf serum. Viable parasites were observed microscopically after seven to 10 days of incubation at 26°C. Parasite load was then determined as the reciprocal of the highest dilution at which promastigotes could be grown in culture at 26°C and detected by microscope.

2.3. Statistical Analyses

All the statistical tests were performed using PRISM software. To measure the correlation between the lesion size obtained either using a plethysmometer or a caliper, the Pearson correlation coefficient r and the p value were used. To evaluate the sensitivity of plethysmometer method versus caliper one, number of variables above or below the linear regression were quantified.

3. Results

3.1. Lesion Size Monitoring

For each tested *Leishmania* isolate, a group of five to six BALB/c mice were infected. Footpad sizes were weekly measured during eight weeks using both the caliper and the plethysmometer. The sizes of the contralateral footpads of each mouse were also measured using both methods in the same day of the former measurement.

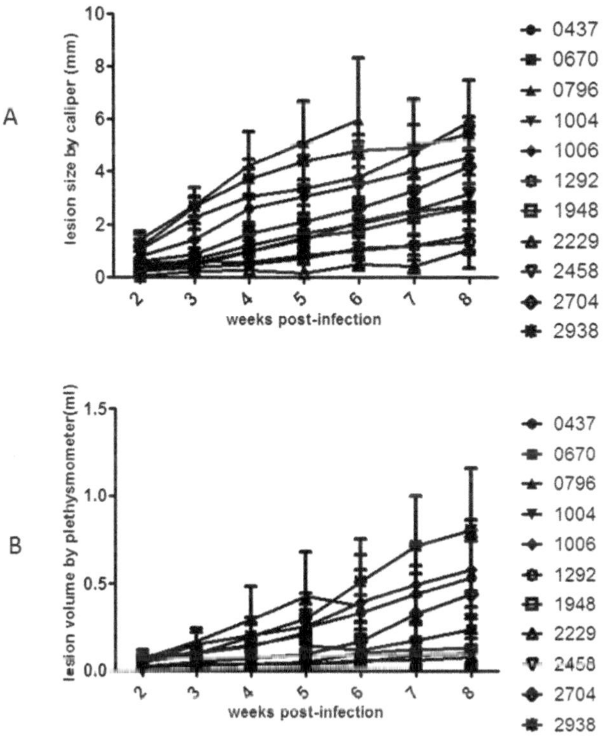

Figure 1. Lesion evolution in BALB/c mice infected with different wild Leishmania major field isolates. Left hind footpad Mice were inoculated subcutaneously with 2×10^6 metacyclic promastigotes. Measurements were performed weekly using a vernier caliper (A) and a plethysmometer (B). Lesion diameter (A) and volume (B) were calculated by subtracting the measure of the contralateral-uninfected footpad using the same tool. Arabic numbers corresponding to each isolate mentions the parasite identification. Results are expressed as the mean lesion size of five to six mice per group ± SD.

As shown in Fig. 1, lesion evolution in each group of mice was measured either with caliper (Panel A) or plethysmometer (Panel B). Results showed a heterogeneous evolution of lesions during the infection course, according to the parasite isolate used. When comparing the two methods for each isolate, we did not notice any important difference according to the lesion evolution. Nevertheless, scale extent seems to be more pronounced at the beginning or the end of infection course, when measures were taken by caliper or by plethysmometer, respectively.

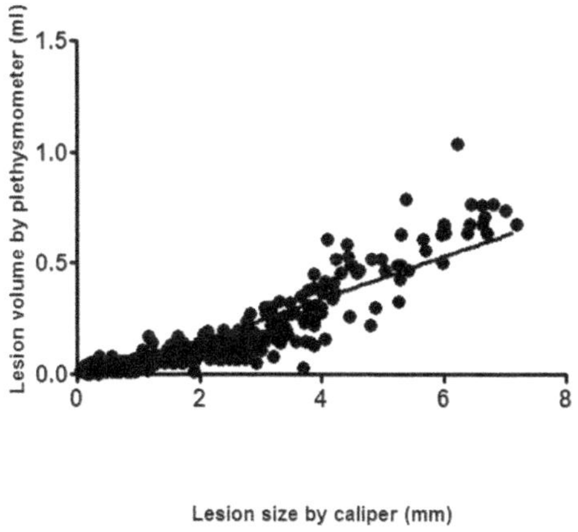

Figure 2. Pair-comparison and linear regression of 362 plethysmometer measurements against their caliper counterparts of lesion sizes during eight-week protocol. Caliper measurements were expressed by mm and plethysmometer measurements were expressed by ml and correspond respectively to the diameter and the volume of each lesion as the difference between the infected and uninfected footpad. Pearson r correlation coefficients were 0.9070 and 0.8227 respectively.

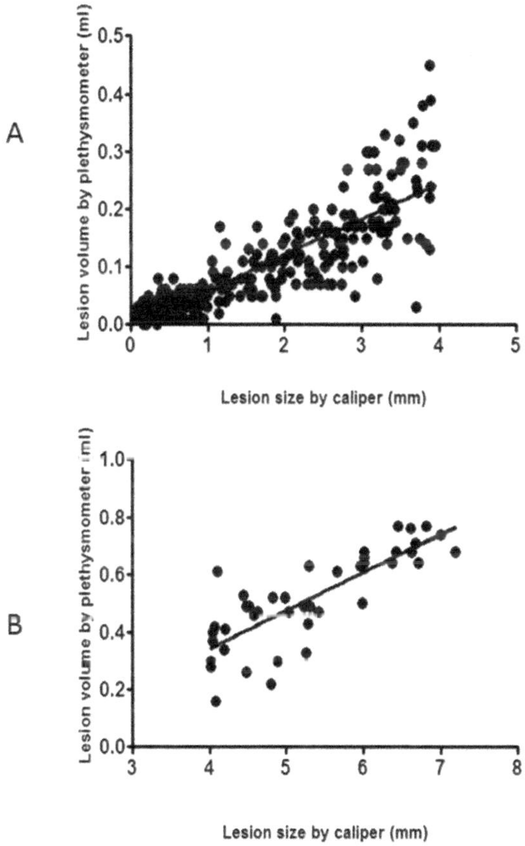

Figure 3. Pair-comparison and linear regression of caliper measurements against their plethysmometer counterparts of lesion sizes depending on their diameter range. Panel A corresponds to lesion diameter < 4 mm (r=0.8578) and panel B corresponds to lesion diameter > 4 mm (r=0.8089). Caliper measurements were expressed by mm and plethysmometer measurements were expressed by ml and correspond respectively to the diameter and the volume of each lesion after calculating the difference between the infected and uninfected footpads.

3.2. Correlation, Sensitivity and Reproducibility Between Plethysmometer and Caliper

Lesion size obtained with plethysmometer and caliper were then pair-compared for each mouse at each time point. The distribution of the total 362 paired-measures was plotted. Results (Fig. 2) showed that global correlation between these paired-measures is statistically significant with a Pearson r coefficient significantly close to 1 (Pearson r=0.9070 and p < 0. 0001). This result witnesses a high correlation between the measures generated using the caliper and those using the plethysmometer.

To assess the sensitivity of each method towards the other, we considered number of points above and below the linear regression curve.

Points above the regression line were more numerous than those below the line (200 versus 162, respectively) indicating that sensitivity is more important by plethysmometer than caliper.

Interestingly, paired-measures' points above the regression line are more numerous when lesion measurements are higher (by both methods) and vice versa. Accordingly, we separated the paired-measures lower or higher than 4 mm as measured by caliper and compared points of each group (range 1 and range 2 respectively, Fig. 3). When comparing paired-measures at range 1, (lower than 4 mm by caliper), Pearson r=0.8578 and p < 0.0001 and when comparing measures at range 2 (higher than 4 mm by caliper), Pearson r=0.8089 and p < 0.0001. Points above the line are more numerous at range 2 (24 out of 42; 57%; Fig. 3, Panel B) than at range 1 (155 out of 313; 49%; Fig. 3, Panel A).

All these results indicate that sensitivity of plethysmometer measurements seems higher than caliper ones with bigger lesions than with smaller ones and vice versa.

To assess reproducibility, we assumed that diameter and volume of each non-infected footpad would be the same during the whole time of experiment. Hence, measures of diameter and volume of contralateral non-infected pads were weakly taken by the same experimenter using both plethysmometer and caliper. Intra-observational variations were 2,5% (2.45 ± 0,06 mm; mean ± SD) in caliper measures and 15,1% (0.13 ± 0.02 ml; mean ± SD) in plethysmometer measures. This result indicates that measures using caliper were more reproducible than those taken with plethysmometer. However, this should be taken with caution since all measures of non-infected footpad are within a range where caliper is more sensitive.

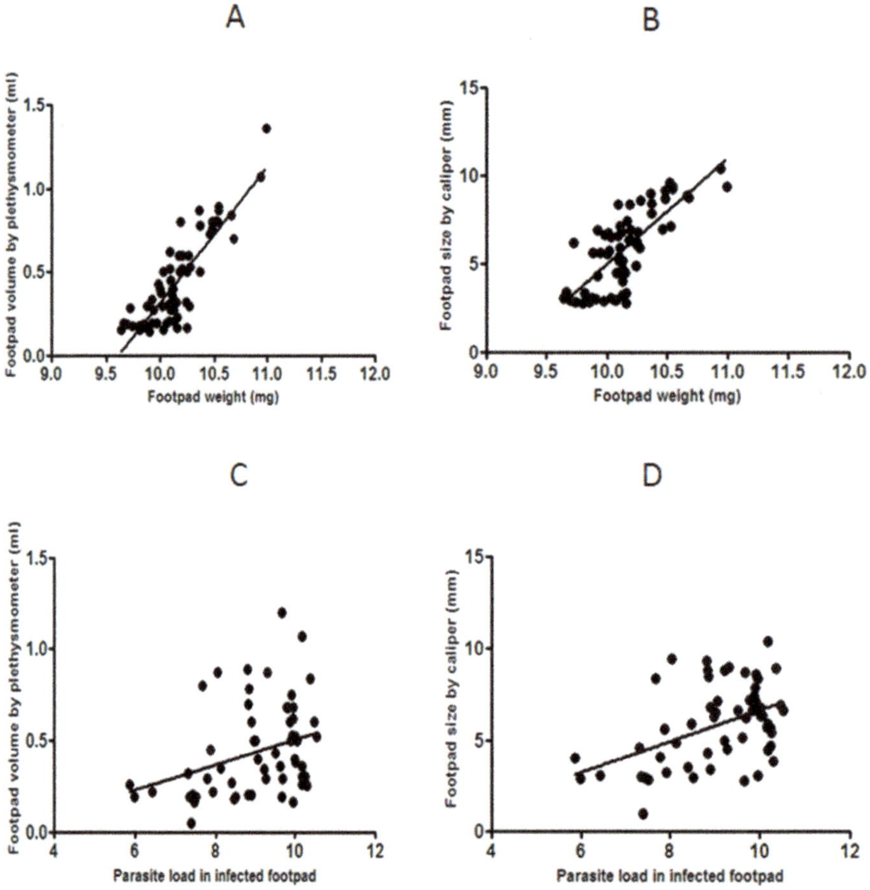

Figure 4. Pair-comparison and linear regression of plethysmometer and caliper measurement of infected footpads size against footpad weight (panels A and B) and parasite load (panels C and D). Panel A corresponds to plethysmometer measurement versus footpad weight (r=0.8515), panel B to caliper measurement versus footpad weight (r=0.7936), panel C to plethysmometer measurement versus parasite load (r=0.3239) and panel D to caliper measurement versus parasite load (r=0.4634).

3.3. Correlation Between Plethysmometer or Caliper Measures and Footpad Weight or Parasite Load

At the end of the eight weeks, mice were sacrificed and the infected feet were excised and weighed. Parasite load was also monitored. The foot weight and the parasite load were used as golden standard measures to evaluate the accuracy of each method. Accuracy can be defined as proximity between the measure of an object and its true value. Indeed, the foot weight is likely reflecting the direct effect of a given isolate on tissue inflammation and lesional extent and the parasite load might be correlated with the apparent lesion size.

As shown in Fig. 4, the volume of the whole infected footpad determined by plethysmometer correlated with footpad weight (Pearson r=0.8515; Fig. 4, panel A) slightly better than the diameter of the whole infected footpad measured with caliper (Pearson r=0.7936; Fig. 4, panel B). When splitting the measurements into two ranges, in those higher than 4 mm by caliper (data not shown), correlations still slightly higher between plethysmometer measurements and footpad weight than those between caliper measurements and footpad weight (Pearson r=0.9436 and 0.8852 respectively). In < 4mm diameters, correlations between plethysmometer measurements and footpad weight are however faintly lower than those between caliper measurements and footpad weight (r=0.8835 and 0.9435 respectively).

When comparing the diameter and volume measures with footpad parasite load, Pearson coefficients are much lower with a slight better correlation with caliper measurements (Pearson r=0.4634; Fig. 4, panel D) then with plethysmometer measurements (Pearson r=0.3239; Fig. 4, panel C). These very low correlations indicate that parasite load cannot be considered, like footpad weight, as a good standard for lesion monitoring.

In conclusion, all these results indicate that measures undertaken either by plethysmometre or caliper are comparable and not revealing notable differences. Nevertheless, when lesions are important, the measures made by plethysmometre are dimly better correlated with infected footpad weight than those undertaken using caliper. However, caliper is better to be used when lesions are small.

4. Discussion

In order to compare two measurement methods for lesion development, Tunisian isolates of *L. major* freshly collected from the field were tested for their experimental pathogenicity in BALB/C mice model. Lesion development was assessed during the infection course using both the caliper and the plethysmometer. Despite the strong correlation between the two methods, power discrimination between the isolates when measures were taken by caliper or plethysmometer was different depending on the lesion size. Indeed, for lesion diameter lower than 4 mm by caliper, plethysmometer is less sensitive but when lesion size is higher than 4 mm, caliper is less sensitive.

Interestingly, when correlating the lesions diameters or volumes obtained by both methods, with total infected foot weight as a standard for lesion development, plethysmometer shows faintly more accurate measures; whereas caliper method seems more accurate when correlating its measures with the total parasite load in infected pads.

These results indicate that both methods could be used, depending on the objectives.

Many studies argued in favor of the use of plethysmometer instead of caliper. As for parasitological studies, cancer studies for instance, require a precise tool to measure tumor volume. Several authors concluded that caliper is inaccurate and encumbered with a significant and size dependent bias compared to other methods [24, 25]. Indeed, and despite its low cost, caliper method was often affected by much error, subjective and inaccurate especially for large tumors which shape differs from small ones [24]. To measure pathogen-induced edema and hyperalgesia during inflammation, other authors used the plethysmometer rather than the caliper for its accuracy [26]. Other physical methods have been shown superior to caliper measurements for determining xenograft tumor volume in mouse models [27].

However, and as far as we know, only one study suggested that the micrometer method, a method comparable to caliper one, could be more sensitive and useful in measuring paw edema in mice than the plethysmometer method, when used to assess the anti-inflammatory activity [28]. Besides the mice models, a recent study presented a precise, complete and noncontact 3D assessment tool for monitoring the evolution of human cutaneous leishmaniasis wounds based on a 3D laser scanner and computer vision algorithms [29]. This proposed 3D assessment tool showed higher accuracy and precision rates than conventional manual methods.

We conclude that use of plethysmometer to measure lesion volume in *Leishmania* mouse model will result in more sensitive measures of volume change at endpoints, especially when lesions are important, like those induced by high virulent strains. However, the caliper method, the current gold standard for lesion measurement in experimental leishmaniasis shows a slight more reproducibility and should be used to monitor lesion size for anti-*Leishmania* vaccines or drugs, where the lesions are expected to be smaller.

5. Conclusion

In conclusion, the use of caliper or plethysmometer for monitoring disease progression in *Leishmania* infected mice should depend mainly on the study goals, having in mind the limitations of each tool and used methodology towards better accuracy. Hence, plethysmometer method showed more sensitivity at the end of experimental protocols when lesion size is important but caliper is more indicated for small lesions.

Acknowledgments

We thank Mr Ammar Marouani and Dr Zakaria Ben

Lasfar, Animal Facilities of the Institut Pasteur de Tunis for their help conducting this study. This work was supported by an NIH/NIAID/DMID Grant Number 5P50AI074178 for and Tunisian Ministry of Higher Education and Research for DL. The funders had no role in study design, data collection and analysis, decision to publish, or preparation of the manuscript.

References

[1] Kebaier C, Louzir H, Chenik M, Ben Salah A, Dellagi K. Heterogeneity of wild Leishmania major isolates in experimental murine pathogenicity and specific immune response. Infect Immun. 2001; 69 (8): 4906-15.

[2] Van Thiel PP, van Gool T, Faber WR, Leenstra T, Kager PA, Bart A. Variation in clinical presentation and genotype of causative Leishmania major strain in cutaneous leishmaniasis in north and south Afghanistan. Am J Trop Med Hyg. 2011; 85 (1): 60-3.

[3] Lima HC, Titus RG. Effects of sand fly vector saliva on development of cutaneous lesions and the immune response to Leishmania braziliensis in BALB/c mice. Infect Immun. 1996; 64 (12): 5442-5.

[4] Rohousova I, Volf P. Sand fly saliva: effects on host immune response and Leishmania transmission. Folia Parasitol (Praha). 2006; 53 (3): 161-71.

[5] Baldwin TM, Elso C, Curtis J, Buckingham L, Handman E. The site of Leishmania major infection determines disease severity and immune responses. Infect Immun. 2003; 71 (12): 6830-4.

[6] Sacks D, Noben-Trauth N. The immunology of susceptibility and resistance to Leishmania major in mice. Nat Rev Immunol. 2002; 2 (11): 845-58.

[7] Soto M, Corvo L, Garde E, Ramirez L, Iniesta V, Bonay P et al. Coadministration of the Three Antigenic Leishmania infantum Poly (A) Binding Proteins as a DNA Vaccine Induces Protection against Leishmania major Infection in BALB/c Mice. PLoS Negl Trop Dis. 2015; 9 (5): e0003751.

[8] Fortin A, Caridha DP, Leed S, Ngundam F, Sena J, Bosschaerts T et al. Direct comparison of the efficacy and safety of oral treatments with oleylphosphocholine (OlPC) and miltefosine in a mouse model of L. major cutaneous leishmaniasis. PLoS Negl Trop Dis. 2014; 8 (9): e3144.

[9] Martinez Salazar MB, Delgado Dominguez J, Silva Estrada J, Gonzalez Bonilla C, Becker I. Vaccination with Leishmania mexicana LPG induces PD-1 in CD8(+) and PD-L2 in macrophages thereby suppressing the immune response: a model to assess vaccine efficacy. Vaccine. 2014; 32 (11): 1259-65.

[10] Meddeb-Garnaoui A, Zrelli H, Dellagi K. Effects of tropism and virulence of Leishmania parasites on cytokine production by infected human monocytes. Clin Exp Immunol. 2009; 155 (2): 199-206.

[11] Soong L, Duboise SM, Kima P, McMahon-Pratt D. Leishmania pifanoi amastigote antigens protect mice against cutaneous leishmaniasis. Infect Immun. 1995; 63 (9): 3559-66.

[12] Brown DR, Swier K, Moskowitz NH, Naujokas MF, Locksley RM, Reiner SL. T helper subset differentiation in the absence of invariant chain. J Exp Med. 1997; 185 (1): 31-41.

[13] Cortez M, Huynh C, Fernandes MC, Kennedy KA, Aderem A, Andrews NW. Leishmania promotes its own virulence by inducing expression of the host immune inhibitory ligand CD200. Cell Host Microbe. 2011; 9 (6): 463-71.

[14] Xu W, Xin L, Soong L, Zhang K. Sphingolipid degradation by Leishmania major is required for its resistance to acidic pH in the mammalian host. Infect Immun. 2011; 79 (8): 3377-87.

[15] Spath GF, Garraway LA, Turco SJ, Beverley SM. The role(s) of lipophosphoglycan (LPG) in the establishment of Leishmania major infections in mammalian hosts. Proc Natl Acad Sci U S A. 2003; 100 (16): 9536-41.

[16] Tomayko MM, Reynolds CP. Determination of subcutaneous tumor size in athymic (nude) mice. Cancer Chemother Pharmacol. 1989; 24 (3): 148-54.

[17] Uzcategui B, Avila D, Suarez-Roca H, Quintero L, Ortega J, Gonzalez B. Anti-inflammatory, antinociceptive, and antipyretic effects of Lantana trifolia Linnaeus in experimental animals. Invest Clin. 2004; 45 (4): 317-22.

[18] Romero-Sandoval EA, Molina C, Alique M, Moreno-Manzano V, Lucio FJ, Herrero JF. Vitamin A active metabolite, all-trans retinoic acid, induces spinal cord sensitization. I. Effects after oral administration. Br J Pharmacol. 2006; 149 (1): 56-64.

[19] Ratnasooriya WD, Deraniyagala SA, Galhena G, Liyanage SSP, Bathige SDNK, Jayakody RAC. Anti-inflammatory Activity of the Aqueous Leaf Extract of Ixora coccinea. Pharmaceutical Biology. 2005; 43 (2): 147-52.

[20] Raut MK, Bhandari SV, Bothara KG, Patil AA, Sarkate AP. Anti-inflammatory, analgesic, ulcerogenic, activities of some new non-acidic diclofenac and 1, 3, 4-oxadiazole derivatives in aanimal models Pharmacologyonline. 2007; 2: 172-86.

[21] Vazquez E, Navarro M, Salazar Y, Crespo G, Bruges G, Osorio C et al. Systemic changes following carrageenan-induced paw inflammation in rats. Inflamm Res. 2015; 64 (5): 333-42.

[22] De Toni LG, Menaldo DL, Cintra AC, Figueiredo MJ, de Souza AR, Maximiano WM et al. Inflammatory mediators involved in the paw edema and hyperalgesia induced by Batroxase, a metalloproteinase isolated from Bothrops atrox snake venom. Int Immunopharmacol. 2015; 28 (1): 199-207.

[23] Benhnini F, Chenik M, Laouini D, Louzir H, Cazenave PA, Dellagi K. Comparative evaluation of two vaccine candidates against experimental leishmaniasis due to Leishmania major infection in four inbred mouse strains. Clin Vaccine Immunol. 2009; 16 (11): 1529-37.

[24] Jensen MM, Jorgensen JT, Binderup T, Kjaer A. Tumor volume in subcutaneous mouse xenografts measured by microCT is more accurate and reproducible than determined by 18F-FDG-microPET or external caliper. BMC Med Imaging. 2008; 8: 16.

[25] Girit IC, Jure-Kunkel M, McIntyre KW. A structured light-based system for scanning subcutaneous tumors in laboratory animals. Comp Med. 2008; 58 (3): 264-70.

[26] Chanana V, Sehgal R, Rishi P. Salmonella typhi iron-regulated outer-membrane proteins cause oedema and hyperalgesia during inflammation induced in a rat model. J Med Microbiol. 2005; 54 (Pt 4): 421-3.

[27] Fiennes AG. Growth rate of human tumour xenografts measured in nude mice by in vivo cast modelling. Br J Surg. 1988; 75 (1): 23-4.

[28] Sharma JN, Samud AM, Asmawi MZ. Comparison between plethysmometer and micrometer methods to measure acute paw oedema for screening anti-inflammatory activity in mice. Inflammopharmacology. 2004; 12 (1): 89-94.

[29] Zvietcovich F, Castaneda B, Valencia B, Llanos-Cuentas A. A 3D assessment tool for accurate volume measurement for monitoring the evolution of cutaneous leishmaniasis wounds. Conf Proc IEEE Eng Med Biol Soc. 2012; 2012: 2025-8.

6

Effects of Gonadotropin Releasing Hormone analogue in Enhancements of Pregnancy in repeat Breeding Dairy Cows in and around Mekelle, Tigray, Ethiopia

Birhanu Hailu[1,*], Berihu Gebrekidan[2], Solmon Raju[2], Alemselam Birhanu[2], Gebrhiwot Tadesse[2]

[1]Samara University, College of Veterinary Medicine, P.O.Box.132, Samara, Ethiopia
[2]Mekelle University, College of Veterinary Medicine, Mekelle, Ethiopia

Email address:
birhailu2002@gmail.com (B. Hailu)

Abstract: Clinical trial was carried out to evaluating the effects of GNRH analogue (buserelin acetate) along with AI in repeat breeding cross breed cows on enhancement of pregnancy. The trial was also aimed at evaluation of dose variation on conception rate. Sixty six cross breed dairy cattle which were apparently healthy, exhibits estrus regularly were selected and assigned randomly in to three equal groups(A,B and C); two treated groups and one control group. Group A (n=22) cattle were injected intramuscularly a 20 µg buserelin acetateat along with AI and Group B (n=22) cattle have injected with dose of 10µg Buserelin acetate. Group C (n=22) cattle were receive no treatment and considered as a control group, given a single service. These cows were examined for pregnancy after three months through rectal palpation. Additional history was taken from herd owners. The pregnancy rates recorded were 68%, 59% and 32% in the cattle grouped with A, B and C respectively. The conception rates of the treated groups exceeds control group by 36% and 27% respectively. Treated groups showed a significant statistical variation ($P<0.05$) as compared to control group. Dose variation between two treated groups has an effect on pregnancy rate with significant variation. Other observed finding was that treated first and second parity cows became more responsive to therapy than those with more than two parity with a significant variation ($P<0.05$). The study revealed that the use of GNRH analogue therapy at the time of AI can enhance pregnancy rate. This would be helpful and cost effective to minimize financial losses incurred from milk production loss, managmental and feed cost. This might be achieved through reducing calving interval and treating repeat breeding cases. The benefit cost ratio indicates that individual cow could benefit small holder farmer by 140 USD within a single month.

Keywords: Crossbred Cattle, Estrus, Repeat Breeding GNRH Analogue, Pregnancy Rates

1. Introduction

Livestock production is one segments of agriculture constituting means of improving living standards of exponentially increasing poor farmers in many regions of developing world (Sere and Steinfeld, 1995; FAO, 2009). Eight-five percent of the Ethiopian people are heavily dependent on the contribution of agriculture with particular emphasis of livestock for multipurpose activity (Tegegn, 1998). Cattle production has been considered as major economic sector and still to be continued in the future in Ethiopia (FAO, 2009). The country has high potential of cattle population (Tegegn*et al.*, 1999). These production sectors can significantly reduce poverty and ensure food security. To get expected productions, improvement in management,environment, genetical, health and reproductive management is mandatory (Azage *et al.*, 1981).

For bringing of changes or upgrading reproductive performance, understanding of reproductive traits is necessary in bovine species (Hoglund, 2013). These traits are; age at first service, number of services per conception, day's open and calving interval and these are bases for profitable dairy cattle and beef cattle production system (Azage *et al.*, 1981 and Stvenson *et al.*, 2000). Otherwise, low reproduction efficiency hinders genetic improvement as local breeds which were not crossed leads to low milk production, long calving interval, late sexual maturity, short lactation length and hence such factors directly affects the livelihoods of farmers and gross domestic product of the nation (Mukosa-Mugerwa *et al*., 1993).

For the development of livestock industry, particularly the dairy farm, it must be highly integrated with the great biotechnological advancements to improve reproduction and genetics of farm animals (Foote, 2002). Artificial insemination technology was come into practices for years ago (Foote, 2002 and Bale, 2003). AI was introduced to our country, some years ago, by the ministry of agriculture and had got wide acceptance by the society with a hope to upgrading the local breeds (Yemane *et al*., 1993). But only knowledge of semen deposition in the reproductive tracts will not result in high conception rate and high milk yield since factors such as female fertility and heat detection accuracy must be considered in conjunction with the AI.

Using this technology, many exotic breeds were crossed with local one with improved potential of milk yield by many folds having good mangemetal situations (Foote, 2002). However, this technology is not without constraints. In contrast to the above condition, major problem observed now days is low conception rate using AI. This was the main problem that needs a solution to increase pregnancy rate in crossbred cattle (Morrel, 2011). According to the available literatures, major reproductive problems identified were, delayed ovulation, anovulation, anestrus, cystic ovaries and early embryonic death which cause cows to show repeated estrus cycle and low conception rate (Maureral, 1985). Such conditions were observed due to hormonal deficiency; GNRH produced by hypothalamus which controls synthesis and release of luteinizing hormone (LH) and follicle stimulating hormone (FSH). These two hormones have combined effects on follicular development, ovulation and corpus lutetium functions (Douglas, 1998).

Many protocols were taken in to consideration to treat reproductive problems associated with such hormonal imbalances (Mwaagna, 2004). One of these techniques were the use of synthetic GNRH analogue that has been used to modify reproductive efficiency of normal as well as repeat breeder dairy cows which has been investigated extensively. Synthetic buserelin acetate has an added advantage of improved half life in the blood circulation, greater stability to enzymatic degradation, increased receptor affinity, prolonged biological potency and less antigenic than the other molecules for repeated use(Cline,2002 and Ehler *et al*.,2013). Exogenous administration of these hormones at different period of estrus of cow may lead to treat disease condition or cysts in the ovary or may rectify the hormonal insufficiency to these cows (Morgan, *et al*., 1993; Bearden and Fuquay, 1997). The GNRH had been used as treatment for fertilization rates, embryonic mortality and as a therapeutic treatment for cystic ovaries (Gustafsson *et al.,* 1986).

In case of Ethiopia and Tigray region in particular, limited knowledge was available about the use of synthetic hormones for treatment of hormonal imbalances and for enhancement of pregnancy rates. No work was done to investigate the effects of GNRH analogue on enhancement of conception rate of cross breed repeat breeders of dairy cattle and therefore the present study was conducted with the aim of enhancing the fertility rates in cross breed cattle with specific objectives of: observing the effects of GNRH analogue (buserellin acetate) on enhancement of pregnancy on treated groups as compared to control and to evaluate the effects of dose variation between treated groups. Finally the study estimates financial benefits obtained from treatment of hormones.

2. Materials and Methods

2.1. Description of the Study Areas

The study was conducted in Tigray regional state;located in northern part of Ethiopia and bordering with Eritrea in the north, Sudan in the west, Afar in the east and Amhara in the southwest. The region extends from 120° 13' to 140° 54' N and from 36° 27' to 40° 18' E. It has seven Administrative Zones and this study was carried out in the capital city of the region which is located at 783 km north of Addis and geographically located 39° 29'E and 13° 3'N longitude. Mekelle is surrounded by south east zone in south and east, Eastern zone from north, central zone from west. It has an average temperature of 20°c and experiences an average annual rain fall of 600 mm. Livelihoods of the people in and around the city depends on trade, civil servants and agricultural practices. Dairy farming is one of the major farming systems practiced in the city. Small holder farmers around the city supply moderate amount of milk to urban dwellers and some of the farmers in the nearby area practice a mixed crop livestock production system. The area is moderately covered with savanna, bushy and low weed vegetations. Both small holder farmers and commercial dairy farms owners were included the study.

2.2. Study Population and Husbandry System

The study was conducted in repeat breeding cross breed dairy herds owned by small holder farmers and commercial dairy farms. These cows were kept in stall facility; fed grass hay, concentrate composed of wheat by products, crop residues, forages and other locally prepared fermented alcohol by products 'atella'. These dairy herds were milked twice per day and vaccinated regularly against common infectious diseases. In general, dairy cows were managed in similar agro ecological and climatic conditions. Artificial insemination was practiced based on the visual observation of standing heat and mucosal discharges by herd attendants.

2.3. Study Design and Selection of Animals

A randomized clinical trial was conducted to study effects of buserelin acetate on enhancement of pregnancy rates and evaluating the effects of doses variation on pregnancy. The study period was ranged from January to April 2010 in and around Mekelle. A total of 66 dairy cows were selected from thirty seven farms for this study. Cows with normal cycling, no clinical abnormalities, failed to conceive after two successive inseminations, not previously assigned for any study and aged from three to ten years were included in the study. Cows that were treated at first AI and back to estrus couldn't be reassigned for the study. The study repeat breeding cross breed dairy cows were selected based on these factors and equally divided in to three groups each consisting of twenty two dairy cows. These animals were randomly assigned into three protocols.

2.4. Study Procedures

The study had three main phases. Phase one: training of thirty seven herd owners or their representatives for having more experience about the symptom and behavioral changes of estrus cycle. Farmers were made aware about mucosal discharges from vulva, restlessness, frequent urination; stand to be mounted and raised tails during estrus exhibition. As soon as such symptoms were observed, they informed to make phones to local inseminator immediately and included in the study. Phase two: based on the above criterion; selection process of animals for the study was carried out and assigned randomly to control and treatment groups. The first group A (n=22) was inseminated along with intramuscular injection of 20 μg (5ml) buserelin acetate. Second group B(n=22) was also inseminated along with injection of 10 μg (2.5 ml) of GNRH analogue. Third group C (n=22) was assigned as a control group, receive no treatments except single AI. Phase three: After cows were followed for 90 days post AI, pregnancy diagnosis was carried out using a rectal palpation in cows' herds with history of failure to return to estrus. The cows were considered as pregnant if we were able to palpate the fetal membrane, amniotic vesicles, cotyledons and fetus otherwise the cows were classified as negative.

2.5. Estimation of Financial Losses and Benefits Obtained after Treatment

Financial losses of single cows per cycle were computing and estimated by considering the following variables. Average enhanced conception rate as result of the treatment, average milk yield per head of cross breed cow, duration of cycle and current market price of one liter of milk. During this financial losses calculation, costs of calf loss, management and feed costs were not considered.

2.6. Data Collections and Statistical Analysis

Study variables were collected from dairy herd owners by asking breed type, insemination and service history, parity, management condition, milk yield, price of milk per liter, time and day of estrus exhibition and previous condition of dairy herds. During this study period, pregnancy diagnosis was made through rectal palpation and positive and negative results were recorded. Some data were collected from farm records about animals' previous milk yield, clinical cases, origin of the animal, replacement herd and breeding type. The experimental study was of a randomized type in which data was collected from treated and controlled study animals. Collected data was fed to Microsoft Excel spread sheet and process of data cleaning, handling, validating and coding was done on this spread sheet. The difference in pregnancy proportion, age and parity between treated groups against control one was compared using descriptive statistics and Pearson's chi-square tests (SPSS16.0; 2005). The significance level of differences was observed at P value of less than 5%.

3. Results

Out of the 66 dairy cows included in the study, 35 cows were found to be pregnant. A total of 15 cows from group A were recorded as pregnant with the conception rate of 68%. In group B, from the 22, 13 of them were conceived with the conception rate of 59% and the remaining 7 were from the control group as indicated in Table-1. Those animals treated with the higher dose of buserelin acetate exceeds in conception rate to second group by 9%. In general, treated groups recorded higher pregnancy rate in comparison with controlled group with average score of 32 % over controlled one and the rest results obtained from each group was indicated in Table-1.

Conception rate of group A (treated) exceeds conception rate of group C (control) by 36% with significant statistical variation (χ^2=4.79, P=0.029). The recorded conception rates of group B was 59% greater than group C by 27 % with significant statistical variation (χ^2=7.108, P=0.008). Comparison between treated groups, Group (A) with higher dose of buserellin acetate scores more conception rate with significant difference as compared to group B which receive half dose of group A. Comparison among the three groups; conception rate in both treated groups were significantly higher than control groups. Overall comparison of treated and controlled group was shown in table-2. Management condition, season and parity variation doesn't show any significant variation in treated groups as compared to controlled group, dairy herds of younger age were found more response to therapy as compared to older treated cows with a statistical significance variation (χ^2 =3.93, P<0.05) (Table-2).

Table 1. *Results of the various protocols with their respective percentages.*

Group	No. animals in each protocol	Type of Protocol	Pregnancy rate
A	22	20μg(5ml) buserelin acetate along AI	15/22 (68%)
B	22	10μg(2.5ml) buserelin acetate along AI	13/22(59%)
C	22	Controlled group(receive no treatment)	7/22(32%)

Table 2. Cross tabulation of the treated groups with the controlled animals.

Cross tabulated groups			Group C Negative	Positive	Total	Significance Level
		Negative	7	0	7	(χ^2=4.79,P=0.029)
A*C	Group A	Positive	8	7	15	
		Total	15	7	22	
			Group C			
		Negative	9	0	9	(χ^2=7.108,P=0.008)
B*C	Group B	Positive	6	7	13	
		Total	15	7	22	
			Group B			
		Negative	7	0	7	(χ^2=14.830,P=0.000)
A*B	Group A	Positive	2	13	15	
		Total	9	13	22	

4. Discussion

Repeat breeding have been a problem dairy farmers, causing economic damage and the present study was carried out to evaluate the effects of buserelin acetate on repeat breeding cross breed cows in association with improvement of pregnancy rate. The study demonstrated that supplementation of buserelin acetate along with AI increase pregnancy rate by 63% as compared to control group. Treatment improves pregnancy rate significantly in the first two groups ($P<0.05$) and comparison between treated groups, the first group with higher dose was observed with conception rate of 68%, exceeds the second group with significant statistical variation ($p<0.05$). This shares similar results with experiments done by Anjum *et al.,* 2010. Improvement in conception rate was also associated with increment of doses of GNRH analogue. This finding was in line with reports by Kharche and Srivastava (2007). This improvement in pregnancy rate may be related to timing of ovulation or synchronization ovulation with insemination and increased progesterone secretion by corpus luteum due to increased LH surge by treatment with GNRH analogue (Karg *et al,* 1980; Mc Dougall *et al.*, 1995).

The present study showed an improvement in conception rate of 36% which is approximately the same to the works of Kharche and Srivastava (2007) that's around 39% using the same analogue and same dose. So, this study supported dose dependent effect of GNRH analogue, done on repeat breeder cross breed cows under different environmental condition and breeding season. This result confirmed the ideas that GNRH analogue can increase conception rate at the time of AI despite the fact that breed type, management, environmental and physiological status of the animals which might be contributing factors towards the differential fertility response to GNRH analogue treatments (Thatcher *et al.,* 1993, Ullah *et al.*, 1996 and Cam et *al.,* 2002). Several works reported that there was an increase in conception rates using GNRH analogue in repeat breeder cows than the control ones (Stevenson *et al.*, 1990). Study by Blowey (1999) also indicated that an improvement of 7% over the controlled groups in the GNRH treated repeated breeder dairy cows. In contrast to the present study, Drew and Peter (1994) stated that administration GNRH analogue 10µg GNRH did not improve fertility at the time of AI.

From the treated 16 first and second parity repeat breeding cows, 13 of them (81%) were found to be pregnant and this difference has a statistical significant variation. Most of animals treated with this protocol show a response indicating that dairy herds need administration of hormones to boost reproduction. This result is in agreement with study by Gustafsson (1986). The overall pregnancy rates were higher in treated than the controlled groups. These results indicates that there is high incidence of reproductive organ disturbances such as ovarian cysts, delayed ovulation, anovulation, anestrous or defective corpus luteum function which could be improved by administration of GNRH analogue. This may also be caused by lack of good management and malnutrition in the study area.

Intramuscular injection of GNRH analogue enhances pregnancy rate that prevents owners from economic losses as a result of prolonged calving interval since cows return to heat repeatedly. This protocol is fair in cost and has fewer tendencies for pharmacological intervention in reproductive tract of the cow as compared to other complicated and expensive protocols. Financial losses of cows per cycle were computing and estimated based on the following parameters. (Average conception rate= 31%, Average milk yield = 14 liters per head, treated cows get conceived over control =21 cows, average number of days per cycle=21days). So, the total financial loss would be computed as: 14 liters of milk per day* 21 days per cycle *21 cows *10 birr = 61,740 Birr or $3118) at which owners going to loss in addition to loss of calf, management and feed costs. From this we can understand that as the cow takes more time, the loss will be more severe. A farmer could loss birr 2940 / $148.48 per cycle from single cow; that highly affects its livelihood. In calculation of benefit cost ratios, it is indicated that farmers would be benefitted if bought GNRH analogue (buserelin acetate) for treatments of repeat breeding dairy cows rather than living with problem. The cost is effective and affordable to farmers to pay 25 to 50 birr (2.20-4.40 $) to the 10 / 20 µg of the hormone rather than losing 140 USD.

5. Conclusion and Recommendation

The finding of our study revealed that the use of GNRH analogue (buserelin acetate) therapy along with AI improved in pregnancy rate in repeat breeding cross breed cows. The scored conception rates were 68% and 59% in the first and the second treated groups respectively as compared to the control groups (32%). This improvement in conception rate indicated that farmers would be benefitted financially as benefit exceeds in the benefit-cost ratios. So, individual house hold was benefitted worth of $ 140 as compared to those control one. Based on these results the following points are recommended.

- The GNRH analogue administration along with AI improved reproductive performance of repeat breeding dairy cows
- Farmers should be aware on beneficial effects of the gonadotropin releasing hormone analogues (buserelin acetate)
- Incensement of dose of buserelin acetate may enhance more conception rates among the repeat breeding dairy cows
- GNRH analogue can be effectively used to overcome the problem of repeat breeding in crossbred cattle dairy cows and farmers could prevent financial losses by using buserelin acetate as an alternative treatment of choice

Acknowledgements

The authors acknowledge to the Ethiopia Ministry of Science and Technology for financial support and to Mekelle University for provision of necessary facilities and administrative work which had remarkable role for the success of research work.

Conflicts of Interest Statements

None of the authors has any financial or personal relationships that could inappropriately influence the contents of the paper.

References

[1] Anjum, I. A., Usmani, R. H., Tunio, M. T. and Abro, S. H.(2010). Improvement of Conception rate in Cross Breed Cattle by Using Gonadotropin Releasing Hormone (GNRH) analogue thereapy. *Agricultura Tropica et Subtropica, 43:1*

[2] Azage, T., Galal, E. and Beyene, K. (1981).A Study on the reproduction of local zebu andF1cross breeds (European Zebu) Cows, Number of services per conception, gestation length and days open till conception. *Ethiopian. J. Agri. Sci* 3:1-14.

[3] Azage, T. and Alemu, G. (1998). Prospect for Urban, Periurban dairy development in Ethiopia. Ethiopian Society of Animal production (ESAP), publication no5 Addis Ababa Ethiopia.

[4] Bale, O. (2003). Artificial Insemination Practice in Nigeria, Nigerian Journal of Animal Production.

[5] Banerjee, G. (1998). A Text Book of Animal Husbandry, 8th edition, Oxford and IBH publishing corporation New Delhi

[6] Bearden, J. and Fuquay, W. (1992). Applied Animal Reproduction, 3rd edition Mississippi State University

[7] Beckers, F., Szenci, O., Takacs, E., Sulon, J. and Sousa, N. (2006). Evaluation of GNRH treatment 12 days post A.I in the reproductive performance of dairy cows. Theriogenology.

[8] Blowey, W. (1999). The repeat breeder cow, 3rd edition, A Veterinary Book for Dairy Farmers.

[9] Cam, M. A. – Kuran, M. Yildiz, S. Selcuk, E. 2002. Fetal growth and reproductive performance in ewes administered GNRH agonist on day 12 post-mating. *Anim. Reprod. Sci.*, vol. 72, p. 73-82.

[10] Cline, A. M., (2002). Efficiency of Synthetic Gonadotropin Releasing Hormone analogue for the control of ovulation during estrus synchronization protocols, Animal Science, Physiology of Reproduction.

[11] Connor, O. (2000). Dairy Integrated Reproductive Management, Pennsy State University.

[12] Dougall, S., Williamson, N. and Macmillan, K. (1995). GNRH induces ovulation of dominant follicle in primiparous dairy cows undergoing anovulatory follicle turn over. *Anim. Reprod. Sci.* 39: 205-214.

[13] Drew, S. and Peters, A. (1994). Veterinary Pharmacology and Therapeutics, Endocrine pharmacology. Vet Rec .134-267.

[14] Ehlers, K., Halvorson, L. and Glob. liber (2013).Gonadotropin Releasing Hormone and Gonadotropin Releasing Hormone Receptors. ISSN, 1756-2228.

[15] FAO. (2000). Food and Agricultural Organization, year book, Rome Italy.

[16] FAO., 2009. Food and Agricultural organization of the United Nations, The State of Food and Agriculture. Livestock, food security and poverty reduction.pp32-50.

[17] Foote, R. (2002). The history of Artificial Insemination, Selected notes and notables, American society of Dairy Sciences

[18] Goley R and Kadu M. (1995). Efficacy of PGF2 α, GNRH and HCG in treatment of repeat breeder cow. *Indian Veterinary Journal* 72: 472-475.

[19] Gustafsson, H,. Larsso, H, Kindah .and A.Madei. (1986). Sequential Endocrine Changes and Behavior during estrus and met estrus in repeat breeder and virgin heifer's *Anim Repro Sci* 10:261.

[20] Hoglund, K. J., (2013), Gene mapping of Reproductive Traits in Cattle, Faculty of Veterinary Medicine and Animal Science, Department of Animal Breeding and Genetics, Uppsala, Sweden

[21] Karg, H., Claus, R., Gunzler, O., Rattenberger, E., Pirchner, F. (1980). Hormonal Recognition of cyclicity and infertility in cows under practical conditions. In proceeding of the 11thWorld congress.Disease of cattle Israel, Pp.885-894.

[22] Karten, M. and River, J. (1986).*Endocr Rev.*7:44-66.Protective effects of analogs of luteinizing hormone-releasing hormone against chemotherapy-induced testicular damage in rats

[23] Kharche, S. and Srivastava, S. (2007). Dose dependent effect of GNRH analogue on pregnancy rate of repeat breeder cross breed cows. Indian Veterinary Research institute *Anim.Repro. Sci*. India.

[24] Markandeya, N. (2006). Approaches to enhance conception rate and embryo survivability, Department of Gynecology and Obstetrics Veterinary College, Reproductive Techniques to augment Fertility in dairy animals. Karnataka Veterinary Animal and Fisheries Sciences University.

[25] Mauurer, R. and Echternkamp S. (1985). Repeat breeder Females in Beef cattle Influences and causes, J.Anim *Sci*, 61:624.

[26] Michael, O, Jeffrey, Stevenson, Brenda, M. and Garth, R. (1993). Administration of GNRH at estrus influences pregnancy rates Serum concentration of LH, FSH estradiol-17 beta, pregnancy specific protein and progesterone, proportion of the luteal cell types and invitro production progesterone in dairy cows. *J Anim Sci 71*:185-198.

[27] Morgan, W. Lean, I. (1993). Gonadotropin Releasing Hormone treatment in cattle a Meta analysis of effects on conception at the time of insemination. *Aust Vet J* 70: 205-9.

[28] Morrel, M., (2011). Artificial Insemination; Current and the Future Trends: Swedish University of Agricultural Science, Uppsala, Sweden

[29] MukasaMugaerwa, E., Agaze, T., Tafese, M and Teklu, Y. (1993). Reproductive Efficiency of Bosindicus (Zebu) cows under Artificial Insemination. *Anim. Reprod Sci* 24: 63-67.

[30] Mwanga, S. E., Zdunczyk, S., and Janowsk, T., (2004). Comparative Efficacy of Hormonal and Non-Hormonal Treatment Methods in Ovarian Afunctions affected dairy cows.

[31] Nagaraja, R. Devaraj, M. (2006). Multi facet Roles of GNRH in Reproduction. Veterinary college, Karnataka Veterinary, animal and Fisheries Sciences University.

[32] Petrie, A. and Watson, P. (2000): Statistics for Veterinary, Revised edition. Blackwel Science Ltd., Osney Mead Oxford OX2 OEL, 25 John Street, London WCIN2 BS.

[33] Schels, H. Mostafawi, D., Morgan, W. (1978). The effect of GNRH on pregnancy rate of artificially inseminated cows.*Vet Rec*; 103: 31-32.

[34] Sere, C. and Steinfeld, H., 1995.World livestock production system, Current status, Issues and Trends pp6-12.

[35] Stevensen, J, Thompson, W. Forbes, G. Lamb, D. Gerieger, L, Corah. (2000). Synchronizing estrus and ovulation in beef cows after combination of GNRH, norgestment and prostaglandin with or without timed ovulation .*J Anim sci*, 78:1747-1758.

[36] Stevenson J .Caller, Scoby.and .Phatak. (1990).Double insemination and gonadotropin releasing hormone treatment of repeat breeding dairy cattle *J. Dairy Sci* 73:1766.

[37] Stojilkovic, S and Catt, K. (1995). *Rec. Prog. Horm. Res 50*: 161-205.

[38] Srivastava, S.K. and Kharche, S. D. (2002). Effect of GNRH on fertility in crossbred cows. *Indian. J. Anim. Sci*. 72:428-430.

[39] Tegegn, T., Alemayehu, A. and Ayele, G. (1999). Cross border livestock trade in Southern and south eastern Ethiopia border lines. OSSREA (organization for social science research in eastern and southern Africa) Development Research report series, Commercial printing enterprises.

[40] Thatcher, W. W., M. Drost, J. D. Savio, K. L. Macmillan, K. L. Entwistle, E. J.-P. Schmitt, R. L. de la Sota, and G. R. Morris.1993. New clinical uses for GNRH and its analogues in cattle. *Anim. Reprod. Sci*. 33:27–49.

[41] Ullah, G., J. W. Fuquay, T. Keawkhong, B. L. Clark, D. E. Pogue,and E. J. Murphey. 1996. Effect gonadotrophin-releasing hormone at estrus on subsequent luteal function and fertility in lactating Holsteins during heat stress. *J. Dairy Sci*. 79: 1950–1953.

[42] Vishwanath R. (2003). Theriogenology, 59:585-598.

[43] Yemane,B.,Chernet,T.,Shiferaw,T.(1993). Improved Cattle breeding, National Artificial Insemination Center, and Addis Abeba, Ethiopia.

7

Dynamics of Parasitaemia in *Trypanosoma evansi* Infection in Donkeys and the Efficacies of Buparvaquone and Isometamidium chloride Treatments

Garba UM[1,*], Sackey AKB[2], Lawal AI[3], Esievo KAN[4]

[1]Veterinary Clinic, Equitation Department, Nigerian Defence Academy, Kaduna, Nigeria
[2]Department of Veterinary Medicine, Faculty of Veterinary Medicine, Ahmadu Bello University, Zaria, Nigeria
[3]Department of Veterinary Parasitology and Entomology, Faculty of Veterinary Medicine, Ahmadu Bello University, Zaria, Nigeria
[4]Department of Veterinary Pathology, Faculty of Veterinary Medicine, Ahmadu Bello University, Zaria, Nigeria

Email address:
garbaum@yahoo.com (G. UM), akbsackeyabuzaria@yahoo.com (S. AKB), lawaidris@yahoo.com (L. AI), kanescokok@yahoo.com (E. KAN)
[*]Corresponding author

Abstract: The aim of this study was to evaluate the efficacies of Buparvaquone (an anti-theilerial drug) and Isometamidium chloride (a standard trypanocide) in the treatment of experimental *Trypanosoma evansi* infection in donkeys. Out of a total of 24 donkeys, 6 were assigned to each of the experimental groups A_1, A_2, A_3 and B at random. About 2.0×10^6 *T. evansi* parasite in 2 mL inoculum was used to infect each of the donkeys in groups A_1, A_2 and A_3 through jugular vein while group B remained as Un-infected control. On day 28 post-infection, animals in groups A_2 and A_3 were treated with Isometamidium chloride and Buparvaquone respectively. Parasitaemia levels were evaluated post-infection and post-treatment using Haematocrit Centrifugation Technique and supported with mice inoculation tests to ascertain effectiveness of treatments. Group means of parasitaemia were presented on graphs. Result showed that parasites were first detectable from peripheral blood of the infected animals from day 3 and by day 4 post-infection all animals were parasitaemic and the levels fluctuated in subsequent days. The infected-untreated group of animals was aparasitaemic on day 100 post-infection onward using haematocrit centrifugation technique test but mice inoculation test detected relapse with death of all mice used due to heavy parasitemia. Similarly, the buparvaquone-treated group was aparasitemic on day 49 post-treatment (corresponding to day 77 post-infection) but mice inoculation test detected relapse of parasitaemia in the group and all mice used also died. Isometamidium-treated animals were negative for parasitaemia for 50 days on mice inoculation test but later on day 100 post-treatment, showed 60% relapse with parasiaemia level of 1^+ in the mice used and they did not die within 48 days of observation. In conclusion, experimental *Trypanosoma evansi* infection in donkeys have pre-patent period of 3-4 days, parasitaemia pattern is undulating and infected-untreated animals became subclinical carriers from day 100 post-infection. The parasites in untreated, carrier animals maintained their virulence and pathogenicity. Buparvaquone on the other hand, depressed parasitaemia but the parasites were virulent and pathogenic to mice. Isometamidium chloride treatment resulted in incomplete clearance of parasitaemia due to *Trypanosoma evansi* and the relapsed parasites were avirulent and apathogenic. This is also the first report on the trial of buparvaquone for anti-*Trypanosoma evansi* effect in donkeys.

Keywords: Buparvaquone, Donkeys, Dynamics, Efficacies, Isometamidium chloride, Parasitaemia, *Trypanosoma evansi*

1. Introduction

In Nigeria, donkeys (*Equus africanus asinus*) are widespread especially in the northern region, where they serve as source of traction power in transport and ploughing for both pastoralists and settled farmers [1]. Coincidentally,

T. evansi infection (surra) is endemic in donkeys in Nigeria [2]. The disease manifests as acute, in which case it is rapidly fatal in camels and horses or chronic form, which may persist for several months or years [3] as in donkeys which usually result in emaciation and death [4].

The causative agent; *T. evansi* belongs to the *Salivaria* section of pathogenic species of *Trypanosoma* and the subgenus, *Trypanozoon* which consists of three major trypanosome species; *Trypanosoma brucei*, *T. evansi* and *T. equiperdum* [5, 6].

The transmission of *T. evansi* among animals is mechanical, by biting flies mainly; *Tabanus sp*, and *Stomoxys sp*, *Haematopota sp*, *Lyperosia sp* and *Chrysops sp* [7]. Transplacental transmission mode has also been reported in donkeys [8].

The control of *T. evansi* infection in animals depends on chemotherapy and chemoprophylaxis relying on diminazene aceturate, quinapyramine, cymelarsan and suramin sodium, but emerging resistance of *T. evansi* strains to available drugs has limited the success of treatments [9, 10].

As part of efforts in the search for drugs with trypanocidal effects, the efficacies of buparvaquone and Isometamidium chloride against experimental *T. evansi* infection in donkeys were evaluated in this study. Buparvaquone is a second-generation injectable hydroxynaphthoquinone compound in aqueous solution with both curative and prophylactic effects against the causative agents of Bovine Theileriosis; *Theileria parva* (*T. parva*), *T. sergenti* and *T. annulata* [11, 12]. Isometamidium chloride belongs to the same chemical group as homidium; the phenanthridine aromatic amidine compounds [13, 10].

2. Materials and Methods

2.1. Location of Research

The Experiment was conducted in the Department of Veterinary Parasitology and Entomology Research Pen, Faculty of Veterinary Medicine, Ahmadu Bello University, Samaru campus, Zaria, North-Western Nigeria. Main campus, Samaru, Zaria, North-Western Nigeria. Main campus in Samaru is located on latitude 11 ° 15'N to 11° 3'N of the equator and longitude 7° 30'E to 7° 45'E of Greenwich Meridian [14].

2.2. Experimental Animals

Twenty four apparently healthy donkeys were purchased from International Livestock Market in Maigatari, Jigawa State, North-Western Nigeria and used for this experiment. The donkeys comprised of 12 males and 12 females, between the ages of 11 to 15 months old. The donkeys' ages were estimated at point of purchase using dental eruption pattern of the incisors teeth as described by Wayne and Melvin [15] and Joe [16].

Four (4) apparently healthy and haemoparasites-free, adult albino Wistar rats, with body weight range of 200g-220g were used as donors for the propagation of *T. evansi* to obtain sufficient inoculum for the experimental infection.

Mice inoculation tests (MIT) were conducted using apparently healthy and haemoparasites-free, adult Wistar mice (100 only) with body weight range of 14g-16g. Two mice were used for each donkey screened, each time, as support test for HCT at pre-infection phase to ensure that they were haemoparasites-free, post-infection and post-treatment to determine relapse, ascertain effectiveness or otherwise of the treatment drugs against *T. evansi* infection. The rats and mice were sourced in batches from Animal Laboratory, Faculty of Pharmaceutical Sciences, Ahmadu Bello University, Zaria.

2.3. Pre-infection Evaluation and Management of Experimental Animals

2.3.1. Housing and Acclimatisation

On arrival in the Department of Veterinary Parasitology and Entomology, A.B.U., Zaria, the experimental donkeys were further examined for signs of disease and external parasites infestations. Topical sweat resistant fly-repellant spray (Endure®, Farnam co. inc., USA) was applied on the animals to keep flies away and then housed in prepared, fly-proof experimental animal pen of the department. Wood shaving was used as bedding material on the floor of the pen; it was mucked daily to remove faecal droppings and changed as soon as the old one was bad. The experimental animals were acclimatised for 14 days [17].

In addition the following samples were collected and examined:

2.3.2. Faecal Sample

About 5g of fecal sample was collected from the rectum of each animal and examined for gastro-intestinal parasites using floatation and sedimentation methods as reported by Charles [18]. The animals were dewormed using Fenbendazole bolus (Fenacure®, Ashish Life Sciences PVT ltd, India) at the dose rate of 10mg/kg bd wt orally, once [19].

2.3.3. Blood Sample

Four millilitres (4ml) of blood was collected from each animal through the jugular vein using 5ml syringe and 18G needle. Three milliliters of the blood was placed in blood sample bottle containing liquid tripotassium salt of Ethylene Diamine Tetra-acetate ($EDTA+K_3$), 1mg/mL of whole blood as anticoagulant [20] and examined immediately for haemoparasites infections using 2 preparations of Wet Blood Film at 40x magnification, HCT and Giemsa Stained thin blood smear as reported by Weiser [21]. An average of 20 microscope fields of the stained thin smear slide was examined.

2.3.4. Animal Inoculation

The balance of 1mL of blood collected from each donkey was transferred into sodium heparin-coated 1mL sterile disposable syringe with 29G x ½ inch needle and 0.5mL of the blood was injected into a mouse intra-peritoneally [17] using 2 representative mice per donkey [3]. The inoculated mice were monitored for haemoparasites on HCT and Wet Film using tail tip blood at 48 hours intervals for 14 days [22], and remained under observation up to 60 days post-inoculation.

2.3.5. Feeding of Experimental Animals

The experimental donkeys were provided with feed daily equivalent to 5% of their mean body weight, in the forms of; Sorghum/Maize stovers and Rhodes grass/groundnuts hay (4:1 ratio), the concentrate feed consisted of a mixture of sorghum grain (500g), dried groundnut cake (130g) and Maize/Wheat bran (2.5kg) per 200-300kg bd wt of animal. Salt lick blocks, rich in dicalcium phosphate and clean drinking water were provided *ad-libitum* as recommended by Aganga *et al* [23].

The albino rats and Wister mice were maintained in separate, labeled cages and were provided with commercially obtained pelletised feed in feeders and clean drinking water in sipper tubes *ad libitum* [17].

2.4. Identification and Grouping of Animals

Serially numbered aluminum plates (about 5g) neck-tags were assigned to the donkeys at random for identification. A sample frame of each gender was prepared and treated one after the other by random picking of animals' numbers and placing in experimental groups A_1, A_2, A_3 and B to obtain a total of 6 animals (3 male and 3 female) in each experimental group. Choice of groups of animals inoculated with *T. evansi* as well as assigning of either Isometamidium chloride or Buparvaquone for group treatment was made at random [24].

The rats and mice were caged according to the group of donkeys they represented. Marks were applied on the various body parts of the rats and mice using permanent marker to reflect the donkey they represented.

2.5. Propagation of Trypanosoma evansi

Trypanosoma evansi (Sokoto isolate) originally isolated from camel and maintained in Wistar rats in the Department of Veterinary Parasitology and Entomology, Ahmadu Bello University, Zaria, was used in this experiment.

The level of parasitemia of the infected Wistar rat was first determined to be +4 (representing greater than 20 parasites per field of microscope after examining 20 fields) on haematocrit centrifugation technique (HCT). One milliliter of parasitaemic blood was collected via ocular vein into heparinised sample bottle and diluted with 1mL phosphate buffered saline glucose solution. About 0.5 mL of the inoculums was inoculated into each of a set of 4 donor rats, intra-peritoneally using sterile 1mL disposable syringe, $25G_X$ $1^1/_2$ inch needle [22, 17].

The donor rats were monitored for parasitaemia levels at 48 hours intervals using Wet Film method. Twelve days post-inoculation, the 4 rats had attained between +2 to +4 (i.e 6-10 to >20 parasites per microscope field). All donor rats were bled and the blood was pooled into a sterile conical flask containing heparin sodium 20 Units/mL of blood. A total of 15mL of pooled blood was obtained and the parasitemia was re-evaluated using haemocytometer [20]. The blood was diluted with phosphate buffered saline glucose solution to obtain an inoculum containing 1.0 $x10^6$ *T. evansi* /mL [22].

2.6. Experimental Infection and Monitoring of Animals

The prepared inoculum was immediately used to infect the experimental animals in groups A_1, A_2 and A_3 at the rate 2mL ($2.0x10^6$ *T. evansi*) per animal through the jugular vein and the day was considered as day0 of infection. Group B animals remained as Un-infected (control) group.

The infected animals were monitored for parasitaemia using ear vein blood. The blood samples were collected once daily from all groups of animals between day1 and day7 post-infection (PI). This was followed by blood collection twice per week between day8 and day 28 PI. The samples were examined using HCT and References and further reading may be available for this article. To view references and further reading you must purchase this article. Giemsa-stained thin blood smears as reported by Elaine and Margi [20]. Levels of parasitemia were scored using the method of Woo [25].

2.7. Treatment of Specific Infected Animals

On day 28 PI, which coincided with the third wave of parasitemia as determined on HCT, animals in groups A_2 and A_3 were treated and the day of first treatment was considered as day 0 of treatment. Group A_1 was Infected but Untreated, A_2 was Infected and treated with Isometamidium (Securidium®, Laprovet, France) 1% solution, 0.5mg/kg bd wt by deep intramuscular injection once [26] while group A_3 was infected and treated with Buparvaquone (Butalex®, Coopers K-brand Ltd, Kenya) 5% w/v, 2.5 mg/kg bd wt by deep intramuscular injection twice at 72 hours apart as recommended by the manufacturers. Animals in group B were uninfected and untreated (Control)

2.7.1. Post-Treatment Monitoring

The experimental donkeys were monitored further for levels of parasitemia for 148 days during which blood samples were collected from all animal groups as follows; once daily between day1 and day 7 post-treatment (PT), twice per week between day 8 and day 28 PT and once per week between day 29 and day 148 PT. The levels of parasitemia were evaluated on HCT and Giemsa-stained thin blood smear and were supported with mice inoculation test.

2.7.2. Animal Inoculation

Mice inoculation test (MIT) was performed for infected-untreated in chronic stage of infection and for the infected, treated groups of donkeys post-treatment as a support for direct microscopic methods in-order to detect any case of subclinical infection. After 10 days or more of sustained aparasitemia from HCT in a group of donkeys, 1mL of blood was collected from each donkey in the group through jugular vein using heparin-coated 2mL syringe 19Gx $1^1/_2$ inch needle.

Half millilitre (0.5mL) of collected blood was sub-inoculated into mouse intra-peritoneally using sterile 27G needles and 2 representative mice per donkey. The mice were identified and monitored for parasitemia using tail blood on HCT and Wet Film at 48 hours intervals [3]. Based the observed aparasitaemic status by groups of animals, MIT was conducted as follows;

Group A_1 (Infected-Untreated) Donkeys: Blood samples were collected from the donkeys in the group on day 110 PI and sub-inoculated into mice.

Group A_2 (Infected, Isometamidium chloride-treated) Donkeys: Mice inoculation test was performed for the group on days 21, 50 and 100 PT.

Group A_3 (Infected, Buparvaquone-treated) Donkeys: Mice inoculation test was conducted for the group on day 59 PT.

3. Data Analysis

Group means of parasitaemia levels in the various stages of the experiment were determined and graphs were prepared for post-infection and post-treatment phases of the experiment using Microsoft Excel 2010 [27].

4. Results

The infection day 0, prepatent-period, undulating parasitaemia and treatment day 28 PI are as presented in Fig. 1.

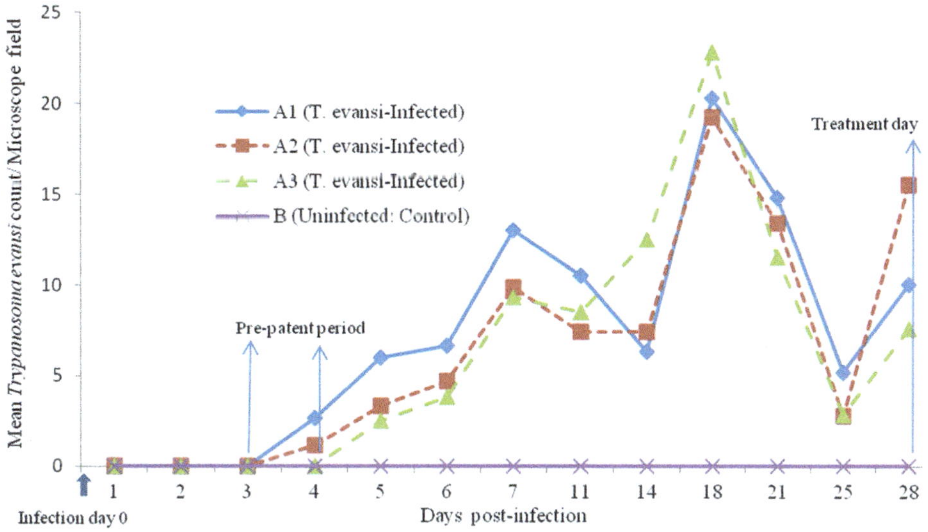

Fig. 1. Mean levels of parasitaemia in donkey experimentally infected with Trypanosoma evansi.

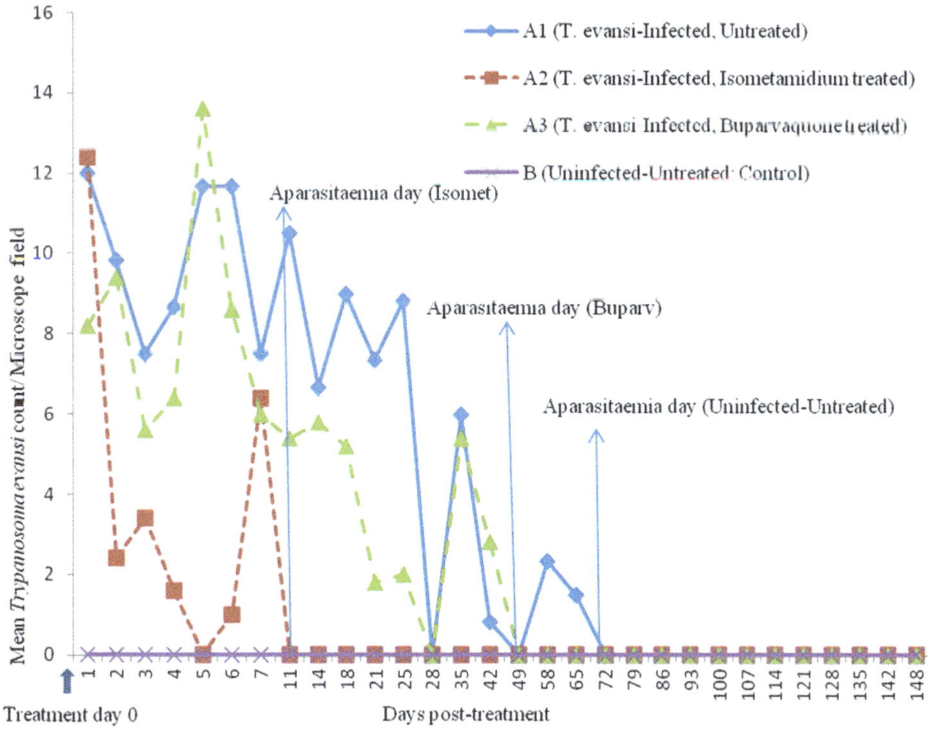

Fig. 2. Mean levels of Trypanosoma evansi observed in experimentally infected donkeys post-treatment.

Group A_1 (Infected-Untreated)

The infected-untreated group of animals maintained an undulating wave of parasitaemia until it became aparasitaemic on HCT examination on day 100 PI, equivalent to day72 PT, (Fig. 2). Mice inoculation test (MIT) conducted on day 110 PI resulted in death of all mice, barely 15 days post-inoculation from heavy parasitemia (+3 and +4/field) on HCT and Wet Film (WF).

Group A_2 (Infected, Isometamidium chloride-treated)

The T. evansi-infected, Isometamidium chloride-treated group of animals had sharp drop in mean parasitaemia on HCT from approximately 12/field on day1 to about 2/field on day 2 PT and they became aparasitaemic on day 11 PT (Fig. 2). Mice inoculation tests on days 21 and 50 were negative but became positive on day 100 PT in 6/10(60%) of mice used representing 3/5(60%) donkeys in the group. The test (MIT) showed that there was no detectable parasitaemia within 50 days PT and that by day 100 PT, subclinical status is detectable in 3/5(60%) of the donkeys treated with isometamidium. The inoculated mice showed only 1 parasite (1+) per microscope field both on Wet Film and HCT during 48 days of post-inoculation observation. The remaining 4 mice were negative both on WF and HCT for the same period of observation (Fig. 2).

Group A_3 (Infected, Buparvaquone treated)

The Infected, Buparvaquone treated group became aparasitaemic on HCT on day 49 PT (Fig. 2). Following MIT on day 59 PT, all inoculated mice tested positive for T. evansi and died by day 23 post-inoculation observation.

5. Discussion

In this study, a pre-patent period (PP) of 3-4 days was observed and could be due to the level of pathogenicity of Sokoto isolate of T. evansi or susceptibility of the animal as determined by immunotolerance of donkeys to T. evansi infection [28, 29].

The trend of parasitaemia in all groups of animals infected with T. evansi was undulating suggesting trypanosomes ability to reside intermittently in intra- or extra-vascular fluids [30] and switches of surface glycoprotein in antigenic variation causing relapses of parasitaemia and remittent clinical signs [31, 32, 33]. The parasitaemia detected from Infected-Untreated group of animals using MIT and the death of all mice as a result of high level of parasitaemia means that untreated donkeys became chronic subclinical carriers of low level, virulent and pathogenic parasites from day 100 PI but detectable on MIT [3]. The negative parasitaemia status (on MIT) exhibited by Isometamidium-treated group of animals for 50 days PT with the later show of relapse on day 100 in 60% of treated animals which did not result in death of any of the inoculated mice suggest that Isometamidium chloride, controlled the T. evansi infection for 50 days as a standard trypanocides reported to have therapeutic and prophylactic effects against T. evansi infection for 2-4 months in cattle [34, 35, 19], that relapse can occur in 60% of treated donkeys from day 100 PT onward and that treatment renders the T. evansi non-pathogenic and avirulent. This can be explained by the report that Isometamidium acts by cleavaging kDNA-topoisomerase complexes, resulting in the disintegration of minicircle network within T. evansi kinetoplast [36] and mechanisms apart from those dependent on kDNA [37]. The show of aparasitaemic status by buparvaquone-treated group earlier than the Infected-Untreated group on HCT, with positive detection when MIT was used and death of all mice used for MIT from heavy parasitaemia suggest depression of parasitaemia due to buparvaquone treatment but the drug did not cure or clear infection and the donkeys were, therefore, chronic subclinical carriers of virulent and pathogenic T. evansi PI.

6. Conclusion

The dynamics of parasitemia in donkeys showed a pre-patent period of 3 to 4 days and was charracterised by an undulating wave. The infected-untreated animals became chronic carriers with parasitaemia that was not detectable on HCT from day 100 PI onward but such parasites, when relapsed or detected using mice inoculation test, were virulent and pathogenic.

Isometamidium chloride 1%, at 1mg/Kg body weight, intramuscularly dosed did not completely clear T. evansi infection in donkeys. Relapse of upto 60% in Isometamidium-treated animals was detected from day 100 post-treatment using the mice inoculation test and the relapsed parasites were avirulent and non-pathogenic because they did not cause death of mice used for test.

Buparvaquone, 5mg/kg body weight, intramuscularly dosed, twice at 3 days apart caused disappearance (depression) of parasitemia due to T. evansi infection from peripheral circulation in donkeys but do not cure infection. The parasites were detected using the mice inoculation test and such parasites were virulent and pathogenic because they caused death of all mice used for test despite exposure to buparvaquone treatment. This is the first report on the trial of buparvaquone for anti-trypanocidal effect.

Acknowledgements

The financial contribution of Niger State Government under the Postgraduate Research Funding Programme is appreciated. Prof. Natala AJ, Head of Department of Veterinary Parasitology and Entomology approved the use of Research Animals Pen and protozoology laboratory. The technical staff of Veterinary Protozoology laboratory, Ahmadu Bello University, Zaria, assisted during laboratory tests.

Ethical Considerations

All procedures on the animals were performed as recommended by the European Union 'Directive 2010/63' contained in the report by Wolfensohn and Lloyd (2013) and approved by the Research and Ethics Committee of Ahmadu Bello University, Zaria, Nigeria.

References

[1] Blench R, de Jode A Gherzi E. Donkeys in Nigeria: history, distribution and productivity. A resource book of the Animal Traction Network for Eastern and Southern Africa (ATNESA). ACP-EU Technical Centre for Agricultural and Rural Cooperation (CTA), Wageningen, The Netherlands. 2013; 244p. ISBN 92-9081-219-2. Retrieved January 01, 2013, from http://www.atnesa.org

[2] Ilemobade AA. Studies on the incidence and pathogenicity of *Trypanosoma evansi* in Nigeria. 11: The pathogenicity of *Trypanosoma evansi* for equine and bovine species. ISCTRC, OAU/STRC. 1971; 105:107-114.

[3] OIE [Office International des Epizootes]. *Trypanosoma evansi* infection (*surra*).Version adopted by The World Assembly of Deligates of the OIE in May 2010. 2010; Chapter 2.1.17. Retrieved November 24, 2012 from, http://www.oie.int/fileadmin/Home/eng/Health_standards/tahm/2.01.17_TRYPANO.pdf

[4] Cadioli FA, Marques LC, Machado RZ, Alessi AC, Aquino LPCT, Baznabe PA. Experimental *T. evansi* infection in donkeys: Haematological, biochemical and histopathological changes. Arquivo Brasileiro de Medicina Veterinaria e Zootecnia. 2006. doi.org/10.1590/S0102-09352006000500008

[5] Kirsten Gillingwater aus Hornussen AG. Discovery of novel active diamidines as clinical candidates against *Trypanosoma evansi* infection, Inaugural dissertation, zur Erlangung der Würde einer Doktorin der Philosophie, vorgelegt der, Philosophisch-Naturwissenschaftlichen Fakultät, der Universität Basel. 2007; 229pp.

[6] WHO [World Health Organisation]. Trypanosomiasis, Human African (sleeping sickness). 2012; Fact sheet No: 259 Updated October 2012, Retrieved May 01, 2013 from, http://www.who.int/mediacentre/factsheets/fs259/en/.

[7] Luckins AG. Trypanosomiasis caused by *Trypanosoma evansi* in Indonesia. J Protozool Res.1999; 144-152.

[8] Kumar R, Kumar S, Virmani N, Yadav SC. Transplacental transmission of Trypanosoma evansi from experimentally infected donkey mare to neonatal foal. J Equine Vet Sci. 2015; DOI: http://dx.doi.org/10.1016/j.jevs.2015.02.004

[9] Zhou J, Shen J, Liao D, Zhou Y, Lin J. Resistance to drug by different isolates of *Trypanosoma evansi* in China. *Acta Tropica.* 2015; 90: 271-275.

[10] FAO (Food and Agriculture Organisation). A field guide for the diagnosis, treatment and prevention of African animal trypanosomiasis. Retrieved September 22, 2012. From, www.///C:/Users/HPUSER/ Documents/trypanosomeschemotherapy.htm.

[11] Dhar S, Malhotra DV, Bhushan C, Gautam OP. Chemoprophylaxis with Buparvaquone against theileriosis in calves. Vet Record. 1987; 120: 375.

[12] Antti M, Tracy G, Jarkko R, Tapio N, Jouko V, Ari K, Simon LC, Tomi J. Synthesis, In Vitro evaluation and antileishmanial activity of water soluble pro-drugs of Buparvaquone. J Med Chem. 2004; 47(1): 188-195.

[13] Anene BM, Onah DN, Nawa Y. Drug resistance in pathogenic African trypanosomes: what hopes for the future? Vet Parasitol. 2001; 96: 83-100.

[14] Abbas II, Arigbede YA. Green area mapping of Ahmadu Bello University Main Campus, Zaria, Nigeria using remote sensing (Rs) and geographic information system (Gis) techniques. *J Geog Regional Plan.* 2012; 5(10): 287-292. DOI: 10.5897/JGRP12.024.

[15] Wayne L, Melvin B. Determining age of horses by their teeth, Extension and Agricultural Information, 1-98 Agriculture Building, Columbia, MO 65211; XPLOR website:.http://extension.missouri.edu/publications/index.aspx . 2000. Accessed 12:30 GMT July 20, 2011.

[16] Joe A. The Donkey Sanctuary. British Veterinary Association. Retrieved February 11, 2012. From, www.bva.co.uk

[17] Wolfensohn S, Lloyd M. (2013). Handbook of Laboratory Animal Management and Welfare. Fourth edition, Wiley-Blackwell Publishing ltd, U.K., 371pp.

[18] Charles M. Internal parasites, External paraspites. In: Charles M.H. and Margi S (Eds) *Laboratory procedures for veterinary technicians.* Fifth edition, Mosby Elsevier Inc., St Louis Missouri. 2007;.pp. 187-252.

[19] YO. Aliu, *Nigerian Veterinary Formulary; Handbook of Essential Veterinary Drugs, Biologics and Pesticide Chemicals* First edition, (Veterinary Council of Nigeria. 2007; p. 67.

[20] Elaine A, Margi S. Hematology and hemostasis. In: Charles M. H. and Margi S. (Eds) *Laboratory Procedures for Veterinary Technicians.* Fifth edition, Mosby Elsevier Inc., St Louis Missouri. 2007; pp. 27-73.

[21] Weiser G. Sample collection, processing and analysis of laboratory service options, In: Mary A. T., Glade W., Robin W. A. and Terry W. C. (Eds) *Veterinary Hematology and Clinical Chemistry,* second edition, Wiley-Black Well, U. K.. 2012; pp. 34-50.

[22] Monzon CM, Mancebo OA, Roux JP. Comparison between 6 parasitological methods for diagnosis of *Trypanosoma evansi* in the subtropical area of Argentina. Vet Parasitol. 1990, 36. 141–146.

[23] Aganga AA, Letso M, Aganga AO. Feeding donkeys, *Livestock* Research for Rural Development, 2000; 12(2): 2000. http://www.cipav.org.co/lrrd/lrrd12/2/agan122.htm. Retrieved on 12/07/12, 1200 GMT

[24] Aviva P, Poul W. Statistics for Veterinary and Animal Science. Third edition (Wiley-Blackwell ltd, UK. 2013; 391pp.

[25] Woo PTK. The haematocrit centrifugation technique for the diagnosis of African trypanosomiasis. Acta Tropica. (1970; 27 (4): 384-386.

[26] Aliu YO. Nigerian Veterinary Formulary; Handbook of Essential Veterinary Drugs, Biologics and Pesticide Chemicals. First edition, Veterinary Council of Nigeria. 2007; p. 67.

[27] Mead R, Curnow RN, Hasted AM. *Statistical Methods in Agriculture and Experimental Biology (Texts in Statistical Science).* Third edition, Chapman and Hall/CRC, UK. 2002; 488pp.

[28] Brun R, Hecker V, Lu V. *Trypanosoma evansi* and *Trypanosoma equiperdum*: Distribution, biology, treatment and phylogenetic relationship (A review), Vet Parasitol. 1998; 79(1998): 95-107.

[29] Herrera HM, Davila AM, Norek A, Abru UG, Souza SS, Andrea PSD, Jansen AM. Enzootiology of *Trypanosoma evansi* in the pantanal. Braz Vet Parasitol. 2004; 125: 263-275.

[30] Sudarto MW, Tabel H, Haines DM. Immunohistochemical demonstration of *Trypanosoma evansi* in tissues of experimentally infected rats and a naturally infected water buffalo (*Bubalus bubalis*). J Parasitol. 1990; 76 (2): 162–167.

[31] Ramirez LE, Wells EA, Betancourt A.. La trypanosomises en los animales domesticos en Colombia (S.L.) Centro International Agricultura Tropical. 1979; 71pp.

[32] Stephen L. Trypanosomiasis: A Veterinary Perspective. Pergamon Press, New York, USA. 1986.

[33] Hutchinson OC, Picozzi K., Jones NG, Mott H, Sharma R, Welburn SC, Carrington M. Variant Surface Glycoprotein gene repertoires in Trypanosoma brucei have diverged to become strain-specific. *BioMed Central Genomics.* 2007; 8: 234. doi:10.1186/1471-2164-8-234.

[34] Touratier L. The advantages of using Isometamidium for the control of animal trypanosomiasis. International Scientific Council for Trypanosomiasis Research and Control. Sixteenth meeting, Yaounde, Cameroon, 1979. OAU/STRC. 1981; 308-316.

[35] Mira SF, Ralph R. Manual of Tropical Veterinary Parasitology. First edition, C.A.B., England. 1989; pp. 181-260.

[36] Shapiro TA, Englund PT. Selective cleavage of kinetoplast DNA minicircles promoted by antitrypanosomal drugs. Proceedings Natl Acad Sci USA. 1990; 87: 950–954.

[37] Kaminsky R, Schmid C, Lun ZR. Susceptibility of dyskinetoplastic *Trypanosoma evansi* and *Trypanosoma equiperdum* to isometamidium chloride. Parasitol Res. 1997; 83: 816-818.

Retrospective Study of Tick-Borne Pathogens and Observation of *Ehrlichia ewingii / Anaplasma phagocytophilum* and Hemotropic *Mycoplasma* spp. in Dogs' Blood Films

Maryam Rassouli[1, 2, *], Ghazaleh Aghazamani[3]

[1]Pathobiology Department, Shahmirzad School of Veterinary Medicine, Semnan University, Semnan, Iran
[2]Pathobiology Department, Faculty of Veterinary Medicine, Semnan University, Semnan, Iran
[3]Shahmirzad School of Veterinary Medicine, Semnan University, Semnan, Iran

Email address:
Mrdvmp@yahoo.com (M. Rassouli), Mrvpar@semnan.ac.ir (M. Rassouli), Ghazale.zamani3@yahoo.com (G. Aghazamani)

Abstract: *Ehrlichia ewingii*, *Anaplasma phogocytophilum* and hemotropic *Mycoplasma* spp. are three bacteria which can infect different dog's blood cells. All of these three pathogens can be transmitted by different ticks and some reservoir hosts also play a role in their transmission. Although *E. ewingii* and *A. phagocytophilum* infect granulocytes and neutrophils of their hosts, respectively, hemotropic *Mycoplasma* spp. can infect reticulocytes. In this research, the previously taken dogs' blood films were collected randomly from different veterinary hospitals of Tehran, the capital of Iran. The blood films were reinvestigated for arthropod-borne diseases. Surprisingly, *E. ewingii*/*A. phagocytophilum* morulae and hemotropic *Mycoplasma* spp. were observed in 18% and 37.7% of samples, respectively. None of these pathogens have been reported in Iran. In addition to the new report, the changes which have been made by these pathogens, their similarities, differences and zoonotic importance are discussed.

Keywords: *Ehrlichia ewingii*, *Anaplasma phagocytophilum*, *Mycoplasma*, Dog, Iran

1. Introduction

Ehrlichiosis is caused by several bacterial species in the genus *Ehrlichia*, pronounced (err-lick-ee-uh) [1], family Anaplasmataceae, order Rickettsiales. They are small, pleomorphic Gram-negative bacteria found in circulating leukocyte or platelets of susceptible mammalian hosts. *Ehrlichia* spp. are tick-borne, obligatory intracellular pathogens. These organisms are often observed in compact colonies or phagosomal inclusions which are named morula [2]. Canine ehrlichiosis is caused by *Ehrlichia canis*. This disease is distributed worldwide and its primary vectors are brown dog tick (*Rhipicephalus sanguineus*) and *Dermacentor variabilis*. This species of *Ehrlichia* commonly infect mononuclear white blood cells [1]. In addition to *E. canis*, *E. chafeensis*, the agent of human monocytic monocytotropic ehrlichiosis (HME) can infect dogs' mononuclear leukocytes. *E. ewingii* causes canine granulocytic ehrlichiosis, this disease is reported in the US and its potential vector is *Amblyomma americanum*. Granulocytes are the most infected cells [1]. *Anaplasma phagocytophilum* is another tick-borne pathogen of family Anaplasmataceae which can be transmitted by different species of *Ixodes* [3]. *A. phagocytophilum* infection was first described in Human. It also can infect horses, ruminants, dogs and cats. Macaques and baboons were infected experimentally [4]. Small mammals can be reservoir of *A. phagocytophilum* [3].

Hemotropic mycoplasmosis (formely, hemobartonellosis) is caused by wall-less Gram-negative bacterial organisms, *Mycoplasma* spp., class Mollicutes. These hemotropic *Mycoplasma* spp. attach and grow on the surface of infected reticulocytes [5]. *Mycoplasma haemocanis* (formely, *Hemobartonella canis*) and *Candidatus* Mycoplasma haematoparvum cause hemotropic mycoplasmosis in dogs. *M. haemocanis* was experimentally transmitted by *R.*

sanguineus [6], transstadial and transovarial transmission in tick has also been described. The infection transmission through blood transfusion from clinically normal carrier dogs has also been reported [3].

Diagnosis of *E. ewingii* is usually based on tick infestation history, observation of its morula in granulocytes, hematological abnormalities and serological findings. Polymerase chain reaction (PCR) is now available [3].

A. phagocytophilum is often pleomorphic organisms are varying in size from 0.2 to 2 µm in diameter. *A.phagocytophilum* inclusions are morphologically similar to *E.ewingii* morula. More diagnostic techniques are needed for their differential diagnosis [3].

Mycoplsma spp. are easily recognized in stained blood films, *M. haemocanis* are usually occur singly with one to four cocci per red blood cell or in doublets, but ring forms and chains have not been described [7], but these bacteria should be differentiated from Basophilic stipplings and Howell-Jolly bodies [3].

Most symptoms of Ehrlichiosis among dogs were described in *E.canis* infection. This disease is divided into acute, subclinical and chronic forms; clinical disease in *E.ewingii* infection is acute rather than chronic [3]. Common clinical signs are fever, depression, anorexia, weight loss, stiffness, joint swelling [8-11], lethargy and CNS signs such as head tilt, tremors and anisocoria [10, 12]. Rarely observed signs include hemorrhage, weight loss, uveitis, pruritis, vomiting, diarrhea and organomegaly [10-13]. The most important laboratory changes can be observed as mild nonregenerative anemia and thrombocytopenia [9, 12, 14].

The symptoms of *A. phagocytophilum* infection are associated with acute phase of the disease and include: fever, lethargy, depression, anorexia, vomiting, diarrhea, musculoskeletal pain (reluctance to move, stiffness, weakness and lameness) [15, 16], polyarthritis [17], vomiting, diarrhea, respiratory signs (coughing, labored breathing) [15, 16, 18, 19]. Organomegaly is also present [15, 16, 20, 21, 22]. In clinical laboratory examinations; mild to moderate thrombocytopenia and nonregenerative normocytic normochromic anemia can be observed [15, 16, 23].

In Canine hemotropic mycoplasmosis, clinical evidences do not develop. It can cause mild to severe regenerative anemia [7]. The severe symptoms are mostly seen in splenectomized dogs, PCR detection is also available [3].

All of these three organisms can potentially be transmitted to human [24, 25], but their zoonotic importance will be discussed later.

2. Materials and Methods

61 blood films were randomly collected from dogs (33 bitches, 28 studs) which were referred to different veterinary hospitals of Tehran, the capital of Iran. Dogs' age and breed were recorded in a few cases. Previously taken blood films were observed again for hemotropic arthropod-borne pathogens. The observed abnormalities were recorded and compared with previous diagnosis. The newly recorded diseases were analyzed among studs and bitches by chi-square test, SPSS software. The breeds and ages were not analyzed because they had not mostly been recorded in the case histories.

3. Results

Hemotropic *Mycoplasma* spp. were observed in 15 samples out of 61 (24.6%) (group A) and *Ehrlichia ewingii*/*Anaplasma phagocytophilum* morulae were observed in 3 blood films out of 61 (4.9%) (group B) and 8 samples out of 61 (13.1%) (group AB) had coinfection of *Mycoplasma* spp. and *E. ewingii*/*A. phagocytophilum* (Figs 1, 2, 3); therefore 11 samples (18%) (5 Bitches, 6 studs) were positive in *E. ewingii*/*A. phagocytophilum* and 23 samples (37.7%) (14 Bitches, 9 studs) were positive in *Mycoplasma* spp. The species of *Mycoplasma* could not be determined because there was no access to the previously referred dogs' whole blood samples and the *E. ewingii*/*A. phagocytophilum* could not be differentiate because the dogs' sera were not available in the referred veterinary hospitals. There was no significant difference between infected studs and bitches ($P>0.05$).

In Diff Quick of group A, in 11 samples mature neutrophils were decreased but band cells increased, the other leukocytes were normal in counting. 2 cases were leukopenic. In 2 cases lymphocytosis was observed in addition to mature neutropenia and band cell increasing. In band cell increasing samples, the band cells of 3 samples was 20%-30%, 9 samples were 10-20% and 1 sample 5-10%. There were toxic changes in addition to left shift in neutrophils. Polychromatophilic macrocytes, hypochromic reticulocytes and anisocytosis were also observed in all samples (Figures 1, 3).

In group B, all of the *E. ewingii*/*A. phagocytophilum* morulae were observed in neutrophil cytoplasms. In Diff Quick, 2 samples were leukopenic whith hypochromatic reticulocytes, demonstrated as discocytes. Poikilocytosis include: discocyte, codocyte, echinocyte, Elliptocte, echinoelliptocyte and shistocyte. In 1 sample lymphopenia with monocytosis was observed. Reactive lymphocytes were also observed in this group (Figures 2, 3).

In group AB: in Diff Quick, 5 samples were leukopenic, 3 cases had mature neutropenia and band cell increasing (1 sample 30-40% and the rest 2 cases 10-20% of the counted leukocytes were band cells). In 1 case in addition to mature neutropenia and band cell increasing, Lymphopenia, monocytosis and reactive lymphocytosis could be observed. Reticulocyte changes include: hypochromasia, anisocytosis and poikilocytosis.

In all leukopenic samples, only neutrophils could be counted in low numbers.

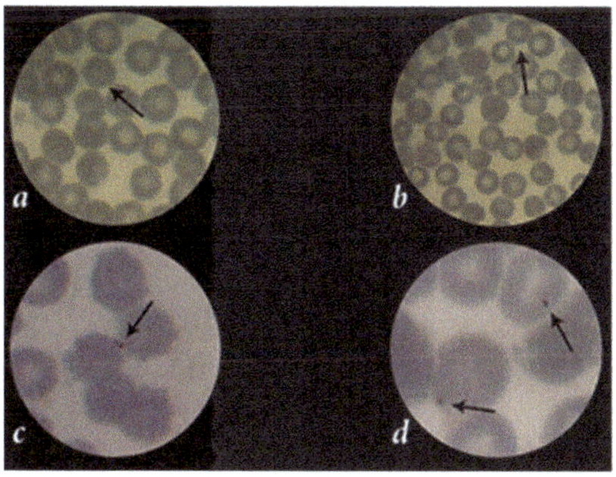

Figure. 1. *a: hemotropic Mycoplasma sp. closed to reticulocyte membrane, black arrow. Note the discocytes, 300X, stained by Giemsa. b: hemotropic Mycoplasma sp. closed to reticulocyte membrane, black arrow. Note the discocytes and hyperchromatic macrocytes, 200X, stained by Giemsa. c: doublet of hemotropic Mycoplasma sp., black arrow, 400X, stained by Giemsa. d: hemotropic Mycoplasma sp. closed to two reticulocyte membranes, black arrows, 500X, stained by Giemsa.*

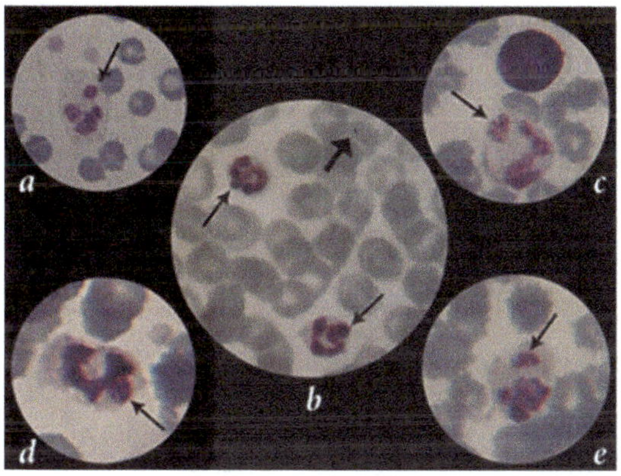

Figure. 2. *a: Ehrlichia ewingii/Anaplasma phagocytophilum inclusion in a neutrophil cytoplasm, black arrow, 300X, stained by Giemsa. b: Ehrlichia ewingii/Anaplasma phagocytophilum inclusion in a neutrophil cytoplasm, black arrow, 400X, stained by Giemsa, c: Basophilic Ehrlichia ewingii/Anaplasma phagocytophilum inclusions on neutrophil neuclei, thin black arrows and hemotropic Mycoplasma sp. closed to reticulocyte membrane, thick black arrow. Note the discocytes and rouleaux. 400X, stained by Giemsa. d: Ehrlichia ewingii/Anaplasma phagocytophilum inclusion in a band cell cytoplasm, black arrow. 500X, stained by Giemsa. e: Ehrlichia ewingii/Anaplasma phagocytophilum inclusion in a neutrophil cytoplasm, 500X, stained by Giemsa.*

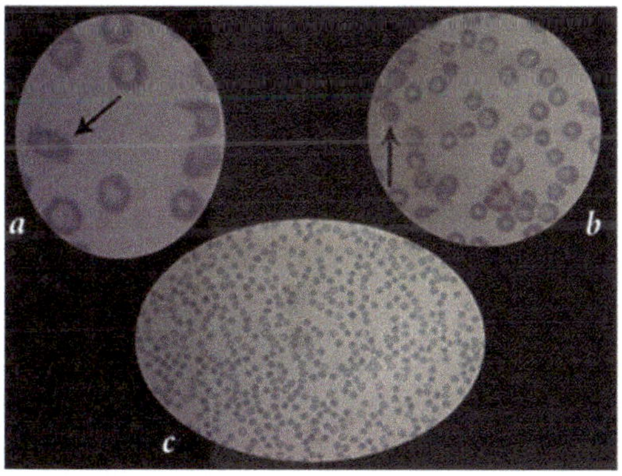

Figure. 3. *a: poikilocytosis, note the echinoelliptocyte, black arrow, 400X, stained by Giemsa. b: hypochromasia, poikilocytosis and anisocytosis. Note the codocyte, black arrow, 200X, stained by Giemsa. c: panleukopenia and hypochromasia, 40X. stained by Giemsa.*

4. Discussion

According to the research, the most important problem among the samples was history taking. Most of them were incomplete. The age and breed of dogs were rarely recorded. In spite of finding some tick-borne diseases, tick infestation history was recorded in only 6 samples. None of these observed abnormalities in the blood films were recorded as a "diagnosed disease" and most of the referred dogs diseases had been diagnosed as viral infections. The concurrent viral infections cannot be rejected but these tick-borne infections (*E. ewingii*/*A. phagocitophilum* and hemotropic *Mycoplasma* spp.) may make the infected dogs susceptible to other infectious diseases such as distemper.

Therefore, it can be concluded that blood films were not used for diagnosis and just taken as a routine procedure from referred dogs.

E. ewingii was endemic in southeastern and south-central of the United States and 26% of shelter dogs were seropositive in endemic areas of the U. S [3, 11]. *E. ewingii* DNA was detected in Cameroon and Brazil [26, 27]. *A. phagocytophilum* is distributed worldwide. In the United States, *A. phagocytophilum* is mostly in western and northern Midwestern states [15, 23, 28]. The range of the seroprevalence in infected dogs can vary widely; in the Europe, the *A. phagocytophilum* seroprevalence may vary from 5% to 70.5% [29-37] and in the United States was from 0.0% to 67.4% [23, 38-40]. In Canada, there was low seroprevalence of *A. phagocytophilum* among dogs which were tested in different provinces (0.09-0.9%) [3, 41]. *A. phagocytophilum* DNA was also detected in Europe and North Africa [3].

Canine hemotropic mycoplasmosis was reported in Europe, especially in its Mediterranean countries [42]. In France 3.3% of examined blood samples were infected with *M. haemocanis* and 9.6% with *Candidatus* M. haematoparvum [43] and high prevalence of this disease was reported among dogs in Africa [44].

None of these diseases has been reported in Iran, so; the importance of our findings is to prove that *E. ewingii*/*A. phagocytophilum* and hemotropic *Mycoplasma* spp. infections are present among dogs in Iran, therefore; further researches are needed to understand the true prevalence, the importance, species diagnosis and the potential vectors of these diseases. Seroprevalnece of *E. canis* has been reported among dogs in different parts of Iran [45,-47]. There is a cross-reactivity between *E. ewingii* and *E. canis* in some serological methods [3]. Therefore some of the reported seropositive samples might be related to *E. ewingii* exposure, but there is not any cross-reactivity between *E. ewingii* and *A. phagocytophilum* [3] and serological tests can well differentiate these infections from each other. In this case, because of retrospective study, the access to referred dogs sera was impossible. In this reserach 23 samples (37.7%) (25.5-50%; 95% confidence interval "CI") were positive in *Mycoplasma* spp. and 11 samples (18%) (8.4-27.6%; 95% CI) were positive in *E. ewingii*/*A. phagocytophilum* which are relatively high. One of the results of the disease unidentification is, no treatment of infected dog will occur and consequently high prevalence of the infection among more ticks and more dogs will be observed.

Amblyomma americanum is the main vector of *E. ewingii* and white-tail deer (*Odocoileus virginianus*) serve as a reservoir for *E. ewingii* in the southern parts of the U.S [48-50]. *E. ewingii* DNA was detected in *D. variabilis and Rh. sanguineus* [14, 51-54]. These species and may be some other ticks are more important in other countries such as Brazil and Cameroon where *E. ewingii* has been detected [26, 27]. Once ticks are infected by *E. ewingii*, they remain infected throughout their life (transstadial transmission) [14, 55]. *A.phagocytophilum* can be transmitted by members of the *Ixodes persulcatus* complex (e.g., *I. scapularis*, *I. pacificus*, *I. ricinus* and *I. persulcatus*) [3, 56]. A minimum required feeding time for *Ixodes* spp. which can transmit *A. phagocytophilum* to susceptible mammalian hosts is 24 to 48 hours [57-59]. *A. phagocytophilum* is able to reside in the salivary glands of unfed *Ixodes* spp. ticks [60]. *R. sanguineus* serves as a vector and reservoir of *M. haemocanis* because of transstadial and transovarial transmission of the organism [3]. Unfourtunately, there is no information of vectors and reservoirs of above pathogens in Iran. *A. americanum* has not been reported in Iran thus, the *E. ewingii* vectors can be the other tick genera. It is also predicted that because of the mean temperature increase in Iran, ticks can be active in more months of the year and thus tick-borne diseases will increase. Therefore, tick control is necessary for pets and farm animals.

Observable changes in blood films were recorded in dogs infected with *E. ewingii*, *A. phagocytophilum* and *M. haemocanis* and listed as below; in *E. ewingii* infection, the most important abnormality is thrombocytopenia but platelet counts are not helpful for diagnosis [9, 10, 12, 14]. Mild anemia and reactive lymphocytosis are observed [10, 11]. Biochemical abnormalities are mild and nonspecific in this disease [3]. Neutrophilic inflammation causes polyarthritis [10]. *E.ewingii* morulae can also be detected in CSF fluid, joint fluid, prostatic fluid or other body fluids [9, 10, 12]. Another problem which is caused by *E. ewingii* is the delay in neutrophil apoptosis. In normal cases neutrophils are in peripheral circulation for only 6 to 8 hours [61], but in some naturally and experimentally infected dogs this time prolonged to 5 days [62]. This phenomenonprovides additional time for the pathogen replication [63, 64]. In this study, in leukopenic cases, just low numbers of neutrophils could be counted. Some of these neutrophils were in abnormal shapes; these neutrophils can be named “old neutrophils”. In canine granulocytic anaplasmosis, mild to moderated nonregenerative anemia and thrombocytopenia are observed [15, 16, 23]. In Diff Quick, both neutrophilia and neutropenia can be recorded, lymphopenia, monocytosis, eosinopenia are also observed. Monocytopenia was reported in some dogs in the US [65, 66]. In hemotropic mycoplasmosis the anemia is regenerative so hematological findings include: reticulocytosis, polychromasia, anisocytosis and presence of Howell-Jolly bodies.

Macrocytosis takes more time to develop [3]. In this case, polychromatophic macrocytes were observed, so this is another reason for chronic forms of these diseases in Iran because of the unidentification.

Neutrophilia, monocytosis and lymphopenia can occur in a response to endogenous or exogenous glucocorticoids in dogs like other animals [67-70]. Potential causes of increased endogenous releasing of glucocorticoids include fever, pain, stress, intense exercise and hyperadrenocorticism [69, 71]. Left shift is often associated with inflammatory conditions. Bacterial infections, among other infectious diseases are more important for left shift occurrence [72, 73]. Glucocorticoids increase lymphocyte sequestration and apoptosis [74-76], some secreted cytokines in bacterial and viral infections also cause lymphopenia [77-79]. Reactive lymphocytes are antigen stimulated lymphocytes which their size and their cytoplasmic basophilia were increased [73]. In this case all of the above abnormalities were observed and mentioned in details in the result section but leukopenia might occur due to chronic *E. ewingii*/*A. phagocytophilum* or other concurrent dignosed diseases like distemper or parvovirus infection! It is also unclear if *E.ewingii*/*A. phagocytophilum* and hemotropic *Mycoplasma* spp. infections can make dogs susceptible to other infections.This question and other ambiguous aspects of these tick-borne diseases must be answered by further reseaches.

No breed predispositions have been reported in *E. ewingii*, *A. phagocytophilum* and *M. haemocanis* infection [15, 16, 30]. There were some reports of coinfection of *A. phagocytophilum* with *Borrelia burgdorferi* in different hosts [80]. *A. phagocytophilum* infected dogs in the US coinfected with other *Anaplasma* spp., *Babesia canis*, *Babesia vinsonii*, *E. canis*, *Rickettsia rickettsia* [3, 81-83]. In this research only coinfection of *E. ewingii*/*A. phagocytophilum* with hemotropic *Mycoplasma* spp. was observed.

The mortality has not been reported in order to *E. ewingii* or *A. phagocytophilum* infection among dogs, thus these diseases are mild or in apparent. *E. ewingii* infection may clear spontaneously within weeks or several months [84]. Two deaths of puppies were reported due to hemotropic mycoplasmosis [3]. *M. haemocanis* could be successfully transmitted congenitally and orally [3, 85] in experimental studies. *M. haemocanis* can cause severe life-threating anemia in splenectomized dogs [3]. According to the results, these diseases have not been diagnosed in Iran, so their mortality rate cannot be estimated.

There are some reports of *E. ewingii* in immunocompromised human [24, 86-88], but there is no report of dog-to-human transmission [3]. *A. phagocytophilum* in human is self-limiting such as dogs [3], but pet animals have an important role in epidemiological aspects of *A. phagocytophilum* in an area [25, 89]. *E. ewingii* and *A. phagocytophilum* infections are also important in sheepdogs because both can also infect small ruminants [90, 91]. *Mycoplasma haemofelis* was detected in an immunocompromised man from Brazil [92]. This case and some similar cases in human [93, 94] suggest vector, bite, or scratch transmission, or handling blood from animals may transmit the infection into human, especially in immunocompromised individuals [3].

E. ewingii can be treated rapidly by suitable antimicrobial therapy. Doxycycline is a choice drug but other tetracycline can also be used [95]. Supportive treatment is necessary in polyarthritis cases [3]. *A. phagocytophilum* responds to doxycycline, rifampin and levofloxacin. Other tetracycline derivatives are also useful [96]. Canine hemotropic mycoplasmosis is never treated completely and after treatment latent infection is still in infected dogs. This disease can be limited by orally administered tetracyclines. Blood transfusion is necessary when the anemia is severe [3].

5. Conclusion

E. ewingii and *A. phagocytophilum* infection make some similar symptoms in infected dogs and their morulae cannot be differentiated in the blood films [3, 21], but fortunately both bacteria are susceptible to tetracyclines [95]. It is recommended that if the morula was observed in the infected dog's blood film, treatment must start immediately either the infectious agent is *E. ewingii* or *A. phagocytophilum* but the laboratory should record the result as *E. ewingii/A. phagocytophilum*. Afterward, if it is necessary, the serum is tested by serological techniques. Greene (2012) also mentioned that differential diagnosis between *E. ewingii* and *A. phagocytophilum* is usually done for zoonotic concern (for the owner or academic importance) [3]. In developing countries such as Iran because all of the veterinary laboratories have not been equipped for serological and molecular tests, the differential diagnosis between *E. ewingii* and *A. phagocytophilum* may get in trouble. In this research the accurate diagnosis of the reported infections didn't occur due to retrospective study limitations which were mentioned above but further researches to complete our findings are necessary.

Acknowledgments

Special thanks to Dr. Fathipour for his help and there is no competing of financial interests exists.

References

[1] Parker, J. N. and Parker, P. M. (2002). The official patient's sourcebook on Ehrlichiosis. ICON Health Publication, San Diego, CA, USA, pp. 11-14.

[2] Williams, J. C. and Kakoma, I. (1990). Ehrlichiosis, a vector-borne disease of animals and humans. Kluwer Academic Publishers. Buston, USA, pp. 1-5.

[3] Greene, C. E. (2012). Infectious diseases of the dog and cat, forth ed. Elsevier Saunders, Saint Louis, Missouri, USA, pp. 227-258, 310-319.

[4] Raoult, D. and Parola, P. (2007). Rickettsial diseases. Informa healthcare, New York, USA.

[5] Peters, I. R., Helps, C. R., McAuliffe, L., Neimark, H., Lappin, M. R., Gruffydd-Jones, T. J., Day, M. J., Hoelzle, K., Willi, B., Meli, M. L., Hofmann-Lehmann, R. and Tasker, S. (2008). RNase P RNA gene (rnpB) phylogeny of hemoplasmas and other *Mycoplasma* species. J. Clin. Microbiol. 46: 1873-1977.

[6] Seneviratna, P., Weerasinghe, N. and Ariyadasa, S. (1973). Transmission of *Haemobartonella canis* by the dog tick *Rhipicephalus sanguineus*. Res. Vet. Sci. 14: 112-114.

[7] Sykes, J. E., Ball, L. M., Bailiff, N. L. and Fry, M. M. (2005). *Candidatus* Mycoplasma haematoparvum, a novel small haemotropic mycoplasma from a dog. Int. J. Syst. Evol. Bact. 55: 27-30.

[8] Bellah, J. R., Shull, R. M., Shull Selcer, E. V. (1986). *Ehrlichia canis*–related polyarthritis in a dog. J. Am. Vet. Med. Assoc. 189: 922-923.

[9] Stockham, S. L., Schmidt, D. A., Curtis, K. S., Schauf, B. G., Tyler, J. W. and Simpson, S. T. (1992). Evaluation of granulocytic ehrlichiosis in dogs of Missouri, including serologic status to *Ehrlichia canis, Ehrlichia equi*, and *Borrelia burgdorferi*. Am. J. Vet. Res. 53: 63-68.

[10] Goodman, R. A., Hawkins, E. C., Olby, N. J., Grindem, C. B., Hegarty, B. and Breitschwerdt, E. B. (2003). Molecular identification of *Ehrlichia ewingii* infection in dogs: 15cases (1997-2001). J. Am. Vet. Med. Assoc. 222: 1102-1107.

[11] Liddell, A. M., Stockham, S. L., Scott, M. A., Sumner, J. W., Paddock, C. D., Gaudreault-Keener, M., Arens, M. Q. and Storch, G. A. (2003). Predominance of *Ehrlichia ewingii* in Missouri dogs. J. Clin. Microbiol. 41: 4617-4622.

[12] Gieg, J., Rikihisa, Y. and Wellman, M. (2009). Diagnosis of *Ehrlichia ewingii* infection by PCR in a puppy from Ohio. Vet. Clin. Pathol. 38: 406-410.

[13] Goldman, E. E., Breitschwerdt, E. B., Grindem, C. B., Hegarty, B. C., Walls, J. J. and Dumler, J. S. (1998). Granulocytic ehrlichiosis in dogs from North Carolina and Virginia. J Vet. Intern. Med. 12: 61-70.

[14] Anziani, O. S., Ewing, S. A. and Barker, R. W. (1990). Experimental transmission of a granulocytic form of the tribe Ehrlichieae by *Dermacentor variabilis* and *Amblyomma americanum* to dogs. Am. J. Vet. Res. 51: 929-931.

[15] Greig, B., Asanovich, K. M., Armstrong, P. J. and Dumler, J. S. (1996). Geographic, clinical, serologic, and molecular evidence of granulocytic ehrlichiosis, a likely zoonotic disease, in Minnesota and Wisconsin dogs. J. Clin. Microbiol. 34: 44-48.

[16] Egenvall, A. E., Hedhammar, A. A. and Bjöersdorff, A. I. (1997). Clinical features and serology of 14 dogs affected by granulocytic ehrlichiosis in Sweden. Vet. Rec. 140: 222-226.

[17] Foley, J. E., Drazenovich, N., Leutenegger, C. M. and Chomel, B. B. (2007a). Association between polyarthritis and thrombocytopenia and increased prevalence of vectorborne pathogens in Californian dogs. Vet. Rec. 160: 159-162.

[18] Pusterla, N., Huder, J., Wolfensberger, C., Litschi, B., Parvis, A. and Lutz, H. (1997). Granulocytic ehrlichiosis in two dogs in Switzerland. J. Clin. Microbiol. 35, 2307-2309.

[19] Carrade, D., Foley, J., Borjesson, D. and Sykes, J. E. (2009). Canine granulocytic anaplasmosis: a review. J. Vet. Intern. Med. 23: 1129-1141.

[20] Maretzki, C. H., Fisher, D. J. and Greene, C. E. (1994). Granulocytic ehrlichiosis and meningitis in a dog. J. Am. Vet. Med. Assoc. 205: 1554-1556.

[21] Kohn, B., Galke, D., Beelitz, P. and Pfister, K. (2008). Clinical features of canine granulocytic anaplasmosis in 18 naturally infected dogs. J. Vet. Intern. Med. 22: 1289-1295.

[22] Granick, J. L., Armstrong, P. J. and Bender, J. B. (2009). *Anaplasma phagocytophilum* infection in dogs: 34 cases (2000-2007). J. Am. Vet. Med. Assoc. 234: 1559-1565.

[23] Beall, M. J., Chandrashekar, R., Eberts, M. D., Cyr, K. E., Diniz, P. P., Mainville, C., Hegarty, B. C., Crawford, J. M. and Breitschwerdt, E. B. (2008). Serological and molecular prevalence of *Borrelia burgdorferi, Anaplasma phagocytophilum*, and *Ehrlichia* species in dogs from Minnesota. Vector. Borne. Zoonotic. Dis. 8: 455-464.

[24] Buller, R. S., Arens, M., Hmeil, S. P., Sumner, J. W., Rikhisa, Y., Unver, A., Gaudreault-Keener, M., Manian, F. A., Liddell, A.M., Schmulewitz, N. and Storch, G.A. (1999). *Ehrlichia ewingii*, a newly recognized agent of human ehrlichiosis. N. Engl. J. Med. 341: 148-155.

[25] Cleaveland, S., Meslin, F. X. and Breiman, R. (2006). Dogs can play useful role as sentinel hosts for disease. Nature. 440: 605.

[26] Ndip, L. M., Ndip, R. N., Esemu, S. N., Dickmu, V. L., Fokam, E. B., Walker, D. H. and McBride, J. W. (2005). Ehrlichial infection in Cameroonian canines by *Ehrlichia canis* and *Ehrlichia ewingii*. Vet. Microbiol. 111: 59-66.

[27] Oliveira, L. S., Oliveira, K. A., Mourao, L. C., Pescatore, A. M., Almeida, M. R., Conceição, L. G., Galvão, M. A. and Mafra, C. (2009). First report of *Ehrlichia ewingii* detected by molecular investigation in dogs from Brazil. Clin. Microbiol. Infect. 15 (suppl 2): 55-56.

[28] Arsenault, W. G. and Messick, J. B. (2005). Acute granulocytic ehrlichiosis in a Rottweiler. Am. Anim. Hosp. Assoc. 41: 323-326.

[29] Pusterla, N., Pusterla, J. B. and Deplazes, P. (1998). Seroprevalence of *Ehrlichia canis* and of canine granulocytic *Ehrlichia* infection in dogs in Switzerland. J. Clin. Microbiol. 36: 3460-3462.

[30] Egenvall, A., Bonnett, B. N., Gunnarsson, A., Hedhammar, A., Shoukri, M., Bornstein, S. and Artursson, K. (2000). Seroprevalence of granulocytic *Ehrlichi*a spp. and *Borrelia burgdorferi* sensu lato in Swedish dogs 1991-94. Scand. J. Infect. Dis. 32: 19-25.

[31] Barutzki, D., De Nicola, A., Zeziola, M. and Reule, M. (2006). Seroprevalence of *Anaplasma phagocytophilum* infection in dogs in Germany. Berl. Munch. Tierarztl. Wochenschr. 119: 342-347.

[32] Solano-Gallego, L., Llull, J., Osso, M., Hegarty, B. and Breitschwerdt, E.B. (2006). A serological study of exposure to arthropod-borne pathogens in dogs from northeastern Spain. Vet. Res. 37: 231-244.

[33] Torina, A. and Caracappa, S. (2006). Dog tick-borne diseases in Sicily. Parasitol. 48: 145-147.

[34] Amusategui, I., Tesouro, M. A., Kakoma, I. and Sainz, A. (2008). Serological reactivity to *Ehrlichia canis, Anaplasma phagocytophilum, Neorickettsia risticii, Borrelia burgdorferi* and *Rickettsia conorii* in dogs from Northwestern Spain. Vector Borne. Zoonotic. Dis. 8: 797-803.

[35] Ebani, V., Cerri, D., Fratini, F., Ampola, M. and Andreani, E. (2008). Seroprevalence of *Anaplasma phagocytophilum* in domestic and wild animals from central Italy. New. Microbiol. 31: 371-375.

[36] Ravnik, U., Tozon, N., Strasek, K. and Avsic Zupanc, T. (2009) Clinical and haematological features in *Anaplasma phagocytophilum* seropositive dogs. Clin. Microbiol. Infect. 15(suppl 2): 39-40.

[37] Santos, A. S., Alexandre, N., Sousa, R., Núncio, M. S., Bacellar, F., and Dumler, J. S. (2009). Serological and molecular survey of *Anaplasma* species infection in dogs with suspected tickborne disease in Portugal. Vet. Rec. 164: 168-171.

[38] Suksawat, J., Hegarty, B. C. and Breitschwerdt, E. B. (2000). Seroprevalence of *Ehrlichia canis, Ehrlichia equi* and *Ehrlichia risticii* in sick dogs from North Carolina and Virginia. J. Vet. Intern. Med. 14: 50-55.

[39] Foley, J. E., Foley, P. and Madigan, J. E. (2001). Spatial distribution of seropositivity to the causative agent of granulocytic ehrlichiosis in dogs in California. Am. J. Vet. Res. 62: 1599-1605.

[40] Foley, J. E., Brown, R. N., Gabriel, M. W., Henn, J., Drazenovich, N., Kasten, R., Green, S.L. and Chomel, B. B. (2007b). Spatial analysis of the exposure of dogs in rural north-coastal California to vectorborne pathogens. Vet. Rec. 161: 653-657.

[41] Gary, A. T., Webb, J. A., Hegarty, B. C. and Breitschwerdt, E.B. (2006). The low seroprevalence of tick-transmitted agents of disease in dogs from southern Ontario and Quebec. Can. Vet. J. 47: 1194-1200.

[42] Willi, B., Novacco, M., Meli, M., Wolf-Jackel, G. A., Boretti, F. S. and Wengi, N. (2010). Haemotropic mycoplasmas of cats and dogs: transmission, diagnosis, prevalence and importance in Europe. Schweiz. Arch. Tierheilkd. 152: 237-244.

[43] Kenny, M. J., Shaw, S. E., Beugnet, F. and Tasker, S. (2004). Demonstration of two distinct hemotropic *Mycoplasmas* in French dogs. J. Clin. Microbiol. 42 (11): 5397-5399.

[44] Barker, E. N., Tasker, S., Day, M. J., Warman, S. M., Woolley, K., Birtles, R., Georges, K. C., Ezeokoli, C. D., Newaj-Fyzul, A., Campbell, M. D., Sparagano, O. A. E., Cleaveland, S. and Helps, C. R. (2010). Development and use of real-time PCR to detect and quantify *Mycoplasma haemocanis* and "*Candidatus* Mycoplasma haematoparvum" in dogs. Vet. Microbiol. 140: 167-170.

[45] Akhtardanesh, B., Ghanbarpour, R., Blourizadeh, H., 2010. Serological evidence of canine monocytic ehrlichiosis in Iran. Comp. Clin. Path. 19: 469–474.

[46] Avize, R., Mosallanejad, B., Razi Jalali, M. H. and Alborzi, A.R. (2010). Seroprevalence of *Ehrlichia canis* in dogs referred toVeterinary Hospital of Shahid Chamran University of Ahvaz, Iran. Arch. Razi. Inst. 65: 1-5.

[47] Ansari-Mood, M., Khoshnegah, J., Mohri, M. and Rajaei, S.M. (2014). Seroprevalence and risk factors of *Ehrlichia canis* infection among companion dogs of Mashhad, North East of Iran, 2009–2010. J. Arthropod. Borne. Dis. 9(2): 184-194.

[48] Beaufils, J. P. (1997). Ehrlichiosis: clinical aspects in dogs and cats. Compend. Cont. Educ. Pract. Vet. 19: 57-61.

[49] Yabsley, M. J., Varela, A. S., Tate, C. M., Dugan, V. G., Stallknecht D. E., Little, S. E. and Davidson, W. R. (2002). *Ehrlichia ewingii* infection in white-tail deer (*Odocoileus virginianus*). Emerg. Infect. Dis. 8: 668-671.

[50] Murphy, G. L., Ewing, S. A., Whitworth, L. C., Fox, J. C. and Kocan, A. A. (1998). A molecular and serologic survey of *Ehrlichia canis, E. chaffeensis*, and *E. ewingii* in dogs and ticks from Oklahoma. Vet. Parasitol. 79: 325-339.

[51] Varela-Stokes, A. S. (2007). Transmission of bacterial agents from lone star ticks to white-tailed deer. J. Med. Entomol. 44: 478-483.

[52] Steiert, J. G. and Gilfoy, F. (2002). Infection rates of *Amblyomma americanum* and *Dermacentor variabilis* by *Ehrlichia chaffeensis* and *Ehrlichia ewingii* in southwest Missouri. Vector. Borne. Zoonotic. Dis. 2: 53-60.

[53] Childs, J. E. and Paddock, C. D. (2003). The ascendancy of *Amblyomma americanum* as a vector of pathogens affecting humans in the United States. Annu. Rev. Entomol. 48: 307-337.

[54] De Shields, A., Borman-Shoap, E., Peters, J. E., Gaudreault-Keener, M., Arens, M. Q. and Storch, G. A. (2004). Detection of pathogenic *Ehrlichia* in ticks collected at acquisition sites of human ehrlichiosis in Missouri. Mo. Med. 101: 132-136.

[55] Varela, A. S., Moore, V. A. and Little, S. E. (2004). Disease agents in *Amblyomma americanum* from northeastern Georgia. J. Med. Entomol. 41: 753-759.

[56] Woldehiwet, Z. (2010). The natural history of *Anaplasma phagocytophilum*. Vet. Parasitol. 167: 108-122.

[57] Hodzic, E., Fish, D., Maretzki, C. M., De Silva, A. M., Feng, S. and Barthold, S. W. (1998). Acquisition and transmission of the agent of human granulocytic ehrlichiosis by *Ixodes scapularis* ticks. J. Clin. Microbiol. 36: 3574-3578.

[58] Katavolos, P., Armstrong, P. M., Dawson, J. E. and Telford, S. R. (1998). Duration of tick attachment required for transmission of granulocytic ehrlichiosis. J. Infect. Dis. 177: 1422-1425.

[59] Des Vignes, F., Piesman, J., Heffernan, R., Schulze, T. L., Stafford, K. C., Fish, D. and (2001).Effect of tick removal on transmission of *Borrelia burgdorferi* and *Ehrlichia phagocytophila* by *Ixodes scapularis* nymphs. J. Infect. Dis. 183: 773-778.

[60] Kidd, L. and Breitschwerdt, E. B. (2003). Transmission times and prevention of tick-borne diseases in dogs. Compend. Cont. Educ. Pract. Vet. 25: 742-750.

[61] Christopher, M. J. and Link, D. C. (2007). Regulation of neutrophil homeostasis. Curr. Opin. Hematol. 14: 3-8.

[62] Xiong, Q., Bao, W., Ge, Y. and Rikihisa, Y. (2008). *Ehrlichia ewingii* infection delays spontaneous neutrophil apoptosis through stabilization of mitochondria. J. Infect. Dis. 197: 1110-1118.

[63] Yoshiie, K., Kim, H. Y., Mott, J. and Rikihisa, Y. (2000). Intracellular infection by the human granulocytic ehrlichiosis agent inhibits human neutrophil apoptosis. Infect. Immun. 68: 1125-1133.

[64] Scaife, H., Woldehiwet, Z., Hart, C. A. and Dwards, S. W. (2003). *Anaplasma phagocytophilum* reduces neutrophil apoptosis in vivo. Infect. Immun. 71: 1995-2001.

[65] Johansson, K. E., Pettersson, B., Uhlen, M., Gunnarsson, A., Malmqvist, M., and Olsson, E. (1995). Identification of the causative agent of granulocytic ehrlichiosis in Swedish dogs and horses by direct solid phase sequencing of the PCR products from the 16S rRNA gene. Res. Vet. Sci. 58: 109-112.

[66] Daniels, T. J., Falco, R. C., Schwartz, I., Varde, S. and Robbins, R. G. (1997). Deer ticks (*Ixodes scapularis*) and the agents of Lyme disease and human granulocytic ehrlichiosis in a New York City park. Emerg. Infect. Dis. 3: 353-355.

[67] Osbaldiston, G. W. and Greve, T. (1978). Estimating adrenal cortical function in dogs with ACTH. Cornell. Vet. 68: 308-309.

[68] Kaufman, J. (1984). Diseases of the adrenal cortex of dogs and cats. Mod. Vet. Pract. 65: 429-434.

[69] Davis, J. M., Albert, J. D., Tracy, K. J., Calvano, S. E., Lowry, S. F., Shires, G. T., and Yurt, R. W. (1991). Increased neutrophil mobilization and decreased chemotaxis during cortisol and epinephrine infusions. J. Trauma. 31: 725-731.

[70] Yamada, R., Tsuchida, S., Hara, Y., Tagawa, M. and Ogawa, R. (2002). Apoptotic lymphocytes induced by surgical trauma in dogs. J. Anesth. 16: 131-137.

[71] Brenner, I., Shek, P. N., Zamecnik, J. and Shephard, R. J. (1998). Stress hormones and the immunological responses to heat and exercise. Int. J. Sports. Med. 19: 130-143.

[72] Kogan, D. A., Johnson, L. R., Jandrey, K. E. and Polard, R. E. (2008). Clinical, clinicopathologic, and radiographic findings in dogs with aspiration pneumonia: cases (2004-2006). J. Am. Vet. Med. Assoc. 233: 1742-1747.

[73] Stevens, A., Lowe, J. S. and Scott, I. (2011). Veterinary Hematology. A Diagnostic guide and color atlas. Elsevier Saunders, Saint Louis, Missouri, USA, pp. 122-174.

[74] Bloemena, E., Weinreich, S., Schellekens, P. T. A. (1990). The influence of prednisolone on the recirculation of peripheral blood lymphocytes in vivo. Clin. Exp. Immunol. 80: 460-466.

[75] Toft, P., Lillevang, S. T., Tonnesen, E., Svendsen, P. and Höhndorf, K. (1993). Redistribution of lymphocytes following *E.coli* sepsis. Scand. J. Immunol. 38: 541-545.

[76] Ammersbach, M. A., Kruth, S. A., Sears, W. and Bienzle, D. (2006). The effect of glucocorticoids on canine lymphocyte marker expression and apoptosis. J. Vet. Intern. Med. 20: 1166-1171.

[77] Ulich, T. R., del Castillo, J., Ni, R. X. and Bikhazi, N. (1989). Hematologic interactions of endotoxin, tumornecrosis factor alpha (TNF alpha), interleukin 1, and adrenal hormones and thehematologic effects of TNF alpha in *Corynebacterium parvum* primed rats. J. Leukoc. Biol. 45: 546-557.

[78] Van Miert, A. S., van Duin, C. T. and Wensing, T. (1992). Fever and acute phase response induced in dwarf goats by endotoxin and bovine and human recombinant tumour necrosis factor alpha. J. Vet. Pharmacol. Ther. 15: 332-342.

[79] Sheridan, W. P., Hunt, P., Simonet, S. and Ulrich, T. R. (1997). Hematologic effects of cytokines. In: Remick DG, Friedland JS, eds. Cytokines in Health and Disease, second ed. Marcel Dekker Inc., New York, USA, pp. 487-505.

[80] Nieto, N. C. and Foley, J. E. (2009). Meta-analysis of coinfection and coexposure with *Borrelia burgdorferi* and *Anaplasma phagocytophilum* in humans, domestic animals, wildlife, and *Ixodes ricinus*-complex ticks. Vector. Borne. Zoonotic. Dis. 9: 93-102.

[81] Du Plessis, J. L., Fourie, N., Nel, P. W. and Evezard, D. N. (1990). Concurrent babesiosis and ehrlichiosis in the dog: blood smear examination supplemented by the indirect fluorescent antibody test, using *Cowdria ruminantium* as antigen. Onderstepoort. J. Vet. Res. 57: 151-155.

[82] Dykstra, E. A., Slater, M. R. and Teel, P. D. (1997). Perceptions of veterinary clinics and pest control companies regarding tick-related problems in dogs residing in Texas cities. J. Am. Vet. Med. Assoc. 210: 360-365.

[83] Kordick, S. K., Breitschwerdt, E. B., Hegarty, B. C., Southwick, K. L., Colitz, C. M., Hancock, S. I., Bradley, J. M., Rumbough, R., Mcpherson, J. T. and MacCormack, J. N. (1999).Coinfection with multiple tick-borne pathogens in a Walker hound kennel in North Carolina. J. Clin. Microbiol. 37: 2631-2638.

[84] Stockham, S. L., Tyler, J. W., Schmidt, D. A. and Curtis, K. S. (1990). Experimental transmission of granulocytic ehrlichial organisms in dogs. Vet. Clin. Pathol. 19: 99-104.

[85] Krakowka, S. (1977). Transplacentally acquired microbial and parasitic diseases of dogs. J. Am. Vet. Med. Assoc. 171: 750-753.

[86] Paddock, C. D., Folk, S. M., Shore, G. M., Machado, L. J., Huycke, M.M., Slater, L. N., Liddell, A. M., Buller, R. S., Storch, G. A., Monson, T. P., Rimland, D., Sumner, J. W., Singleton, J., Bloch, K. C., Tang, Y. W., Standaert, S. M. and Childs, J. E. (2001). Infections with *Ehrlichia chaffeensis* and *Ehrlichia ewingii* in persons coinfected with human immunodeficiency virus. Clin. Infect. Dis. 33: 1586-1594.

[87] Thomas, L. D., Hongo, I., Bloch, K. C., Tang, Y. W. and Dummer, S. (2007). Human ehrlichiosis in transplant recipients. Am. J. Transplant. 7: 1641-1647.

[88] Ganguly, S. and Mukhopadhayay, S. K. (2008). Tick-borne ehrlichiosis infection in human beings. J. Vector. Borne. Dis. 45: 273-280.

[89] Duncan, A. W., Correa, M. T., Levine, J. F. and Breitschwerdt, E. B. (2005). The dog as a sentinel for human infection: prevalence of *Borrelia burgdorferi* C6 antibodies in dogs from southeastern and mid-Atlantic States. Vector. Borne. Zoonotic. Dis. 5: 101-109.

[90] Dumler, J. S., Barbet, A. F., Bekker, C. P. J., Dasch, G. A., Palmer, G. H., Ray, S. C., Rikihisa, Y. and Rurangirwa, F. R. (2001). Reorganization of genera in the families Rickettsiaceae and Anaplasmataceae in the order Rickettsiales: unification of some species of *Ehrlichia* with *Anaplasma, Cowdria* and *Ehrlichia*, and *Ehrlichia* with *Neorickettsia*, descriptions of six new species combinations and designation of *Ehrlichia equi*, and "HGE agent" as subjective synonyms of *Ehrlichia phagocytophila*. Int. J. Syst. Evol. Microbiol. 51: 2145-2165.

[91] Loftis, A. D., Levin, M. L. and Spurlock, J. P. (2008). Two USA *Ehrlichia* spp. cause febrile illness in goats. Vet. Microbiol. 130: 398-402.

[92] Dos Santos, A. P., Dos Santos, R. P., Biondo, A. W., Dora, J. M., Goldani, L. Z., de Oliveira, S. T., de Sá Guimarães, A. M., Timenetsky, J., de Morais, H. A., González, F. H. D. and Messick, J. B. (2008). Hemoplasma infection in HIV-positive patient Brazil. Emerg. Infect. Dis. 14: 1922-1924.

[93] Yuan, C. L., Liang, A. B., Yao, C. B., Yang, Z. B., Zhu, J. G., Cui, L., Yu, F., Zhu, N. Y., Yang, X. W. and Hua, X. G. (2009). Prevalence of *Mycoplasma suis (Eperythrozoon suis)* infection in swine-farm workers in Shanghai, China. Am. J. Vet. Res. 70: 890-894.

[94] Sykes, J. E., Lindsay, L. L., Maggi, R. G. and Breitschwerdt, E. B., (2010). Human coinfection with *Bartonella henselae* and two hemotropic *Mycoplasma* variants resembling *Mycoplasma ovis*. J. Clin. Microbiol. 48: 3782-3785.

[95] Quinn, P. J., Markey, B. K., Leonard, F. C., Fitz Patrick, E. S., Fanning, S. and Hartiga, P. J. (2011).Veterinary microbiology and microbial disease, second ed. Wiley-Blackwell, London, UK, pp. 1048-1076.

[96] Maurin, M., Bakken, J. S. and Dumler, J. S. (2003). Antibiotic susceptibilities of *Anaplasma* (*Ehrlichia*) *phagocytophilum* strains from various geographic areas in the United States. Antimicrob. Agents. Chemother. 47: 413-415.

Manipulation of Fertility in Crossbred Dairy Cattle Using Controlled Internal Drug Release Device Combined With Prostaglandin and Equine Chorionic Gonadotrophin

Alemselam Birhanu Mekonnin[1, *], A. Forbes Howie[1], Christopher C. Harlow[1], Goitom Gidey[2], Desalew Tadesse Tegegne[2], Gidena Desta[2], Tadesse Gugsa[3], Berihu Gebrekidan[2], Gebregiorgis Ashebir[2], Simon C. Riley[1]

[1]MRC Centre for Reproductive Health, The Queen's Medical Research Institute College of Medicine and Veterinary Medicine, University of Edinburgh, Edinburgh, United Kingdom

[2]College of Veterinary Medicine, Mekelle University, Mekelle, Ethiopia

[3]Tigray Regional State Agriculture Bureau, Tigray, Mekelle, Ethiopia

Email address:

a.b.mekonnin@sms.ed.ac.uk (A. B. Mekonnin)

[*]Corresponding author

Abstract: Simplifying and improving our understanding of the protocols for inducing or synchronizing estrus is important for improving management of dairy cattle. This study evaluated the estrus response and conception rate of crossbred (Holstein Friesian X Zebu) dairy cows (n=75) and heifers (n=47) assigned to a 10-day controlled internal drug release (CIDR) device – prostaglandin F2-alpha (PGF2α) – equine chorionic gonadotrophin (eCG) based estrus synchronization protocol. Animals were assigned to three groups (a) anestrus (n=62), (b) repeat-breeders (n=11) and (c) silent estrus (n=46), according to their reproductive history, per rectal palpation, and progesterone concentrations determined by On-Farm enzyme-linked immunosorbent assays (ELISA) in milk (lactating cows) or serum (dry cows and heifers). For each animal, a CIDR device (containing 1.38g progesterone) was inserted into the vagina and allowed to remain in-situ for 10 days. On Day 8 after device insertion, a dose of 500µg of PGF2α was administered intramuscularly (IM). On Day 10 (device removal), 500 IU of eCG was given IM. Animals were inseminated or mated 48 and 72 hrs post device removal. Pregnancy was assessed 20-24 days post insemination by measurement of progesterone in milk/serum and pregnancy was confirmed by per rectal palpation and/or ultrasonography 44-90 days post insemination. Overall estrus response and conception rates were 97.5% and 78.3%, respectively, with no significant differences in parity, pre-treatment reproductive status and farming system (smallholder vs organized commercial farms). Conception rate after induced/synchronized estrus was 82.9% and 72.1% in cows and heifers, respectively, with an overall calving rate of 94.4%. In conclusion, the present study has shown high estrus response and conception rate in crossbred dairy cattle using this CIDR - PGF2α - eCG based estrus synchronization protocol. Application of this protocol is highly recommended to enhance fertility of dairy cattle in the study area, and this could readily be applied to other regions.

Keywords: Cattle, CIDR, eCG, Estrus, Fertility, PGF2α, Synchronization

1. Introduction

Ethiopia possesses the tenth largest cattle population in the world, and the largest in Africa. Despite this, productivity and reproductive performance of its indigenous and crossbred (Holstein Friesian X Zebu) cattle herd is poor [1, 2]. Efficient reproduction underpins a profitable dairy industry [3] and producing one calf per year per cow is an important step in achieving this. Cows must get pregnant and maintain the pregnancy with parturition 270 days post service/AI, and wait for a period of 40-50 days (voluntary waiting period) to be successfully inseminated again [4]. This results in one calf per year per cow with regular availability and increased milk production in the dairy farm, together with the provision of replacement heifers. However, there are a number of factors affecting reproduction in dairy cattle, particularly in the tropics, where both reproductive performance as well as milk production of local (Zebu) and crossbred, including Holstein Friesian, is regarded as poor. The main reasons are poor nutritional status, estrus detection, AI technique or breeding management and postpartum uterine disease and calf suckling [5]. Anestrus and repeat-breeding are the major problems affecting the reproductive performance of crossbred dairy cattle in Ethiopia [6]. Both anestrus and repeat-breeding lead to a longer calving interval. In smallholder farms, most cows including crossbreeds, fail to calve every 12 to 13 months after the first calving [6, 7]. Puberty in crossbred (Zebu x Holstein-Friesian/HF) heifers is usually 24 months [8], and heifers are also reported to be older at first calving [1, 2, 6].

A successful breeding program must incorporate efficient and accurate detection of estrus, proper semen handling techniques, and timely AI [9]. Failure of proper estrus detection is the most common problem in dairy cattle breeding programs [9, 10] resulting in loss of lifetime milk yield, a decrease in number of calves born per lifetime, excessive days open, and an increase in reproductive culling [9]. As the accuracy and efficiency of estrus detection declines, it is important to incorporate estrus synchronization/induction and timed AI into the breeding management program [11]. Estrus synchronization can avoid or reduce the need for estrus detection, and increases the fertility and productivity of cattle [12]. Furthermore, estrus synchronization facilitates planning of AI, shortens first day service in postpartum cows, reduces the calving interval and helps to maintain uniform calf crops and replacement heifers [12, 13].

Current world-wide research is focused on the development of methods that effectively synchronize estrus by decreasing the period of time over which estrus is detected, hence facilitating the use of fixed time AI [14]. Progesterone based estrus synchronization protocols are more advantageous than others. A controlled internal drug release (CIDR) based estrus synchronization protocols have been widely studied [15, 16], and are more preferable than using prostaglandin (PGF2α) alone, due to ineffectiveness of PGF2α to induce cyclicity/ estrus in animals that do not have a corpus luteum (CL), nor does it exert an effect on follicular wave [17]. Most successful estrus synchronization protocols have been developed in *Bos taurus* cattle, however in *Bos indicus* breeds, utilization of same synchronization protocols results in low to unacceptably low pregnancy rates [15, 18].

It has been demonstrated that CIDR can be maintained in the vagina for a longer period of 14 days [19], however, intravaginal devices maintained over 12 days reduces fertility by causing aged follicles [20, 21, 22]. Promising developments have been shown by reducing the time of keeping CIDR devices in the vagina to 4 [23] or 5 days [15, 24], although estrus response and conception rates are not consistent even after the use of the standard 7-day CIDR regime [3, 25, 26] which could be due to environmental, management, breed and other factors. Yet, a recent report showed a similar pregnancy success when CIDR was maintained for 5 days, 6 days and 14 days in heifers [27]. Moreover, another recent study that compared between 7 and 9 days CIDR inserts on estrus response and fertility in dairy cattle has shown a similar effect between the two protocols [28]. Others have suggested that keeping intravaginal devices for a period of 10 to 12 days has no negative effect on fertility and recommended for use in controlled breeding programs in cattle [20, 22, 25].

In view of the poor estrus detection and reproductive performance of crossbred dairy cattle in the Ethiopia [1, 2, 6, 29, 30], it is necessary to establish an estrus synchronization program that can operate under any reproductive condition (anestrus and cycling) as a management tool to enhance their fertility and productivity. The objective of the present study was to evaluate the reproductive performance of crossbred dairy cattle following treatment with a 10-day CIDR in combination with PGF2α and eCG.

2. Materials and Methods

2.1. Study Area

The proposal was presented to key stakeholders and livestock experts and approved by The Government of National State of Tigray Bureau of Agriculture and Rural Development, Tigray, Ethiopia. It was conducted from November 2013 to December 2014 in and around Mekelle, the largest city in northern Ethiopia, and the capital city of Tigray, which is located at 39° 29`E and 13° 30` N at an altitude of 2000 m.a.s.l. The climate of the study area conforms to that of Ethiopian Highlands. The mean annual rainfall is 619mm, and is bimodal with a short rainy season occurring from March to May and another from middle September to February. The annual minimum and maximum temperature is 11.8°C and 29.9°C, respectively [31].

2.2. Study Farms and Animals

Crossbred dairy cattle owned by smallholder farms and organized commercial farms were included in this study. Cattle in both farm types were fed grass hay or straw, concentrate composed of wheat by products, crop residues and local beer residue (Attela). However, cows in organized commercial farms were supplemented with green fodder, such as fresh grass, alfalfa, elephant grass, lucinia and suspania, they received regular watering; and, the farms had better breeding records and housing condition. A total of 122 dairy cattle (75 cows with a mean age of 6.6 years old and >60 days postpartum and 47 heifers with a mean age of 3.1 years old) from smallholder farmers and organized commercial farms, with an average body condition score (BCS) of 3.1 (on a scale of 1-5) [32] were assigned in the study. Reproductive organs of the study animals were assessed for genital tract pathology using per rectal palpation, and only apparently health animals were included in the study. Study animals were assigned into three groups prior to treatment as (a) anestrus (non-cycling, n=67), (b) repeat-breeders (normally cycling and observed estrus, but never conceived despite multiple inseminations, n=11), and (c) silent estrus (cycling but no visible estrus signs, n=44) according to their reproductive history, two equivalent on-farm progesterone assays, dipstick (Progesterone Rapid, Ridgeway Science Ltd, Gloucestershire, UK) in milk (cows) or Target Progesterone ELISA (Biometallics Inc, New Jersey, USA) in serum (heifers) and per rectal palpation. Progesterone assays were carried out twice at 11 days interval immediately after breeding history was recorded, which was immediately followed by per rectal examination of ovarian and uterine conditions [30].

2.3. Study Design

The perineal region of each animal was thoroughly washed with water, an Eazi-Breed CIDR™ (CIDR®, Pfizer Ltd, Kent, UK) device, containing 1.38g of progesterone, was inserted into the vagina and allowed to remain in-situ for 10 days. On the 8th day after device insertion, a dose of 500µg PGF2α (Estrumate, Schering-Plough Animal Health Corp, Summit, Germany) was administered intramuscularly (IM). On the day of device removal (Day 10), 500 IU (Equine chorionic gonadotropin (eCG) (Intervet UK Ltd, Walton, UK) was injected IM. The estrus response was compared according to parity (cows vs heifers), pre-treatment group (anestrus, repeat-breeders and silent estrus) and farming systems (smallholder vs organized commercial farms). Animals were inseminated using frozen semen or naturally mated twice at 48 and 72 hrs post device removal. Animals were examined for presence of pregnancy 20-24 days (average of 21 days) post insemination by on-farm milk (lactating cows) progesterone test using Dipstick or on-farm serum (dry cows and heifers) progesterone test using Target progesterone kits, and pregnancy was confirmed by per rectal palpation/ ultrasonography (KX5200V, Kaixin®, Xuzhou Kaixin Electronic Instrument Co., Ltd, Xuzhou, Jiangsu, China) 44-90 days post insemination/mating. Conception rate was compared according to the variables above and between breeding methods (AI vs natural mating). Data were analysed using Fisher's exact test and Chi-square test using GraphPad Prism (GraphPad Software, Inc, CA, USA). Differences were considered significant when $p < 0.05$.

3. Results

The overall estrus response and conception rate in the present study was 97.5% and 78.3%, respectively. There was similar estrus response between cows and heifers (Table 1). Although, the estrus response of cattle to CIDR - PGF2α - eCG treatment, based on observed estrus behaviour recorded by the farmers, was 97.5%, the remaining animals 3/122 (2.5%) that did not exhibit external symptoms, were deemed fit for insemination as their cervices were open, as evidenced by the AI gun easily passing through to deposit semen in the uterine body. This brought the estrus response to 100%. Subsequently, three (2.5%) animals (two cows and one heifer did not retain their CIDR. Of 119 animals in estrus, 115 (96.6%) were inseminated or naturally mated, however four (3.4%) were not bred due to various reasons including animals being unable to be inseminated or mated.

The conception rate in cows and heifers was 82.9% and 72.1% respectively, which was not significantly different ($p > 0.05$) (Table 1). Similar conception rates were found between anestrus, repeat-breeders and normally cycling-but silent estrus/unobserved by the farmers (Table 2). Natural mating resulted in a higher conception rate than AI, but the difference was not significant (Table 3). The farming system did not affect estrus response or conception rate (Table 4).

Two cows and one heifer gave birth to twin calves, while the remaining deliveries were singletons. Of 90 pregnant cows/heifers 85 (94.4%) successfully calved, and there was no effect of parity (Table 1), pre-treatment reproductive status (Table 2), breeding method (Table 3) or farming system (Table 4). Pregnancy loss occurred in 4/90 (4.4%) animals: three cows (3/59, 5.1%) and one heifer (1/31, 3.2%). These losses occurred in one cow in a smallholder farm with the remaining losses of two cows and one heifer in organized commercial farms where animals were bred by AI. There was also death of a pregnant cow (1/90, 1.1%) in one of the organized commercial farms due to lumpy skin disease.

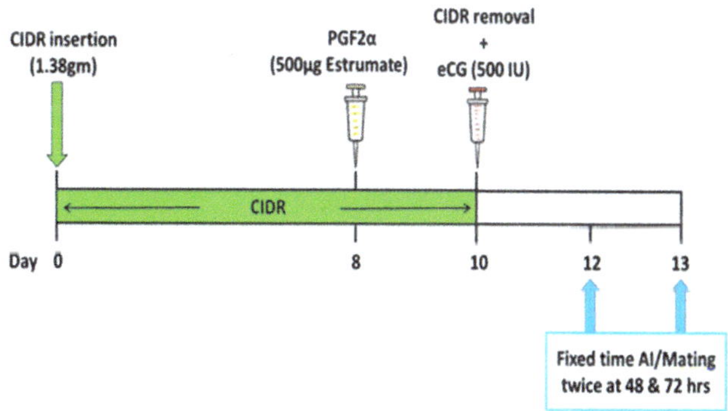

Figure 1. Schematic representation of treatment regime.

Table 1. Estrus and conception status of cows and heifers treated with CIDR - $PGF_{2\alpha}$ - eCG combination estrus synchronization protocol.

Observations	Treated animals		
	Total*	Cows*	Heifers*
No. treated	122 (100)	75 (100)	47 (100)
No. in estrus	119 (97.5)	73 (97.3)	46 (97.9)
Number mated/ inseminated	115 (96.6)	72 (98.6)	43 (93.5)
No. conceived at induced/synchronized estrus	90 (78.3)	59 (82.9)	31 (72.1)
No. calved	85 (94.4)	56 (94.9)	29 (93.5)

*Values in parentheses are percentages.

Table 2. *Fertility status of cows and heifers post CIDR - PGF2α - eCG combination treatment on the basis of pre-treatment reproductive history and status.*

Observation	Total*	Anestrus*	Repeat-breeders* (Observed estrus)	Silent estrus/ unobserved estrus*
No. of animals mated/ inseminated	115/122	62/67 (92.5)	11/11 (100)	42/44 (95.4)
Conception rate (% pregnant/ AI or mated)	90 (78.3)	48 (77.4)	8 (72.7)	34 (81.0)
No. calved	85 (94.4)	44 (91.7)	7 (87.5)	34 (100)

*Values in parentheses are percentages.

*Silent/unobserved estrus: cattle in this group were reported by the farmers as anestrus, however on-farm progesterone tests along with per rectal palpation confirmed them cycling.

Table 3. *Fertility status of cows and heifers following estrus synchronization/induction on the basis of breeding methods.*

Observation	Total*	Breeding Method	
		AI*	Natural mating*
No. of animals mated/inseminated	115	95 (100)	20 (100)
No. conceived at induced/synchronized estrus	90 (78.3)	72 (75.8)	18 (90)
No. calved	85 (94.4)	68 (94.4)	17 (94.4)

*Values in parentheses are percentages.

Table 4. *Fertility status of cows and heifers treated following estrus synchronization/induction on the basis of farming system.*

observations	Total	Smallholder farms	Organized commercial farms
No. treated	122	34	88
No. inseminated	115	33	82
No. pregnant	90 (78.3)	24 (72.7)	66 (80.5)
No. calved	85 (94.4)	22 (91.7)	63 (95.4)

*Values in parentheses are percentages.

4. Discussion

A simple procedure that uses solely CIDR inserts without any combination treatment on the initial day was performed in this study. This is unlike previous reports [26, 33] that used CIDR in combination with a Co-Synch or Ovsynch protocol (gonadotrophin-releasing hormone (GnRH)- PGF2α-GnRH combination protocol) whereby GnRH is administered simultaneously with CIDR on the initial day, which has been demonstrated to be effective. Progesterone delays the time of estrus after natural or induced luteolysis and extends the oestrous cycle by preventing the occurrence of spontaneous estrus [34]. Administration of PGF2α on Day 8 of CIDR insertion was intended to cause regression of the CL and to bring the animals into estrus 1-3 days post treatment. The PGF2α reduces the risk of continued progesterone production by a functional CL after device removal [35]. eCG has both follicle stimulating hormone (FSH) and luteinizing hormone (LH) like activity in bovine [36], but with more of FSH activity [37]. Therefore, administration of eCG on the day of device removal stimulates follicular development, final maturation of the dominant follicle, initiation of ovulation and CL formation [36, 38]. Furthermore, in the present study three animals gave birth to twin calves, which could be due to administration of gonadotrophins, such as eCG that can cause superovulation [39].

In the present study the retention of CIDR exceeded 97% which is comparable with previous reports [25, 40], although, others reported no CIDR loss [21]. Animals which did not show external symptoms of estrus, but when inseminated had open cervices evidenced when the AI gun was easily and smoothly passed through the cervix is suggestive of silent estrus post CIDR treatment. In agreement with our finding, a previous report showed that 2% of CIDR treated heifers had a palpable CL, although they were not observed in estrus [25]. All animals which were reported by the farmers as anestrus, but confirmed cycling by the on-farm progesterone tests, showed external symptoms of estrus when subjected to the present estrus synchronization protocol, which indicates poor estrus detection. Furthermore, all anestrus (except 3 with just their cervical os opened) and repeat-breeder cattle, including those with silent/unobserved estrus showed external symptoms of estrus following estrus synchronization. CIDR treatment in anovulatory and anestrus cows/heifers re-establishes the hypothalamic responsiveness to estradiol produced from the dominant follicle. It also normalizes the duration of the luteal phase [41], and increases estradiol responsiveness in behavioural centres of the brain [42, 43] thereby increasing the proportion of cattle expressing behavioural estrus in conjunction with ovulation [44, 45].

The high estrus response and conception rate in the present study is possibly due to the exclusion criteria such as unacceptable BCS, assessment of pre-treatment reproductive condition of animals as unfit for estrus synchronization (having unhealthy and small sized reproductive tract and organs), and the use of double insemination or mating at 48 and 72 Hrs. Previous reports have shown that BCS and uterine infections are among the factors that reduce fertility [46]. Despite the difference in reproductive status of animals (anestrus/cycling) prior to CIDR insertion, a high estrus response was found in both cows and heifers in the present study. This is in agreement with previous studies that reported a 100% estrus response using a 7-day CIDR and eCG injection in 30 anestrus Zebu breed cows [47], a 100% response in 73 crossbred cows with unknown ovarian cyclicity using a 7-day CIDR in combination with PGF2α and GnRH [3] and a 100% response in anestrus Sahiwal (Zebu) cows when used a 9-day CIDR in combination with eCG injection one day prior to CIDR removal and hCG at the time of AI [48]. Conversely, the present study improved on other studies that reported 79.5% and 87.5% estrus response using 7-day and 9-day CIDR, respectively in combination with PGF2α in 128 Holstein Friesian / crossbred dairy cows [28], 86.7% using Ovsynch + CIDR in 55 repeat-breeder Holstein Friesian cows [26], 80% in 5 normally cycling Aceh cattle in Indonesia using CIDR-B + PGF2α [16] and *Bos indicus* and other cattle breeds [12, 15].

There were similar conception rates between anestrus, repeat-breeder and silent estrus crossbred dairy cattle in this study, with a high overall conception rate (78.3%) similar to reports in anestrus Zebu breed cows (70%) in India [47]. The present study has shown a better conception rate than reports in crossbred cattle (40.9%) in the tropics [3], in Holstein Friesian/crossbred cows (45.5%) [28], in *Bos indicus* cattle [15] and in beef cattle in USA [12], and in beef heifers (54.5/55.5%) using 14-day/ 5-dayCIDR protocols [49] that reported lower pregnancy rates, 54.5% and 55.5%, when used long and short term CIDR protocols, respectively. Moreover, the present study has shown better conception rate in repeat breeder cows/heifers than previous reports in South Korea [26] and Japan [33]. Conversely, conception rate in the present study was lower than previous reports that used CIDR treatment in Aceh cattle (100%) in Indonesia [16]. However, their study was only in 5 cattle; therefore, higher conception rate may reflect their small sample size. Nevertheless, conception rate can be affected by factors such as nutrition, breed, postpartum interval, and geographic location [50, 51].

The conception rate in cows (82.9%) was slightly higher, but not significant, than in heifers (72.1%) in the present study. Contrary to our findings, a previous report showed higher conception rate in heifers (67.9%) than cows (53.1%) [52]. The present study recorded lower pregnancy loss (5.1%) in cows compared with previous reports where the loss in cows was 20% when PGF2α/ progestins was used [53]. Infectious diseases, and non-infectious factors such as poor management systems, milk yield, parity, BCS, ambient temperature [54] can cause pregnancy loss.

By way of direct comparison, the estrus response recorded in the present study was higher than our recent report that used single or double administration of PGF2α with simultaneous administration of GnRH [55]. The present study had a higher (78.3%) conception rate than our recent report in same study area when repeat-breeder crossbred dairy cattle were subjected to 20μg or 10μg GnRH (Buserelin acetate) (68%) [29]. Furthermore, the present study has shown a higher conception rate than was observed in the large scale controlled reproduction program in Tigray region that used PGF2α (31.5%) in local/ crossbred dairy cattle [56]. This may be due to progesterone having a positive effect in inducing/ synchronizing estrus in anestrus and cycling cattle, whereas PGF2α has no effect on anestrus cattle. AI technicians lack the experience and skills to effectively diagnose cyclicity of animals through palpation of the ovaries per rectum [57, 58], so non-cycling animals may have been included in the PGF2α based breeding program. In this current study the on-farm progesterone assay confirmed the presence of CL, though our CIDR based estrus synchronization can be used at any stage of the estrous cycle, including in anestrus animals and prepubertal heifers.

Although farmers were advised to record animals in estrus, all animals were inseminated or naturally mated at a fixed time. This did not affect pregnancy regardless of pre-treatment reproductive status of animals, breeding method, farming system or parity. This was similar to a previous report in cows and heifers, although they reported comparatively lower overall pregnancy rate than the present findings [13]. Some farmers in the study area prefer to have their own bull to using AI services due to numbers of reasons discussed in our recent reports [6, 58]. Conception rate did not vary between breeding methods (AI vs bull) in the present study, yet a higher conception rate was found in animals bred with natural mating/bull than with AI, which could be due improper insemination. We recently evaluated the quality of frozen semen (sperm motility and viability) in the study area, and it was within the normal range [58]. In the present study, double inseminations at 48 and 72 hrs has resulted in improved pregnancy rate in all animal groups (anestrus, repeat-breeding and silent/unobserved estrus), in contrast to a previous report indicating the use of double insemination did not bring any significant difference in pregnancy rates compared to single insemination in repeat-breeder dairy cattle in other treatment regime [59]; it has also been proposed that double insemination can improve pregnancy by 5-10% [35].

Application of a progesterone (CIDR) based estrus synchronization programme is highly recommended to enhance fertility of dairy cattle. Furthermore, the expense of hormones required for estrus synchronization (US $18.60/per animal: CIDR, US $11.16 + PGF2α, US $4.03 + eCG, US $3.41/animal) used in this study is less than the cost farmers spend feeding anestrus and repeat-breeder cows, with an estimated loss of production cost of US $148.48 per cycle from single cow [29] for extended periods of time. This excludes the labour costs. In anestrus cattle, the cost of this estrus synchronization protocol can be further reduced to US $14.57, as PGF2α is not necessary in the absence of CL. Additionally, the prospect of reusing a used CIDR device [60] makes the protocol worthwhile.

5. Conclusion

The present study has shown a high estrus response, conception rate and calving rate in cows and heifers assigned to progesterone (CIDR) - PGF2α - eCG based estrus synchronization protocol irrespective of pre-treatment reproductive condition, farming system and breeding methods. This study also confirms the effectiveness and affordability of the protocol. Thus, the protocol is recommended to enhance fertility of dairy cattle in the study area and other part of the country and improve the livelihood of the farming community.

Acknowledgments

The authors would like to thank MRC Centre for Reproductive Health, College of Medicine and Veterinary Medicine, University of Edinburgh, United Kingdom for supporting ABM and funding the study. Special thanks are also offered to the College of Veterinary Medicine, Mekelle University, Ethiopia for the offer of transportation facilities and other support. Authors would like to thank Tigray Regional State Agriculture Bureau for facilitating the support team. Finally, the authors would like to express their deepest gratitude to the farmers, AI technicians and veterinarians for their willingness and co-operation during the study.

References

[1] Kumar, N. and Tkui, K. (2014). Reproductive performance of crossbred dairy cows in Mekelle, Ethiopia. *Sci. J. Anim. Sci.* 3(2): 35-40.

[2] Kumar, N., Abadi, Y., Gebrekidan, B. and Woldearegay, Y. H. (2014). Productive and Reproductive Performance of Local Cows under Farmer's Management in and around Mekelle, Ethiopia. *IOSR-JAVS* 7(5): 21-24.

[3] Dickson, N., Siew N., Singh-Knights, D., Bourne G. and Knights, M. (2012). Technical and Economic Outcome Using Various Timed Artificial Insemination Protocols in Dairy Cattle in the Tropics. *J. Anim. Prod. Adv.* 2(1): 490-499.

[4] Perez-Marin, C., Moreno, M. and Calero, G. (2012). Clinical approach to the repeat breeder cow syndrome. (Ed. Perez-Marin C). *A Bird's-Eye View of Veterinary Medicine*, 337-362.

[5] Dubuc, J. (2011). Postpartum Uterine Diseases: Prevalence, Impacts, and Treatments. *WCDS Advances in Dairy Technology*. 23: 255-267.

[6] Mekonnin, A. B., Harlow, C. R., Gidey, G., Tadesse, D., Desta, G., Gugssa, T. and Riley, S. C. (2015a). Assessment of Reproductive Performance and Problems in Crossbred (Holstein Friesian X Zebu) Dairy Cattle in and around Mekelle, Tigray, Ethiopia. *J. Anim. Vet.* 3(3): 94-101.

[7] Shiferaw, Y., Tenhagen, B. A., Bekana, M. and Kassa. T. (2003). Reproductive performance of crossbredd cows in different production systems in the central highlands of Ethiopia. *Trop. Anim. Health and Prod.* 35: 551-561.

[8] Duguma, B., Kechero, Y. and Janssens, G-P. J. (2012). Productive and Reproductive Performance of Zebu X Holstein-Friesian Crossbred Dairy Cows in Jimma Town, Oromia, Ethiopia. *Global Veterinaria* 8(1): 67-72.

[9] Walker, W. L., Nebel, R. L. and McGillard, M. L. (1996). Time of ovulation relative to mounting activity in dairy cattle. *J. Dairy Sci.* 79: 1555-1561.

[10] Hansar, E., Lemma, A. and Yilma, T. (2014). Pre-service ultrasonic and manual evaluation of the reproductive organs of dairy cows presumed to be in estrus. *Springer Plus* 3: 529.

[11] Nebel, R. and DeJarnette, M. (2015). Dairy cow synchronization protocols. Select Sirs. Available at: http://www.selectsires.com/resources/fertilitydocs/dairy_cow_synch_protocols.pdf. (Accessed 20 September 2015).

[12] Larson, J. E., Lamb, G. C., Stevenson, J. S., Johnson, S. K., Day, M. L., Geary, T. W., Kesler, D. J., DeJarnette, J. M., Schrick, F. N., DiCostanzo, A. and Arseneau, J. D. (2006). Synchronization of estrus in suckled beef cows for detected estrus and artificial insemination and timed artificial insemination using gonadotropin-releasing hormone, prostaglandin F, and progesterone. *J. Anim. Sci.* 84: 332-342.

[13] Lamb, G. C, Dahlen, C. R., Larson, J. E., Marquezini, G. and Stevenson, J. S. (2010). Control of the estrous cycle to improve fertility for fixed-time artificial insemination in beef cattle: a review. *J. Anim. Sci.* 88(13 Suppl): E181-192.

[14] Patterson, D. J. Mallory, D. A. Nash, J. M. Martin, N. T. and Smith, M. F. (2011). Strategies to optimize use of AI in cow/calf production systems: focus on fixed-time AI protocols for cows *Proceedings, Applied Reproductive Strategies in Beef Cattle* – Northwest, September 30 - October 1, 2011; Boise, ID, USA.

[15] Williams, G., Stanko, R., Allen, C., Cardoso, R., Prezotto, L., Thorson, J., and Amstalden. M. (2011). Evidence that prostaglandin administration at the onset of a 5-day CO-Synch + CIDR synchronization protocol markedly improves fixed-time AI pregnancy rates in *Bos indicus*-influenced cattle. *J. Anim. Sci.* 89 (E-Suppl. 1): 264.

[16] Siregar, T. N., Hamdan, H., Riady, G., Panjaitan, B., Aliza, D., Pratiwi, E. F., Darianto T., and Husnurrizal (2015). Efficacy of Two Estrus Synchronization Methods in Indonesian Aceh Cattle. *Inter. J. Vet. Sci.* 4(2): 87-91.

[17] DeJarnette, M. (2015). Ovsynch, Co-synch, Presynch and Kitchensynch: how did breeding cows get so complicated? *Select Sires.* pp. 1-6. Available at: http://www.selectsires.com (Accessed 2 September 2015).

[18] Yelich, J. V. and Bridges, G. A. (2012). Synchronization response: Bos taurus vs. Bos indicus cattle. A review. *Beef Improvement Federation (BIF) Research Symposium and Annual Meeting,* April 18-21, 2012, Houston, Texas, USA.

[19] Powell, J. G., Lester, T. D., Reynolds, J. L., Davis, A. J., Hornsby, J. A. and Rorie, R. W. (2012). Comparison of a 5- or 14-day CIDR-based estrous synchronization protocols with sorted semen in beef heifers. *AAES Research Series 606.* pp. 51-53.

[20] Maurer, R. E., Webel, S. K. and Brown, M. D. (1975). Ovulation control in cattle with progesterone intravaginal device (PRID) and gonadotropin releasing hormone (GnRH). *Ann. Biol. Anim. Bioch. Biophys.* 15: 291-296.

[21] Macmillan, K. L. and Peterson, A. J., (1993). A new intravaginal progesterone releasing device for cattle (CIDR-B) for oestrous synchronization, increasing pregnancy rates and the treatment of postpartum anoestrus. *Anim. Reprod. Sci.* 33: 1-25.

[22] Gordon, I. (1999). Artificial control of oestrus and ovulation. In: I. Gordon (ed.) Controlled reproduction in cattle & buffaloes. CAB Int. Publ., Wallingford, UK, pp. 133-166.

[23] Palomares, R. A., Fishman, H. J., Jones, A. L., Ferrer, M. S., Jenerette, M. and Vaughn A. (2015). Comparison of 4- versus 5-day Co-Synch þ controlled internal drug release (CIDR) þ timed artificial insemination protocols in dairy heifers. *Theriogenology* 84: 868-874.

[24] Bridges, G. A., Helser, L. A., Grum, D. E., Mussard, M. L., Gasser, C. L. and Day, M. L. (2008). Decreasing the interval between GnRH and PGF2alpha from 7 to 5 days and lengthening proestrus increases timed-AI pregnancy rates in beef cows. *Theriogenology* 15: 843-851.

[25] Broadbent, P. J., Tregaskes, L. D., Dolman, D. F., Franklin, M. F. and Jones, R. L. (1993). Synchronlzatlon of estrus in embryo transfer recipients after using a combination of PRID or CIDR-B plus PGF2α. *Theriogenology* 39: 1055-1065.

[26] Kim, U. H., Suh, G. H., Hur, T. Y., Kang, S. J., Kang, H. G., Park, S. B., Kim, S. H. and Kim, I. H. (2007). Comparison of two types of CIDR-based timed artificial insemination protocols for repeat breeder dairy cows. *J. Reprod. And Develop.* 53: 639-645.

[27] Bridges, G. A., Lake, S. L., Kruse, S. G., Bird, S. L., Funnell, B. J., Aries, R., Walker, J. A., Grant, J. K. and Perry, G. A. (2014). Comparison of three CIDR-based fixed-time AI protocols in beef heifers. *J. Anim. Sci.* 92: 3127-3133.

[28] Romano, J. E. and Fahning, M. L. (2013). Comparison between 7 vs 9 days of controlled internal drug release inserts permanency on oestrus performance and fertility in lactating dairy cattle. *Ital. J. Anim. Sci.* 12(e63): 390-394.

[29] Hailu, B., Gebrekidan, B., Raju, S., Birhanu, A. and Tadesse, G. (2015). Effects of Gonadotropin Releasing Hormone Analogue in Enhancements of Pregnancy in Repeat Breeding Dairy Cows in and around Mekelle, Tigray, Ethiopia. *Anim. Vet. Sci.* 3(1): 12-17.

[30] Mekonnin, A. B. Harlow, C., Howie, F., Gidey, G., Tadesse, D., Desta, G., Ashebir, G., Gebrekidan, B., Gugsa, T. and Riley, S. C. (2015b). Assessment of major reproductive problems and reproductive status of crossbred (Holstein Friesian X Zebu) dairy cattle in and around Mekelle, Tigray, Ethiopia. *Society for Reproduction and Fertility annual conference*, 19-22 July 2015, Oxford, UK.

[31] BoPED (2011). Bureau of Planning and Economic Development: Tigray, Ethiopia.

[32] DEFRA (2001). Condition scoring of dairy cows: Action on animal health and welfare. The Department for Environment, Food and Rural Affairs, UK.

[33] Kawate, N., Watanabe, K., Urnaka, K., Takahashi, M., Inaba, T. and Tamada, H. (2011). Comparison of plasma concentration of estradiol 17β and progesterone, and conception in dairy cows with cystic ovarian diseases between Ovsynch and Ovsynch plus CIDR timed protocols. *J. Reprod. Develop.* 57: 267-272.

[34] Lucy, M. C., Billings, H. J. Butler, W. R. Ehnes, L. R. Fields, M. J. Kesler, D. J. Kinder, J. E. Mattos, R. C. Short, R. E. Thatcher, W. W. Wettemann, R. P. Yelich, J. V. and Hafs. H. D. (2001). Efficacy of an Intravaginal Progesterone Insert and an Injection of PGF2a Synchronizing Estrus and Shortening the Interval to Pregnancy in Postpartum Beef cows, Peripubertal Beef Heifers, and Dairy Heifers. *J. Anim. Sci.* 79: 982-995.

[35] EBLEX, (2014). Artificial insemination (AI) and oestrus synchronisation of beef cattle. *Better Returns Program (BRP).* pp. 1-12. http://beefandlamb.ahdb.org.uk/wp/wp-content/uploads/2014/07/BRP-plus-artificial-insemination090714.pdf. (Accessed 12 September 2015).

[36] Racowsky, C. (1991). Gamete resources: origin and production of oocytes. (Eds. Pedersen RA., McLaren A, First, NL). Animal applications of research in mammalian development. Current communications in cell and molecular biology 4, 26-38, Cold Spring Harbor Laboratory Press, New York, USA.

[37] Gospodarowicz, D. (1972). Purification and physiochemical properties of pregnant mare serum gonadotropin (PMSG). *Endocrinology* 91: 101-106.

[38] Sá Filho, O. G, Meneghetti, M., Peres, R. F., Lamb, G. C. and Vasconcelos, J. L. (2009). Fixed-time artificial insemination with estradiol and progesterone for Bos indicus cows II: strategies and factors affecting fertility. *Theriogenology* 72: 210-218.

[39] Tegegne, A., Franceschini, R. and Sovani, S. (1994). Superovulatory response, embryo recovery and progesterone secretion in Boran (Full-size image (<1 K)) cows after treatment with either Pergovet or Pluset. *Theriogenology* 41(8): 1653-1662.

[40] Grant, E. (2006). Understanding CIDR. National Association of Animal Breeders. Accessed at: http://beefmagazine.com/mag/beef_understanding_cidr (Accessed 10 September 2015).

[41] Garcia-Winder, M., Lewis, P. E., Deaver, D. R., Smith, V. G., Lewis, G. S. and Inskeep, E. K. (1986). Endocrine profiles associated with life span of induced corpora lutea in postpartum beef cows. *J. Anim. Sci.* 62: 1353-1362.

[42] Rosenberg, M., Kaim, M., Herz, Z. and Folman, Y. (1990). Comparisons of methods for synchronization of estrous cycle in dairy cows. 1. Effects on plasma progesterone and manifestation of estrus. *J. Dairy Sci.* 73(10): 2807-2816.

[43] Fike, K. E., Day, M. L, Inskeep, E. K., Kinder, J. E., Lewis, P. E., Short, R. E. and Hafs, H. D. (1997). Estrus and luteal function in suckled beef cows that were anestrous when treated with an intravaginal device containing progesterone with or without a subsequent injection of estradiol benzoate. *J. Anim. Sci.* 75(8): 2009-2015.

[44] McDougall, S., Burke, C. R., Macmillan, K. L. and Williamson, N. B. (1992). The effect of pretreatment with progesterone on the oestrous response to oestradiol-17β benzoate in the post-partum dairy cow. *Proc. N.Z. Soc. Anim. Prod.* 52: 157-160.

[45] Gasser, C. L. (2013). Joint Alphapharma – Beef Species Symposium, considerations on puberty in replacement beef heifers. *J. Anim. Sci.* 91: 1336-1340.

[46] McNally, J. C., Crowe, M. A., Roche, J. F., Beltman, M. E. (2014). Effects of physiological and/or disease status on the response of postpartum dairy cows to synchronization of estrus using an intravaginal progesterone device. *Theriogenology* 82(9): 1263-1272.

[47] Singh, H., Luthra, R. A., Khar, S. K. and Nanda, T. (2006). Oestrus Induction, Plasma Steroid Hormone Profiles and Fertility Response after CIDR and eCG Treatment in Acyclic Sahiwal Cows. *Asian-Aust. J. Anim. Sci.* 19(11): 1566-1573.

[48] Virmani, M., Malik, R. K., Dalal, D. S., Singh, P. and Vikash (2013). Comparing efficacy of different hormonal protocols for induction of cyclicity in postpartum anestrus Sahiwal cows. *Haryana Veterinarian* 52: 121-123.

[49] Kasimanickam, R., Schroeder, S., Hall, J. B. and Whittier, W. D. (2015). Fertility after implementation of long- and short-term progesterone-based ovulation synchronization protocols for fixed-time artificial insemination in beef heifers. *Theriogenology* 83: 1226-1232.

[50] Gordon, I. (1996). Controlled reproduction in cattle and buffaloes. CAB International. Wallingford, UK.

[51] Lamb, G. C., Stevenson, J. S. Kesler, D. J. Garverick, H. A. Brown, D. R. and Salfen, B. E. (2001). Inclusion of an intravaginal progesterone insert plus GnRH and prostaglandin F2α for ovulation control in postpartum suckled beef cows. *J. Anim. Sci.* 79: 2253-2259.

[52] Colazo M. G., Kastelic, J. P, Whittaker, P. R., Gavaga, Q. A., Wilde, R., Mapletoft, R. J. (2004). Fertility in beef cattle given a new or previously used CIDR insert and estradiol, with or without progesterone. *Anim. Reprod. Sci.* 81: 25-34.

[53] Smith, M. W. and Stevenson. J. S. (1995). Fate of the dominant follicle, embryonal survival, and pregnancy rates in dairy cattle treated with prostaglandin F2α and progestins in the absence or presence of a functional corpus luteum. *J. Anim. Sci.* 73: 3743-3751.

[54] Zobel, R., Rkalcic, S., Pipal, I. and Buic, V. (2011). Incidence and factors associated with early pregnancy losses in Simmental dairy cows. *Anim. Reprod. Sci.* 127: 121-125.

[55] Mekonnin, A. B, Tadesse, G., Bitsue, H. K. and Khar, S. K. (2016). Efficacy of a Modified GnRH-PGF Combination for 2 Estrous Synchronization in Dairy Cattle. *Global Veterinaria* 16(2): 200-205.

[56] Giday, J. (2014). Livestock development in Tigray, an overview of past and current development efforts. Livestock Development and Animal Health Services Main Department, Tigray BoARD, Mekelle, Tigray, Ethiopia. A report presented at International Conference on Enhancing Economic Growth and Public Health through Livestock Development and One Health Approach (Mekelle, Ethiopia).

[57] Lobago, F. (2007). Reproductive and lactation performance of dairy cattle in the Oromia Central Highlands of Ethiopia with special emphasis on pregnancy period. Doctoral thesis Swedish University of Agricultural Sciences, Uppsala.

[58] Ashebir, G., Birhanu A. and Gugsa, T. (2016). Status of artificial insemination in Tigray Regional State, "Constraints and acceptability under field condition". *J. Dairy Vet. Anim. Res.* 3(3): 00078. DOI: 10.15406/jdvar.2016.03.00078.

[59] Stevenson, J. S., Call, E. P. Scoby, R. K. and Phatak, A. P. (1990). Double insemination and gonadotropin releasing hormone treatment of repeat-breeding dairy cattle. *J. Dairy Sci.* 73: 1766.

[60] Abdallah, H. and Abd El Rahim, A. (2014). Efficiency of previously used CIDR stored for a prolonged period. *Adv. Anim. Vet. Sci.* 2(9): 508-515.

Gross and Histo-Pathological Changes in Japanese Quail (*Coturnix Coturnix Japonica*) Experimentally Infected with *Salmonella Enterica* Serovar Gallinarum

Barde Israel Joshua[1, *], Bale James Olaniyi Olabode[2], Oladele Sunday Blessing[2], Fatihu Mohammed Yakassai[2], Kumbish Peterside Rinle[1], Chukwu Doris Isioma[1], Rimfa Amos Gambo[1], Akanbi Babatunde Olatunde[1], Moses Gyang Davou[1], Ahmed James Saidu[1], Okewole Philip Ademola[1]

[1]Department of Central Diagnostic Laboratory, National Veterinary Research Institute, Plateau State, Nigeria
[2]Department of Veterinary Pathology, Ahmadu Bello University, Zaria, Kaduna State, Nigeria

Email address:
israelbarde@yahoo.com (B. I. Joshua)

Abstract: A total of 160 (108 males and 52 females) Japanese quails (Coturnix coturnix japonica) were used for the experiment. The quails were obtained at the age of four weeks from the Poultry Division of the National Veterinary Research Institute (NVRI), Vom, Plateau State, Nigeria. They were randomly selected and assigned into four groups (A, B, C and D) of forty quails each. Groups A, B and C were infected with Salmonella enterica serovar Gallinarum per os at the dose of 10^6, 10^4 and 10^2, respectively, while group D served as the control. Mortality rate ranged from 30% to 35%. Grossly, congestion of the liver, lung and ovarian follicle were generally observed in all the infected groups. Also bronzed liver, hepato-splenomegaly, swollen and congested kidney and ascites were observed. Histopathological lesions included; congestion and cellular infiltration of various organs (liver, lung and heart), as well as hepatic vacuolation and hemorrhages. The high mortality rate, gross and histo-pathological findings in this study demonstrate that Japanese quails (Coturnix coturnix japonica) are highly susceptible to Salmonella enterica serovar Gallinarum

Keywords: Gross Histopathology, Japanese- Quail, *Salmonella* Gallinarum

1. Introduction

The genus *Salmonella* is a member of the Family *Enterobacteriaceae* and consists of Gram-negative, non-spore forming bacilli (Popoff *et al.*, 2003).*Salmonella enterica* serovar Gallinarum (*Salmonella* Gallinarum) is a non-motile host adaptive *Salmonella* that causes fowl typhoid (FT), a severe systemic disease responsible for heavy economic losses to the commercial poultry industry through morbidity, mortality and pathological lesions (Parmer and Davies, 2007).With the continuous expansion of poultry farming in Nigeria, FT has become endemic in poultry resulting in heavy economic losses through mortality and pathogical lesions (Agbaje *et al.*, 2010). Quails are ideally suited for avian research, because of their small size and require little cage space for rearing. They are easy to raise and are suitable for genetic studies since they rapidly attain sexual maturity (Haruna *et al.*, 1997). Quails are hardy birds which thrive very well in cages and are relatively inexpensive to maintain. They are birds that every household can keep without stress (Huss *et al.*, 2008).Although quail farming contributes to the alleviation of protein- deficiency in the diets of people in developing countries, they have largely been neglected as a livestock species due to their small size. Most farmers have focused mainly on chicken production. Thus, the potential contributions of quail to food production have been greatly ignored and or underestimated by policy makers in the agricultural sector in these countries. Nigerians are interested in quail production especially for medicinal reasons and so quail farming should be encouraged with a special focus on the traditional subsistence rearing system as practiced by resource-limited farmers (NVRI, 2008).

There is a scarcity of information on microscopic lesions of FT in chickens and quails, and most of the lesions described are from field cases which may be complicated by other bacterial and or viral agents in chickens and to a lesser extent quails (Chadfield *et al.,* 2003).Japanese quails have received less attention relative to other poultry species by researchers (Agrey *et al*., 2003).The Japanese quail has the potential of filling the gap in the protein needs of Nigerians, it is therefore important to investigate diseases that can interfere with production such as FT in order to determine effective control measures. Quail meat and eggs are known for high quality protein, high biological value and low caloric value, thus making them good choices for hypertension prone individuals (NVRI, 2008).

This study evaluated the gross and histopathological changes in Japanese quail *(Coturnix coturnix japonica)*infected with *Salmonella enterica* serovar Gallinarum (*Salmonella* Gallinarum)in Zaria, Kaduna State , Nigeria.

2. Methodology

2.1. Area of Study

The study was carried out in Zaria, Kaduna State, which is located within the Northern Guinea Savannah Zone of Nigeria, between latitude 7° and 11°N, and longitude 7° and 44°E. The average rainfall of this zone ranges from 1,000 to 1,250 mm annually, and the average temperature ranges from 17°C to 33°C (Saidu *et al*., 1994).

2.2. Experimental Birds

A total of 160, four-week old Japanese quails (108 males and 52 females) were obtained from the Poultry Division of National Veterinary Research Institute, Vom, Nigeria and used for the experiment. They were randomly selected and divided into four groups (A, B, C and D) of 40 birds each; with 27 males and 13 females in group A, 23 males and 17 females in group B, 29 males and 11 females in group C as well as group D.

2.3. Housing and Feeding

The quails were allowed to acclimatize for two weeks. The quails were kept in mesh cages of 120 × 140 × 120 cm in size in an enclosed house with the litter changed every week throughout the experimental period.The quails were fed for two weeks on commercial chick mash, after which they were fed commercial layer mash throughout the remaining period of the research which lasted 120 days. They were fed and provided with water *ad libitum* during this period.

2.4. Bacteriological Monitoring Before Infection

Before infection, cloacal swabs were collected from all the quails in order to confirm if they were free from *Salmonella* organism. This was done by pre-enrichment of the swab samples in buffered peptone water, followed by plating on MacConkey agar (MCA) and blood agar (BA) using standard laboratory methods (Parmer and Davies, 2007).

2.5. Source of Organism and Infectivity Procedure

The bacterium, Salmonella enterica serovar Gallinarum, was obtained from the bacterial culture bank of the Central Diagnostic Laboratory, National Veterinary Research Institute, Vom, Nigeria. The Salmonella isolate was from a day old chick that died from a natural infection of Salmonella Gallinarum. The lyophilized bacterium from the culture bank was reactivated by sub-culturing on blood agar (BA) and MacConkey agar (MCA). The resulting colonies were examined for their features, colour and morphology and tested for Gram-reaction (Gram-negative). Three colonies were scooped and inoculated into 20 ml of nutrient broth and incubated for 24 hours at 37oC after which a ten-fold dilution was carried out in test tubes. The colony counts from the test tubes were determined. To obtain the number of organisms that were inoculated into the quails, the number of organisms was multiplied by volume and by the dilution factor (CFU= No. of colony × Volume × Reciprocal of Dilution factor) (Miles and Misra, 1938). Challenge of the quails was done orally using sterile syringes.Group A quails received a dose of 1×10^6 organisms/0.2 ml of nutrient broth, group B quails received a dose of 1×10^4 organisms/0.2 ml of nutrient broth, while group C quails received a dose of 1×10^2 organisms/0.2 ml of nutrient broth.Group D served as control and were not challenged with the bacterium, but were given bacteria-free nutrient broth in accordance with the method of Miles and Misra (1938).

2.6. Pathological Examinations

Mortality was recorded. A detailed post-mortem examination was performed on dead birds, and on birds surviving to the end of the experiment, following euthanasia by cervical dislocation. Gross lesions were observed, recorded and photographed. Samples of the liver, spleen, heart, small and large intestines, lung, ovary, pancreas and caecal tonsil showing gross lesions werecollected and fixed in10% buffered neutral formalin for at least 48 hours. Following fixation, the tissues were trimmed, placed in cassettes and dehydrated in graded concentrations of alcohol (70%, 80%, 90% and 100%) using an automatic tissue processor (STP 120). The tissues were cleared with xylene, embedded in molten paraffin wax block and labelled appropriately (Oladele *et al.,* 2008).The tissue paraffin blocks were sectioned at 5μm thick, using a microtome. The sectioned tissues were mounted on a grease-free, clean glass slide, dried at room temperature and stained with haematoxylin and eosin (H & E) stains. The slides were evaluated using light microscope at ×40 and ×100 magnifications in order to determine any pathological changes. Photomicrographs of lesions from the different organs were taken, transferred to a computer and labelled appropriately (Hossain *et al.*, 2006).

3. Results and Discussion

Mortality was observed in all infected groups (A, B and C), with mortality rates of 35%, 30% and 30%, respectively (Table 1). No mortality was recorded in group D (control).

Table 1. *Mortality pattern of Japanese quails after infection with Salmonella enterica serovar Gallinarum.*

Day after infection	Mortality rate per group			
	Group A (10^6)	Group B (10^4)	Group C (10^2)	Group D (control)
5	3	-	-	-
7	4	3	3	-
8	3	3	3	-
9	2	1	2	-
10	1	2	1	-
11	1	1	1	-
15	-	1	-	-
18	-	1	1	-
20	-	-	1	-
Total	14 (35%)	12(30%)	12(30%)	-

Table 2. *Gross lesions in different groups of quails experimentally infected with Salmonella enterica serovar Gallinarum.*

Number and percentage of birds with lesions in each infected group				
	Group			
Organ/Lesion	A (10^6)	B (10^4)	C (10^2)	D (control)
Liver				
Hepatomegaly	5(12.5%)	5(12.5%)	4(10%)	0
Congestion	19(47.5%)	26 (65%)	17(42.5%)	0
Bronze discoloration	2(5%)	1(2.5%)	1(2.5%)	0
Friable	-	-	2(5%)	0
Lung				
Congestion	19(47.5%)	26(65%)	17(42.5%)	0
Edema	3(7.5%)	6(15%)	5(12.5%)	0
Spleen				
Spleenomegaly	6(15%)	4(10%)	3(7.5%)	0
Kidney				
Swelling	-	1(2.5%)	-	0
Ovarian Follicle				
Egg yolk peritonitis	1(2.5%)	1(2.5%)	-	0
Congestion	1(2.5%)	2(5%)	1(2.5%)	0
Peritoneum				
Hydroperitoneum (ascites)	1(2.5%)	-	-	0

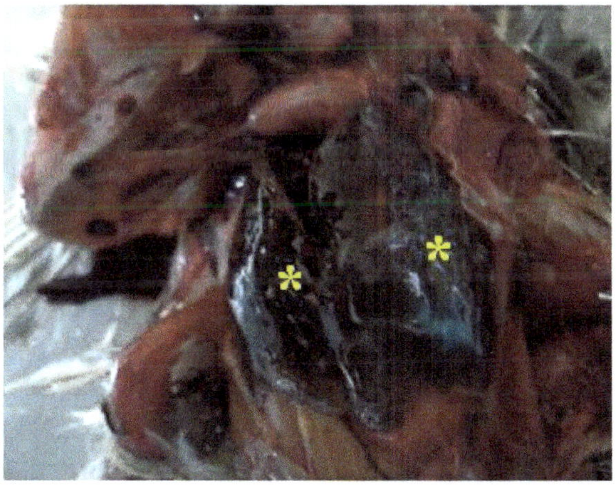

Plate I. *Japanese quail (Coturnix coturnix japonica) experimentally infected with 10^4 of Salmonella enterica serovar Gallinarum.Note hepatomegaly and bronze liver (*)*

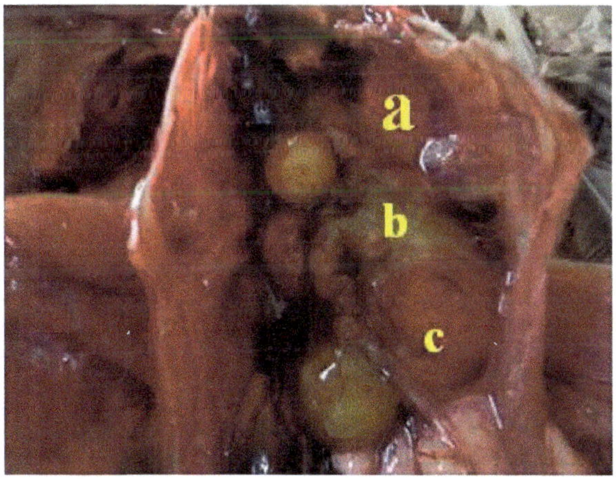

Plate II. *Japanese quail (Coturnix coturnix japonica)experimentally infected with$10^6$of Salmonella enterica serovar Gallinarum. Note congested lung (a), egg yolk peritonitis (b) and congested ovarian follicle (c).*

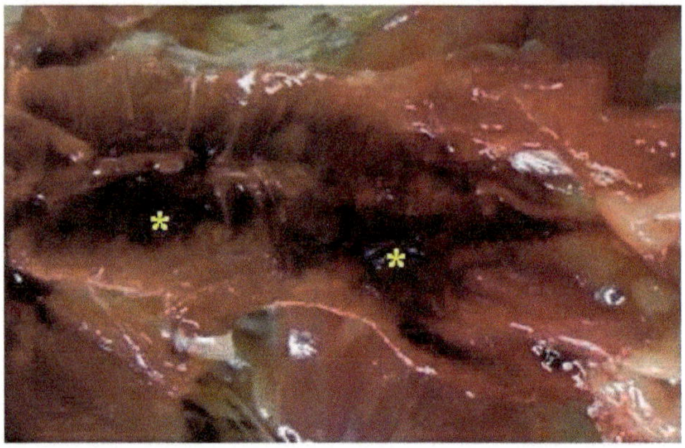

Plate III. *Japanese quail (Coturnix coturnix japonica) experimentally infected with 10^6 of Salmonella enterica serovar Gallinarum. Note enlarged and congested kidneys (*).*

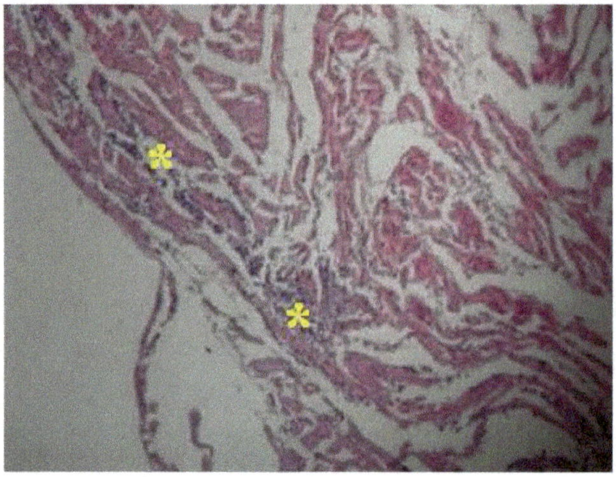

Plate IV. *Photomicrograph of the heart of Japanese quail (Coturnix coturnix japonica) experimentally infected with10^6 of Salmonella enterica serovar Gallinarum Note: Generalized cellular infiltration.*

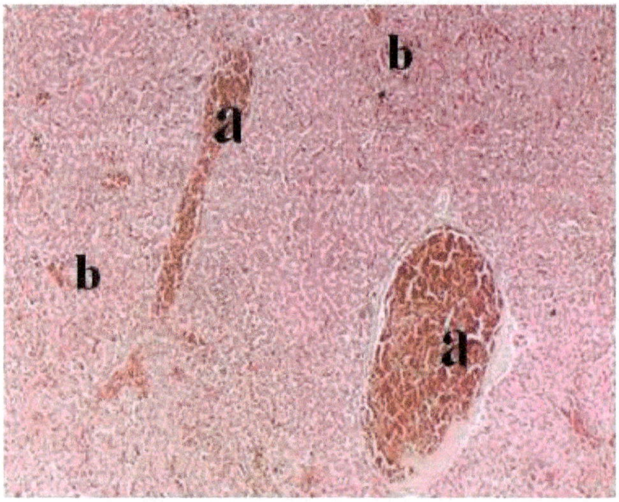

Plate V. *Photomicrograph of the liver of Japanese quail (Coturnix coturnix japonica) experimentally infected with 10^6 of Salmonella enterica serovar Gallinarum. Note severe congestion (a) and haemorrhages(b). H &E. ×40.*

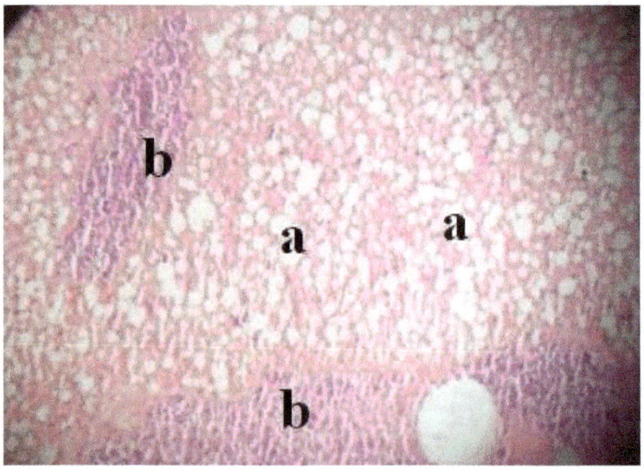

Plate VI. *Photomicrograph of the liver of Japanese quail (Coturnix coturnix japonica) experimentally infected with 10^6 of Salmonella enterica serovar Gallinarum. Note generalized vacuolation due to fatty infiltration (a) and cellular infiltration (b). H & E. ×100.*

A mortality rate of 30-35% was recorded in this study, which is a little lower but still significant as that in chickens (10- 93%) reported by Shivaprasad (1996). The mortality in this study was mostly that of sudden death, suggesting that the infection might have been peracute to acute. The mortality started five days post-infection and persisted tillday twenty.The high mortality recorded in this experiment indicated that Japanese quails are also susceptible to Salmonella enterica serovar Gallinarum similar to the chickens.The gross lesions and histopathological findings observed in Japanese quails (*Coturnix coturnix japonica*) in this study were consistent with previous studies in chickens (Garcia *et al.*, 2010). The gross lesions of hepatomegaly, splenomegaly, swollen kidneys, congested liver, lung and ovarian follicle, bronze liver, egg yolk peritonitis, edematous lung and hydroperitoneum (ascites),observed in this study were also similar to those in chickens reported by previous researchers (Beyaz *et al.*, 2010; Garcia *et al.*, 2010). The gross lesions are highly indicative of septicaemic infection. The histopathological findings (cellular infiltration of the liver and heart, vacuolation of hepatocytes and congested liver and lung) in this study were also similar to previous works in chickens (Hossain *et al.*, 2006; Nwiyi and Omadamiro, 2012).This is the first time these findings were reported in quails in Zaria, Kaduna State, Nigeria to the best of our knowledge.The organism was isolated from the liver, spleen, heart and intestine of the quails at the end of the experiment; implying a septicemic condition.

4. Conclusion

This study demonstrates that Salmonella Gallinarum caused a septicaemic disease with distributionof the organism in major organs and characterized by high mortality, congestion and enlargement of various organs in Japanese quails (Coturnixcoturnix japonica). Other pathological findings, such as bronze liver,hepatomegaly, splenomegaly and congested liver, lung and ovarian follicle in this study indicated that Salmonella Gallinarum produces a disease similar to that in chickens.

Recommendations

Vaccinating Japanese quails reared in the country is highly recommended as a preventive measure against fowl typhoid.Farmers keeping quails should adhere to strict biosecurity measures as means of prevention and control of fowl typhoid in quail farm.

References

[1] Agbaje, M., Davies, R., Oyekunle, M.A., Ojo, O.E., Fasina, F.O.andAkinduti, P.A. (2010). Observation on the occurrence and transmission pattern of Salmonella gallinarum in commercial poultry farms in Ogun State, South Western Nigeria. African Journal of Microbiology Research, 4(9):796-800.

[2] Agrey, S.E., Ankra-Badu, B.A. and Marks, H.L. (2003).Effect of long-term divergent selection on growth characteristic in Japanese quail. Poultry Science, (82): 538- 542.

[3] Beyaz, L., Atasever, A., Aydin, F., Gumusoy, K.S.andAbay, S.(2010). Pathological and clinical findings and tissue distribution of Salmonella gallinarum infection in turkey poults. Turkish Journal of Veterinary and Animal Sciences, 34: 101-110.

[4] Chadfield, M.S., Brown, D.J., Aabo, S., Christensen, J.P. and Olsen, J.E. (2003). Comparison of intestinal invasion and macrophage response of Salmonella gallinarum and other host adapted Salmonella entericaserovars in the avian host. VeterinaryMicrobiology, 92: 49 – 64.

[5] Garcia, K.O., Santana, A.M., FreitasNeto, O. C., Berchieri Jr. A. and Fagliari, J. J. (2010). Experimental infection of commercial layers using a Salmonella entericaserovarGallinarum strain: blood serum component and histopathological changes. Brazilian Journal of Veterinary Pathology, 3(2): 111-117.

[6] Haruna, E.S., Musa U., Lombin, L.H., Tat, P.B., Shamaki, P.D., Okewale, P.A. and Molokwu, J.U. (1997). Introduction of quail production in Nigeria. Nigerian Veterinary Journal, 18:104-107.

[7] Hossain, M.S., Chowdhury, E.H., Islam, M.M., Haider, M.G. and Hossain, M.M. (2006). Avian Salmonella infection: isolation and identification of organisms and histopathologicalstudy.Bangladesh Journal of Veterinary Medicine, 4: 7-12.

[8] Huss, D., Poynter, G. and Lansford, R. (2008). Japanese quail (Coturnixcoturnix japonica) as a laboratory animal model. Department of Biology, Biological Imaging Centre, California Institute of Technology, Pasadena. CA. USA. Laboratory Animal(NY),37(11):513-519.

[9] Miles, A. A and Misra, S A. (1938). The estimation of bacterial power of the blood.Journal of Hygiene, 38:732.

[10] National Veterinary Research Institute (2008). Quail production in the tropics: National Veterinary Research Institute, Vom, Nigeria, 75-92.

[11] Nwiyi, P. and Omadamiro, O. (2012). Seroprevalence and Isolation of Chicken Infected with Salmonella: Haematological and Pathological Evaluation. Journal of Animal and Feed Research, 2(6): 483-487.

[12] Oladele, S.B., Enoch, I and Ibrahim, N.D.G. (2008). Changes in histopathology, haematocrit, haemoglobin, haemagglutination inhibition antibody titre and total protein of Japanese quails (Coturnixcoturnix japonica) administered different doses of Newcastle disease virus. Journal of Animal and Veterinary Advances, 7(4):418-424.

[13] Parmer, D.and Davies, R. (2007). Fowl typhoid in small backyard laying flock. The Veterinary Record, 160:348

[14] Popoff, M.Y., Bockemuhl, J. and Gheeshing, L.L. (2003). Antigenic Formulas of the SalmonellaSerovars, 8th revision. WHO Collaborating Centre for Reference and Research on Salmonella. Supplement 2001 (No: 45) to the Kauffmann-White Scheme Research in Microbiology, 154: 173-174.

[15] Saidu, L., Abdu, P.A., Umoh, J.U. and Abdullahi, U.S. (1994). Diseases of indigenous chicken. Bulletin Animal Health Production in Africa, 42: 19 – 23.

[16] Shivaprasad, H.L. (1996). Pullorum Disease and Fowl Typhoid. Calneck BIN (ed). Disease of poultry .Tenth Edition. Pp 82-96. Iowa State University Press.

Effects of a single dose of ethanol on survival rate and angiogenesis of chick embryo

Zulifqar Ali Laghari[1, *], Ayaz Ali Samo[1, *], Baradi Waryani[2], Zameer Ali Palh[2 *], Khalid Hussain Lashari[2], Ghulam Murtaza Mastoi[3], Gulshan Ara Sahato[2], Tahira Jabeen Ursani[4]

[1]Department of Physiology, University of Sindh, Jamshoro, Sindh, Pakistan
[2]Department of Fresh Water Biology and fisheries, University of Sindh, Jamshoro, Sindh, Pakistan
[3]Centre for Environmental Sciences, University of Sindh, Jamshoro, Sindh, Pakistan
[4]Department of Zoology, University of Sindh, Jamshoro, Sindh, Pakistan

Email address:
zameer_ali110@hotmail.com (Z. A. Palh), kh_lashari@yahoo.com (K. H. Lashari)

Abstract: The developing Chick has been widely used as a model organism for research studies in developmental biology. Various aspects of ethanol (EtOH) toxicity during embryonic development have been documented in experimental studies. The studies on chick embryo address the effects of EtOH on craniofacial abnormalities and angiogenesis. The purpose of this study was to assess the effects of a single dose of ethanol on survival rate and angiogenesis of chick embryos during early stages of development. Chick eggs were incubated at 37°C in the humidified incubator, after 72 hours of incubation these eggs were removed from incubator, and treated with a single doses of 1%, 5%, 10%, 13% and 15% EtOH. The effects on survival rate and angiogenesis were recorded on ethanol treated chick embryos. The survival rate was slightly reduced with 1% and 5% EtOH, however with increasing dose of 10% the survival rate was reduced to 64% and at 15% EtOH complete death was observed. Our results also indicate that treatment of EtOH with 1% and 5% did not have any obvious effects on vessels formation in comparison with the BSS treated embryos. However, treatment of chick embryo with 10%, 13% and 15% EtOH severely inhibited the blood vessels formation.

Keywords: Chick Embryo, Angiogenesis, EtOH

1. Introduction

Ethanol (EtOH) is the main component of the alcohol. Alcohol is consumed frequently irrespective of gender. Some females consume alcohol even in pregnancy, which might result into Fetal Alcohol Syndrome (FAS) (Popova, Lange et al. 2011; Lange, Shield et al. 2013). Individuals suffering from FAS exhibit the spectrum of defects including Physical and Mental retardation, cognitive, behavioral and learning disabilities with identifiable facial dysmorphology (Popova, Lange et al. 2011; Lange, Shield et al. 2013). A number of studies report the use of animal models in the understanding of complexity of FAS and effects of EtOH on various developmental defects have been extensively studied on different animal models including mice (Nakatsuji and Johnson 1984), chick (Tufan, Abban et al. 2007), *Xenopus* (Nakatsuji 1983) and zebrafish (Bilotta, Barnett et al. 2004).

The chick has been widely used as a model organism for research studies in developmental biology (Eckstein, Shibley et al. 1997; Pourquie 2004; Biau, Bayle et al. 2007). Various aspects of EtOH toxicity during embryonic development have been documented in experimental studies (Gu, Bailey et al. 2005; Tufan, Abban et al. 2007). Studies carried out on chick embryo address the effects of EtOH on craniofacial abnormalities (Smith 2008) and angiogenesis (Gu, Bailey et al. 2005). Several studies suggest that EtOH affects the body weight, length and head circumference of chick embryo (Chaudhuri 2004; Kamran, Khan et al. 2011). In addition, it has been shown that microphthalmia may be caused due to EtOH toxicity (Kennelly, Brennan et al. 2011). Some other studies report the negative effects of EtOH on cranial neural crest cells (Smith 1997; Garic-Stankovic, Hernandez et al.

2005). These studies suggest that EtOH causes severe effects on nervous system, and it also causes the decrease in weight and length of embryo. EtOH has been reported as the leading cause of death in humans (Spies, Sander et al. 2001; Ginter and Simko 2008). Model organism has been used to study the survival rate of EtOH treated embryos (Chaudhuri 2004; Kamran, Khan et al. 2011). The treatment of chick embryo with EtOH has been reported to decrease the survival rate in chick embryo (Chaudhuri 2004; Kamran, Khan et al. 2011)

Chorioallantoic membrane (CAM) is formed by the fusion of the chorion and allantoic membrane (Ribatti 2008). This membrane is rich vascular network, which serves as respiratory organ of embryo (Ribatti 2008). Chorionallantoic memrane has been widely used for studying the angiogenesis of chick embryo (Ribatti, Gualandris et al. 1997; Ribatti 2008). CAM is formed on day 7 of incubation. EtOH has been reported to affect the process of angiogenesis in CAM assay using chick embryo as model organism (Richardson and Singh 2003; Ribatti 2012). CAM assay is also used in tumor cell invasion and metastasis (Cimpean, Ribatti et al. 2008; Deryugina and Quigley 2008); this is an easy, quick and inexpensive method to study angiogenesis.

Also, yolk sac blood vessels system, which surrounds the early stage embryo, has also been studied to understand angiogenesis (Rosenbruch and Holst 1990; He, Li et al. 2013). In addition, yolk sac blood vessels system is also used to study the cardiovascular system of early chick embryo (He, Li et al. 2013; Karunamuni, Gu et al. 2014). Several studies report an increase in angiogenesis using CAM assay after treatment with EtOH (Gu, Bailey et al. 2005), however, decrease in angiogenesis has been reported on wound healing (Radek, Matthies et al. 2005; Radek, Kovacs et al. 2008) and yolk sac blood vessels system of early staged chick embryos (Karunamuni, Gu et al. 2014). In an elegant study, it was reported that moderate dose of EtOH has positive effects on development of embryo particularly on vasculature of embryo (Gu, Elam et al. 2001). These studies suggest that EtOH might cause an increase or decrease in angiogenesis, depending on EtOH dose and type of blood vessel system.

The chick is the convenient model, which allows us to directly visualize the effects of EtOH on chick development, which enhances our understanding about Fetal Alcoholic Syndrome. Keeping this view in mind, we carried out a study to find out the effects of various concentration of EtOH on survival rate of chick embryo at early stages of development. In addition, we have also set up experiments on early staged chick embryo to assess the effects of various concentrations of EtOH on yolk sac blood vessels, which surround the developing embryo.

2. Methodology

Chick eggs were obtained from Poultry Institute of Karachi. These eggs were divided into control and treated groups, for each set of treatment 6 eggs were incubated and the experiment was repeated thrice. Chick eggs were incubated at 37 centigrade in the humidified incubator. After 72 hours of incubation (HH stage 19) these eggs were removed from incubator and the egg shell was rinsed with 70% EtOH. A small hole was created on the shell of egg and 3 ml of albumin was removed using syringe. Normally developed embryos were used for experiments and all malformed embryos were excluded. The stages of chick embryo development were determined using Hamburger-Hamilton stages (HH). Chick embryos were treated with 1%, 5%, 10%, 13% and 15% EtOH dissolved in Balanced Salt Solution (BSS) (invitrogen). Control embryos were treated with BSS only. 1 ml of different concentrations of ethanol solutions were poured on the developing embryos, after treating the embryos with a single dose of various concentrations of ethanol solutions, the window of eggs was sealed with transparent tap and the eggs were incubated for 48 hours at 37 centigrade. Preparation of solutions, the dissection procedure and treatments of embryos with various solutions were carried out in biosafety cabinet under aseptic conditions.

The sealed window was open after 48 hours and heart beat of embryos were observed to assess the survival rate. Vessels formation was also observed under microscope and photos were also taken using Digital Camera. Embryos were dissected out and washed with Phosphate buffer saline solution (PBS). Observations were made for any noticeable morphological abnormalities of treated and untreated embryos.

3. Results

Treatment with EtOH affected the survival rate and vascular development of embryos in a dose dependent manner. Figure 1 shows the survival rate of embryos. Only slight difference was observed in the survival rate of chick embryo treated with 1 and 5% of EtOH compared with control (Figure 1), however with increasing dose till 10% EtOH the survival rate was reduced to 64%. At 13 % EtOH survival rate was reduced to half 48%, and at 15 % EtOH complete death was observed.

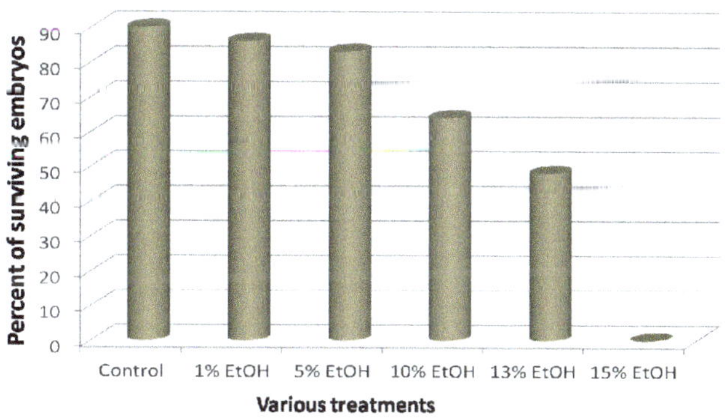

Figure 1. Diagrammatic representation of effects of single dose various concentration of EtOH on survival rate of chick embryos.

EtOH has been reported to negatively and positively affect angiogenesis. In order to find out whether EtOH can affect the angiogenesis we treated the 3 days old chick embryos with a single dose of various concentrations of EtOH. Figure 2 shows that treatment of EtOH with 1% and 5% did not have any obvious effects on vessels formation (Figure 2 B, C) in comparison with the BSS treated (control) embryos (Figure 2 A). However, 10% EtOH severely inhibited the blood vessels formation (Figure 2 D) and treatment of embryos with 13% and 15% EtOH caused severe effects on vessels formation (Figure 2 E-F). At 15% EtOH vessels were fragmented and embryos turned into the pool of blood (Figure 2 F).

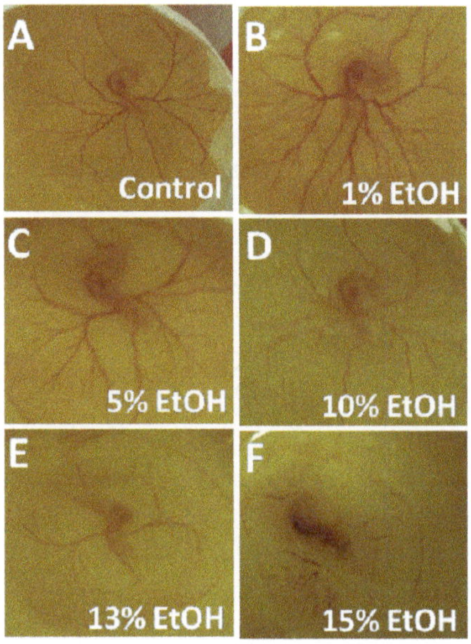

Figure 2. *Effects of EtOH on angiogenesis of 5 days old chick embryos.*

4. Discussion

The data we represent here shows that EtOH affects the survival rate of early stage chick embryos; we have shown that the lethal dose for chick embryo is 15%, our results are not in agreement with the study where it has been shown that 15% EtOH caused the death of 43% chick embryo at various stages (Chaudhuri 2004). The difference in finding is due to the fact that we have used a different strategy to treat the embryos with EtOH.

We have found the slight difference in reduction of the length of embryos; these findings are consistent with already published findings but not consistent with the study where they have reported significant difference in weight and height of embryo (Gilani and Persaud 1992; Kamran, Khan et al. 2013). This might be due to the fact that we are studying the early development of chick embryo. Another difference is we have not used the EtOH vapors but we have directly poured various concentrations of EtOH on early stage chick embryos.

EtOH has been reported to increase the angiogenesis using CAM assay (Gu, Bailey et al. 2005; Tay, Heng et al. 2012). The results we represent indicate that moderate dose of EtOH does not affect vessels formation and heart development, which is in agreement with published study (Gu, Elam et al. 2001). However, higher dose at 10% EtOH inhibit angiogenesis. Inhibition of angiogenesis has also been reported in studies carried out on chick embryo and on wound healing (Radek, Matthies et al. 2005; Radek, Kovacs et al. 2008). This suggests that EtOH inhibit the angiogenesis at higher doses. We have found that at 13% EtOH the severe inhibition of the heart is observed. Some other studies have also reported the inhibition of heart at later development of chick embryo (Karunamuni, Gu et al. 2014). This confirms the role of EtOH in inhibition of heart development. The percentage of EtOH >13% shows marked inhibition of vasculature (Figure 2 E), these results suggest that EtOH might affect the formation of vessels at early stages of chick development.

5. Conclusion

In conclusion, this study demonstrates that the treatment of chick embryo with EtOH at early stages causes decrease in survival rate of chick embryos. This study also suggests that EtOH is harmful for blood vessels, which supply embryo with nutrients at the early stages of development. Collectively, the date provides an insight into the understanding of effects produced by EtOH.

References

[1] Biau, S., S. Bayle, et al. (2007). "The chick embryo: an animal model for detection of the effects of hormonal compounds." Anal Bioanal Chem 387(4): 1397-403.

[2] Bilotta, J., J. A. Barnett, et al. (2004). "Ethanol exposure alters zebrafish development: a novel model of fetal alcohol syndrome." Neurotoxicol Teratol 26(6): 737-43.

[3] Chaudhuri, J. D. (2004). "Effect of a single dose of ethanol on developing skeletal muscle of chick embryos." Alcohol 34(2-3): 279-83.

[4] Cimpean, A. M., D. Ribatti, et al. (2008). "The chick embryo chorioallantoic membrane as a model to study tumor metastasis." Angiogenesis 11(4): 311-9.

[5] Deryugina, E. I. and J. P. Quigley (2008). "Chapter 2. Chick embryo chorioallantoic membrane models to quantify angiogenesis induced by inflammatory and tumor cells or purified effector molecules." Methods Enzymol 444: 21-41.

[6] Eckstein, L. W., I. A. Shibley, Jr., et al. (1997). "Changes in brain glucose levels and glucose transporter protein isoforms in alcohol- or nicotine-treated chick embryos." Brain Res Dev Brain Res 103(1): 59-65.

[7] Garic-Stankovic, A., M. R. Hernandez, et al. (2005). "Ethanol triggers neural crest apoptosis through the selective activation of a pertussis toxin-sensitive G protein and a phospholipase Cbeta-dependent Ca2+ transient." Alcohol Clin Exp Res 29(7): 1237-46

[8] Ginter, E. and V. Simko (2008). "Ethanol and cardiovascular diseases: epidemiological, biochemical and clinical aspects." Bratisl Lek Listy 109(12): 590-4.

[9] Gu, J. W., A. P. Bailey, et al. (2005). "Ethanol stimulates tumor progression and expression of vascular endothelial growth factor in chick embryos." Cancer 103(2): 422-31.

[10] Gu, J. W., J. Elam, et al. (2001). "Moderate levels of ethanol induce expression of vascular endothelial growth factor and stimulate angiogenesis." Am J Physiol Regul Integr Comp Physiol 281(1): R365-72

[11] He, R. R., Y. Li, et al. (2013). "A new oxidative stress model, 2,2-azobis(2-amidinopropane) dihydrochloride induces cardiovascular damages in chicken embryo." PLoS One 8(3): e57732.

[12] Kamran, K., M. Y. Khan, et al. (2011). "Teratogenic effects of ethanol vapour exposure on chick embryos." J Pak Med Assoc 61(4): 328-31.

[13] Kamran, K., M. Y. Khan, et al. (2013). "Ethanol vapour induced dilated cardiomyopathy in chick embryos." J Pak Med Assoc 63(9): 1084-8.

[14] Karunamuni, G., S. Gu, et al. (2014). "Ethanol exposure alters early cardiac function in the looping heart: a mechanism for congenital heart defects?" Am J Physiol Heart Circ Physiol 306(3): H414-21.

[15] Kennelly, K., D. Brennan, et al. (2011). "Histological characterisation of the ethanol-induced microphthalmia phenotype in a chick embryo model system." Reprod Toxicol 32(2): 227-34.

[16] Lange, S., K. Shield, et al. (2013). "Prevalence of fetal alcohol spectrum disorders in child care settings: a meta-analysis." Pediatrics 132(4): e980-95.

[17] Nakatsuji, N. (1983). "Craniofacial malformation in Xenopus laevis tadpoles caused by the exposure of early embryos to ethanol." Teratology 28(2): 299-305.

[18] Nakatsuji, N. and K. E. Johnson (1984). "Effects of ethanol on the primitive streak stage mouse embryo." Teratology 29(3): 369-75.

[19] Popova, S., S. Lange, et al. (2011). "Fetal alcohol spectrum disorder prevalence estimates in correctional systems: a systematic literature review." Can J Public Health 102(5): 336-40.

[20] Pourquie, O. (2004). "The chick embryo: a leading model in somitogenesis studies." Mech Dev 121(9): 1069-79.

[21] Radek, K. A., E. J. Kovacs, et al. (2008). "Acute ethanol exposure disrupts VEGF receptor cell signaling in endothelial cells." Am J Physiol Heart Circ Physiol 295(1): H174-84.

[22] Radek, K. A., A. M. Matthies, et al. (2005). "Acute ethanol exposure impairs angiogenesis and the proliferative phase of wound healing." Am J Physiol Heart Circ Physiol 289(3): H1084-90.

[23] Ribatti, D. (2008). "Chick embryo chorioallantoic membrane as a useful tool to study angiogenesis." Int Rev Cell Mol Biol 270: 181-224.

[24] Ribatti, D. (2012). "Chicken chorioallantoic membrane angiogenesis model." Methods Mol Biol 843: 47-57.

[25] Ribatti, D., A. Gualandris, et al. (1997). "New model for the study of angiogenesis and antiangiogenesis in the chick embryo chorioallantoic membrane: the gelatin sponge/chorioallantoic membrane assay." J Vasc Res 34(6): 455-63.

[26] Richardson, M. and G. Singh (2003). "Observations on the use of the avian chorioallantoic membrane (CAM) model in investigations into angiogenesis." Curr Drug Targets Cardiovasc Haematol Disord 3(2): 155-85.

[27] Rosenbruch, M. and A. Holst (1990). "The chick embryo yolk-sac blood vessel system as an experimental model for irritation and inflammation." Toxicol In Vitro 4(4-5): 327-31.

[28] Smith, S. M. (1997). "Alcohol-induced cell death in the embryo." Alcohol Health Res World 21(4): 287-97.

[29] Smith, S. M. (2008). "The avian embryo in fetal alcohol research." Methods Mol Biol 447: 75-84.

[30] Spies, C. D., M. Sander, et al. (2001). "Effects of alcohol on the heart." Curr Opin Crit Care 7(5): 337-43.

[31] Tay, S. L., P. W. Heng, et al. (2012). "The chick chorioallantoic membrane imaging method as a platform to evaluate vasoactivity and assess irritancy of compounds." J Pharm Pharmacol 64(8): 1128-37.

[32] Tufan, A. C., G. Abban, et al. (2007). "The effect of in ovo ethanol exposure on retina and optic nerve in a chick embryo model system." Reprod Toxicol 23(1): 75-82.

12

Epididymal Sperm Maturation in Bats with Prolonged Sperm Storage

Rodríguez-Tobón Ahiezer[1], León-Galván Miguel A.[2], Arenas-Ríos Edith[3]

[1]Postgraduate in Experimental Biology, Autonomous Metropolitan University–Iztapalapa, Iztapalapa, México
[2]Department of Biology, Autonomous Metropolitan University–Iztapalapa, Iztapalapa, México
[3]Department of Biology of Reproduction, Autonomous Metropolitan University–Iztapalapa, Iztapalapa, México

Email address:
ahiezerrod@yahoo.com.mx (Rodríguez-Tobón A.), león@xanum.uam.mx (León-Galván M. A.), editharenas2000@yahoo.com.mx (Arenas-Ríos E.)

Abstract: Epididymal sperm maturation is the process through which sperm acquire the potential to fertilize the egg. For most mammals, studies report that this process is completed before the sperm enter the cauda region of the epididymis; however, in some bat species, such as the Mexican big-eared bat (*Corynorhinus mexicanus*), this does not occur, as the process does not end until the sperm are inside the cauda of the epididymis, and thus is associated with a long storage period.

Keywords: Epididymis, Epididymal Sperm Maturation, Prolonged Sperm Storage, Bats

1. Introduction

The sperm are formed in the testes during spermatogenesis, but are not yet capable of fertilizing an oocyte as they continue to experience structural, physiological and biochemical changes or modifications after leaving the seminiferous tubules [1]. Later, in the epididymis, the sperm undergo a process called epididymal sperm maturation through which they acquire a marked increase in motility strength, lose the cytoplasmic droplet, increase their surface charge, show changes in lipid composition and, in some species, experience a massive remodeling of the acrosome form [2-10]. Together, all these changes prepare the sperm for capacitation and the acrosome reaction, which are necessary to obtain the ability to fertilize an oocyte [1, 6, 10-13].

The epididymis is a simple, though somewhat convoluted, tubule that can measure from 3-to-80 m depending on the species [1, 14]. In most cases, it has three clearly-differentiated anatomical regions: a) the initial segment, or caput, that receives the sperm and testicular fluid from the testicular efferent vessels; b) the corpus, which is narrower and connects to the final region; and, c) the cauda, which is of globular appearance and is responsible for storing the sperm until ejaculation [1, 6, 10, 13].

One of the most important functional characteristics of the epididymis involves secretion of specific proteins. This function is spatially-restricted to very specific segments of the organ, because each section of the epididymis is further divided into intra-regional segments bordered by connective tissue septa (CTS) [15]. Accordingly, in addition to providing support and stability to the organ itself, the CTS provide the microenvironment that the sperm require, given that gene expression and protein synthesis differ among the three regions [1, 15, 16].

It has been reported that sperm maturation takes place between the caput and corpus of the epididymis, and that the mature sperm are then stored in the cauda until ejaculation [10, 17-21]. This idea that the sperm of many mammalian species achieve maturity before reaching the caudal region emerged over 70 years ago (see Amman and Schanbacher [22]); however, recently-discovered morphophysiological evidence from the vespertilionid Mexican big-eared bat (*Corynorhinus mexicanus*) strongly suggests that the epididymal sperm maturation process requires an unusually long time compared to that reported for other mammals, and is not completed until the sperm are in the cauda. This process also appears to be associated with longer sperm storage time [23]. For these reasons, the objective of the present study was to identify the basic aspects of this process of epididymal sperm maturation in species of bats that have been described as having prolonged sperm storage in the epididymis.

2. Biochemical Basis of Epididymal Sperm Maturation

During maturation, the spermatozoa undergo intracellular changes in their calcium concentration, cyclic adenosine monophosphate content (cAMP), and tyrosine phosphorylation patterns, all of which are essential for the development of coordinated movement [20, 24-26]. The sperm's forward movement depends primarily on the mitochondrial function [20]; however, in order for the sperm to develop the ability to move progressively through the epididymis and later recognize the oocyte in the female genital tract, they must first go through a protein activation process, which is known as tyrosine phosphorylation [27-29].

2.1. Tyrosine Phosphorylation

Protein phosphorylation is a post-translational event that allows the cell to control several processes, including growth, the cell cycle, cytoskeleton assembly, and the modulation of ion transport, which function as adjustment mechanisms of biological activity [27-29]. In eukaryotic cells, most phosphorylations occur in serine (Ser) and threonine (Thr) protein residues and, though to a lesser degree, in those of tyrosine (Tyr). In mammalian sperm, it has been possible to determine that this occurs in a similar fashion, with a phosphorylation ratio of approximately 1000/100/1 for Ser, Thr and Tyr, respectively [27, 29]. The phosphorylation condition is controlled by the activity of protein kinases and phosphatases, where the former add a phosphate group and the latter remove it [27-29]. Studies have shown that phosphorylation of tyrosine residues is particularly important in sperm capacitation [27, 29], and is associated with the process of epididymal maturation, where certain phosphorylation/dephosphorylation events take place (which allow the spermatozoon to turn its function on, or off, like a "switch"), involving primarily the sperm flagellum proteins that participate in the acquisition of motility and the ability to fertilize the oocyte [29, 30].

However, studies of tyrosine phosphorylation have been conducted mainly in species in which the sperm maturation process is seen to end before the spermatozoa enter the epididymal cauda. In the case of *C. mexicanus*, it has been determined that tyrosine phosphorylation increases in sperm obtained from the cauda [31], clearly indicating that the sperm maturation process continues there. And this finding, in turn, may be related to the time that the sperm are stored in the cauda. However, the signaling pathways that allow tyrosine phosphorylation require the participation of certain molecules, such as cholesterol, calcium (Ca^{2+}), bicarbonate ions, progesterone, gamma-aminobutyric acid, and reactive oxygen species (ROS), among others [29, 32-34].

2.2. Involvement of Reactive Oxygen Species (ROS) in Sperm Maturation

Oxygen is essential for all aerobic organisms since it is the main source of energy acquired through oxidative metabolism. However, oxygen consumption generates various derivatives, including active forms of peroxidized oxygen metabolites and molecules, which together are known as reactive oxygen species (ROS) [34]. The ROS that result from the excitation of O_2 form singlet oxygen or transfer 1, 2 or 3 electrons to O_2 to form the superoxide anion ($.O_2$-), hydrogen peroxide (H_2O_2), and the hydroxyl radical (.OH-), respectively [34, 35]. ROS are not necessarily toxic to the cell, for their toxicity depends on their concentration and the context in which they are produced [36]. Indeed, we now know that ROS are essential to the physiology of sperm in relation to such processes as maturation and capacitation [9, 12, 30, 34, 36-43].

Our working group has determined that ROS production in the epididymal sperm of *C. mexicanus* bats may well be involved in the sperm maturation process in the cephalic epididymis region. Moreover, ROS production persists in sperm obtained from the caudal region, suggesting and confirming the results reported by Cervantes et al. [23] In this mammal, unlike reports on other species, the sperm maturation process is completed in the caudal region [44]. In addition, ROS production does not depend on the activity of an NADPH oxidase which, apparently, is absent or inactive [44]. This finding suggests the involvement of cytochrome B5 reductase [33, 45]. Therefore, ROS production in the epididymal sperm of *C. mexicanus* could be of mitochondrial origin; alternatively, it would be necessary to confirm DUOX activity, as reported by Baker et al. [46].

Fortunately, the seminal plasma and sperm contain a whole battery of ROS scavengers, including such enzymes as superoxide dismutase (SOD), catalase (CAT), and glutathione peroxidase (GPX), as well as various substances whose activity is linked to CAT and SOD, such as α-tocopherol, ascorbic acid, glutathione, pyruvate, taurine, hypotaurine, and albumin, which imbues them with the ability to regulate ROS growth [36, 47-53]).

There are studies of the participation of the antioxidant enzymes CAT, SOD and GPX in *C. mexicanus* that have measured the enzyme activity found in the epididymis, including the mechanism that modulates ROS during maturation and prolonged sperm storage, two patterns of enzymatic activity that appear according to the phase of the epididymal reproductive cycle. CAT activity in the epididymis is particularly high throughout the reproductive cycle, while SOD activity is present during sperm transit from the testes to the epididymis, and sperm maturation, but is almost completely absent from the cephalic and caudal epididymal regions during the storage period [54]. GPX activity, meanwhile, is low during the testicular phase but high between the different segments of the epididymis (*i.e.*, caput, corpus and cauda) during maturation [54]. This activity pattern seems to be specifically controlled and differentiated in relation to the compartmentalization of the epididymal functions [44].

3. Prolonged Sperm Storage in the Epididymis

An unusual reproductive particularity in mammals, which has been reported for some bat species, is prolonged gamete storage. Though this feature occurs primarily in females in the form of delayed ovulation in relation to coupling time, cases of prolonged sperm storage have also been identified in the males of some species. In these cases, the epididymis (especially the caudal region) is the organ responsible for this function [55, 56].

The question of prolonged sperm storage in bats has been addressed since 1860, and this phenomenon has been identified in at least 43 species [55-59]. One of the first studies to show that the sperm of bats is capable of fertilization even after a prolonged storage period was conducted by Wimsatt and Folk in the 1940s (cited by Crichton [55]). Today we know that some bats of the Vespertilionidae and Rhinolophidae families show a temporal asynchrony in the development and functioning of the male reproductive organs [60]. Specifically, the development of the testes and the process of spermatogenesis take place mainly in the summer months, while the maximum development of the epididymis and accessory sex glands, the expression of libido, and mating, do not occur until the autumn [56, 61-64]. This asynchrony results in an unusually long period of sperm storage in the epididymis, which may extend for several months after the testes have completely regressed [55]. Indeed, the sperm in the epididymis of some bat species are stored for months, but remain viable for 4-to-10 months, depending on the species and environmental conditions [65-67].

It was long considered that the phenomenon of prolonged sperm storage in bats was limited to species living in temperate and cold zones, and was attributable to the low ambient temperatures that, in turn, caused a decrease in the availability of the insects that constitute the principal source of food for those animals. As a result, those bats experienced prolonged periods of adaptive hypothermia that extended throughout the winter season [61, 68, 69]. However, later studies of bats from warmer climes where this phenomenon is also present indicated that prolonged storage is not related to low ambient temperatures [56, 60], though it is important to clarify that the species reported actually inhabit temperate environments because they live at high altitudes. Currently, there are reports that provide additional support for this view, since they have found regulating mechanisms that maintain sperm structurally and functionally viable during prolonged storage periods due to certain morphophysiological aspects that depend on the epididymal environment [66, 67].

Bats that have prolonged sperm storage typically enter into a state of lethargy early in the winter season. In this condition, individuals drastically reduce their metabolic functions and body temperature, which leads to a decrease in cellular activity and in several central functions related to reproductive processes, such as hormone production and the ability of target organs to respond to hormonal stimulation [70]. With regards to this interesting phenomenon, there are two important parameters that must be taken into account; the first is the time that the sperm remain in storage; the second is the conservation of such characteristics as viability, integrity, and the ability to perform forward movement and achieve effective fertilization. One proposal to explain how the sperm of hibernating bat species remain structurally and functionally viable for long periods in the caudal region of the epididymis was advanced by Crichton et al. [66], who determined that the epididymal fluid obtained from micropunctures of the caudal region maintain high levels of osmolarity as the storage season progresses, a condition that may favor long-term storage. Those authors [66, 67] further reported a close relation among the epididymal epithelial cells of the pallid bat (*Antrozous pallidus*), the northern long-eared bat (*Myotis septentrionalis*), and the little brown bat (*Myotis lucifugus*), all of which form what may be called a blood-epididymal barrier, particularly during the period of sperm storage.

This phenomenon, together with the generation of a hyperosmolar environment in the lumen of the epididymal tubule, was suggested as the conditions that could cause a certain degree of dehydration of some spermatozoa and, therefore, their immobilization. Here, the cell quiescence due to reduced respiration would conserve energy and preserve viability by preventing the onset of progressive movement by the spermatozoids. Hence, lowering the osmolarity of the epididymal lumen allows the sperm to completely recover their motility and, as a result, their fertilization capacity. However, the effect of the hyperosmolar environment on sperm physiology remains to be tested with further studies.

A subsequent study by the same research group hypothesized that the plasma membrane of the sperm of the vespertilionid bat *Myotis velifer* apparently has greater resistance to factors such as detergents for example that are known to destabilize the sperm membrane of other mammals. At the conclusion of their experiments, however, they determined that there was no difference in terms of membrane resistance to the agents they tested. Therefore, long-term sperm survival could not be attributed to the high resistance of the plasma membrane [71].

4. Maturation and Prolonged Storage in Mexican Big-Eared Bats (*Corynorhinus mexicanus*)

Another proposal to consider relates long-term sperm storage to the epididymal maturation process. In the case of the vespertilionid Mexican big-eared bat, in addition to being a species that manifests asynchrony in the development of the male's sexual functions [56, 61-64], it also maintains the sperm in the epididymis for up to 5 months after the testes have fully regressed [60].

Studies of the weight, histology and morphometric variation of the epididymal tubule of *C. mexicanus* revealed that in addition to the asynchrony of the male's sexual functions, an apparent asynchrony among epididymal regions also occurs (caput-cauda), as the caput presents growth peaks in September (due to the presence of sperm), while the cauda peaks in October ($90.3x10^6$). Observations revealed that, anatomically-speaking, the caput of the epididymis is smaller in size than the cauda, a situation that indicates a clear asynchrony of one month between the development of these two regions [60, 72, 73].

Sometime later, Cervantes et al. [23] conducted a study in which they analyzed separately the three regions of the epididymis (caput, corpus and cauda) of *C. mexicanus*. They determined that spermatozoa levels in the corpus and caput never exceeded 30×106, while data for the cauda showed a level of 77.2×106. Sperm were no longer observed in the cephalic region in early October, nor in the body at the end of that month, when sperm concentrations in the cauda were high. In addition, the presence of the cytoplasmic droplet was high in the sperm obtained from the caudal region in September (19.7%), but showed a steady decrease until yielding zero values in late October (1.7).

Upon testing the maturational status of the sperm cells of *C. mexicanus* obtained from the three different regions of the epididymis by analyzing sperm capacitation and the *in vitro* acrosome reaction, those researchers found that the capacitation values from early September were 6% for the corpus and 16% for the cauda, but that they increased in October to 19.4% and 33.2%, respectively. In the case of the acrosome reaction for the same time period, the initial values found were 7.6% and 12.0% for the body and tail, respectively, with a subsequent increase to 22.2% and 32.3%, respectively. These results led them to conclude that the cauda region was not simply a sperm reservoir [74], but that in this species it is the region where sperm maturation may be completed, quite independent of the function of the testes. These findings are most interesting when we recall that the epididymis is androgen-dependent, and that the testicles of these bats have undergone complete involution, so it would seem that they have no additional effect on the epididymis [60] and that the complete differentiation of the spermatozoids could not take place there [1].

In order to strengthen support for the proposal that in *C. mexicanus* sperm maturation ends in the caudal region, Rodríguez-Tobon et al. [73] conducted studies of the morphology and ultrastructure of the spermatozoa of this species. They found a high frequency of cytoplasmic droplet in the middle section of the spermatozoa. In addition to identifying morphological changes in the different cell types of the epididymis of *C. mexicanus*, they also observed that both principal and clear cells are present in all three epididymal regions [73], and are related to the process of sperm maturation, since those cells are characterized by their highly-developed endocytic and secretory machinery and, moreover, show structural and functional differences in each region of the epididymis [1, 75].

Therefore, the presence of principal and clear cells throughout the epididymal tubule is evidence that the maturation process continues from the moment the sperm enter the head region of the epididymal tubule in late August, until such time as the storage period in the caudal region ends; a period that is necessary to complete the process of sperm maturation [73].

5. Conclusions and Prospects for Epididymal Sperm Maturation in *C. mexicanus*

Several authors have explored the mechanisms by which sperm reach maturity in the epididymis, however recent studies of the *C. mexicanus* bat have opened a new perspective to consider in relation to epididymal maturation. The fact that in this species sperm maturation is completed in the caudal epididymis region and is related to prolonged storage times leads to new considerations, given that this species is also characterized by temporal asynchrony in the development and functioning of the male's reproductive organs.

Studying the wide variety of proteins that may be secreted by the epithelial tissue of the epididymal tubule is essential to achieving a better understanding of the maturation process, since many of these proteins propitiate changes in the movement of the flagella and the subsequent recognition of the oocyte. Research into how proteins are incorporated into the spermatozoids is also essential, especially the possible role of the epididimosomes as elements in the pathway that transports them from the epididymal tissue.

Analyzing the parameters of motility using a computerized system (Computer-Assisted Sperm Analysis, or CASA) and gaining a better understanding of the various components and regions that integrate the sperm plasma membrane along the epididymal duct as the spermatozoids pass through the various organs of the male genital tract, will allow us to determine the functional status of the cells at each stage. Finally, reports in the literature affirm that the ROS in sperm allow the activation of proteins involved in flagellar movement, but additional studies are required in order to ascertain exactly what occurs in bat species characterized by long storage periods of the spermatozoids in the caudal region of the epididymis.

References

[1] Bernard Robaire, B.T.H., and Marie-Claire Orgebin-Crist, *The Epididymis*, in *Knobil and Neill's Physiology of Reproduction*, J.D. Neill, Editor. 2006.

[2] Fournier-Delpech, S., et al., *Epididymal sperm maturation in the ram: motility, fertilizing ability and embryonic survival after uterine artificial insemination in the ewe.* Ann. Biol. anim. Bioch Biophys, 1979. 19(3A): p. 597-605.

[3] Brown, D. and R. Montesano, *Membrane specialization in the rat epididymis. I. Rod-shaped intramembrane particles in the apical (mitochondria-rich) cell.* J Cell Sci, 1980. 45: p. 187-98.

[4] Hinrichsen, M.J. and J.A. Blaquier, *Evidence supporting the existence of sperm maturation in the human epididymis.* J Reprod Fertil, 1980. 60(2): p. 291-4.

[5] Awano, M., A. Kawaguchi, and H. Mohri, *Lipid composition of hamster epididymal spermatozoa.* J Reprod Fertil, 1993. 99(2): p. 375-83.

[6] Cooper, T., *Epididymis*, in *Encyclopedia of reproduction*, J.D.N. E. Knovil, Editor. 1999. p. 1-17.

[7] Huang, Y., Y.W. Chung, and P.Y. Wong, *Potassium channel activity recorded from the apical membrane of freshly isolated epithelial cells in rat caudal epididymis.* Biol Reprod, 1999. 60(6): p. 1509-14.

[8] Legare, C., et al., *Effect of vasectomy on P34H messenger ribonucleic acid expression along the human excurrent duct: a reflection on the function of the human epididymis.* Biol Reprod, 2001. 64(2): p. 720-7.

[9] Vernet, P., et al., *Analysis of reactive oxygen species generating systems in rat epididymal spermatozoa.* Biol Reprod, 2001. 65(4): p. 1102-13.

[10] Sullivan, R., G. Frenette, and J. Girouard, *Epididymosomes are involved in the acquisition of new sperm proteins during epididymal transit.* Asian J Androl, 2007. 9(4): p. 483-91.

[11] Oko, R., et al., *The cytoplasmic droplet of rat epididymal spermatozoa contains saccular elements with Golgi characteristics.* J Cell Biol, 1993. 123(4): p. 809-21.

[12] Aitken, R.J., et al., *Relative impact of oxidative stress on the functional competence and genomic integrity of human spermatozoa.* Biol Reprod, 1998. 59(5): p. 1037-46.

[13] Setchell, B. and W. Breed, *Anatomy, Vasculature, and Innervation of the Male Reproductive Tract*, in *Physiology of reproduction*, E. Knobil and D. Neill, Editors. 2006, Academic Press: USA. p. 587-596.

[14] Robaire, B. and R.S. Viger, *Regulation of epididymal epithelial cell functions.* Biology of Reproduction, 1995. 52(2): p. 226-236.

[15] Turner, T.T., et al., *Association of segmentation of the epididymal interstitium with segmented tubule function in rats and mice.* Reproduction, 2003. 125(6): p. 871-8.

[16] Aitken, R.J., et al., *Proteomic changes in mammalian spermatozoa during epididymal maturation.* Asian J Androl, 2007. 9(4): p. 554-64.

[17] Belleannee, C., et al., *Purification and identification of sperm surface proteins and changes during epididymal maturation.* Proteomics, 2011. 11(10): p. 1952-64.

[18] Belleannee, C., et al., *Identification of luminal and secreted proteins in bull epididymis.* J Proteomics, 2011. 74(1): p. 59-78.

[19] Baker, M.A., et al., *Proteomic insights into the maturation and capacitation of mammalian spermatozoa.* Syst Biol Reprod Med, 2012. 58(4): p. 211-7.

[20] Contri, A., et al., *Characteristics of donkey spermatozoa along the length of the epididymis.* Theriogenology, 2012. 77(1): p. 166-73.

[21] Dacheux, J.L., et al., *The contribution of proteomics to understanding epididymal maturation of mammalian spermatozoa.* Syst Biol Reprod Med, 2012. 58(4): p. 197-210.

[22] Amann, R.P. and B.D. Schanbacher, *Physiology of male reproduction.* Journal of animal science, 1983. 57 Suppl 2: p. 380-403.

[23] Cervantes, M.I., et al., *Spermatozoa epididymal maturation in the Mexican big-eared bat (Corynorhinus mexicanus).* Syst Biol Reprod Med, 2008. 54(4-5): p. 196-204.

[24] White, D.R. and R.J. Aitken, *Influence of epididymal maturation on cyclic AMP levels in hamster spermatozoa.* Int J Androl, 1989. 12(1): p. 29-43.

[25] Yeung, C.H., G.F. Weinbauer, and T.G. Cooper, *Responses of monkey epididymal sperm of different maturational status to second messengers mediating protein tyrosine phosphorylation, acrosome reaction, and motility.* Mol Reprod Dev, 1999. 54(2): p. 194-202.

[26] Vijayaraghavan, S., et al., *A Role for Phosphorylation of Glycogen Synthase Kinase-3α in Bovine Sperm Motility Regulation.* Biology of Reproduction, 2000. 62(6): p. 1647-1654.

[27] Tardif, S., et al., *Capacitation is associated with tyrosine phosphorylation and tyrosine kinase-like activity of pig sperm proteins.* Biol Reprod, 2001. 65(3): p. 784-92.

[28] Urner, F. and D. Sakkas, *Protein phosphorylation in mammalian spermatozoa.* Reproduction, 2003. 125(1): p. 17-26.

[29] Naz, R.K. and P.B. Rajesh, *Role of tyrosine phosphorylation in sperm capacitation/acrosome reaction.* Reprod Biol Endocrinol, 2004. 2: p. 75.

[30] Lewis, B. and R.J. Aitken, *Impact of epididymal maturation on the tyrosine phosphorylation patterns exhibited by rat spermatozoa.* Biol Reprod, 2001. 64(5): p. 1545-56.

[31] Rodríguez-Tobón, A., et al., *Tyrosine phosphorylation as evidence of epididymal cauda participation in the sperm maturation process of the Corynorhinus mexicanus bat.* , in *Acta Zoologica-stockholm, In press*. 2015.

[32] Baldi, E., et al., *Intracellular calcium accumulation and responsiveness to progesterone in capacitating human spermatozoa.* J Androl, 1991. 12(5): p. 323-30.

[33] Baker, M.A., et al., *Analysis of the mechanism by which calcium negatively regulates the tyrosine phosphorylation cascade associated with sperm capacitation.* J Cell Sci, 2004. 117(2): p. 211-22.

[34] Chabory, E., et al., *Mammalian glutathione peroxidases control acquisition and maintenance of spermatozoa integrity.* J Anim Sci, 2010. 88(4): p. 1321-31.

[35] Turrens, J.F., *Mitochondrial formation of reactive oxygen species.* The Journal of Physiology, 2003. 552(2): p. 335-344.

[36] de Lamirande, E., et al., *Reactive oxygen species and sperm physiology.* Rev Reprod, 1997. 2(1): p. 48-54.

[37] Bauskin, A.R., I. Alkalay, and Y. Ben-Neriah, *Redox regulation of a protein tyrosine kinase in the endoplasmic reticulum.* Cell, 1991. 66(4): p. 685-96.

[38] Aitken, R.J., et al., *Redox regulation of tyrosine phosphorylation in human spermatozoa and its role in the control of human sperm function.* J Cell Sci, 1995. 108 (5): p. 2017-25.

[39] Leclerc, P., E. de Lamirande, and C. Gagnon, *Regulation of protein-tyrosine phosphorylation and human sperm capacitation by reactive oxygen derivatives.* Free Radic Biol Med, 1997. 22(4): p. 643-56.

[40] Caselli, A., et al., *The inactivation mechanism of low molecular weight phosphotyrosine-protein phosphatase by H2O2.* J Biol Chem, 1998. 273(49): p. 32554-60.

[41] Aitken, R.J., *Possible redox regulation of sperm motility activation.* J Androl, 2000. 21(4): p. 491-6.

[42] Baker, M.A. and R.J. Aitken, *The importance of redox regulated pathways in sperm cell biology.* Mol Cell Endocrinol, 2004. 216(1-2): p. 47-54.

[43] Ford, W.C., *Regulation of sperm function by reactive oxygen species.* Hum Reprod Update, 2004. 10(5): p. 387-99.

[44] Arenas-Ríos, E., *Enzimas anti-especies reactivas de oxígeno, como reguladores en los procesos de espermatogénesis maduración y almacenamiento prolongado de espermatozoides en el murciélago Corynorhinus mexicanus.* . 2009, Universidad Autónoma Metropolitana México.

[45] Baker, M.A., et al., *Identification of cytochrome-b5 reductase as the enzyme responsible for NADH-dependent lucigenin chemiluminescence in human spermatozoa.* Biol Reprod, 2005. 73(2): p. 334-42.

[46] Baker, M.A., et al., *Identification of gene products present in Triton X-100 soluble and insoluble fractions of human spermatozoa lysates using LC-MS/MS analysis.* Proteomics Clin Appl, 2007. 1(5): p. 524-32.

[47] Alvarez, J.G. and B.T. Storey, *Role of superoxide dismutase in protecting rabbit spermatozoa from O2 toxicity due to lipid peroxidation.* Biol Reprod, 1983. 28(5): p. 1129-36.

[48] Nissen, H.P. and H.W. Kreysel, *Superoxide dismutase in human semen.* Klinische Wochenschrift, 1983. 61(1): p. 63-65.

[49] Alvarez, J.G., et al., *Spontaneous lipid peroxidation and production of hydrogen peroxide and superoxide in human spermatozoa. Superoxide dismutase as major enzyme protectant against oxygen toxicity.* J Androl, 1987. 8(5): p. 338-48.

[50] Alvarez, J.G. and B.T. Storey, *Role of glutathione peroxidase in protecting mammalian spermatozoa from loss of motility caused by spontaneous lipid peroxidation.* Gamete Res, 1989. 23(1): p. 77-90.

[51] Jeulin, C., et al., *Catalase activity in human spermatozoa and seminal plasma.* Gamete Res, 1989. 24(2): p. 185-96.

[52] Halliwell, B. and J.M.C. Gutteridge, *Free Radicals in Biology and Medicine.* 2007: Oxford University Press.

[53] Zini, A., E. de Lamirande, and C. Gagnon, *Reactive oxygen species in semen of infertile patients: levels of superoxide dismutase- and catalase-like activities in seminal plasma and spermatozoa.* Int J Androl, 1993. 16(3): p. 183-8.

[54] Arenas-Ríos, E., et al., *Superoxide dismutase, catalase, and glutathione peroxidase during epididymal maturation and prolonged storage of spermatozoa in the Mexican big-eared bat (Corynorhinus mexicanus).* Canadian Journal of Zoology, 2005. 83(12): p. 1556-1565.

[55] Crichton, E.G. and P.H. Krutzsch, *Reproductive Biology of Bats.* 2000: Elsevier Science.

[56] Krutzsch, P.H., *The Reproductive Biology of the Cave Myotis (Myotis velifer).* Acta Chiropterologica, 2009. 11(1): p. 89-104.

[57] Sharifi, M., et al., *Evidence of sperm storage in Pipistrellus kuhlii (Chiroptera: Vespertilionidae) in western Iran.* Folia Zoologica, 2004. 53: p. 1–6.

[58] Sharifi, M., V. Akmali, and G. Rostam, *Evidence of sperm storage in Myotis capaccinii (Chiroptera: Vespertilionidae) in western Iran.* . Journal of Veterinary Research, 2008. 63(2): p. 63–67.

[59] Wang, Z., et al., *Epididymal sperm storage in Rickett's big-footed bat (Myotis ricketti).* Acta Chiropterologica, 2008. 10(1): p. 161-167.

[60] León-Galván, M.A., et al., *Male reproductive cycle of mexican big-eared bats, corynorhinus mexicanus (chiroptera: vespertilionidae).* The Southwestern Naturalist, 2005. 50(4): p. 453-460.

[61] Gustafson, A.W., *Male reproductive patterns in hibernating bats.* J Reprod Fertil, 1979. 56(1): p. 317-31.

[62] Krishna, A. and K. Singh, *The relationship between testicular activity, accessory sex glands, and circulating steroid concentration during the reproductive cycle in a male Indian vespertilionid bat, Scotophilus heathi.* Canadian Journal of Zoology, 1997. 75(7): p. 1042-1050.

[63] Krishna, A. and K. Singh, *Changes in the thyroid gland during the reproductive cycle of the male vespertilionid bat, Scotophilus heathi.* Revista Brasileira de Biologia, 1998. 58: p. 707-716.

[64] Krishna, A. and K. Singh, *Asynchrony of the reproductive organs of the male vespertilionid bat, Scotophilus heathi: role of gonadotrophins.* Acta Theriologica 1999. 44(2): p. 123-131.

[65] Racey, P.A., *The prolonged storage and survival of spermatozoa in Chiroptera.* J Reprod Fertil, 1979. 56(1): p. 391-402.

[66] Crichton, E.G., et al., *Unique features of the cauda epididymidal epithelium of hibernating bats may promote sperm longevity.* Anat Rec, 1993. 237(4): p. 475-81.

[67] Crichton, E.G., et al., *Hyperosmolality and sperm storage in hibernating bats: prolongation of sperm life by dehydration.* Am J Physiol, 1994. 267(5-2): p. R1363-70.

[68] Krutzsch, P.H., *Male reproductive patterns in nonhibernating bats.* J Reprod Fertil, 1979. 56(1): p. 333-44.

[69] Jolly, S.E. and A.W. Blackshaw, *Prolonged epididymal sperm storage, and the temporal dissociation of testicular and accessory gland activity in the common sheath-tail bat, Taphozous georgianus, of tropical Australia.* J Reprod Fertil, 1987. 81(1): p. 205-11.

[70] Wimsatt, W., *Some problems of reproduction in relation to hibernation in bats.* . Bulletin of the Museum of Comparative Zoology Harvard 1960. 124: p. 249-267.

[71] Crichton, E.G., P.H. Krutzsch, and R. Yanagimachi, *Stability of the sperm plasma membrane of hibernating bats (Myotis velifer) compared with other mammals.* J Reprod Fertil, 1993. 97(1): p. 1-4.

[72] León-Galvan, M.A., et al., *Prolonged storage of spermatozoa in the genital tract of female Mexican big-eared bats (Corynorhinus mexicanus): the role of lipid peroxidation.* Canadian Journal of Zoology, 1999. 77(1): p. 7-12.

[73] Rodríguez-Tobón, A., *Análisis macro y micro estructural del epidídimo en relación con la maduración y almacenamiento de espermatozoides en el murciélago estacional Corynorhinus mexicanus.* . 2011, Universidad Autónoma Metropolitana México.

[74] Holland, M.K., J.T. Vreeburg, and M.C. Orgebin-Crist, *Testicular regulation of epididymal protein secretion.* J Androl, 1992. 13(3): p. 266-73.

[75] Robaire, B., B. Hinton, and C. Orgebin-Crist, *The Epididymis: From Molecules to Clinical Practice: From Molecules to Clinical Practice: a Comprehensive Survey of the Efferent Ducts, the Epididymis and the Vas Deferens.* 2001: Springer US.

13

Distribution and Seroprevalence of PPR Virus in Chad During 2004 - 2014

BIDJEH Kebkiba[1,*], BAN-BO Bebanto Antipas[2], MAHAMAT Fayiz Abakar[1], ASSANDI Oussiguere[1], ASSANE Kembe[1], TCHARI Doungous[1], KEILAR Aurelie[1], TAÏTOUIN Sounkreo[3]

[1]Department of Animal Health, Livestock Research Institute for Development, N'Djamena, Chad
[2]Department of Faculty of Exact and Applied Sciences, University of N'Djamena, N'Djamena, Chad
[3]Epidemiology Unit, Directorate of Veterinary Services, N'Djamena, Chad

Email address:
bidjehkebkiba@yahoo.fr (B. Kebkiba)

Abstract: Peste des petits ruminants (PPR) is an acute febrile viral disease of goats and sheep characterized by mucopurulent nasal and ocular discharge, erosive and necrotizing stomatitis, enteritis and pneumonia. It is widespread, virulent and devastating causing significant impacts to the economy, food security and livelihoods of poor marginalized farmers. This study focused on clinical observations of 233 suspected cases of PPR and provided detailed information on the prevalence of antibodies against the PPR virus in sera from 986 small ruminants and 31 from camels. Most of specimens for this study were obtained from the slaughterhouse in N'Djamena. Sera for the detection of antibodies against the PPR virus were not necessarily representative of the target population, even if they were from a larger number of regions. According to information provided by the epidemiological surveillance field agents, the foci of the disease were more severe in goats than in sheep and the outbreaks frequency was higher during the Cold dry season (December to June) than during the other months of the year. Analysis of 1017 sera collected in small ruminants and camels revealed that the prevalence of antibodies against the PPR virus was 34.48%. The prevalence of antibodies against the PPR virus varied by species (goats, 15.21%, sheep, 19.25% and camels, 0%), age groups and geographic areas. The rate of infection by the PPR virus was higher in the sheep population (34. 67%) than in goats (27.37%). The study showed seroprevalence higher in sheep than in goats. In contrast, no serum from camels revealed positive vis-à-vis the PPR virus. Another serological survey would need to be undertaken in the population of camels in order to clarify their role in the epidemiology of PPR.

Keywords: PPR, Virus, Serum, Sheep, Goats, Camels, Chad

1. Introduction

Peste des petits ruminants (PPR) is a disease of small ruminants widespread [26, 27], virulent and devastating causing significant impacts to the economy, food security and livelihoods of marginal farmers in Africa and south Asia. It is an important concern for food security and poverty alleviation. The disease is caused by a *morbillivirus* [9] closely related to rinderpest virus eradicated worldwide in 2011. PPR is considered as one of the most damaging animal diseases in Africa, the Middle East and Asia. It is also one of the priority diseases identified in the World 5-year Action Plan (2013-2017) of the FAO-OIE Global Framework for the Progressive Control of Transboundary Animal Diseases (GF-TADs).

Formerly it was supposed to be confined in West Africa, but now rampant in Oman [27], Sudan and the United Arab Emirates [8]. The isolation of the virus in the gazelle *(Gazella dorcas)* poses the problem of the role of wildlife in the epidemiology of this disease [13]. It was described for the first time in 1942 by Gargadennec and Lalanne in Ivory Coast [6]. The disease is characterized by fever, the onset of clinical signs, state of exhaustion, hyperthermia, oculo-nasal discharge, oral lesions, breathing difficulty with cough, foul-smelling diarrhea, and ends in many cases by the death of the animal [28].

In Chad, the disease is endemic and causes significant economic losses each year related to high morbidity (90%) and mortality (80%) in infected goats and sheep [2,23].

This disease is particularly prevalent in areas where the conditions are ripe for hatching and remain in the animals whose maintenance is usually not satisfactory. This is the case in Chad where the disease has long time existed [22, 23].

All African countries located between the Sahara and the equator in the Atlantic Ocean to the Red Sea, are in the endemic area of PPR [20]. North Africa, excepted Egypt and Morocco, is not affected by PPR virus. It is the same for Southern Africa.

In Chad, the population of small ruminants has been no mass vaccination campaign against the disease. Yet the suspicion of the existence of the disease confirmed by serological surveys [22] and then by the isolation of the pathogen [3] requires a prophylactic action throughout the national territory. If the research has been undertaken in the meantime on small ruminants, there is no information related to the sensitivity of the Chadian camels to PPR virus. In the light of the information available in Ethiopia and Sudan, a serological survey is needed to determine the status of Chadian camels vis-à- vis the PPR virus.

Pneumonia episodes of camels found in Sudan and confirmed as PPR [17] reinforce the first viral identification work in Ethiopia where was observed an emerging disease of camels, characterized by a fever and respiratory syndrome with very high morbidity and variable mortality. The similarity of these syndromes with those of the PPR pushed research towards *morbillivirus* of ruminants, peste des petits ruminants and rinderpest virus [24]. This pathology of camel has since been confirmed in Sudan as the PPR [17].

This pathology similar to rinderpest clinically and antigenically [12,18, 12] reveals of paramount importance and growing *because the* economic losses associated with high morbidity (about 100%) and mortality (about 90%) in infected goats and sheep are considerable. The pathogen is a virus belonging to family *Paramyxoviridae and* the genus *Morbillivirus* [10]. The PPR virus was isolated for the first time in cell culture of sheep kidney by Gilbert et al. (1962) [11]. For a long time the virus was considered as a mutant of rinderpest virus adapted to small ruminants and which has lost its pathogenicity in this adaptation process for cattle. But soon after, with the development of molecular biology technologies, it has been shown that the PPR virus is a separate entity, but closely related antigenically to Rinderpest virus [7, 10].

The purpose of this work is to know the distribution of PPR in the Republic of Chad and present the seroprevalence of PPR in the areas of concentration of small ruminants in the country in order to provide basic information for launching a mass vaccination campaign against this formidable virus.

2. Materials and Methods

Sera were collected from sheep (548), goats (438) and camels (31). To obtain the serum, blood was collected from the jugular vein in dry tubes " *venoject* » then left at room temperature for 2 hours. After the clots are detached from the tube wall and removed. After removing the clots, the contents of the tubes are transported to the laboratory in cold where the serum is obtained by centrifugation at 3000 rev / min for 15 minutes. The sera are then frozen at minus 20 $^{\circ C}$ until further use.

This study focused on suspected cases of PPR based on clinical signs. Information on suspicions were provided by field workers involved in the of epidemiological surveillance network of animal diseases in Chad abbreviated REPIMAT [14]. The study provided also detailed information on the prevalence of antibodies directed against the PPR virus. Most clinical indications for this study were obtained from 11 regions out of 23 that account Chad (Map 1). These are the following areas: Chari-Baguirmi, Hadjer-Lamis, Mayo-Kebbi East and West, Tandjilé, Logone Oriental Mandoul, Moyen chari, Guera, Wadi-Fira and Ouaddaï. Sera were collected mainly from the slaughterhouse in N'Djamena. Analysis of sera was performed by competitive ELISA according to the protocol specified by the manufacturer. The ELISA kit used for this work is that marketed by *IDvet.* It was kindly provided by the International Atomic Energy Agency (IAEA).

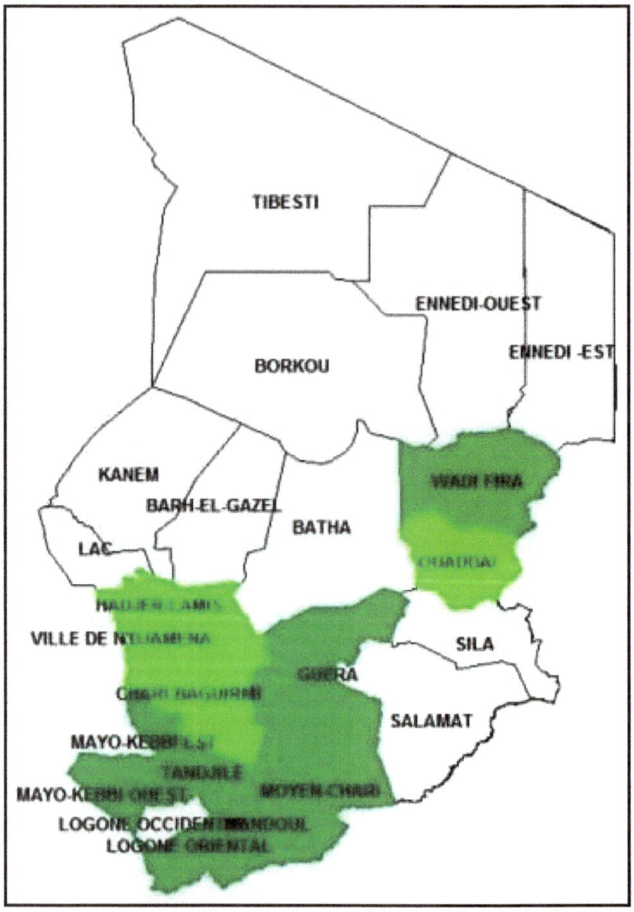

Figure 1. *Administrative division of Chad: The colored areas indicate areas where there has been suspected the PPR virus.*

Information relating to the PPR was collected from 2004 to 2014 in the field through epidemiological surveillance agents trained on the recognition of clinical signs of the disease. Samples taken during these suspicions were sent to the laboratory for diagnostic confirmation.

3. Results

Table 1 shows the number of suspected cases of the disease by region and year. From this table we can see that it is mostly in 2010 and 2011 when there were more suspicions of the disease. According to field workers, clinical signs are mostly seen on goats and lesser extent on sheep. These suspicions are based mainly on clinical signs of disease, but all are not confirmed by the laboratory for various reasons: Non-compliant and / or poorly preserved specimens.

Table 1. *Distribution of suspected cases of PPR by year and region.*

Period (years)	Number of suspicions	Localities (regions)	Laboratory confirmation
2004	27		02C
2005	15	Logone Oriental, Mandoul, Chari- Baguirmi, Ouaddai Tandjilé, Guera	01C
2006	06	Logone Oriental, Chari-Baguirmi, Hadjer- Lamis	NC
2007	18	Wadi -Fira, Mandoul, Hadjer-Lamis	01C
2008	14	Mandoul, Hadjer- Lamis, Wadi- Fira	14C
2009	08	Mandoul, Hadjer-Lamis, Lac, Logone Oriental, Wadi-Fira	03C
2010	66	Moyen Chari, Mandoul, Hadjer-Lamis	11C
2011	45	Hadjer -Lamis	02C
2012	28	Ouaddaï, Chari-baguirmi, Mandoul, Logone Oriental	01C
2013	03	Moyen Chari, Tandjilé	NC
2014	03	Hadjer - Lamis Tandjilé	03C
Grand Total	233		38

Sources : Epidemiological surveillance network of animal diseases in Chad (REPIMAT)
Legends : NC = no confirmed ; C = confirmed

As it can be seen in Map 1, a total of 11 regions out of 23 (18, 18%) in the country are affected by the disease. These regions are located in the eastern, central, south and southwest of the country.

Out of 233 suspicion cases recorded from 2004 to 2014, only 38 (16, 30%) were confirmed by the laboratory.

In total 1017 sera with 548 from sheep, 438 from goats and 31 from camels were collected at the slaughterhouse in N'Djamena. The analysis of these sera showed a prevalence rate of 34.48% in small ruminants which 19.26% for sheep and 15.21% for goats.

Considering the number of sera collected from sheep and goats, we observe the PPR prevalence rate of 34.67% and 27.37% respectively. No camel serum was positive vis-à-vis the PPR virus.

4. Discussion

The data collected from the field indicate that the clinical signs are mostly seen on goats. This is explained by the fact that the goats are more sensitive to the PPR virus than sheep. These observations are similar to those described by Bidjeh et al. (1995) [3] and Lefèvre et al. (1990)[16].

According to the annual reports of the Ministry of Livestock [8], frequency of occurrence of outbreaks of PPR is often seen between December and June. These observations support those reported by Wosu et al. (1990) [29] and Ban-bo et al. (2014) [4] indicating that the incidence of PPR is higher during the cold dry season (December and January) that during the rainy season.

From 2004 to 2014, 233 suspected PPR cases have been recorded by the REPIMAT of which 38 (16, 30%) were confirmed by the laboratory diagnosis. The small laboratory confirmation rate mentioned here would be due to non-availability of diagnostic reagents in the laboratory or inadequate or non-compliance samples collected in the field. Often the samples arrive at the laboratory in state of putrefaction, which does not allow the smooth running of the diagnosis. Hence the need to train field workers not only on the recognition of the disease, but also on how to perform the sampling, preservation and sending them to the laboratory.

This study showed a global seroprevalence of 34. 48%, with 34.67% for sheep, 27.37% for goats and 0% for camels. These results are different from those obtained by Lancelot [15] in sahelian zone of Chad indicating a global seroprevalence varying between 50 and 80%. But it was similar to those mentioned by Chauhan et al. (2005)[5], Singh et al. (2009)[26] and Abraham et al. (2005)[1] and Shaila et al (1989) [25]. These authors noted that the prevalence of PPR virus is higher in sheep than in goats. This is due to the fact that goats are more sensitive to the virus and making a severe form of the disease die quickly before developing antibodies against the virus.

Of 31 sera collected on camels, none was positive vis-à-vis the PPR virus. This result differs from that reported by Abraham et al. (2005)[1]; Ozkul et al. (2002)[21] and Megersa et al. (2012)[19], who detected antibodies directed against the PPR virus in camels. The explanation that can be given to this result of 0% prevalence of PPR in camels is that these animals were perhaps not in contact with the virus because out of an area where the disease does has not yet appeared; it can also be due to the low number of samples collected.

5. Conclusion

The information collected in the field from 2004 to 2014 showed that PPR has spread across much of territory of Chad. However, it remains endemic in central, eastern and southern part of countries.

The study showed a higher seroprevalence in sheep than in goats. By cons, no sera of camels were positive vis-à-vis the PPR virus.

Another serological survey would need to be undertaken in the population of camels in order to clarify their role in the epidemiology of PPR.

Acknowledgments

The authors would like to thank the International Atomic Energy Agency (IAEA) for graciously providing the ELISA kit that allowed the analysis of sera. They thank sincerely all the IRED technicians, who far and near, have contributed to the success of this study.

Our thanks also go to the site of the Directorate of Veterinary Services and REPIMAT agents, who kindly provided us with the information collected in the field.

We express our deep gratitude to the General Director of the Livestock Research Institute for Development (IRED).

References

[1] G. Abraham, A. Sintayehu, G. Libeau, E. Albina, F. Roger, Y. Laekemariam, D. Abaynech, K.M. Awoke, Antibody Against seroprevalence PPR virus in camels, cattle, goats and sheep in Ethiopia, Preventive veterinary medicine, 2005 (70), pp. 51-57.

[2] K. Bidjeh and M. Ouagal, Case PPR reported in several monitoring stations both in the Sahelian zone as Sudan, REPIMAT Bulletin, 1998 (7), pp.3.

[3] K.Bidjeh, P. Bornarel, M. Imadine and R. Lancelot, First isolation in Chad virus PPR. Rev. Elev. Med. Vet. Pays Trop., 1995, vol.48 (4), pp.295-300.

[4] Ban- bo Bebanto Antipas, Mian-Oudanang Koussou, Mopate Logténé Youssouf, Nakour Nargaye and Brahim Guihini. Knowledge of animal diseases and control methods at the Grand Kanem in Chad. Journal of Research in Biology, 2014, vol.4 (5), pp. 1387-1396

[5] C. Chauhan, Hemendra Singh Kher , K.R. Kaushal, Epidemiology of PPR in sheep and goats by serological, molecular and isolation methods in Gujarat, India, Advances in Animal and Veterinary Sciences, 2014, vol.2 4 (1), pp. 92-198.

[6] L. Gargadennec and A Lalanne, La peste des petits ruminants. Bull. Serv. Zoot. Epiz Afr. Occ. Fr., 1942 (5), pp.16-21.

[7] A. Diallo, T. Barrett, Mr. Barbon, Subbarao SM, W.P. Taylor, Differentiation of rinderpest and peste des petits ruminants viruses using cDNA clones Specific. ,J. vir. Methods, 1989 (23), pp. 127-136.

[8] Veterinary Services Department. Annual Report 2011, pp. 53.

[9] C.W. Furley, W.P.Taylor and T. U. Obi, An outbreak of PPR in a zoological collection. Vet. Record, 1987 (121), pp.443-447.

[10] E.P.J. Gibbs, W. P.Taylor, M.J. Lawman, J. Bryant, Classification of PPR virus as the fourth member of the genus Morbillivirus of. Intervirology ,1979 (11), pp.268-274.

[11] Y.Gilbert , J. Monnier, Adaptation of PPR virus to tissue cultures. Rev. Elev. Med. Vet. pays Tropicaux ,1962 (15), pp. 321-335.

[12] F.M. Hamdy, S.S. Breese, C.J. Deboer, Immunological relashionship between rinderpest and peste des petits ruminants viruses. Proc. 79 th Meet. US. Anim. Health Assoc., 1976, pp.168-179.

[13] F.M. Hedjer, I.T.R. Barnett and D.F. Gray, Some virus diseases of domestic animals in the Sultanate of Oman. Tropical Animal Health and Production, 1980 (12), pp.107-114.

[14] P. Hendrikx, K. Bidjeh, K. Ganda, M. Ouagal, H. Ali,M. Saboun, A. Maho, O.A. Idriss, Epidemiological surveillance network of animal diseases in Chad. Scientific and Technical Review of the OIE ,1997, pp.3-12.

[15] R. Lancelot, Enquête éco pathologique sur les maladies respiratoires des chèvres au Tchad, de la Recherche au développement. Capricorne , 1993, vol.7, pp.2-3.

[16] P.C. Lefèvre and A. Diallo. Peste des Petits Ruminants, Scientific and Technical Review of the Office International Des Epizooties, 1990, vol. 9 (4), pp.935- 950.

[17] A. I. Khalafalla, I .K. Saeed, Y. H. Ali, M.B. Abdurrahman, O. Kwiatek, G. Libeau; Z. Abbas, A.A. Obeida, A outbreak of PPR in camels in the Sudan, Acta Trop., 2010 (116), pp.161-165.

[18] P. Mornet, J. Orue, Y. G. Gilbert, Thiery, M. Sow, Peste des petits ruminants in French West Africa, its relations with rinderpest. Rev. Elev. Med. Vet. Pays Trop., 1956, (9) pp.313 - 342.

[19] B. Megersa and D.Biffa et al., Epidemic characterization and modeling within herd transmission dynamics of an emery Transboundary camel disease epidemic in Ethiopia, Tropical animal health and production, 2012, (44) pp. 1643-1651.

[20] F. Njeumi, Current scenario and control initiatives for PPR at global, regional and Countries levels according to the risk factor and socioeconomic impact. In: proceedings of the second regional conference on progressive control of PPR in south Asia, Khathamandu, Nepal, 19- 20 December 2013.

[21] A. Ozkul, Y. Akca, F. Alkan, T. Barrett, T. Karaoglu, S.B. Gagalp, J. Anderson, K. Yesilbag, C. Cokcaliskan, A. Gencay, Prevalence, distribution and host range of PPR virus, Turkey. Emerg. Infect. Dis., 2002(8), pp.708-712.

[22] A. Provost and Joubert, Peste des petits ruminants. Annual report laboratory Farcha, 1973, pp.106- 108.

[23] Y. Maurice, A. Provost and Y. C. Bourdin, PPR does exist in Central Africa ? In proceedings 40th General Conference of the Committee of the OIE report, 1972, (202), pp.9.

[24] F. Roger, A. Diallo, L. Yiggezu, M. C. Hurrard, G. Libeau, G. Y. Mebratu and B. Faye, Investigation of a new pathological conditions of camels in Ethiopia, Camel J. Pract. Res., 2000 (2), pp.163-166.

[25] M.S. Shaila, V. Purushothaman et al., PPR of sheep in India. Veterinary Record, 1989 (125) pp.602.

[26] R.K .Singh, V. Balamurugan et al., Possible control of PPR in India, Technical aspects, Vet Ital., 2009(45), pp. 449-462.

[27] W.P. Taylor, The distribution and Epidemiology of PPR: In Proceeding of 4 th International Conference of Institutions for Tropical Veterinary Medicine, Orlando Florida May 9-13, 1983.

[28] P. Wohlsein and J. Saliki, Rinderpest and peste des petits ruminants virus: Plague of wide and small ruminants : Biology of animal infections, Academic Press: London, UK, 2006, pp.69-85.

[29] L.O. Wosu, I. Okiri and P. A. Enwezor, Optimal time for vaccination Against PPR in goats in the humid tropical region in southern Nigeria: In proceedings of the first biennial conference of the African small ruminant research network. AICC, Arusha, Tanzania, 1990.

Molecular detection of some virulence genes in salmonella spp isolated from food samples in Lagos, Nigeria

Stella Ifeanyi Smith[1,*], Muinah Adenike Fowora[1], Adedamilola Atiba[2], Joseph Anejo-Okopi[3], Tina Fingesi[2], Mary Ehi Adamu[2], Emmanuel Adedayo Omonigbehin[1], Margaret Iteun Ugo-Ijeh[1], Moses Bamidele[2], Peter Odeigah[2]

[1]Molecular Biology and Biotechnology division, Nigerian Institute of Medical Research Yaba, Lagos, Nigeria
[2]Cell Biology and Genetics department, University of Lagos, Akoka, Lagos, Nigeria
[3]Microbiology department, University of Jos/Jos University Teaching Hospital, AIDS Prevention Initiative in Nigeria department, Jos, Nigeria

Email address:
stellaismith@yahoo.com (S. I. Smith)

Abstract: Food-borne salmonellosis is the most prevalent disease and major source of *Salmonella* spp in humans and its detection particularly in developing countries is quite cumbersome and time consuming. Molecular methods for its detection as well as the genotypic diversity of some of the genes responsible for *Salmonella* virulence are necessary. The aim of the study was to screen for *Salmonella* spp using the 16S rRNA, to determine whether the *inv*A gene is specific for *Salmonella* detection as well as virulence genotyping of some genes present in *Salmonella* spp (*inv*A, *sit*C and *spv*A, *spv*B and *spv*C) from food samples in Lagos, Nigeria. All 76 isolates tested positive for 16S rRNA gene while 53 (69.7%) were positive for *salm*3 *and salm*4 (389 bp) gene. PCR analysis of the *inv*A gene (284bp) showed that 73 (96.1%) were positive, 38 (50%) of the isolates were positive for *sit*C gene while none were positive for *spv*A and *spv*B and with the multiplex –PCR of *inv*A/*spv*C gene 25 (33%) were positive for *inv*A (244 bp) gene and none positive for *spv*C gene. The use of *invA* gene for *Salmonella* detection in our food samples is recommended however for most of our isolates the virulence genes were not detected.

Keywords: Detection, Food Samples, PCR, *Salmonella*, Virulence Genes

1. Introduction

Salmonella spp are bacteria that cause salmonellosis, and are also common causes of human foodborne outbreaks and diseases in developed and developing countries with attendant public health problem (1, 2). Salmonellosis affects 1.3 billion people worldwide each year with an estimated 3 million annual deaths from non-typhoidal salmonelloses (NTS) (3). The disease outcomes is due to exposure to *Salmonella* spp which ranged from mild symptoms to severe disease cases and sometimes fatal. *Salmonella* spp are carried by a range of domestic animals including birds and some wild animals. *Salmonella* spp have been widely isolated from raw meats, poultry and poultry products, milk and milk products and the enviroment (4),In addition outbreaks have also been associated with poor cooking, reheating of foods, and improper handling of food by food preparers. Representing 30.4% of all *Salmonella* strains isolated from humans, *Salmonella enterica* serotype Typhimurium was the second most commonly isolated *Salmonella* serotype in the Republic of Ireland (5).

Although *Salmonella* gastroenteritis is generally a self-limiting illness, severe cases may require antimicrobial therapy. Food contamination with antibiotic-resistant bacteria can be a major threat to public health, as the antibiotic resistance determinants can be transferred to other pathogenic bacteria, potentially compromising the treatment of severe bacterial infections. The prevalence of antimicrobial resistance among foodborne pathogens has increased during recent decades (6). This increase is attributed to the selection pressure created by using antimicrobials in food-producing animals, in addition to the unregulated use of antibiotics by humans in developing countries (7). The pathogenicity of NTS is attributed to identified virulence genes which has an association with antibiotic resistance (8).

In developing countries poor sanitary conditions appear to be the main risk factor for the transmission of *Salmonella* spp (9). Majority of Nigerians live below poverty level and patronize low cost foods such as those sold in bukas. However, the hygiene conditions of those bukas are not near standard hygiene practices, and this facilitates transmission of NTS infections among the food consumers. The conventional cultural method of detection of *Salmonella* in food is problematic, cumbersome and time consuming. To overcome this problem, molecular based PCR technique which is rapid, specific and more sensitive has been developed (10, 11). The use of amplification of DNA by PCR method is a revolutionary tool in diagnosis of pathogenic organisms (12, 11). Several virulence genes which are target genes for PCR amplification of *Salmonella* species including *invA, sitC, spv*A, *spv*B and *spvC*, have been used to detect as well as screen for genotypic virulence in *Salmonella* isolates from environmental and food samples (13, 8). Information on the use of PCR target genes to identifity the NTS from foods and food samples is lacking in Nigeria. The study is aimed at using PCR *inv*A virulenes genes to confirm the presence of *Salmonella* spp isolated from food samples as well as to screen our local isolates for some of the virulence genes (*sit*C and *spv*A, *spv*Band *spv*C).

2. Materials and Methods

A total of 189 isolates suspected to be *Salmonella* spp (from previous work on the identification of *Salmonella* from food samples using the REVEAL Kit (Neogen Corp. US), were cultured from meat samples on Salmonella-Shigella agar for 24 hours and pure colonies were obtained and identified using biochemical test as earlier described (4).

2.1. DNA Extraction

From the isolates, DNA was extracted by the boiling method and briefly, 1.5ml of the sample in broth was centrifuged at 10,000rpm for 5 minutes. The supernatant was discarded and the pellets were washed twice with sterile water. After this, 200µl of sterile water was added to the pellets, the pellets were vortexed to homogenize and boiled in a dry bath at 100°C for 10 minutes. This was followed by vortexing and centrifugation at 12,000rpm for 5 minutes. The supernatant containing the DNA was transferred to another tube and stored at -20°C. The concentration and purity of the extracted DNA was estimated using a Nanodrop spectrophotometer.

2.2. DNA Primers

The primers consist of 16S rRNA (574 bp), *salm* 3 and *salm* 4 (389 bp), *inv*A gene (284 bp), *sit*C (768 bp), *spv*A (604 bp) and *spv*B (1063 bp) and multiplex PCR (*inv*A/*spv*C gene: 244 bp and 571 bp). The primer sequences and their corresponding genes are shown in Table 1.

2.3. DNA Amplification

The reaction for all the PCR was carried out in a 25µl reaction mixture containing 1x PCR buffer (Promega, UK), 1.5mM Magnesium Chloride, 200µM of each dNTP, 20pMol of each primer, 1.25U Taq DNA polymerase (Promega, UK). The DNA was diluted to give a final concentration of between 10- 200ng/µl and 1µl of this was used in the PCR and the amplification was carried out in an Eppendorf Mastercycler Gradient (Eppendorf, Hamburg). The 16S rRNA gene, the PCR conditions were 3 min at 95^{0}C, followed by 30 cycles of 30 s at 95^{0}C, 30s at 54.1^{0}C and 1 min at 72^{0}C and final extension for 10 min at 72^{0}C. For the *salm* 3 and *salm* 4 primer, the PCR conditions were initial denaturation of 5 min at 95°C, followed by 35 cycles of 1 min at 95°C, 1 min at 65°C and 1.5 min at 72°C and final extension 10 min at 72°C. The *inv*A gene, the PCR conditions were initial denaturation of 1 min at 95°C, followed by 35 cycles of 1 min at 94°C, 1 min at 56°C and 1 min at 72°C and final extension of 10 min at 72°C.The results of the two *inv*A gene primers (*salm*3 and *salm*4, with *inv*A) were tested using the Chi-square analysis (one-tailed) as well as checking for the positive predictive value (PPV), negative predictive value (NPV), sensitivity and specificity with culture as the gold standard. The idea was to actually predict the best *inv*A gene that could be used to detect *Salmonella* species from our food samples. AS for the *sit*C primer, the PCR conditions were 3 min at 94^{0}C, followed by 30 cycles of 2 min at 94^{0}C, 1 min at 55^{0}C and extension for 1min at 72^{0}C for 1min and final extension for 5 min at 72^{0}C. As for the multiplex PCR (*inv*A/*spv*C) primer, the PCR conditions were 1 min at 94 ^{0}C, followed by 30 cycles of 30 s at 94 ^{0}C, 30 s at 56 ^{0}C, 2 min at 72^{0}C and final extension of 10 min at 72^{0}C. The PCR conditions for the *spv*A and *spv*B primers were; 5 min at 94^{0}C followed by 30 cycles of 30s at 94^{0}C, 30s at 60^{0}C, 1 min at 72^{0}C and then a final extension for 5 min at 72^{0}C. The PCR products were separated on a 1.5% agarose gel at 80 Volts and 50bp DNA ladder was used as molecular weight marker. The primer sequences and their corresponding genes are shown in Table 1.

3. Results

Only 76 (40.2%) of the 189 isolates were confirmed to be *Salmonella* spp using biochemical testing, out of these 53 (69.7%) of the isolates were confirmed as *Salmonella* spp using the *salm*3and *salm*4 primer set (Fig1). A total of 73 (96.1%) of the isolates were confirmed to be *Salmonella* spp using the *invA* primer set (Fig 2). Table 2 shows a comparison between the sensitivity, specificity, positive and negative predictive values of *invAF and invAR* with *salm* 3 and *salm* 4 primer sets. Chi square analysis between the two primers show there is statistical significance with a p-value of 0.019, $P<0.05$. Fig 3 shows the PCR amplification of 16S rRNA *Salmonella* spp. A total of 38 (50%) isolates were positive for the *sit*C gene (Fig 4) while the multiplex PCR of *inv*A/*spv*C genes showed that only 25(33%) were positive for the *inv*A gene and none was positive for the *spv*C gene.

Table 1. *Primer sequences and their corresponding genes*

Primer	Target gene	Sequence	Amplified fragment size (bp)
16S rRNA	Genus specific	5'-TGT TGT GGT TAA TAA CCG CA -3' 5'-CAC AAA TCC ATC TCT GGA -3'	571
Salm3/salm4	*inv*A	5'-GCTGCGCGCGAACGGCGAAG-3' 5'-TCCCGCCAGAGTTCCCATT-3	389
InvF/invAR	*inv*A	5' -ACA GTG CTC GTT TAC GAC CTG AAT -3' 5' -AGA CGA CTG GTA CTG ATC GAT AAT-3'	284
*Sit*C 3'	*sit*C	5'-CAG TAT ATG CTC AAC GCG ATG TGG GTC TCC- 5'- CGG GGC GAA AAT AAA GGC TGT GAT GAA C-3'	578
spvA	*spv*A	5'-GTC AGA CCC GTA AAC AGT-3' 5'-GCA CGC AGA GTA CCC GCA-3'	604
spvB	*spv*B	5'- ACG CCT CAG CGA TCC GCA -3' 5' – GTA CAA CAT CTC CGA GTA -3'	1063
Multiplex			
*inv*A/*spv*C		5'-ACA GTG CTC GTT TAC GAC CTG AAT-3' 5'-AGA CGA CTG GTA CTG ATC TAT -3'	244
*inv*A+*spv*C		5' GTC CTT GCT CGT TTA CGA CCT GAA T 3' 5' TCT CTT CTG CAT TTC GTC A 3'	571

Table 2. *Comparison between salm3/4 and invA genes in detection of Salmonella spp from foods*

	Sensitivity	Specificity	PPV	NPV
Salm ¾	70 (53/76)	100 (113/113)	100 (53/53)	83 (113/136)
Inv A	96 (73/76)	100 (113/113)	100 (73/73)	97 (113/116)

Culture is taken as the gold standard

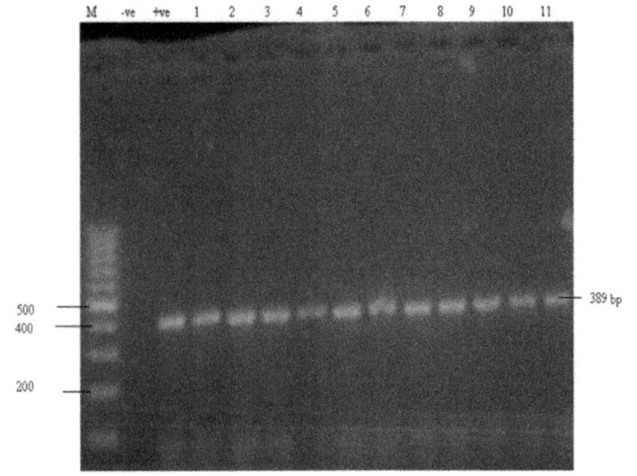

Fig 1. PCR amplification of invA genes of Salmonella spp using salm3 and salm4 gene primer Lanes M: 100 bp ladder; Lanes 1-11 PCR products (389 bp) of salm3/4 from Salmonella spp, lane –ve and +ve is the negative and positive controls respectively.

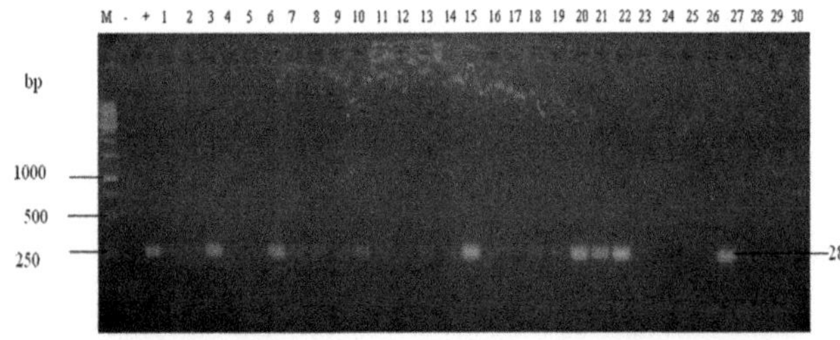

Fig 2. PCR amplification of invA genes of Salmonella spp using invA primers Lanes M: 100 bp ladder; Lanes 1-30 PCR products (284 bp) of invA primers from Salmonella spp, lane – and + is the negative and positive controls respectively. Some lanes show no amplification and were negative for this gene (24 – 26).

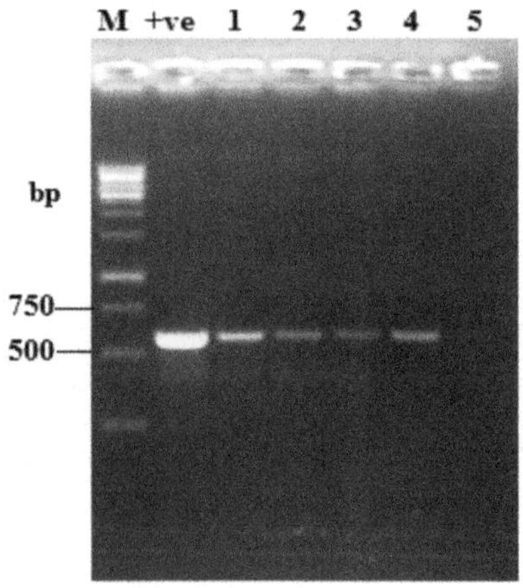

Fig 3. PCR amplification products of 574-bp DNA of 16Sr RNA gene of Salmonella spp. Lane M = 1 kb ladder, Lane (+) = positive control, Lane 5(-) =Negative, 1-4 positive.

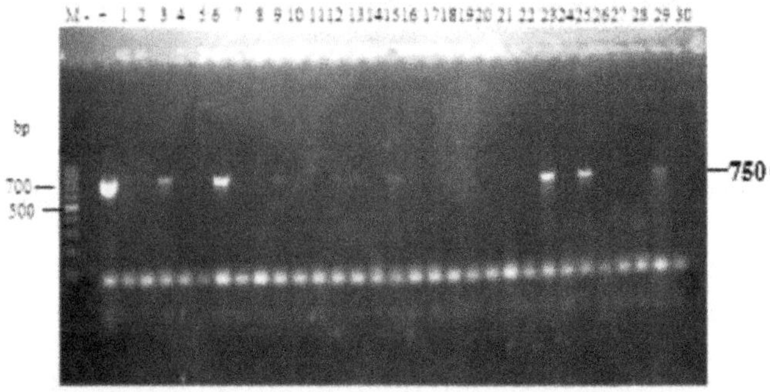

Fig 4. PCR amplification products of 750-bp DNA fragment of the sitC gene in Salmonella spp from food samples .Lane M = 100 base pair marker, Lane – = negative control, Lane + = positive control

4. Discussion

The prevalence of the virulence gene *inv*A from *Salmonella* spp in food samples presents a public health risks and often times result to food industry losses. The detection of *Salmonella* spp in the developing countries is usually difficult involving cultivation and identification of the organism from humans, food samples and environmental samples. The traditional cultural methods of isolating *Salmonella* spp are usually time consuming and laborious. Until recently researchers tried to establish a more rapid method, which could reduce the man-hours of *Salmonella* identification procedures from different ranges of samples. The use of primer set *invA*/*inv*E for confirmation of isolated *Salmonella* spp from turkeys came as relief from time waste on this identification procedures (14, 15). This effort was followed by the proposal of Ferretti *et al.* (16) for rapid detection method of *Salmonella* serotypes from samples within 12 hours using primers *salm*3and*salm*4 and *invA* gene. The *Salmonella invA* gene codes for the protein in the inner membrane which helps the organism to invade the host epithelial cell. The *invA* gene contains sequences unique to *Salmonella* spp and has proved appropriate for specific targets in various diagnostic and research laboratories (17). The use of *Salmonella* specific PCR with primers *invA* is rapid, sensitive and more specific for detection of *Salmonella* in many food samples. The amplification of *invA* gene has been validated as a standard for detection of invasion gene from *Salmonella* spp (12).

This study involves the use of PCR virulence genes which amplifies a 389 bp fragment within the conserved *inv*A gene (*salm*3and *salm* 4) of *Salmonella* spp as well as *inv*A that amplifies 284 bp to confirm the virulence and presence of *Salmonella* spp isolated from food samples. The results of the PCR on *inv*A genes showed that the primer set *inv*AF and *inv*AR that amplified 284 bp fragment (96.1%) was more discriminatory than the *salm* 3 and *salm* 4 primer set that amplified the 389bp (69.7%) fragment and the *inv*A gene was more sensitive than salm3/4 as well as its ability to detect more negative results in comparison to the latter, although both showed 100% PPV and specificity. A recent study from Korea had the same prevalence with the *inv*A gene (284 bp) of 96% (18), but their prevalence with *sit*C genes differed as they had higher prevalence of 96% compared to ours of 50%. Our result supports the ability of the two primer sets (*salm* 3/*salm* 4 and invA) to confirm the presence of virulence gene in *Salmonella* spp. Although the *salm*3 and *salm*4 primer set has been suggested to be useful for direct detection of *Salmonella* spp as well as excellent correlation with the conventional method (16) our results do not confirm that. Our findings however suggest that the primers are specific for detection of *Salmonella* spp, but *invA and invA* primers was found to be more sensitive (96.1%) compared to *salm*3 and *salm*4 (Table1) in the detection of *Salmonella spp* which corroborates the earlier reported study (19, 20). Our report with *inv*A gene (284bp) was also corroborated by a recent study from Nigeria on *Salmonella* spp isolated from cow raw milk and milk products in which *inv*A (284 bp) was prevalent in 100% of their isolates (21). This means that the use of *invA* gene (host invasion) can greatly reduce the reports of false-negative experienced in most laboratories (22). In monitoring some virulence genes such as those that code for iron transport (*sit*C) and the *Salmonella* virulence plasmids (*spv*A, *spv*B and *spv*C), our results showed that whereas half of the isolates encode genes for iron transport, none of our isolates carried the *spv*A, *spv*B and *spv*C genes. This report corroborated with arlier the study (23) in which *inv*A, *sef* genes were detected in their isolates from butcher shops in Brazil, and none of the isolates carried the *spv*C gene. To further corroborate the results of our study and that of Cossi *et al.* (23), 17 virulence genes were studied including *sit*C, *inv*A and *spv*B, none were positive for *spv*B in both food and environmental isolates (24). In a related study out of 17 virulence genes tested, 14 *Salmonella* isolates were positive with the exception of *spv*B, *cdt*B and *pef*A of which *pef*A and *spv*B were plasmid encoded (25). However, from this study only the *spv*B, *pef*A had lower prevalence (5% and 3.75% respectively) while other more common ones such as the *inv*A had 100% prevalence (13). This suggests the possibility that our local food isolates studied did not have virulence genes (*spv*A, *spv*B and *spv*C) located on the plasmids but could be chromosomally located as the latter three genes are for *Salmonella* virulence plasmids. The other possibility could be due to the fact that not all isolates contain virulence plasmids as lower proportions were reported in some reports for the plasmid virulence genes (26, 27, 13,18). In contrast Amini *et al.* (8) reported that the *spv* genes were prevalent in 88.6% for poultry, 90% for humans and 100% for bovine, although all isolates were S. Enteritidis, while other study reported moderate prevalence (42.85%) of the *spv*C gene in their commercial food stuffs (28). However, other reports have confirmed the ubiquitous distribution of virulence genes amongst *Salmonella* spp irrespective of the host (25). The PCR method using target gene remains a suitable molecular tool to diagnose *Salmonella* in human, animal and plant products (8, 19). These findings have important health implications to the entire populace considering the high prevalence of virulence genes in food samples studied and it also underscores the need for rapid identification of *Salmonella* virulence genes using the PCR method.

In conclusion, most of our food isolates harbored *invA* virulence gene and this has its economic and public significance for the country. Consequently, it is necessary to consider food hygiene programs to prevent health hazards and economic loss due to increasing morbidity and mortality associated with salmonellosis with possible antibiotic resistance. Rapid detection of *Salmonella* spp by PCR of *inv*A genes is recommended, although all our isolates did not harbor the *spv* genes. Further analysis on accurate distribution of virulence genes is important to help us develop accurate preventive measures against *Salmonella* spp in Nigeria.

Abbreviations

NTS: Non Typhoidal Salmonella, invA: invasion gene A, sitC: salmonella iron transport, spv: Salmonella plasmid virulence, salm: Salmonella, pefA: plasmid encoded fimbriae A

Acknowledgements

This study was funded by International Foundation for Science (IFS) grant noE/4020- given to SIS.

References

[1] Alvarez, A. M. Integrated approaches for detection of plant pathogenic bacteria and diagnosis of bacterial diseases. Ann. Rev. Phytopath. 42: 339-366. 2004.

[2] Amini, K., Salehi, T. Z., Nikbakht, G., Ranjbar, R., Amini, J and Ashrafganjooei, S. B. Molecular detection of *invA* and *spv* virulence genes in *Salmonella enteritidis* isolated from humans and animals in Iran. *Afr. J. Microbiol. Res*. 4: 2202 - 2210. 2010.

[3] Bennett, A. R., Greenwood, D., Tennant, C., Banks, J. G and Betts, R. P. Rapid and definitive detection of *Salmonella* in foods by PCR. Lett. Appl. Microbiol. 26:437-441. 1998.

[4] Chiu, C. H., Wu, T. L., Su, L. H., Chu, C., Chia, J. H., Kuo, A, J., Chien, M. S and Lin, T. Y. The emergence in Taiwan of fluoroquinolone resistance in *Salmonella* enterica serotype *Choleraesuis*. N. Eng. J. Med. 346: 413-419. 2002.

[5] Chiu, C.H. and Ou, J.T. Rapid identification of *Salmonella* serovars in faeces by specific detection of virulence genes, *inv*A and *spv*C, by an enrichment broth-multiplex PCR combination assay. J. Clin. Microbiol. 34: 2619 -2622. 1996.

[6] Cossi, M. V., Burin, R.C., Lopes, D.A., Dias, M. R., Castilho, N.P., de ArrudaPinto P. S. and Nero L. A. Antimicrobial resistance and virulence profiles of *Salmonella* isolated from butcher shops in Minas Gerais, Brasil. J. Food Prot. 76: 1633-1637. 2013.

[7] Darwin, K. H. and Miller V.L. Molecular basis of the interaction of *Salmonella* with the intestinal mucosa. Clin. J. Microbiol. 12: 405-428. 1999.

[8] Das, A., Hari, S. S., Shalini, U., Ganeshkumar, A. and Karthikeyan, M. Molecular Screening of Virulence Genes from *Salmonella enterica* Isolated from Commercial Food Stuffs. Biosciences Biotechnology Res. 9: 363-369. 2012

[9] Das, S., Singh, S., McClelland, M., Forst, S. and Gyaneshwar, P. Characterization of an Acid-Inducible Sulfatase in *Salmonella enteric* Serovar *Typhimurium*. Appl. Environ. Microbiol.79: 03707-03712. 2013.

[10] Dione, M. M., Ikmapayi, U., Saha, D., Mohammed, I. N., Adegbola, A. R., Geerts, S., Leven, M and Antonio, M. Antimicrobial resistance and virulence genes of non-typhoidal *Salmonella* isolates in the Gambia and Senegal. J. Infect. Dev. Ctries. 5: 765-775. 2011.

[11] Dorji, T.M., Mamata, G., Hyang-Mi, N., Chan, M.D., Suk-Chan. J. and Suk-Kyung, L. Antimicrobial susceptibility and virulence characteristics of Salmonella enteric Typhimurium isolates from healthy and diseased pigs in Korea. J. Food Prot. 9: 1481- 1486. 2014.

[12] Ferretti, R., Mannazzu, L., Cocolin, L., Comi, G. and Clementi, F. Twelve-hour PCR-based method for detection of *Salmonella* spp in food. Appl. Environ. Microbiol. 74: 977-978. 2001.

[13] Gorman, R., Bloomfield, S. and Adley, C. C. A study of cross-contamination of food-borne pathogens in the domestic kitchen in the Republic of Ireland. Int. J. Food Microbiol.76: 143-50. 2000.

[14] Guo, L., Killfer, J., Kenny, P. B. and Amick-Morri, J. D. Use of arbitrarily primed Polymerase chain reaction to study *Salmonella* ecology in a turkey production. Environ. Poult Sc.78: 24-31. 1999.

[15] Karmi, M. Detection of virulence genes (*inv*A) in *Salmonella* isolated from Meat and Poultry Products. Int. J. Genetics 3: 7-12. 2013.

[16] Li, Q., Skyberg, .J A., Fakhr, M. K., Sherwood, J.S., Molan, L.K. and Logue, C.M. Antimicrobial susceptibility and characterization of *Salmonella* isolates from processed Bison Carcasses. Appl Environ Microbiol 72: 3046- 3049. 2006.

[17] Malorny, B., Hoorfar, J., Bunge, C. and Helmuth, R. Multicenter validation of the analytical accuracy of *Salmonella* PCR: towards an international standard. App. Environ. Microbiol. 69: 290-296. 2003.

[18] Mezal, E. H., Stefanova, R. and Khan, A.A. Isolation and molecular characterization of *Salmonella* enterica serovar Javiana from food, environmental and clinical samples. Int. J. Food Microbiol. 164: 113 -118. 2013.

[19] Oluduro, A. O., Thonda, O.A. and Kolawole, D.O. Phenotypic and Molecular Characterization of Salmonella serotypes in cow milk and milk products in Nigeria. Afr. J. Biotechnology 13: 3774 -3789. 2014.

[20] Pan, T. M. and Liu, Y. J. Identification of Salmonella enteritidis isolates by polymerase chain reaction and multiplex polymerase chain reaction. J. Microbiol. Immun. Infect. 35: 147-151. 2002.

[21] Ramya, P., Madhavarao, T. and Rao, L. V. Study on the incidence of *Salmonella enteritidis* in poultry and meat samples by cultural and PCR methods. Vet. World5: 541-545. 2012.

[22] Salehi, T. Z., Mahzounieh, M. and Saeedzadeh, A. Detection of *InvA* Gene in Isolated *Salmonella* from Broilers by PCR Method. *Int. J. Poultry Sc*. 4: 8, 557-559. 2005.

[23] Schneder, A., Gronewald, C., Fandke, M., Kurth, B., Barkowski, S. and Berghof-ager, K. Real-time detection of the genus *Salmonella* with the Light Cycler system. Biochem. J. 4: 19-21. 2002.

[24] Skyberg, J.A., Logue, C.M. and Nolan, L.K. Virulence genotyping of *Salmonella* spp with multiplex PCR. Avian Dis. 50: 77- 81. 2006.

[25] Smith, S. 1., Opere, B., Fowora, M., Aderohunmu, A., Ibrahim, R., Omonigbehin, E., Bamidele, M. and Adeneye, A. Molecular characterization of *Salmonella* spp directly from snack and food commonly sold in Lagos, Nigeria. Southeast Asian J. Trop. Med. 43: 718-23. 2012.

[26] Swamy, S.C., Barnhart. H., Lee, M.D. and Dreesen, D.W. Virulence determinants *inv*A and *spv*C in salmonellae isolated from poultry products, wastewater and human sources. Appl. Environ. Microbiol. 62: 3768 -3771. 1996.

[27] Todd, E. C. D., Greig, J. D., Bartleson, C. A and Michaels, B. S. Outbreaks where food workers have been implicated in the spread of foodborne disease. Part 4. Infective doses and pathogen carriage. J. Food Prot. 71: 2339-2373. 2008.

[28] Van den Bogaard, A. E and Stobberingh, E. E. Epidemiology of resistance to antibiotics. Links between animals and humans. Int. J. Antimicrob. Agents14: 327-35. 2000.

15

Investigation of Rotavirus Infection in Calves with Diarrhea in Northeast Turkey

Volkan Yilmaz

Department of Virology, Faculty of Veterinary Medicine, University of Kafkas, Kars, Turkey

Email address:
volkankara1980@hotmail.com

Abstract: Rotavirus is the most common cause of severe diarrhea in newborn calves. In this study, it was aimed to investigate frequency of Rotavirus infections in calves in Kars region in Northeast Turkey by feces sampling 112 diarrheic calves of 0-6 months old. Feces samples were tested for Rotavirus antigen by Enzyme Linked Immunosorbent Assay (ELISA). Of the 112 feces samples examined by ELISA 10 samples were identified as positive (8.92%). At the molecular stage, reverse transcription polymerase chain reaction (RT-PCR) technique was used to determine the presence of Rotavirus nucleic acid by using specific generic primers for VP6 genetic regions in feces samples. The 10 samples that were rotavirus antigen positive by ELISA were also positive on RT-PCR technique. The proportion of positivity in feces samples suggested that rotavirus infections are common in the Kars region in Northeast Turkey.

Keywords: Calves, Diarrhea, ELISA, RT-PCR

1. Introduction

Factors that cause diarrhea include viruses, bacteria, protozoa, poor hygiene, lack of colostrum consumption and insufficient diet. These factors can cause diarrhea together or by themselves. One of the main viral factors that cause diarrhea in calves is rotaviruses. Rotaviruses are the important etiological agents of acute viral gastroenteritis in young ones of many species of animals and human. Rotavirus infections cause major economic losses in neonates of many domestic animals [23]. Rotaviruses are classified in the genus *Rotavirus* of the subfamily *Sedoreovirinae* in the family *Reoviridae* are characterized by segmented genomes comprising of 11 segments of double stranded RNA contained within a triple layered protein shell composed of a core, inner capsid and outer capsid. Three structural proteins, VP1, VP2 and VP3, form the core of the rotavirus particle. The group specificity of the virus is determined by epitopes on the VP6 protein and based on it; rotaviruses can be divided into seven distinct groups (A - G) [10, 15, 19, 25].

Electron microscopy, latex agglutination, polyacrylamide gel electrophoresis and antigen ELISA techniques are used to diagnosed the Rotavirus infections [4, 5, 6, 12]. When there is a need to examine a large number of samples, latex agglutination and ELISA is a rapid and inexpensive solution. The specificity and sensitivity of these tests is over 90%. The reverse transcription polymerase chain reaction (RT-PCR) is also employed using generic or type-specific primers prepared for various types of viruses [2, 13, 16, 24].

The goal of this study was to obtain information about the presence, viroprevalence of rotavirus infections, which have not been previously reported in calves raised in the region of Kars, Northeast Turkey. The data that was obtained showed that the proportion of positivity in feces samples suggested that rotavirus infections are common in the Kars region in Northeast Turkey.

2. Materials and Methods

2.1. Feces Samples

Feces samples were collected from 112 calves with diarrhea in private small scale production units (< 20 cattle) in the Kars District of Turkey (Figure 1). All calves were taken colostrums and between 0-6 months. Samples were collected during the first days of the disease. Feces samples were stored in -80°C until used.

2.2. ELISA

A commercial ELISA kit (Rotavirus Elisa Kit Cat.Nr.Bio

K 067, Jemelle-Belgium) detecting rotavirus antigen in feces samples was used in the study according to the manufacturer's instructions. After incubation at room temperature (20 to 25°C) for 10 minutes, the process was finished by adding 50 µl stop solution (1M phosphoric acid) to all wells. Optical densities were measured with an ELISA reader at 450 nm absorbance, according to the instructions in the test procedure. Samples giving values equal to or greater than 0.150 were accepted as positives and values less than 0.150 as negatives.

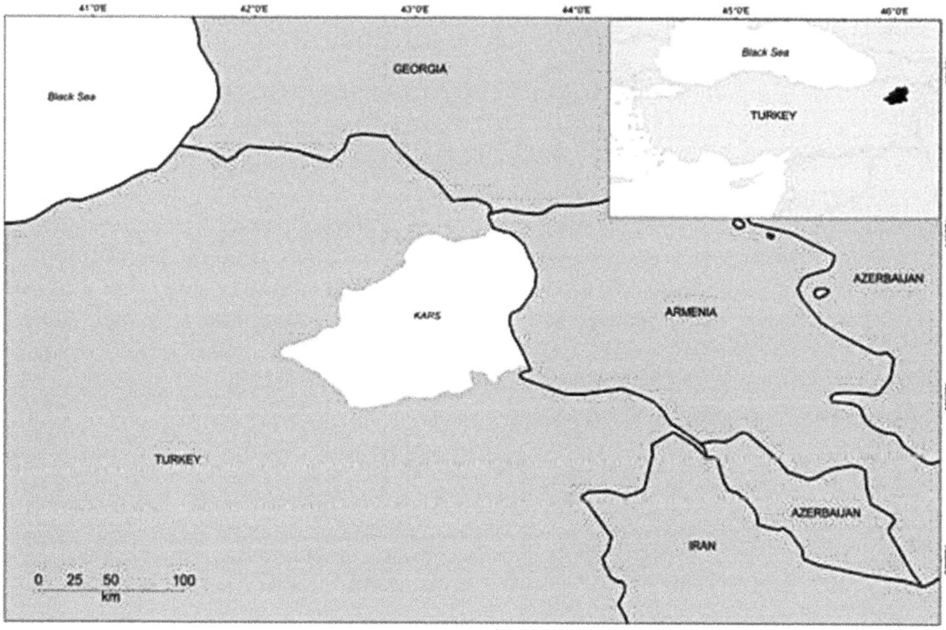

Fig. 1. Geographical positioning of the Kars region in which the study was performed.

2.3. RNA Extraction and Reverse Transcriptase Polymerase Chain Reaction (RT-PCR)

From fecal samples, viral RNA was extracted using a Viral Nucleic Acid Extraction Kit (Vivantis, Malaysia), according to the manufacturer's recommendation. The follow-up cDNA synthesis was carried out using a first strand cDNA synthesis Kit (Fermentas, Lituhania) as described by the manufacturer's protocol, using random primers. The reaction mixture was incubated first at 25°C for 10 mins, followed by a second incubation at 42°C for an hour and then 70°C for 10 min, for inactivation on Moloney murine leukaemia virus reverse transcriptase (MMLV-RT). Amplification of cDNAs by PCR was performed using the primer pairs VP6. The primer VP6-F (5′- GAC GGV GCR ACT ACA TGG T -3′) and primer VP6-R (5′- GTC CAA TTC ATN CCT GGT GG 3′) primers flank a 379 bp DNA fragment for rotavirus [22]. PCR was carried out in a total volume 50 µL containing 5 µL of cDNA to the master mix, 4.5 µL of 10 X reaction buffer (100 mM Tris-HCl pH 8.3 and 500 mM KCl), 2 µL of 50 mM $MgCl_2$, 20 pmole from of each of the primers, 1 µL of 10 mM dNTP mix, and 0.2 µL of 5 IU Taq DNA polymerase (MBI, Fermentas, Lithuania), 35.3 µL of RNAse free distiled water. The PCR was initiated by a single denaturation step at 94°C for 2 min, followed by 35 cycles of 1 min at 94°C, annealing at 55°C for 1 min. The mixture was then incubated, as a single step, for 1 min at 72°C and 7 min at 72°C for final extension. Ten microlitres of each PCR product were analyzed on 1% agarose (Prona, Spain) gel containing ethidium bromide (Sigma, USA).

3. Results

Of the 112 feces samples examined by ELISA 10 samples were identified as positive (8.92%). The 10 samples that were rotavirus antigen positive by ELISA were also positive on RT-PCR technique. In this study, the presence of rotavirus antigen were determineted between the ages 0-15 days in diarrheic calves. Distributions antigen positive samples with ELISA and RT-PCR according to ages were shown in Table 1.

Table 1. Distributions antigen positive samples with ELISA and RT-PCR according to age.

Age (days)	No. of calves with diarrhea (0-15 days)	Positive	Positive (%)
0-5	14	5	35.71
5-10	6	3	50.00
10-15	11	2	18.18

4. Discussion

Rotavirus is the major cause of acute gastroenteritis in newborn calves. Rotavirus infection is non-viremic, have very short incubation period, and manifests profuse diarrhea and severe dehydration in neonates [13]. Rotavirus causes significant economic losses for cattle farms due to death or weight loss in infected animals, the cost of veterinary services and other reasons.

Numerous studies [7, 9, 11, 17, 18, 20, 21, 27, 30, 31, 32] conducted with regard to the rotavirus infection in Turkey and around the world have demonstrated that the infection is widespread in populations of cattle. These studies have reported that incidence of rotavirus infection varies between 10–62.5% in cattle. This study is the first one to determine the viroprevalence of rotavirus in calves with diarrhea in the Kars District of Turkey. The location for the study was chosen because Kars is located in the middle of an animal transit route between North-East Anatolia and Caucasus functioning as a bridge between Asia and Europe. Yildirim et al. [32] determined rotavirus seropositivity rates in cattle as 29.3% in the same region where this study was conducted. They examined total 498 cattle serum samples collected from northeast Turkey by virus neutralisation test and found 146 out of 498 cattle blood samples positive.

Fecal contamination plays an important role in transmission of rotavirus infection. Rotavirus spread too much with feces. Both healthy animals and calves with diarrhea spread too much spread rotavirus antigen [26]. Many methods are used to determined the presence of rotavirus antigen. ELISA, Polyacrylamid Gel Electrophoresis (PAGE), Latex Agglutination (LA), Electron Microscopy (EM), Immunofluorescence (IF) and Immunoperoxidase (IP) are most widely used methods [12, 28, 29]. ELISA is a simple, sensitive, specific and rapid test; it used widely calves with diarrhea in feces for the determination of rotavirus. ELISA had the advantage of being inexpensive for examination of many samples and has the probability of being much more sensitive. Recently, RT-PCR, using the VP4 or VP7 gene primers, is much widely used for detection of animal rotaviruses [1, 3, 18, 24]. Also, semi-nested or multiplex RT-PCR are being developed. Besides the sequencing of the outher capsid genes has also helped in differentiating various rotavirus isolates [28]. Using antigen ELISA and RT-PCR depending on the amplification of the VP6 gene of rotavirus, feces samples of calves with diarrhea collected from farm in Turkish Republic of Northern Cyprus were checked by Alkan et al. [3]. In the study, the aetiological agent was tested by RT-PCR with generic and type-spesific to the genome segments encoding VP4 and VP7 of rotavirus. It was determited that the rotavirus circulating within the farm belongs to G6 and P [11] genotype in the study. In this study, RT-PCR technique was used to determine the presence of rotavirus nucleic acid by using specific generic primers for VP6 genetic regions in feces samples. The 10 samples that were rotavirus antigen positive by ELISA were also positive on RT-PCR technique.

In this study, of the 112 feces samples tested by ELISA 10 samples were detected positive (8.92%). This percentage is lower than the percentages found in studies conducted in past years [8, 14]. This situation can explain that the ages of calves higher than these studies. These studies showed mostly between the ages of 0-15 days. Although, feces samples of calves of 0-6 months old were tested by ELISA in this study, the presence of rotavirus antigen were determineted between the ages 0-15 days in calves. Similarly, Robaiee and Farwachi [4] were detected rotavirus antigen in neonatal calves, aged between 8-15 days by antigen ELISA. They examined a total of 220 feces samples collected from both diarrheic (n=110) and non- diarrheic (n=110) neonatal calves, aged between 1– 30 days from different part of Mosul city, Iraq. In the study, rotavirus infection was found in n=17 (15.5%) of 110 diarrheic calves and only 5 feces samples (4.5%) from 110 non-diarrheic animals.

5. Conclusion

The virological data that were collected in this study indicate the presence of rotavirus infection in calves with diarrhea in the Kars District of Turkey. An evaluation of the data leads us to the conclusion that a vaccination program needs to be implemented to bring rotavirus infections under control. Furthermore, genomic identification of the rotavirus isolates obtained from this study will play an important role in future studies on protection and control strategies to combat and prevent the spread of infection.

References

[1] A. A. ALFIERI, M. E. PARAZZI, E. TAKIUCHI, K. MEDICI, et al. Frequency of group a rotavirus in diarrheic calves in Brazilian cattle herd, 1998-2002. *Trop. Anim. Health Pro.* 2006, 38, 521-526.

[2] F. ALKAN, V. GULYAZ, M. O TIMURKAN, S. IYISAN, et al. A large outbreak of enteritis in goat flocks in Marmara, Turkey, by G8P [1] group A rotaviruses. *Ach Virol.* 2012, 157: 1183-1187.

[3] F. ALKAN, M. O. TIMURKAN, I. KARAYEL. The Molecular Characterization and Detection of Group A Rotavirus From Calves with Diarrhea in Turkish Republic of Northern Cyprus. *Kafkas. Univ. Vet. Fak. Derg.*, 2015, 21 (1): 127-130.

[4] I. A. AL-ROBAIEE, M. I. AL-FARWACHI. Prevalence of rotaviral infection in diarrheic neonatal calves in Mosul city, Iraq. doi: 10.5455/vetworld.2013.538-540.

[5] Y. AL-YOUSIF, J. ANDERSON, C. CHARD-BERGSTROM, A. BUSTAMANT, et al. Evaluation of a latex agglutination kit (virogenrota test) for detection of bovine rotavirus in fecal samples. *Clin. Diagn. Lab. Immunol.* 2001, 8(3): 496-498.

[6] M. ARENS, E. M. SWIERKOSZ. Detection of rotavirus by hybridization with a nonradioactive synthetic DNA probe and comparison with commercial enzyme immunoassays and silver-stained polyacrylamide gels. *J. Clin. Microbiol.* 1989, 27(6): 1277–1279.

[7] E. F. BARBOSA, H. C. P. FIGUEIREDO, A. M GARCIA, Z. I. P LOBATO, et al. Group A rotavirus in calves in Minas Gerais State, Brazil. *Ciencia. Rural.* 1998, 28, 435–439.

[8] I. BURGU, Y. AKCA, F. ALKAN, A. OZKUL, et al. Yeni doğan ishalli buzağılarda rotavirusların Elektron Mikroskopi (EM), Enzyme Linked Immunosorbent Assay (ELISA) ve Polyacrylamide Gel Electrophoresis (PAGE) teknikleri ile çabuk teşhisi ve antijenik karakterizasyonu. *AU. Vet. Fak. Derg.* 1995, 42: 491-498.

[9] M. A. CABALAR. serologic study of rotavirus infection in some dairy cattle herds in Van province. *YYÜ Vet Fak Derg* 2004, 15 (1-2): 33-35.

[10] E. B. CARSTEN. Ratification vote 10 taxonomic proposals to the İnternational Committe on taxonomy of viruses 2009. *Arch. Virol.* 2010, 155, 133-146.

[11] R. S. CHAUHAN, N.P. SINGH. Epidemiology of rotavirus infection in calves in India. *Int. J. Anim. Sciences,* 1996, 11, 221–223.

[12] S. K. DASH, A. TEWARI, A. GOEL, A. K. BHATIA. Detection of Rotavirus fromdiarrhoeic cow calves in Mathura. *India. Vet. World,* 2011, Vol. 4(12): 554-556.

[13] K. DHAMA, R. S CHAUHAN, M. MAHENDRAN, S. V. S MALIK. Rotavirus diarrhoea in bovine and other domestic animals. *Vet. Res. Commun.* 2009, 33: 1-23.

[14] M. EKIK. Konya bölgesinde yeni doğan ishalli buzağılardan rotavirus antijenlerinin belirlenmesi ve annelerinden rotavirus antikorlarını tespiti. SU Sağ. Bil. Enst., PhD. Thesis, Konya. 2002.

[15] M. K. ESTES, A. Z. KAPIKIAN. Rotaviruses. In, Knipe DM, Howley PM (Eds): Field's Virology. 1917-1974, Williams and Williams, Philadelphia, 2007.

[16] E. FALCONE, M. TARANTINO, L. DI TRANI, P. CORDIOLI, et al. Determination of bovine rotavirus G and P serotypes in Italy by PCR. *J. Clin. Microbiol.* 1999, 37: 3879-3882.

[17] K. FUKAI, T. SAKAI, H. KAMATA, H. Distribution of G serotypes and P genotypes of bovine group A rotavirus isolated in Japan. *Aust. Veter. J.,* 1998, 76, 418–422.

[18] L. GARAICOECHEA, K. BOK, L. R. JONES, G. COMBESSIES, et al. Molecular characterization of bovine rotavirus circulating in beef and dairy herds in Argentina during a 10-year period (1994–2003). *Vet. Microbiol.,* 2006, 118, 1–11.

[19] S. GAZAL, A. K. TAKU, B. KUMAR. Predominance of rotavirus genotype G6Pin diarrhoeic lambs. *The Vet J.* 2011, 193, 299-300.

[20] S. O. GUMUSOVA, Z. YAZICI, H. ALBAYRAK, Y. MERAL. Rotavirus and coronavirus prevalence in healthy calves and calves with diarrhea. *Medycnya. Weterinaria.* 2007 63, 62–64.

[21] A. H. HUSSEIN, E. CORNAGLIA, M. S. SABER, Y. EL-AZHARY. Prevalence of serotypes G6 and G10 group A rotaviruses in dairy calves in Quebec. *Can. J. Vet. Res.,* 1995 59, 235–237.

[22] M. ITURRIZA-GOMARA, C. WONG, S. BLOME, U. DESSELBERGER et al. Molecular characterization of VP6 genes of human rotavirus isolates: Correlations of genogroups with subgroups and evidence of independent- segregation. *J. Virol.* 2002, 76: 6596-6601.

[23] A. Z. KAPIKIAN, R. M. CHANOCK. Rotaviruses. Fields Virology, 4th ed. Lippincott Williams and Wilkins, Philadelphia, 1996. pp: 1657-1708.

[24] M. H. KHAFAGI, M. A. MAHMOUD. Prevalence of rotavirus infections in small ruminants. *Global Veterinaria.* 2010, 4: 539-543.

[25] J. MATTHIJNSSENS, M. CIARLET, S. M. MCDONALD, H. ATTOUIH, K. BANYAI, et al. Uniformity of rotavirus strain nomencuature proposed bythe Rotavirus Classification Working Group (RCWG). *Arch. Virol.,* 2011, 156, 1397-1413.

[26] A. MAYAMEEI, G. MOHAMMADI, S. A. YAVARI, E. FISHERY, et al. Evaluation of relationship between rotavirus and corona virus infection with calf diarrhea by capture ELISA. *Comp. Clin. Pathol.* 2010, 19: 533-557.

[27] G. PISANELL, V. MARTELLA, U. PAGNINI, L. DEMARTINO LORUSSO, et al. Distribution of G (VP7) and P (VP4) genotypes in buffalo group A rotaviruses isolated in Southern Italy. *Vet. Microbiol.* 2005, 110, 1–6.

[28] N. REIDY, G. LENNON, S. E. FANNING, E. POWER, et al. Molecular characterization and analysis of bovine rotavirus strains circulating in Ireland 2002–2004. *Vet. Microbiol.* 2006, 117, 242–247.

[29] A. D. STEELE, A. GEYER, G. H. GERDES. Rotavirus infections. In: Coetzer, J.A.W. and Tustin, R.C. (eds), Infectious diseases of Livestock, Oxford University Press, Southern Africa, 2004, 1256–1264.

[30] P. VENDE, R. KAROUM, G. MANET, C. RIZET, et al. Molecular epidemiology or bovine rotaviruses from the Charolais area. *Vet. Res.,* 1999, 30, 451–456.

[31] K. VERDIER KLINGENBERG, L. SVENSSON. Group A rotavirus as a cause of neonatal calf enteritis in Sweden. *Acta Vet. Scan.,* 1998, 39, 195–199.

[32] Y. YILDIRIM, S. BILGE DAGALP, M.T. TAN A.T. KALAYCIOGLU. Seroprevalence of the Rotavirus and Corona Virus Infections in Cattle. *J. Anim. Vet. Adv.* 2008, 7: 1320-1323.

Sheep Infection by *Haemonchus* Species: Effect on Haematocrit and Evaluation of the FAMACHA© Method in Arsi Negele District, Oromia, Ethiopia

Guash Abay[1,*], Tilaye Demissie[2], Amene Fekadu[3], Teshale Teklue[4]

[1]Abergelle Agricultural Research Center, Abyi-Adi, Ethiopia
[2]Addis Ababa University, Addis Ababa, Ethiopia
[3]Hawassa University, Hawassa, Ethiopia
[4]Mekelle Agricultural Research Center, Mekelle, Ethiopia

Email address:
guashaba81@gmail.com (G. Abay)

Abstract: Infection with *Haemonchus* species in sheep at Arsi- Negele district was determined by differential third-stage larvae and the objective was to evaluate the validation of FAMACHA© chart in the diagnosis of *Haemonchus* infection. The animal's anemia level was determined by using the FAMACHA© method and their corresponding PCV (packed cell volume) were determined by haematocrit centrifugation method. The color of the ocular membrane of all animals was scored 1 to 5 using the FAMACHA© card and blood samples were collected from each animal for determination of PCV. Fecal samples also collected from sampled animals tested for fecal egg counts (FEC), and fecal culture for identification of third stage larvae of *Haemonchus* species. All sheep studied were negative for *Fasciola* and were not heavily infested by lice and ticks. A highly significant negative correlations [(R-square = 0.28, Coef. = -0.78); (R-square= 0.58, Coef= -0.34)] was observed between *Haemonchus* larvae and PCV, and PCV and eye color respectively. Positive correlations [(R-square= 0.19, Coef. = 1.53); (R-square=0.274, Coef= 0.05)] was observed between FAMACHA© score and *Haemonchus* infection, and FAMACHA© score and egg per gram of faces (EPG) respectively. The PCV of the *Haemonchus* positive sheep had a strong negative correlation with the EPG (R-square=0.53, Coef= -0.023). We evaluated the validity of FAMACHA© eye scoring to measure severely infested sheep and got strong correlation among FAMACHA© eye scoring, PCV and Fecal culture positivity. As a conclusion the FAMACHA© anaemia scoring guide can be used to treat only severely anemic sheep and hence reduce mass treatment and this reduce chance of drug resistance.

Keywords: Arsi-Negele, FAMACHA, FEC, *Haemonchus*, PCV, Sheep

1. Introduction

There are about 25.5 million sheep and 24.06 million goats in the country playing an important role in the livelihood of resource-poor farmers [1]. Unlike the large potential of small ruminants in the country their productivity is low. The major constraints of small ruminant production in Ethiopia are diseases, feed shortage and poor management.

Helminthosis has nationwide distribution and is also considered as one of the major setbacks to livestock incurring huge indirect and direct losses in the country [2]. A loss of US $81.8 million is reported annually due to helminth parasites in Ethiopia [3]. The blood feeding nematode, *Haemonchus* species, is among the most important gastrointestinal parasite of sheep. This parasite, besides its, pathologic significance has a very important position from epidemiological point of view in that it is a parasite of tropical, subtropical and temperate regions of the world [4].

The control of gastro-intestinal parasites of livestock in Ethiopia is based on only the use of anthelmintics. Anthelmentics are imported in bulky by the government, individuals and privates, and distributed all over the country and used voraciously by every individual including farmer. The use of anthelmintics at regular intervals for an extended period and treating by mass when one animal shows any clinical sign has resulted in the development of resistance of nematodes to one or more available drugs, for instance against benzimidazoles [5]. There is no field diagnostic technique introduced in Ethiopia but the FAMACHA© system can help in the reduction of drug resistance by treating those only unable to cope with current *Haemonchus* species challenge on pasture, by using clinical anaemia as the determinant. Although FAMACHA© is a novel system of treating only animals with clinical signs and then reducing the chance of development of drug resistance it was checked in developed countries like South Africa, and U.S.A at bigger farm levels and comparatively at net environment, it was not practiced in countries like Ethiopia where mixed parasitc infection, and where traditional feeding practice is followed. So the objectives of this work were to evaluate the effect of haemonchosis on haematocrit value and eye mucous membrane for decision making of individual animal treatment and evaluation of the importance of the FAMACHA© system in Ethiopia in field diagnosis.

2. Material and Methods

2.1. Study Area Description

The study was carried out in and around Arsi-Negele district peasant associations found around Arsi-Negele town from November 2011 to April 2012. The district is located at an altitude of 1500 to 2300 meters above sea level in the longitude $7^0 20'$N and latitude of 38^0 40'E. The district has an estimated 379,645, cattle population, 111,062 sheep, 151,353 goats, 14,114 horses, 1,455 mules, 27,971 donkeys, 103,206 poultry and 3,450 bee hives [6].

2.2. Study Animals

Privately owned sheep flocks were included in the study. The flocks were taken out in the morning for grazing on communal land, road sides and brought back to their holding in the evening. The small ruminants were grazed together with cattle in the open spaces. Different sheep flocks were visited on weekly basis during which 400 sheep (227 Female and 173 Male) were randomly selected from which sample has been collected. Animals free of Fasciola, tick and lice infestation based on the faecal examination and inspection respectively were included in this study.

2.3. Study Design and Sampling Technique

A cross-sectional study was followed and animals were randomly selected. Sex, age, eye mucous membrane and body condition of randomly selected animals was recorded. The eye mucous membrane color was compared to the FAMACHA© card and was recorded, and 5 ml blood was collected from the jugular vein in vacutainers with anticoagulant (EDTA) after preparing the sites. During sampling general information related to grazing, housing, breeding condition, deworming practice and other factors were collected for each sampled animal.

2.4. Sample Size Determination

To maximize the number of animals and to evaluate the system at the prevalence level the sample size was determined using the formula given by [7]:

$$N = \frac{1.96^2 (P)(1-P)}{d^2} \tag{1}$$

Where; N= sample size, 1.96= the value of z at 95% confidence level, P= expected prevalence, d= desired absolute precision level at 95% confidence level

Expected prevalence of 50% were considered as there was no previous study in the area and 5% absolute precision, the minimum sample size calculated was 384. Therefore about 400 sheep of all age group were selected from study sites.

2.5. Sample Collection

2.5.1. Blood Sample Collection

Blood samples were taken in EDTA coated vacutainer tubes from the jugular vein to determine PCV. The blood samples were taken to the laboratory of veterinary parasitology and pathology, school of veterinary medicine and PCV were determined immediately after arrival using the micro-haematocrit method.

2.5.2. Fecal Sample Collection

Fecal samples were collected per-rectum using a disposable plastic gloves in universal while blood sample collection and labeled and kept cool before transportation to the laboratory using ice box on the same day of collection and were processed immediately.

The positive samples were subjected to fecal culture for investigating the infective larvae. Fecal sample that were positive *Fasciloa* egg were discarded.

2.6. Laboratory Investigation

2.6.1. Packed Cell Volume Determination

At the laboratory PCV was determined and the level of anemia was recorded for each animal according to [8].

2.6.2. Egg per Gram of Faeces Determination

A modified McMaster technique was used to determine fecal egg counts according to [9].

2.6.3. Ova Culture

After screening for *Fasciola* and FECs the feces were cultured for L_3 of *Haemonchus* species at a temperature of approximately 25^0c according to [9].

2.6.4. Identification of Haemonchus Species Third Stage Larvae

The identification was conducted based on the distinguishing features such as the shape of the "head" (cranial extremity) of the larvae or the length of the sheath "tail" (the extension of the sheath from the tip of the larval caudal extremity to the tip of the tail of sheath) [10].

3. Data Analysis

Data were subjected to stata-11 software. Correlations between PCV and eye mucous membrane color, PCV and FEC, and eye mucous membrane color and FEC were compared at p<0.05.

4. Result

Out of the 400 fecal cultured 151(37.75%) were purely positive for *Haemonchus* and 52 were positive for *Haemonchus* and other nematodes. Based on results of faecal cultures, *Haemonchus* species was the primary gastrointestin al nematode infecting sheep.

4.1. Effect of Haemonchus Larvae on Packed Cell Volume

In the present study the minimum observed PCV was 10% and the maximum 43.5% with the mean PCV 24±0.43%. A highly significant negative correlation (R^2 = 0.28, Coef. = -0.78, P<0.001) was observed between *Haemonchus* larvae and PCV as indicated in Table 1. Many lower haematocrit values (PCV) were registered during periods of heavier *Haemonchus* infection that is when many animals were positive and the lowest PCV values were also recorded for *Haemonchus* positive animals than other nematode positive animals. That means more animals with *Haemonchus* positive were identified with lower haematocrit (PCV) value than negative animals.

4.2. Effect of Haemonchus Larvae on Eye Color

There was significant positive correlation between the eye color score (FAMACHA© score) and *Haemonchus* infection in the study area as indicated in Table 1(R^2= 0.19, Coef. = 1.53, P<0.001.There was a positive correlation between *Haemonchus* larvae and eye score meaning animals that were positively cultured for *Haemonchus* showed severe anemia (5 score) and anemia (4 score) compared to animals that were positive to other nematode parasites. During high *Haemonchus* infection (short rainy season/when many animals were culture positive) the percentage of sheep with FAMACHA© scores of 4 and 5 were increased, and vice versa. Some animals were culture positive for *Haemonchus* but the FAMACHA© score were score 1, score 2 and/or score3 (not signs of anemia), this may be due to pre-patent period of infection, or due to low worm burden or host-resistance to GI helminthes. There were also few animals that were *Haemonchus* negative on culture but with FAMACHA© score fall in 3, 4 and 5. This may be due to nutritional deficiencies.

Table 1. *Frequency of animals with Haemonchus species positive with ranges of PCV and FAMACHA© score in sheep in Arsi-Negele districts.*

	PCV values			Eye mucous membrane color				
H.larvae	PCV<19	PCV20-29	PCV>30	Ec1	Ec2	Ec3	Ec4	Ec5
Positive	54	74	23	37	10	18	21	65
negative	9	75	142	140	20	20	14	38

Keys: Ec= eye color

4.3. Packed Cell Volume and Eye Color (FAMACHA©-categories)

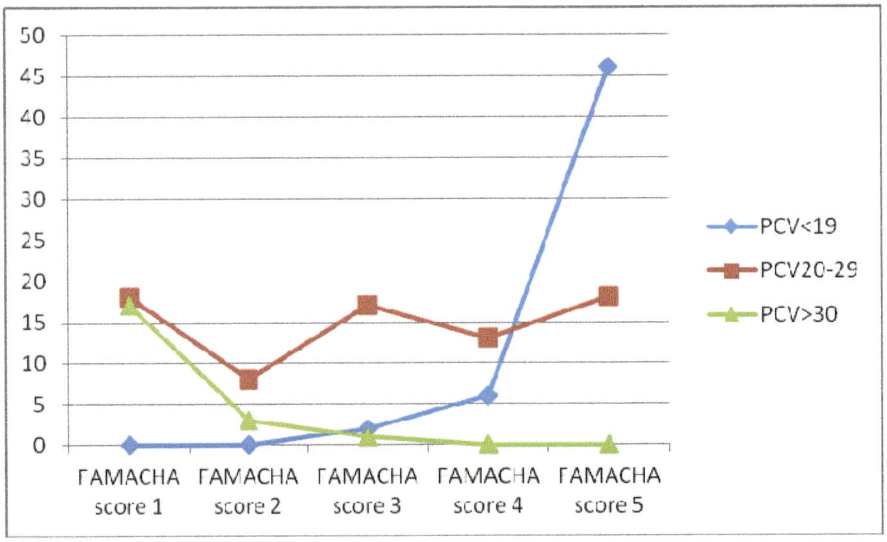

Figure 1. *Correlation between PCV and FAMACHA© score; indicates that FAMACHA© eye color scoring of 3, 4 and 5 measured many animals with PCV values less than 19.*

To evaluate the correlation between the amount of red blood cells and the colour of the conjunctiva, the PCV of blood samples and FAMACHA© scores were simultaneously and independently determined. There was an agreement too between the lower haemtocrits and paler mucous membrane scored according to FAMACHA© method. The correlations between PCV and eye color were strong and negative (R^2= 0.58, Coef= -0.34, P<0.001) for sheep in the study area as indicated in Fig.1, that is as the eye color score approaches score 5 (severe anemia) the PCV level dropped the lowest values (PCV<19). The FAMACHA© categories of score 4 and 5 or sometimes category score of 3 were considered positive for anemic animals, and categories one and two or sometimes three, were considered negative.

4.4. Quantitative Fecal Examination

The McMaster technique was used to determine the number of EPG revealed an overall mean EPG of 1584 with minimum and maximum count of 50 and 7,450 respectively. There was a significant association between the mean EPG and eye color score.

4.4.1. Fecal Egg Count and Packed Cell Volume

There was a strong negative correlation between the PCV of the *Haemonchus* positive sheep and the EPG (R^2=0.53, Coef= -0.023, P<0.001) as indicated in Fig.2. That is, during high EPG the lower PCV value was recorded. Many animals were anemic and severe anemic for *Haemonchus* positive animals, and EPG of these animals was also higher than animals positive for other nematodes.

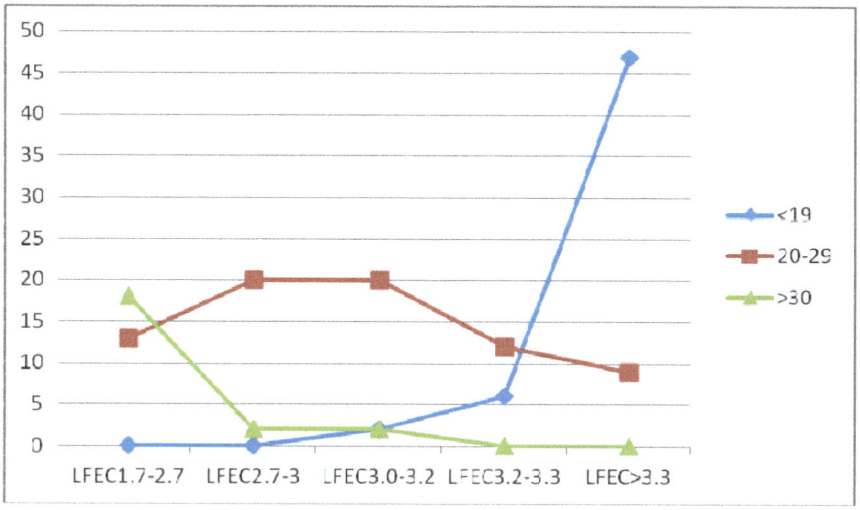

Figure 2. *Correlation between PCV and FAMACHA© score; indicates that FAMACHA© eye color scoring of 3, 4 and 5 measured many animals with PCV values less than 19.*

4.4.2. Faecal Egg Count and Eye Color (FAMACHA©) Categories

To evaluate the correlation between FAMACHA© scoring and the number of excreted eggs for pure culture positive sheep (culture negative for other nematodes) the FAMACHA©-scores and the EPG were independently recorded.

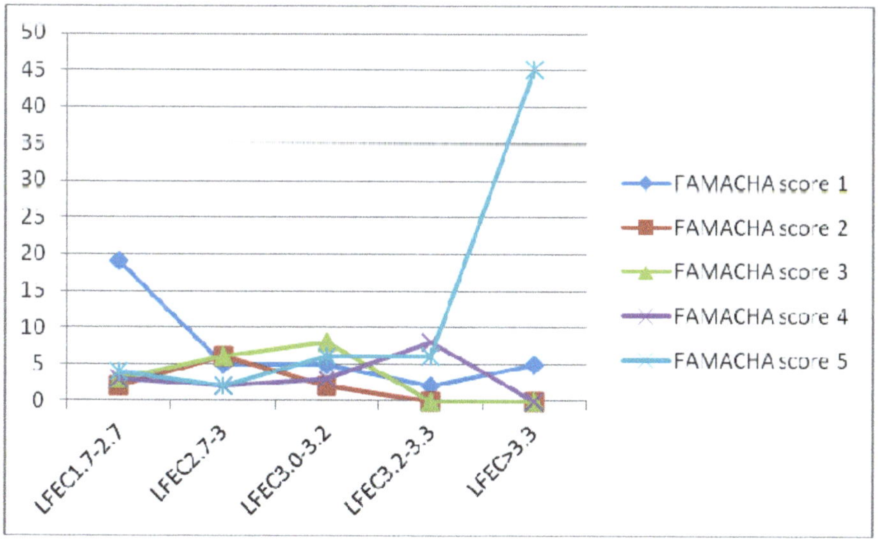

Figure 3. *Correlation between EPG and eye color; indicates that LFEC>3.3 measures many animals with FAMACHA© score 5.*

For FAMACHA© category 3, the EPG ranges was between 1050 EPG and 1500 EPG, for category 4 ranges between 1550 EPG and 2000 EPG and for category 5 a FEC was greater than 2000 EPG. The frequencies of FEC categories for each FAMACHA©-score are presented in figure 5. The result elucidated a relationship between EPG level and eye mucous membrane color (FMACHA© score). The FAMACHA© score had a strong positive correlation (R=0.274, P<0.001) with EPG as indicated in Fig. 3 i.e. the percentage of sheep with FAMACHA© scores of 3, 4 and 5 increased as the EPG for *Haemonchus* positive animals increased than EPG for other nematodes. Results revealed that in sheep with an EPG level of 1050-2000, most of the animals fell in category 3, 4 with pink and pink white eye color. Similarly, with EPG level above 2000 animals fell in category 5, having white eye color showing sever anemic condition.

5. Discussion

In this study 37.8% of the 400 animals were positive to Haemonchus infection as to cultured faeces for throughout the study periods and this was in agreement with [10]. In the study area just like other parts of the country antihelmintics were used frequently and almost for animals visiting the clinic. Multiple-drug resistant nematodes especially to *Haemonchus* species have been reported in many areas of the world and *Haemonchus* species were known for developing drug resistant [11, 13-15] to the extent that total anthelmintic failure is seen as a real possibility in some situations.

In present work the PCV of the study sheep had a strong negative correlation with the FAMACHA© eye colour scores and this agreed with the findings of [16], found that strong negative correlations (R^2 = –0.72, P<0.0001) for the FAMACHA© eye color and PCV. Thus, the FAMACHA© anaemia scoring guide can measure significant number of sheep positive for *Haemonchus* and anemic and severely anemic and thus can be utilized as procedure for the indirect diagnosis of haemonchosis if other causes of anemia were minimum. In the present study the FAMACHA© score had a strong positive correlation with EPG that is the percentage of sheep with FAMACHA© scores of 3, 4 and 5 increased as the EPG increased, and this was in line with the finding of [17]. [17] States that animals with high FAMACHA© scores generally had high FECs, and vice versa. However, the prolificacy of worms can be affected by many factors such as season and host immunity, so repeated measures should be taken.

When PCV fell below 19%, FEC were higher than 1050EPG and the majority of FEC were above 2000EPG and this was agreed with the finding of [4, 5, 14, 16-18]. Such an association might allow drawing some conclusions on the intensity of infection with *Haemonchus* species as *Haemonchus* species are prolific egg layers than other nematodes.

Targeted or selective application of anthelmintic treatment might be an important tool to keep susceptible GIN strains in livestock and to delay the development of antihelmintic resistance. The accuracy and feasibility of FAMACHA© was tested in 400 sheep in Arsi-Negele districts and such method [19] can be used by the farmers themselves by checking their animals for signs of anaemia.

6. Conclusion and Recommendations

The PCV and FECs, FECs and eye mucous membrane color (FAMACHA© score) were significantly associated in the study sheep flock. Based on the results of this work it can be concluded that the FAMACHA© method can be used as quick, simple and cheap alternative for an integrated control of nematode parasites, particularly when *Haemonchus* species is the primary pathogen which would result in reducing the frequency of anthelmintic treatments which in turn result in reduced chance of drug resistance. Based on the above the following recommendations are forwarded;

- Still now there are few works on the validation of FAMACHA© chart in Ethiopia so FAMACHA© eye color evaluation that covers the large parts of the country should be done and results should be pooled together, evaluated and broad conclusions should be drawn on the use of FAMACHA© system.
- There was agreement too between the lower haematocrits and paler mucous membranes scored according to the FAMACHA© method. The use of this system may be recommended as part of an integrated approach to worm control in sheep kept in the resource-poor areas studied.

Acknowledgments

Our acknowledgment goes to all members of Hawassa University School of Veterinary Medicine parasitology laboratory workers for allowed me to use all the available facilities.

References

[1] CSA, 2013. Central statistics for livestock population in Ethiopia. Addis Ababa, Ethiopia

[2] Kumsa B. and Wossene A. 2006. Abomasal nematodes of small ruminants of Ogaden region, Eastern Ethiopia. Prevalence, worm burden and species composition, *Revue Med. Vet, 157:27-32.*

[3] Demelash B., Yilma J. and Hassen C. 2006. Ovine helminthosis is major health constraints to productivity of sheep in Ethiopia. Faculty of Veterinary Medicine, Hawassa University, Hawassa, Ethiopia, pp. 65-90.

[4] Chaudary F.R., Khan M.F. and Qayyum M. 2007. Prevalence of *Haemonchus contortus* in naturally infected small ruminants grazing in the Potohar area of Pakistan. *Pakistan vet. J, 27:73-79.*

[5] Woldemariam D.L. 2005. Nematode Prevalence, helminth management practices and anthelmintic resistance in small ruminants in the mid rift valley of Ethiopia. University of Pretoria, Faculty of veterinary sciences, Pretoria, South Africa, Pp.2-3, 29, 60.

[6] Arsi-Negele beureau of agriculture and rural development, 2013.

[7] Thrusfield M. 2008. Sampling in Veterinary epidemiology. 2nd ed, Blackwell science, London. Pp.198

[8] Hansen J. and Perry B. 1994. The epidemiology, diagnosis and control of helminth parasites of ruminants. 2nd ed, Nairobi, Kenya: ILRAD (international laboratory for research on animal diseases).

[9] Hendrix C.M. and Robinson E. 2012. Diagnostic parasitology for veterinary technicians. 4th ed, Mosby, USA, Pp.54.

[10] MAFF (Minstry of Agriculture, Fisheries and Food), 1997. Manual of Veterinary parasitological laboratory techniques. Tech.Bull, NO. 18, Her Majesty's stationery office, London, Pp.129.

[11] Zeryhun T. 2011. Helminthosis of sheep and goats in and around Haramaya, Southeastern Ethiopia. Journal *of Vet. Med. and Animal Health, 4:48-55.*

[12] Burke J.M., Kaplan R.M., Miller J.E., Terrill T.H., Getz W.R., Mobini S., Valencia E., Williams M.J., Williamson L.H. and Vatta A.F. 2007. Accuracy of the FAMACHA© system for on-farm use by sheep and goat producers in the southeastern United States. *Vet. Parasitol, 147:89-95.*

[13] Chandrawathani P., Yusoff N., Wan L.C., Ham A. and Waller P.J. 2004. Total anthelmintic failure to control nematode parasites of small ruminants on government breeding farms in Sabah East Malaysia. *Vet. Res. Comm, 28: 1–11.*

[14] Kaplan R.M., Burke J.M., Terrill T.H., Miller J.E., Getz W.R., Mobini S., Valencia E., Williams M.G., Williamson L.H., Larsen M. and Vatta A.F. 2004. Validation of the FAMACH© eye color chart for detecting clinical anemia in sheep and goats on farms in the Southern United States. *Vet. Parasitol, 123: 105-120.*

[15] Kumsa B. 2004. Study on Ogaden small ruminant haemonchosis: morphological characterization and susceptibility to Albendazole and Tetramisole. Msc thesis, school of veterinary medicine, Addis Ababa University, Addis Ababa, Ethiopia.

[16] Menkir S. 2007. Helminth Parasites of Sheep and Goats in Eastern Ethiopia: Epidemiology, and Anthelmintic Resistance and its Management. Doctoral thesis, Faculty of Veterinary Medicine and Animal Science, Swedish University of Agricultural Sciences, Uppsala, Sweden.

[17] Scheuerle M. 2009. Anthelmintic resistance of *Haemonchus contortus* and the FAMACHA© method as a tool to delay the development of anthelmintic resistance. 1st ed. vvb laufersweiler verlag, pp.4.

[18] Saddiqi H. 2010. Evaluation of some indigenous breeds of sheep for natural resistance against *Haemonchus contortus* infection. Doctoral thesis, Faculty of Veterinary science, University of Agriculture Faisalabad, Pakistan.

[19] VanWyk J.A. 2001. Refugia – overlooked as perhaps the most potent factor concerning the development of anthelmintic resistance. *Onderstepoort J. Vet. Res, 68: 55-67.*

17

Gamma Glutamyl Transpeptidase Activity Determination in Epididymis of *Corynorhinus mexicanus* Bat Throughout Its Annual Cycle

Arenas-Ríos Edith[1,*], Rosado Adolfo[1], Rodríguez-Tobón Ernesto[2], Rodríguez-Tobón Ahiezer[3], León-Galván Miguel Ángel[4]

[1]Department of Biology of Reproduction, Autonomous Metropolitan University–Iztapalapa, Iztapalapa,México
[2]Masters in Biology of Reproduction ,Autonomous Metropolitan University–Iztapalapa, Iztapalapa,México
[3]PhD in Experimental Biology, Autonomous Metropolitan University–Iztapalapa, Iztapalapa,México
[4]Department ofBiology, AutonomousMetropolitanUniversity–Iztapalapa, Iztapalapa,México

Email address:
editharenas2000@yahoo.com.mx (Arenas-Ríos E.), adolfo.rosado@gmail.com (Rosado A.), rotoern@hotmail.com (Rodríguez-Tobón E.), ahiezerrod@yahoo.com.mx (Rodríguez-Tobón A.), leon@xanum.uam.mx (León-Galván M. Á.)

Abstract: GGT initiates the degradation of both oxidized and reduced glutathione at the cell surface by cleaving the unique gamma glutamyl bond. The successive hydrolysis of oxidized or reduced CysGly by aminopeptidase or dipeptidase releases Gly, and cysteine/cysteine is recovered for intracellular synthesis of glutathione. In addition, GGT plays a major physiological role in providing cysteine to cells for GSH synthesis and protein synthesis, thereby playing a major role in antioxidant defense and normal growth. GGT is present in the epididymis, principally in caput. The catalytic activity of GGT is highest in the proximal epididymal regions and decreases toward the distal regions; participating in the epididymal sperm maturation process.In most mammals, epididymal sperm maturation takes place in a period not exceeding ten days, ending in the distal part of the corpus of the epididymis, before reaching the caudal region, which is responsible only for sperm storage; however, in *C. mexicanus* the epididymal sperm maturation ends in caudal epididymal region.For this reason, the main goal of the present study was to determine the relationship between the GGT activity through the caput and caudal epididymal regions, throughout annual cycle of *Corynorhinus mexicanus* bat.We found that the GGT activity appears to be important for epididymal sperm maturation in *C. mexicanus* bat in cephalic region, and important for protection against ROS epididymal caudal region.

Keywords: Bats, Gamma Glutamyl Transpeptidase, Epididymis, Sperm Maturation, Glutathione

1. Introduction

The gamma glutamyl transpeptidase(GGT; EC 2.3.2.2) is an enzyme found in mammals [1, 2]; initiates the degradation of both oxidized and reduced glutathioneat the cell surface by cleaving the unique gamma glutamyl bond.The successive hydrolysis of oxidized or reduced CysGly by aminopeptidase or dipeptidase releases Gly, and cysteine/cysteine is recovered for intracellular synthesis of glutathione (GSH)[3].

Has been confirmed that GGT plays a major physiological role in providing cysteine to cells for GSH synthesis and protein synthesis, thereby playing a major role in antioxidant defense and normal growth [4-12].

GGT is present in the epididymis,principally in caput [13]. The catalytic activity of GGT is highest in the proximal epididymal regions and decreases toward the distal regions [14, 15].

Once the spermatozoa are formed during spermatogenesis and pass to the epididymis, they will carry on morphological and biochemical changes known as epididymal sperm maturation [16], *i.e.*the potential to acquire rectilinear and vigorous movement, to interact with zona pellucida and to fertilize the oocyte [17].

During sperm maturation, in addition to a major role as an antioxidant and in eliminating toxic compounds, GSH has been implicated in prooxidation processes in various cells, via GGT dependent catabolism [18, 19]. Modulating effects of GSH catabolism have been observed on components of signal transduction pathways, such as those involving cell surface receptors and factors within the sperm cell itself and/or in the epididymis may control sperm protein thiol (PSH) oxidation[18-20].

In most mammals, epididymal sperm maturation takes place in a period not exceeding ten days, ending in the distal part of the corpus of the epididymis, before reaching the caudal region, which is responsible only for sperm storage [21].

However, the Vespertilionidae bat *Corynorhinus mexicanus*(Allen, 1916) provides an interesting experimental model for the epididymal study, because it presents prolonged storage of sperm in the epididymal cauda for several months after the spermatogenesis and regression of testes.

September is the beginning of sperm epididymal storage, therefore since October, there are no new contributions of sperm cells from the testis, and cells remain viable until the copulating season which occurs during November[22, 23]. Earlier research conducted by our group has suggested that in this species the sperm maturation has to be finished in the caudal region of the epididymis and should be dependent on storage time[24].

For this reason the main goal of the present study was to determine the relationship between the GGT activity through the caput and caudal epididymal regions, throughout annual cycle of *Corynorhinus mexicanus* bat.

2. Materials and Methods

2.1. Reagents and Solutions

All chemicals and reagentsusedwereof thehighest analytical gradeand most of them were purchasedfrom Sigma(St.Louis MO)

2.2. Ethics Statement

Corynorhinus mexicanus is not listed as an endangered species in the Norma Oficial Mexicana NOM-059-ECOL-2010 SEMARNAT-2010 for the protection of native wild species of México[25]. All protocols for the capture and handling of the live animals, as well as the euthanasia procedure used in this study were conducted in strict accordance with the guidelines established by the American Society of Mammalogists for the use of wild mammals in research [26], and were approved by the Ethics Committee of our institution. The capture of specimens studied were approved by the scientific collector's license FAUT-0159 issued to Dr. Miguel Angel León Galván, by the Dirección General de Vida Silvestre de México (an agency of SEMARNAT).

2.3. Capture of Animals

Three adult males of *C. mexicanus* were captured fortnightly from September to October 2011 using a expand hand-net (Bioquip Tropic net) in a tunnel where they take refuge. This tunnel is located in central México (19°37′14″N, 98°02′02″W; 3320 m altitude). Capture regime includes the period when spermatozoa reach the caput region of the epididymis and the period of sperm storage before the mating season starts[22, 24].

Bats were always captured before or as they left their roost. To ensure adult status of bats, only those animals with complete ossification of the cartilaginous epiphyseal growth plates of the fourth metacarpal–phalangeal joint were selected [22]. In order to ensure the age category and the reproductive condition of the individuals included in this study, according to the report in León-Galván*et al.*[22]; Arenas-Ríos *et al.*, [27]; and Cervantes *et al.*[24], the following variables were determined: body weight registered using an Ohaus® (Ohaus Corporation NJ) portable electronic balance (±0.01 gr); forearm length measured with a Vernier caliper (±0.1 mm); and the external aspects of the sexual organs.

2.4. Epididymides Obtention

The animals for each determination were captured on the same day. Immediately after decapitation, the epididymides of the bat were externalized through an incision of the interfemoral skin and tunica vaginalis that covers it, cleared of fat and connective tissue, and dissected. Caput and cauda segments of the epididymides were isolated according to the procedure described by Arenas-Ríos *et al.*[27] and Cervantes et al.[24].

Both epidydimal segments of the same region (right and left caput and cauda) were pooled and frozen in liquid nitrogen (−170 °C) until utilized. Caput and cauda segments of the epididymides were thawed to 4 °C in ten volumes of cold HEPES buffer (0.1 M, pH 7.4) and homogenized in a Potter– Elvehjem type, glass–glass homogenizer. The obtained homogenates were centrifuged for 10 min at 5000 ×g, the precipitates were discarded and all enzymatic activities were measured in the supernatants [27].

2.5. Gamma Glutamyl Transpeptidase Determinations

GGT (EC 2.3.2.21) activity was determined by the method of Yash and Tapani[28], using p-nitroanilide as substrate. Activity is expressed as nmoles of p-nitroaniline produced per min.

The activity of all enzymes tested was calculated either as specific activity, i.e. units of enzyme activity per mg of tissue protein, and as total activity, i.e. units of enzyme activity per total wet weight of the organ.

Some preliminary enzyme determinations were done to ensure appropriate maintenance of enzyme activity after freezing and thawing and to test kinetic conditions. In addition, to ensure zero order kinetics, all enzyme assays were run in duplicate utilizing one and twice the amount of homogenate. All those unusual assays in which duplicates were not satisfactory were repeated using smaller amounts of homogenate.

Total protein content for the determination of the specific activities of the enzymes was measured using a commercially available bi-cinchoninic acid protein assay kit (Pierce, Rockford, IL, USA).

2.6. Statistical Analysis

Comparisons among groups were made with one-way ANOVA [29] followed by the Bonferroni post hoc test. Homogeneity of variances was tested by Bartlett and Levene tests [29]. Differences were considered statistically significant when pb0.05.

Realization of this work, including the use and handling of animals, was reviewed and approved by the Consejo Divisional de Ciencias Biológicas y de la Salud (Biology and Health).

Sciences Divisional Board) of the Universidad Autónoma Metropolitana- Iztapalapa. Animals were cared for in accordance to the "Guidelines for the capture, handling, and care of mammals" as approved by the American Society of Mammalogist (Animal Care and Use Committee, 1998).

3. Results

In total 41 adult male bats were used. Mean body mass was 7.5303 (range 7.07-8.0 g) and the mean forearm length was 41.8623 (range 41.37-42.65 mm). Testes were permanently inguinal, and the epididymides, were always bound to the testicles. The epididymis recrudescence occurs in August, with their highest weight in September-October (Fig. 1). Afterwards epididymis weights decreases slowly, reaching their lowest values until March. The separate regions

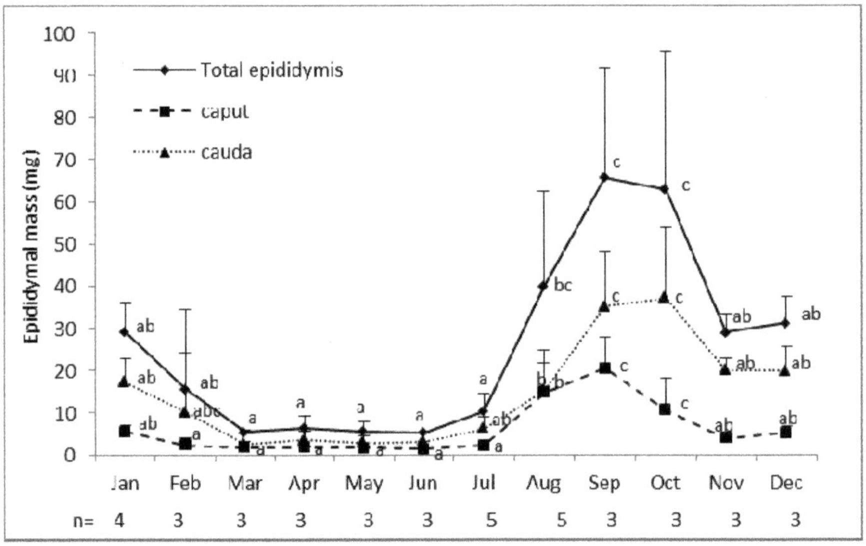

Figure 1.Changes in epididymal mass of Corynorhinus mexicanus bat during annual cycle. The epididymal segments were obtained after ligation of epididymides at the deferent-cauda, cauda-corpus, corpus-caput. For simplicity, we report only the mean ± DS mass of one reproductive organ or epididymal region per bat, using all bats in the sample, and the values in the base indicate the number of bats. Different letters indicate statistically significant differences (P < 0.05) between values in the same trace (ANOVA plus Bonferroni post hoc test)

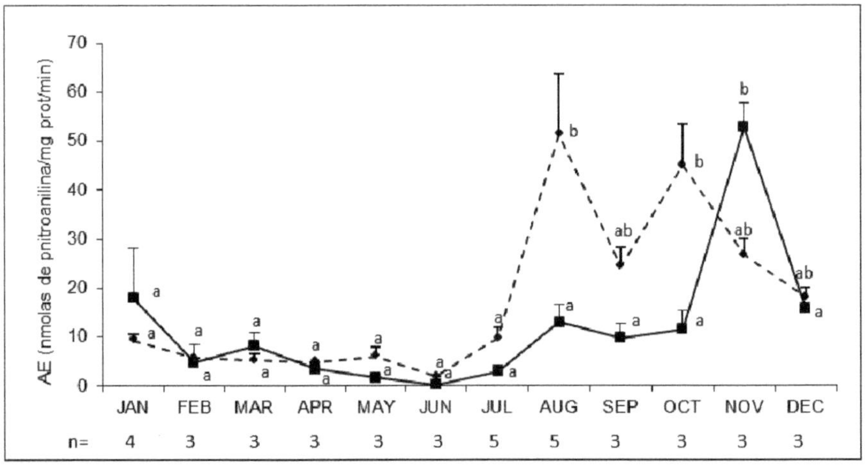

Figure 2.Activity of GGT in the epididymides of C. mexicanus bats captured monthly during the annual reproductive cycle; (A) Activity of the enzyme from caput; (B) Activity of the enzyme from cauda. Activity of the enzyme expressed as specific activity, i.e. units of enzyme activity per mg of tissue protein. Data indicate Mean±SEM. Numbers indicate the number of bats. Different letters indicate the existence of statistical significant differences between values in the same trace (ANOVA plus Bonferroni post hoc test).

4. Discussion

The Mexican big-eared *Corynorhinus mexicanus*bat, is an endemic species of Mexico, living in temperate zones. It takes a lethargy type "daily torpor" during the cold season, so it has no need to migrate away from their breeding site. Females are seasonal monoestric, observing their mating period principally during November [30, 31]. The Males also have one annual reproductive cycle, with a temporal asynchrony between testis and epididymis; therefore, prolonged sperm storage in epididymis [22, 24, 27].

The testicular development in *C. mexicanus* bat, begins in May reaching its maximum weight in August, and returning to its lowest values in October [32]. The histological data indicate that from November to April testicles have no spermatogenic activity. The seminiferous tubules regressed and Sertoli cells found significantly decreased in number and some show vacuolar degeneration [30].

On the other hand, the maximum epididymis development is in September; a month after the testicle reached its highest values; however, downsizing in the epididymis is observed gradually from December to February, it shows a great development in the caudal region of the epididymis, being evident since September and continuing until January, showing great development in the caudal epididymal region, being evident since September and continuing until January. The record of the presence of epididymal spermatozoa in this specie, was observed from late August until January [31, 33]. In the cephalic region, a clear decrease in sperm concentration was reported in late October [33], which coincides with the weight decrease of this region, while on the same date, a clear tendency to increase sperm concentration in the caudal region was reported [33]. León-Galván et al [22] propose, that increased size of epididymis, the abundant pampiniforme venous plexus system [34] and the absence of hair in this area, could function as an important element and cooling device as part of protection mechanisms of sperm in the sperm long period of storage, along with the participation of antioxidant enzymes: superoxide dismutase, catalase and glutathione peroxidase may be modulating the production of reactive oxygen species (ROS) [27].

However, it has been reported that, unlike other mammalian species in *C. mexicanus*, the epididymal sperm maturation ends in caudal region [24, 35], showing that it is the month of October, the most important, as it was in that month, in which, an important tyrosine phosphorylation of protein in sperm increase, was detected [35], and it is from this date, that sperm were found with the ability of capacitation and to experience acrosome reaction [24, 35].

As mentioned before, GGT is present in the epididymis, mainly in the head region [13], being the high catalytic activity of GGT in proximal epididymal region, and decreases in the distal region [14, 15]. In the present study, it was found that GGT activity is high in the cephalic region, on dates in which sperm are present in the epididymis, something equivalent to what was reported in rat, where they found that GGT concentration was low in immature rats and increased in sexual maturity of rats. This associated with decreased GSH and L-glutamic acid accumulation levels, which is thought, they could play an important role at the time of the sperm arrival, participating in the epididymal sperm maturation process [28].

GSH Modulators catabolism effects, have been observed in components of signal transduction pathways, such as control of protein oxidation of thiol groups, in epididymal sperm [18-20].

However, if the sperm maturation in *C. mexicanus* bat ends in the caudal region, and this must be accomplished before mating season (November), the results found in this study about the GGT activity, suggest that; the effects associated with GGT activity and related with epididymal sperm maturation, in *C. mexicanus* bat, are only important in the cephalic region [3-12, 18, 19]. In the caudal region, GGT could be involved, only in antioxidant protection of tissue and sperm cells against the attack of ROS [4-12, 27].

It has been reported that, the catalytic activity of GGT is androgen dependent [36]. However, we found an important activity of GGT, even on dates when the testicle reportedly no longer presents activity [22, 23], so this last point deserves to be studied deeply.

Acknowledgments

We would like to acknowledge the entire research group: Morphophysiology and Biochemistry of Sperm (Universidad Autónoma Metropolitana, Iztapalapa) and MarioGabriel Hidalgo. This work was partially financed by CONACYT (Mexico) grants 0105961/M10-A02; UAM-I-CA-136, SEP-PROMEP and scholarship number 233313 to AR.

References

[1] T. Kasai, and P.O. Larsen, "Chemistry and Biochemistry of γ-Glutamyl Derivatives from Plants Including Mushrooms (Basidiomycetes), in Fortschritte der Chemie organischer Naturstoffe / Progress in the Chemistry of Organic Natural Products", W. Herz, H. Grisebach, and G.W. Kirby, Editors. Springer: Vienna, 1980, pp. 173-285.

[2] Taniguchi, N. and Y. Ikeda, gamma-Glutamyl transpeptidase: catalytic mechanism and gene expression. Adv Enzymol Relat Areas Mol Biol, 1998. 72: p. 239-78.

[3] Kinlough, C.L., et al., Gamma-glutamyltranspeptidase: disulfide bridges, propeptide cleavage, and activation in the endoplasmic reticulum. Methods Enzymol, 2005. 401: p. 426-49.

[4] Barrios, R., et al., Oxygen-induced pulmonary injury in gamma-glutamyl transpeptidase-deficient mice. Lung, 2001. 179(5): p. 319-30.

[5] Chevez-Barrios, P., et al., Cataract development in gamma-glutamyl transpeptidase-deficient mice. Exp Eye Res, 2000. 71(6): p. 575-82.

[6] Harding, C.O., et al., Mice with genetic gamma-glutamyl transpeptidase deficiency exhibit glutathionuria, severe growth failure, reduced life spans, and infertility. J Biol Chem, 1997. 272(19): p. 12560-7.

[7] Jean, J.C., et al., gamma-Glutamyl transferase (GGT) deficiency in the GGTenu1 mouse results from a single point mutation that leads to a stop codon in the first coding exon of GGT mRNA. Mutagenesis, 1999. 14(1): p. 31-6.

[8] Jean, J.C., et al., Gamma-glutamyl transferase deficiency results in lung oxidant stress in normoxia. Am J Physiol Lung Cell Mol Physiol, 2002. 283(4): p. L766-76.

[9] Kumar, T.R., et al., Reproductive defects in gamma-glutamyl transpeptidase-deficient mice. Endocrinology, 2000. 141(11): p. 4270-7.

[10] Levasseur, R., et al., Reversible skeletal abnormalities in gamma-glutamyl transpeptidase-deficient mice. Endocrinology, 2003. 144(7): p. 2761-4.

[11] Lipton, A.J., et al., S-nitrosothiols signal the ventilatory response to hypoxia. Nature, 2001. 413(6852): p. 171-4.

[12] Pardo, A., et al., Bleomycin-induced pulmonary fibrosis is attenuated in gamma-glutamyl transpeptidase-deficient mice. Am J Respir Crit Care Med, 2003. 167(6): p. 925-32.

[13] Kohdaira, T., et al., Distribution of gamma-glutamyl transpeptidase in male reproductive system of rats and its age-related changes. Andrologia, 1986. 18(6): p. 610-7.

[14] DeLap, L.W., S.S. Tate, and A. Meister, gamma-glutamyl transpeptidase and related enzyme activities inthe reproductive system of the male rat. Life Sci, 1977. 20(4): p. 673-9.

[15] Agrawal, Y.P., T. Peura, and T. Vanha-Perttula, Distribution of gamma-glutamyl transpeptidase in the mouse epididymis and its response to acivicin. J Reprod Fertil, 1989. 86(1): p. 185-93.

[16] Sullivan, R., G. Frenette, and J. Girouard, Epididymosomes are involved in the acquisition of new sperm proteins during epididymal transit. Asian J Androl, 2007. 9(4): p. 483-91.

[17] Lewis, B. and R.J. Aitken, Impact of epididymal maturation on the tyrosine phosphorylation patterns exhibited by rat spermatozoa. Biol Reprod, 2001. 64(5): p. 1545-56.

[18] Filomeni, G., G. Rotilio, and M.R. Ciriolo, Cell signalling and the glutathione redox system. Biochem Pharmacol, 2002. 64(5-6): p. 1057-64.

[19] Paolicchi, A., et al., Glutathione catabolism as a signaling mechanism. Biochem Pharmacol, 2002. 64(5-6): p. 1027-35.

[20] Accaoui, M.J., et al., Gamma-glutamyltranspeptidase-dependent glutathione catabolism results in activation of NF-kB. Biochem Biophys Res Commun, 2000. 276(3): p. 1062-7.

[21] Bernard Robaire, B.T.H., and Marie-Claire Orgebin-Crist, The Epididymis, in Knobil and Neill's Physiology of Reproduction, J.D. Neill, Editor. 2006.

[22] León-Galván, M.A., et al., Male reproductive cycle of mexican big-eared bats, corynorhinus mexicanus (chiroptera: vespertilionidae). The Southwestern Naturalist, 2005. 50(4): p. 453-460.

[23] Arenas-Ríos, E., et al., Superoxide dismutase, catalase, and glutathione peroxidase in the testis of the Mexican big-eared bat (Corynorhinus mexicanus) during its annual reproductive cycle. Comparative Biochemistry and Physiology Part A: Molecular & Integrative Physiology, 2007. 148(1): p. 150-158.

[24] Cervantes, M.I., et al., Spermatozoa epididymal maturation in the Mexican big-eared bat (Corynorhinus mexicanus). Syst Biol Reprod Med, 2008. 54(4-5): p. 196-204.

[25] SEMARNAT, NORMA Oficial Mexicana NOM-059-SEMARNAT-2010, Protección ambiental-Especies nativas de México de flora y fauna silvestres-Categorías de riesgo y especificaciones para su inclusión, exclusión o cambio-Lista de especies en riesgo. 2010: México.

[26] Sikes, R.S. and W.L. Gannon, Guidelines of the American Society of Mammalogists for the use of wild mammals in research. Journal of Mammalogy, 2011. 92(1): p. 235-253.

[27] Arenas-Ríos, E., et al., Superoxide dismutase, catalase, and glutathione peroxidase during epididymal maturation and prolonged storage of spermatozoa in the Mexican big-eared bat (Corynorhinus mexicanus). Canadian Journal of Zoology, 2005. 83(12): p. 1556-1565.

[28] Agrawal, Y.P. and T. Vanha-Perttula, Gamma-glutamyl transpeptidase, glutathione, and L-glutamic acid in the rat epididymis during postnatal development. Biol Reprod, 1988. 38(5): p. 996-1000.

[29] Sokal, R.R. and F.J. Rohlf, Biometry. 1995: W. H. Freeman.

[30] López-Wilchis, R., Fisiología de Plecotus mexicanus (Chiroptera vespertilidae) en el estado de Tlaxcala, in UNAM. 1989, UNAM: México.

[31] León-Galvan, M.A., et al., Prolonged storage of spermatozoa in the genital tract of female Mexican big-eared bats (Corynorhinus mexicanus): the role of lipid peroxidation. Canadian Journal of Zoology, 1999. 77(1): p. 7-12.

[32] León-Galván, M.A., Espermatogénesis en el murciélago Corynorhinus mexicanus, participación de la muerte celular por apoptosis, in Ciencias Biológicas y de la Salud. 2008, Universidad Autónoma Metropolitana-Iztapalapa: México.

[33] Arenas-Ríos, E., Enzimas anti-especies reactivas de oxígeno, como reguladores en los procesos de espermatogénesis maduración y almacenamiento prolongado de espermatozoides en el murciélago Corynorhinus mexicanus. 2009, Universidad Autónoma Metropolitana México.

[34] Cooper, T., Epididymis, in Encyclopedia of reproduction, J.D.N. E. Knovil, Editor. 1999. p. 1-17.

[35] Rodríguez-Tobón, A., et al., Tyrosine phosphorylation as evidence of epididymal cauda participation in the sperm maturation process of the Corynorhinus mexicanus bat. , in Acta Zoologica-stockholm, In press. 2015.

[36] Palladino, M.A. and B.T. Hinton, Developmental regulation of expression of multiple gamma-glutamyl transpeptidase mRNAs in the postnatal rat epididymis. Biochem Biophys Res Commun, 1994. 198(2): p. 554-9.

18

Effect of Traditional Cattle Farming Systems on Farmer Knowledge, Cattle Performances and Agribusiness Potential in West New Guinea-Papua Barat Province, Indonesia

Deny A. Iyai[1, 2], Desni T. R. Saragih[1], Frandz P. Rumbiak[1]

[1]Department of Animal Production, Faculty of Animal Sciences, Papua University, Jl, Gunung Salju, Amban, Manokwari, Papua Barat Province, Indonesia

[2]Perumahan Dosen, Papua University, Jl, Tugu Jepang, Amban, Manokwari, Papua Barat, Indonesia

Email address:

da.iyai@yahoo.com (D. A. Iyai)

Abstract: Cattle have been long time introduced in Papua. However adaptation to raise cattle has been unpredictable. An explorative field study using participatory analysis was done in fifteen villages to comprehensively understand the dynamic of cattle performances. Cattle farming system was classified in to three sizes, i.e. small-medium- and large systems. Analyses of data were using Anova and Kruskal-Wallis. The finding of this research was that the three cattle farming sizes were similar in many components of good agricultural practices ($p>0.05$). No wide gap was found in line with farmers, cattle and economical performances. Tropical livestock unit of West New Guinea was low and has possibility to be increased due to agribusiness potential. Lack of good agricultural practices should be narrowed down by better services of government and other related stakeholders.

Keywords: Cattle, Farmer Performances, Traditional Farming System, Agribusiness, West New Guinea

1. Introduction

Cattle is one of the exotic and conventional animal agriculturesin Asia (Devendra, 2007), Indonesia (Utomo danWidjaya, 2007) and Papua (Hartono and Widayatl, 2011). Its rank is in the third place after pigs, and native chicken. During the Ducth administration several animal agricultures had been introduced since 1963, such as pigs, rabbit, chicken, and dairy cattle. In alternated administration of Ducth to Indonesia, several animal agricultures have been introduced since 1972, i.e. Bali cattle, goat, and duck. Under Indonesia administration as well livestock projects were established by designing several relevant and related programs (Bahri *et al.*, 2004). Programs a suchwere president aid, low developed villages program (Kusnadi, 2008), and direct community aid. Since then, less information concerning cattle farming productivity has been reported yet. This induces development of livestock farming systems are growing behind national average productivity. Figures of cattle population in Papua Barat and Manokwariare 37.212 head and 20.829 head. Due to the third places of cattle, local Papuan farmers raise cattle with low effort and support by using their local resources. It is predicted that their livelihood improved slower than that of non Papuan ethnic (transmigrates). The cattle which are raised by each farmer in Papua Barat is less than counted by Hartono and Widayati (2011). Unskilled and less experiences of local Papuan farmers bring difficulty and unease to raise cattle. Therefore although it has been long time since introduced, adaptation to raise cattle is still unpredictable. Due to unskilled raising cattle, local Papuan is prone to keep cattle with low even no external and internal inputs. This in turn induces declined productivity of farmers and cattle performances. Because of introduce with less even no extension program, local Papuan farmers have no experiences. This is a common situation experienced by Papuan livestock farmers (Supriadi, 2008). They even do not know what does nutrition composition offered for cattle (Haryanto, 2009; Nulik and Hau, 2005) and what management is needed to raise cattle (Sudaryanto and Jamal, 2000). The latter becomes so important and plays a role in designing and applying resources. Several livestock farming systems have been identified by Iyai and Chrisostomus (2013) and the focus of this article is on traditional cattle farming systems. The objective of this study was to picturing performances of several classes of cattle farming systems in Manokwari. This study was done to specifically seekhow well traditional cattle farming systems run their farms using inputs, outputs and what happen in the process inside the farms (Sudaryanto and Jamal, 2000).

2. Materials and Methods

An explorative-field case study was done in Manokwari regency and involved six districts, i.e. Northern Manokwari district, Eastern Manokari District, Western Manokwari district, Warmare district, Prafi district and Masni district. Manokwari regency, which has a total area of 14.445 km^2, possesses a population of around 161.000 inhabitants with a density of 11.51 heads km^{-1}, and is located at 132°30' – 134°45' East Meridian and 0°20' – 2°25' South latitude.

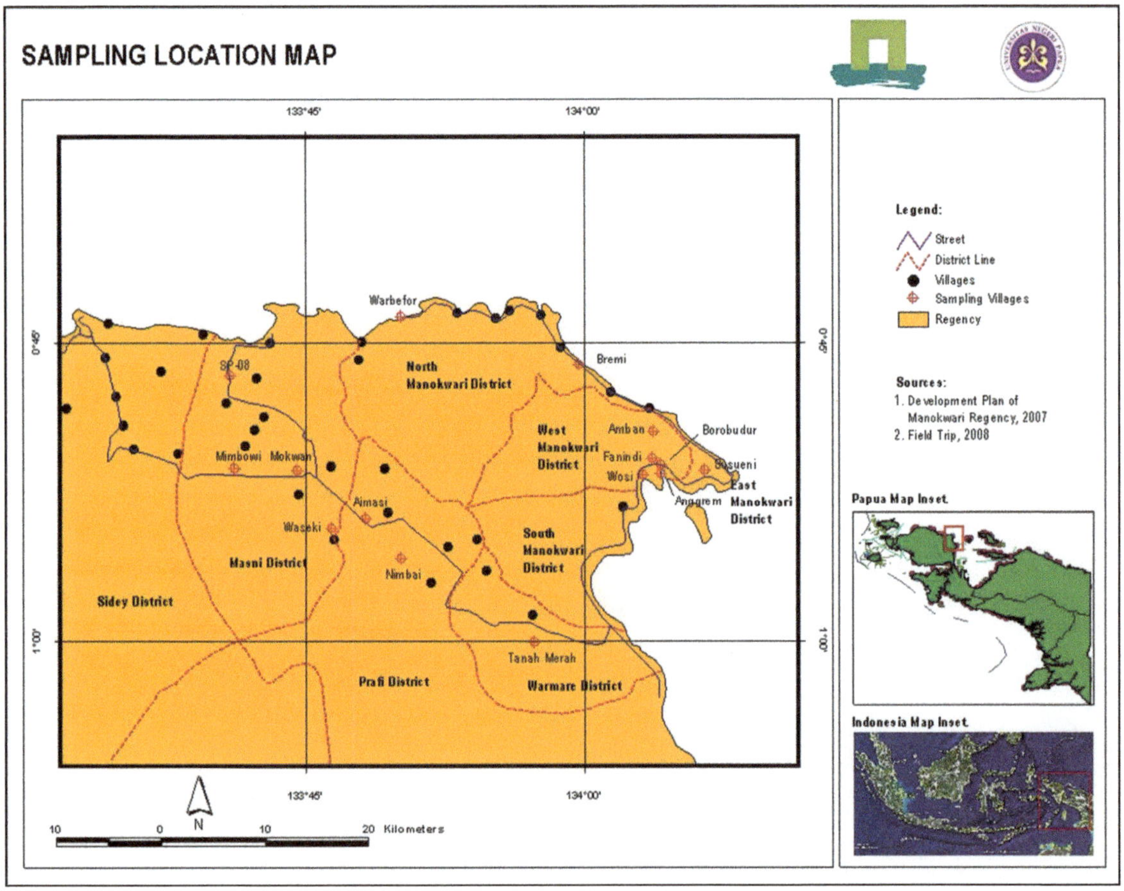

Figure 1. *Sampling location of cattle farmers' survey in Manokwari, Papua barat-West New Guinea.*

The population in Manokwari is growing in both urban and rural areas, especially in transmigration areas, such as Prafi and Masni districts. Respondents chosen were guided by local extensionists, originated from 14 villages, i.e..Warbefor, Bremi, Susweni, Amban, Fanindi, Tanah Merah, Nimbai, Aimasi, Mokwam, Mimbowi, SP-08, Wosi, and Waseki. Several villages and chosen using snowball sampling method.

Research approach was Participatory situation analysis (PSA) applied to approach livestock farmers (Conroy, 2005). Interviews using questionnaires were done to collect information from whole selected farmers. Queries of 36 opened and closed semi-structured questions were asked to the farmers, i.e. characteristics of the farmers, characteristic of farming performances, and characteristic of cattle production and reproduction performances.Allocated time was around 70 minutes. This field work was done in 15 days.

Parameters used to measure objectives of this study were ages (y),experience (y), household member (head/hh), livelihood, education, work hours, selection, mating sign, pregnant detection, provided forage, grass quality, offered forages, cattle housing, disease knowledge, prevention, utilization, kind of product, herd size, parental stock (head), mating period, forage frequency, sold cattle, and statistic vital consisted of height at withers (cm), body length (cm), heart girth (cm) and body weight (kg).

Qualitative and quantitative data were entered in Excel 2010. Several qualitative data, i.e. livelihood, education, selection, mating sign, pregnant detection up to kind of product were made using coding scales. Classification was based on the three sizes of cattle farming systems in three agroecological zones of Manokwari i.e. coastal, and lowland

Manokwari. Mathematical formula then was $Yij = \mu + \alpha i + \varepsilon ij$, where Yij is variable responses. μ is overall mean, αi is effect of farming system sizes, i.e.1 is small-scale, 2 is medium-scale and 3 is large-scale cattle farming systems, and εij is errors with normal distribution, N (0, I).Test for data normality was made using Kolmogorov-Smirnov and Shapiro-Wilk. Data are normally distributed if p-value of tested variables are higher than 0.05 ($p>0.05$).

Analysis of data for normally distributed parameters was made using One-Way Anova (Ott and Longnecker, 2001). Analysis of data using SPPS version 18.0., was used. Data normally distributed were ages of farmers, and price-adult cattle. After test for data normality, several data were found with not normally distributed. Non normality data were livelihood, education, working hours, selection, mating sign, pregnant detection, provided forages, grass quality, offered forages, cattle housing, knowledge diseases, diseases prevention, utilization and kind of product. Each variable was then transformed using Square root (sqrt). The formula of square root (sqrt) transform is $(Y + 1/2)^{1/2}$ which was made to obtain normalityof data. Non parametric data then analyzed using Kruskal-Wallis (H). The formula of Kruskal-Wallis (1952) is equal to $H=\frac{1}{S^2} \times \left[\sum_i \frac{R_i^2}{r_i} - \frac{N(N+1)^2}{4}\right]$. For knowing which samples were significant difference ($p<0.05$), post-hoc analysisusing Scheffewas done (Ott and Longnecker, 2001). Mental model of cattle farming systems were drawn using Microsoft Visio version 15.0.

3. Results and Discussions

3.1. Farmers Performance

Age of cattle farmers in Manokwari was at productive ages and similar between the scales ($p>0.05$). Large-scale farmers might have been raising cattle first followed by medium and small-scales. Therefore they were developed in time. It was also found in experiences. Although not significant ($p>0.05$), it was linear with the ages that larger-scale farmers have higher experiences compared to medium and small-scales. Family number living in each household was also similar ($p>0.05$). Large-scale farmers had higher number compared to medium and small-scales. In Thailand, most farmers were grouped into moderate livestock farmers (Suppadit *et. al.*, 2006). The ordinary livelihood of the cattle farmers in Manokwari were limited to as farmers and few found making private works. Small shops are commonly found in Manokwari. In general education background of the farmers was in level of elementary school. Education in Thailand had impact on good agricultural practices (GAPs) of cattle farmers in Thailand (Suppadit *et. al.*, 2006). Working time of the farmers allocated to tethered cattle was less than three hours. It means that cattle were released in several communal land and under secondary forest and palm oil trees.

Table 1. *Performances of traditional cattle farmers in Manokwari, Papua Barat.*

Farmers' Performances	Scale of groups								p
	Small (n=20)		Medium (n=17)		Large (n=7)		Total (N=44)		
	Mean	SD	Mean	SD	Mean	SD	Mean	SD	
Ages (y)[1]	41.2	11.9	45.6	7.6	47.9	12.7	44.9	10.7	NS
Experience (y)[1]	10.00	5.4	13.1	5.8	14.57	7.3	11.9	6.0	NS
Family (head)[1]	4.5	1.0	4.4	1.4	5.3	1.8	4.6	1.3	NS
Livelihood[2]	1.0	0.2	1.0	0.0	1.0	0	1	0.1	NS
Education[2]	2.1[a]	1.2	1.3[b]	0.8	1.0[c]	0	1.6	1.0	0.00
Workingtime (h)	1.1[a]	0.3	1.6[b]	0.5	1.6[b]	0.5	1.4	0.5	0.03
Farmers' knowledge									
Selection[2]	1.2[a]	0.4	1.6[b]	0.5	1.9[c]	0.4	1.5	0.5	0.00
Mating sign[2]	1.9	0.3	1.8	0.3	2.0	0.0	1.9	0.2	NS
Pregnant Detection[2]	1.3	0.5	1.2	0.4	1.1	0.4	1.2	0.4	NS
Provided forage[2]	1.1	0.3	1.4	0.5	1.4	0.5	1.3	0.4	NS
Grass Quality[2]	1.6	0.5	1.7	0.4	2.0	0.0	1.7	0.4	NS
Cattle housing[2]	1.1	0.2	1.1	0.2	1.0	0.0	1.1	0.2	NS
Disease knowledge[2]	1.2	0.4	1.1	0.3	1.1	0.4	1.2	0.4	NS
Diseases prevention[2]	1.7	0.5	1.7	0.5	1.3	0.5	1.6	0.5	NS
Utilization[2]	1.1[a]	0.2	1.5[b]	0.5	1.3[c]	0.5	1.2	0.4	0.01
Kind of product[2]	1.1	0.2	1.3	0.7	1.0	0.0	1.1	0.5	NS

[1)]Anova (F-test), $p<0.05$, [2)]NPar-test=Kruskal-Wallis (H), $p<0.05$. NS: Not Significant. Different superscripts indicated significant difference at $p<0.05$.

Selection of the cattle as breed was not almost done by farmers. Identification of mating time was also very limited only in few farmers as well as pregnant detection. The knowledge of farmers in raising cattle had notsufficient enough as recruited in management of livestock.

Some farmers applied offered forages for cattle and most cattle farmers did not provide forages.

The quality of grasses planted by farmers had low nutrient contents. Semi-natural grasses have low nutrient contents (Niemela *et. al.*, 2008). Experiences shown by

Central Java's farmers using paddy leaves. They were then made improvement by applying ammonization and fermentation for increase nutrient quality of paddy leaves (Nurcholidah *et. al.*, 2013; Muslim, 2006). Cattle farming systems in Manokwari have been kept mostly without houses, free-range cattle farming systems. It is similar in Kenya as reported by Ohaga *et. al.*, (2007). Cattle farmers had no sufficient knowledge in livestock diseases. While in Kenyan as reported by Ohaga *et. al.* (2007), diseases of livestock was Trypanosomosis, East Coast Fever, Anasplasmosis, Helminthosis, Anthrax, Food and Mouth Disease. However, Helminthosis could have huge infestation under tropical systems in Indonesia. Therefore, prevention of diseases had seldom done. Kenyan farmers had recognized diseases compared to West Papuan farmers. Utilization of cattle were done by selling and drought animal. Cattle have been seldom used as animal traction. In contrary, Kenyan livestock farmers have been intensively using cattle as animal traction (Ohaga *et. al.*, 2007). Kind of cattle products in Manokwari were meat, skin and feces.Skin was processed as fast food (in Bahasa called Kerupuk). Bio-fuel was extensively applied by many farmers in Papua (Widodo and Hendriadi, 2005). Other utilization of cattle product is bio-fertilizer which was intensively applied by crop farmers in Upland (Thanner *et al.*, 2001), Middle Java (Nurcholidah *et. al.*, 2013) and as well as Mid-Hill Nepal (Thanner and Tanner, 2002).

3.2. Cattle Performance

Herd size of cattle raised by farmers in Manokwari was significant difference ($p<0.000$). Small-scale farmers in average had only kept 2.5±0.9 head/hh. In one hand, medium and large-scale cattle farmers had doubled subsequently, i.e. 6.5±0.8 head/hh and 12.9±1.6 head/hh. Bali cattle werea commonly local breed introduced and raised in West New Guinea Papua. The herd size kept by farmers in Manokwari was lower than in Jawa Tengah/Centre of Java (Nurcholidah *et. al.*, 2013), i.e.14.6 livestock unit. In the Mid-Hill Nepal herd size in terms of Tropical Livestock Unit was 4-6 unit (Thorne and Tanner, 2002). Widayati and Suawa (2007) grouped cattle farmers in Sarmi-Papua into three classes, i.e. farmer with keeping cattle 1-2 head/hh, 3-6 head/hh and 7-10 head/hh. In Thailand farm size become significant component determining cattle performance (Suppadit *et. al.*, 2006). In Kenya as reported by Ohaga *et. al.* (2007), livestock herd size was relatively varied, i.e. 2-23 head/hh (median of 2).

Table 2. *Cattle performances in Manokwari, Papua Barat.*

Performance Cattle	Scale of groups						Total (N=44)		p
	Small (n=20)		Medium (n=17)		Large (n=7)				
	Mean	SD	Mean	SD	Mean	SD	Mean	SD	
Herd size (head)[1]	2.5^a	0.9	6.5^b	0.8	12.9^c	1.6	5.7	3.8	0.00
Parental stock (head)[1]	2.4	0.3	2.3	0.2	2.7	0.1	2.4	0.3	NS
Mating period (d)[1]	66.7	17.32	69	22.4	56.4	16.8	65.9	19.4	NS
Forage freq(times)[1]	2.4	0.5	2.3	0.5	2.6	0.5	2.4	0.5	NS
Offered Forages[2]	1.1^a	0.2	1.1^b	0.2	2.0^c	0.0	1.2	0.4	0.00

[1)]Anova (F-test), $p<0.01$, NS: Not Significant. Different superscripts indicated significant difference at $p<0.05$.

Parental stock of the cattle kept by farmers in Manokwari was slightly similar amongst the three scales ($p>0.05$), i.e. 2 livestock unit. Parental stock becomes much more important in designing future livestock development in Indonesia (Ilham, 2007). This should be done to improve genetically quality cattle. Mating period of cattle entering reproduction cycle was similar between the three systems ($p>0.05$). Forage frequency was practiced similar in the whole cattle farming scales ($p>0.05$). Due to free-range cattle farming systems adopted by traditional cattle farmers, forages offered to the cattle were less than that expected. Tropical forages grown commonly under agro-ecological zones in Manokwari were *Themeda arguens*, *Paspalum conjugatum*, *Digitaria* sp, *Imperata cylindrica*, *Cyperus rotundus* dan *Eleusine indica*. Wastes from agricultural crops should be utilized as applied by cattle farmers in East Java (Winarso *et. al.*, 2005). Therefore alternative forages should be prepared for the cattle such as reported by Kusnadi, (2008), Devendra and Sevilla, (2002) in Asia. Cattle farming system in West New Guinea needs some improvement. Nulik and Hau (2005) in East Nusa Tenggara had shown their research for improving local forages to high quality nutrient. Local forages applied were *Glirisedia sepium*, *Leucaena leucocephala* and *Sesbania glandiflora*. Those forages were made in the shapes of cube and pellet. The cube was the preferred one compared to pellet with sufficient nutrient quality. Best practices applying forages for livestock was reported in East Java (Anggraeni *et. al.*, 2006; Anggraeni *et. al.*, 2008). Therefore, Bahri (2004) recommended several issues to be promoted for improving cattle farming systems in Indonesia, i.e. breeds, feeds, policy, veterinary and food security and post-harvesting.Theses underlined issues were also suggested by Ilham (2007), national livestock feeds and cattle breeds.

3.3. Economical Performances

Agribusiness of cattle farms was measured in net benefits earned by cattle farmers. The calves, weaned calves, grower and adult cattle were varied sold. The prices of young steer cattle were in the ranges of 4 to 5 million rupiahs (US$400-

500).The prices of young heifer grower cattle were in the ranges of 4 (US$410-470). In Indonesia the prices are made based commonly on the simple mathematical formulae, i.e. Cattle prices=weight of cattle × 0.50 × the prices per kg meat.

Table 3. Agribusiness of traditional cattle farming system in Manokwari, Papua Barat.

Economic Performance(IDR)*	Scale of groups						Total (N=44)		p
	Small (n=20)		Medium (n=17)		Large (n=7)				
	Mean	SD	Mean	SD	Mean	SD	Mean	SD	
Male calf[1]	5352000	949720	5264700	615360	4785710	128637	5215900	898300	NS
Female calf[1]	4125000	930120	4794110	662820	4357140	110733	4420450	901280	NS
Young steer[1]	1190000	335449	1129411	211437	1114285	260950	1154545	277408	NS
Young heifer[1]	8900000	836660	8794110	685990	8928570	838080	8863630	765260	NS
Adult steer[1]	1925000	410231	2058823	511198	1714285	367099	1943181	452074	NS
Adult heifer[1]	1425000	276966	1405882	272650	1371428	309377	1409090	274343	NS

[1)]Anova (F-test), $p<0.05$, $p<0.05$. NS: Not Significant. *IDR.10.000=USD 1.

No differences ($p>0.05$) were found in prices of sold cattle in Manokwari. It means that the prices of sold cattle in Manokwari were very much controlled by the farmers and the middle men. Middle man had high benefit compared to cattle farmers (Widayati and Suawa, 2007). Although, it is traditional market, the farmers and buyers were put many effort to keep cattle prices.Similar information was also reported by Priyanti *et. al.* (1997) in Lampung. The small-scale cattle farms tend to sell cattle in high prices to gain fresh money as capitals for farm continuity. While the other two cattle farming were lower than that of small-scale. It is therefore, Adnyana (2000) cited by Sudaryanto and Jamal (2000) developed agribusiness of cattle in Indonesia. Other record of economical aspect was informed by Winarso *et. al.* (2005) in Eastern Java-Indonesia. Income from beef raising cattle had significant impact on good agricultural practices (GAPs) in Thailand (Suppadit *et. al.*, 2006). Good agricultural practices were also successful experienced by South Sulawesi's farmers (Basuno and Sehaeti, 2007). They said that GAPs are very much determined by available and ready human resources capacities. In conclusion of Winarso *et. al.* (2005), integration of livestock and farm agribusiness is the success story of beef cattle development in East Java.

4. Conclusions

Farmers performances will have severe determinant factor in shaping cattle farming system. Integration of livestock with farming business needs further collaboration. Breeds and feeding are the first two components for further improvement. Forages with low nutrient content would need feeding technology such as ammonization and fermentation. Good Agriculture Practices (GAPs) will be determined by available and capability of human resources. Extension is a small technical aspect that need further activities run under traditional cattle farming systems.

Acknowledgment

Authors thanked Dadan, S. Pt. for sharing data of cattle performances in Manokwari. Special thanks were given to the whole cattle farmers as participants during field visits in several villages both in coastal and lowland agro-ecological zones of Manokwari.

References

[1] Anggraeni, Y. N., U. Umiyasih, D. Pamungkas dan Aryogi. 2006. Potensi bahan pakan Inkonvensional Asal Limbah Pertanian dan Perkebunan di Beberapa Kabupaten di Jawa Timur. Seminar Nasional Teknologi Peternakan dan Veteriner. Hal.: 891-899.

[2] Anggraeni, Y. N. dan U. Umiyasih. 2008. Evaluasi Potensi Pakan Asal Limbah Tanaman Pangan dan Limbah Perkebunan di Daerah Prioritas Kawin Alam Pendukung Program P2SDS. Seminar Nasional Teknologi Peternakan dan Veteriner. Hal. 304-311.

[3] Bahri, S., B. Setiadi, I. Inounu. 2004. Arah penelitian dan pengembangan Peternakan Tahun 2005-2009. Seminar nasional teknologi peternakan dan veteriner 2004. P. 6-10.

[4] Basuno, E. and R.N. Suhaeti. 2007. Analisis bantuan pinjaman langsung masyarakat (BPLM); kasus pengembangan usaha ternak sapi di provinsi Sulawesi Selatan. Analisis kebijakan pertanian. Vol 5. No. 2., Juni 2007.p: 150-166.

[5] Bradford, G.E. 1999. Contribution of animal agriculture to meeting global human food demand. Livestock production science 59 (1999) 95-112.

[6] Conroy, C. 2005. Participatory livestock research; a Guide. ITDG publishing. Warwickshire. UK.

[7] Devendra, C. 2007. Perspectives on animal production systems in Asia. Livestock science 106 (2007) 1-18.

[8] Devendra, C. and C.C. Sevilla. 2002. Availability and use of feed resources in crop animal systems in Asia. Agricultural systems 71 (2002) 59-73.

[9] Devendra, C. and D. Thomas. 2002. Smallholder farming systems in Asia. Agricultural systems 71 (2002) 17-25.

[10] Diwyanto, K., B. R. Prawiradiputra dan D. Lubis. 2001. Integrasi Tanaman Ternak dalam Pengembangan Agribisnis yang Berdaya Saing, Berkelanjutan dan Berkerakyatan. Seminar Nasional Teknologi Peternakan dan Veteriner 2001. Hal.: 17-26.

[11] Hartono, S. and T.W. Widayati. 2013. An alternative approach to meet beef self-sufficiency in West Papua. J. Indonesian Trop. Anim. Agric. 36 (3) September. Diponegoro University, Semarang.

[12] Ilham, N. 2007. Alternatif kebijakan peningkatan pertumbuhan PDB Subsektor peternakan di Indonesia. Analisis kebijakan pertanian. Vol. 5. No. 4. Desember 2007. Hal.: 335-357.

[13] Indraningsih, R. Widyastuti, Y. Sani. .... Limbah Pertanian dan Perkebunan Sebagai Pakan Ternak; Kendala dan Prospek. Lokakarya Nasional Ketersediaan IPTEKS dalam pengendalian penyakit strategis pada ternak ruminansia besar. Hal.: 99-105.

[14] Iyai, D.A. dan H. Y. Chrisostomus. 2013. Scoping, Pemodelan dan Kuantifikasi Sistim-Sistim Peternakan Terpadu di Manokwari, Papua Barat. Laporan Penelitian. Fakultas Peternakan Perikanan dan IlmuKelautan. UniversitasNegeri Papua. Manokwari.

[15] Kusnadi, U., S. Iskandar, dan M. Sabrani. 1993. Research methodology for crops-animal systems in Hilly Areas of Indonesia. (Ed). C. Devendra dan C. Sevilla. Proceedings of an International Workshop. Crop-Animal Interaction. IRRI Discussion Paper Series No. 6. IRRI Philippines.

[16] Kusnadi, U. 2008. Inovasi teknologi peternakan dalam sistim integrasi tanaman-ternak untuk menunjang swasembada daging sapi. Jurnal pengembangan inovasi pertanian. 1 (3): 189-205.

[17] Muslim, C. 2006. Pengembangan sistim integrasi padi-ternak dalam upaya pencapaian swasembada daging di Indonesia: Suatu tinjauan evaluasi. Analisis kebijakan pertanian. Vol. 4. No. 3. September 2006. Hal. 226-239.

[18] Niemela, M., A. Huuskonen, S. Jaakola, E. Joki-Tokola, and M. Hyvarinen. 2008. Coastal meadows as pastures for beef cattle. Agriculture, Ecosystem and Environment 124 (2008) 179-186.

[19] Nulik, J., D.K. Hau. 2005. Pembuatan dan pemanfaatan pakan awet pada ternak sapi bali timor. Seminar nasional teknologi peternakan dan veteriner 2005.

[20] Nurcholidah, A. Sodiq, K. Muatip. 2013. Kinerja usaha peternakan sapi potong sebelum dan setelah mengikuti program Sarjana Membangun Desa Periode 2008-2012. Jurnal ilmiah peternakan 1 (3): 1183-1191.

[21] Ohaga, S.O., E.D. Kokwaro, I.O. Ndiege, A. Hassanali, R.K. Saini. 2007. Livestock farmer's perception and epidemiology of bovine trypanosomiasis in Kwale District, Kenya. Preventive veterinary medicine. 80 (2007) 24-33.

[22] Ott, R.L. and M. Longnecker. 2001. An introduction to statistical methods and data analysis. 5thEdition.Texas A & M University. Wadsworht Group USA.

[23] Priyanti, A., T.D. Soedjana, R. Matondang, P. Sitepu. 1997. Estimasi sistim permintaan dan penawaran daging sapi di provinsi Lampung. Jurnal Ilmu Ternak dan Veteriner. Vol. 3. No.2. Tahun 1998.

[24] Sudaryanto, T. dan E. Jamal. 2000. Pengembangan agribisnis peternakan melalui pendekatan Coorporate Farming untuk mendukung ketahanan pangan nasional. Seminar nasional peternakan dan veteriner. p: 35-47.

[25] Supriadi, H. 2008. Strategi kebijakan pembangunan pertanian di Papua Barat. Analisis kebijakan pertanian. Vol. 6 No. 4.Desember 2008: 352-377.

[26] Suppadit, T., N. Phumkokrak, P. Poungsuk. 2006. Adoption of Good Agriculture Practices For Beef Cattl Farming of Beef cattle raising farmers in Tambon Hindard, Dan Khunthot District, Nakhon Rachasima Province, Thailand. KMITL. Sci. Tech. J. Vol. 6. No.2. Juli-Des. 2006.

[27] Tanner, P.J., S.J. Holden, E. Owen, M. Winugroho, M. Gill. 2001. Livestock sustaining intensive smallholder crop production through traditional feeding practices for generating high quality manure-compost in Upland Java. Agriculture, Ecosystems and Environment. 84 (2001) 21-30.

[28] Thorne, P.J. and C.J. Tanner. 2002. Livestock and nutrient cycling in crop animal systems in Asia. Agricultural systems 71 (2002) 111-126.

[29] Utomo, B.N. and E. Widjaja. 2007. Integrasi ternak sapi bali dengan perkebunan kelapa sawit; 1. Introduksi teknologi inseminasi buatan dan sinkronisasi estrus untuk meningkatkan reproduktifitas ternak. Seminar nasional teknologi peternakan dan veteriner.

[30] Widayati, T.W. and E. K. Suawa. 2007. Pengembangan agribisnis peternakan sapi potong melalui perbaikan manajemen mikro di kabupaten Sarmi-Papua. Seminar nasional teknologi peternakan dan veteriner.

Epidemiological Status of Contagious Bovine Pleuropneumonia in Southern Zone of Tigray Regions, Northern Ethiopia

Teshale Teklue[1,*], Temesgen Tesfay[2], Tsigabu Nirayo[3], Birhanu Hailu[4], Solomon Wayu[2], Tesfay Atsbha[2]

[1]Mekelle Agricultural Research Center, Mekelle, Ethiopia
[2]Alamata Agricultural Research center, Alamata, Ethiopia
[3]Axum Agricultural Research Center, Axum, Ethiopia
[4]Samara University, College of Veterinary Medicine, Department of Veterinary Epidemiology and Preventive Medicine, Samara, Ethiopia

Email address:
teshale12@gmail.com (T. Teklue), teshalearaya@yahoo.com (T. Teklue)

Abstract: A cross sectional study was conducted from December 2012 to May 2013 to determine the epidemiological status of CBPP in southern zone of Tigray region, Northern Ethiopia. Purposive sampling was used in selection of districts, peasant association and farmers for interview and random sampling was used in selection of animals for serum collection. The questionnaire was provided to 109 informative farmers by face to face interview to know the general animal diseases in the zone and specifically about CBPP. About 26.6 % of the farmers mentioned CBPP as one of the major cattle diseases in the zone. Serum samples from 384 animals were collected to determine the sero-prevalence using complement fixation test. The overall he overall sero-prevalence was 11.9 % ranging from zero (0%) to 28% across different districts. There was no significant ($p<0.05$) association of sero-prevalence to age and sex groups but was significantly ($p< 0.05$) associated to the agro ecology and implies a great attention at the mid highland and lowland. The present work highlights a need to scheme and implement control measures directing at preventing further spread and lowering the prevalence of the disease in the zone through the use of better and coordinated vaccination program with great emphasis to animal movement routes.

Keywords: Epidemiology, Cattle, CBPP, Southern Zone of Tigray

1. Introduction

Agriculture is the mainstay of Ethiopia's economy providing 47% of the Gross Domestic product (GDP), employment to 85% of the population whereas industry contributes about 5% and services 10% (4) Livestock contributes about 25% to agricultural and 61% of total export (14). Ethiopia is one of the top ranking countries in Africa and among the first ten in the world in terms of livestock resource. Investment opportunities are potentially attractive for modern commercial livestock breeding, production and processing of meat, milk and eggs (http://www.africa-do-business.commention 05.06.2014).

Ethiopia possesses the highest number of livestock in Africa with an estimated 53.99 million cattle, 25.5 million sheep and 24.06 million goats (7). However, the productivity of this livestock sector is lower than the potential level of the African production average. Traditional methods of animal husbandry render the output per unit of domestic breed of livestock to be too low (6). The major biological constraints contributing to low productivity include low genetic potential of the animals, poor nutrition and prevailing diseases (2,3). Among the prevalent diseases Foot and mouth Disease (FMD), Contagious Bovine Pleuropneumonia (CBPP), lumpy skin disease, trypanosomiasis, external parasites and tick borne diseases are main animal health problems in animal health context.

Contagious bovine pleuropneumonia is a highly infectious

cattle disease, which is caused by *Mycoplasma mycoides* subspp *mycoides* SC (small colony, bovine biotype). It is the most economically important disease worldwide (18) and causes high morbidity and mortality losses to cattle (20). Contagious bovine pleuropheumonia is considered as one of the main stumbling blocks to the growth of the livestock industry on the African continent. Yearly losses directly or indirectly due to CBPP in Africa estimated to be is around two billion US dollars (27). Next to the eradication of rinderpest, CBPP is prime concern in African continent (1). It is one of the major threat in Ethiopia hindering and challenging the livestock production system (11, 10 and 12).

Even though there had been many research works in southern zone of Tigray region, there is limited information about the epidemiological status of the CBPP but there are frequent reports of the disease and this study was conducted to assess the epidemiological distribution of the disease in the zone across the different ecology and districts to implement continuous and tighten control and prevention measures both at farming level and outlet as well as inlet markets.

2. Material and Methods

2.1. Study Area Description

The study was conducted in Southern zone of Tigray Regional State, Northern Ethiopia. The zone is located at 660km North of Addis Ababa, capital of Ethiopia and 120 km South of Mekele, capital city of the Tigray regional state. Geographically it is located at 12^0 15'and 13^0 41' north latitude and 38° 59'and 39° 54'east longitude, constituting an area of 9,446 km^2. The zone consists of five administrative districts; the districts are namely Raya Alamata, Alaje, and Endamohoni, Ofla, and Raya azebo under different agro ecological zones. The study area has a total human population of 1,004,558 (12, 4813 from urban and 879,745 from rural) (5). The livestock population consists of 699,559 cattle, 269,098 sheep, 398,503 goats, 950 horses, 160,761 donkeys, 2,154 mule, 13,0303 camel, 845,548 poultry and 52,699 beehives (7). Livestock production is a major component of the livelihood system and provides draught power, food and income.

2.2. Study Animals

Herds of cattle managed under the traditional extensive production system were included in this study. Animals were randomly selected and all animals greater than six month in age were selected for serum collection. All animals from which blood samples were collected were apparently healthy and with no history of vaccinations to CBPP.

2.3. Study Design

A cross-sectional type of study was conducted from December 2012 to May 2013 in the four districts of southern zone of Tigray region. At the beginning of the study momentary description and discussion about the study was done with the district animal health experts (9) and all data were collected accordingly.

2.4. Data Collection

2.4.1. Questionnaire

Four districts were selected purposively from the five districts of the zone and from each districts, two peasant associations were included based on number of livestock population and ease of access for transportation (9). The study was done on eight peasant association and a total of 109 farmers were interviewed to collect the community perception. The farmers were selected purposively with the community animal health workers that own livestock species and expected to have experience about animal health. A detailed, organized and structured questionnaire were prepared and administered in person to farmers in an interview to obtain base line information on the existing diseases of ruminants according to the farmers. The questionnaire were pre-tested in the field and adjusted as required, translated into local language in a simple way that the farmers can understand. Main disease of cattle with local name, risk factors, and new diseases observed as well as transmission perceptions were collected as base line to know importance of CBPP in comparison with other cattle diseases in the farming community.

2.4.2. Sample Size and Serum Collection

Sample size was determined according to Thrusfield (21) formula and serum from 384 animals were collected randomly from the purposively selected peasant associations for serum collection considering 50% prevalence since there was no previous study specifically in the study area. Blood sample was collected aseptically from the jugular vein in 10ml to obtain serum. The serum was kept at-20^0C until serological testing (16). Data on sex, age, herd size, animal management, and agro climate of the area were collected along with sampling.

2.5. Laboratory Analysis

All sera collected were subjected to Complement Fixation Test (CFT) for the detection of contagious bovine pleura pneumonia antibodies according to OIE (15).

2.6. Data Analysis

Data of both community perception and biological collected was stored in the Microsoft Excel spread sheet program and analyzed using SPSS (19) The community perception was described by frequencies and the sero-prevalence was estimated by dividing the number of CFT positive animals by the total number of animals tested. Chi-square test was utilized to quantify the relationship between the sero-prevalence with categorical variables (districts), age, sex and agro-ecology. Fisher's exact test was utilized when the outcome variable was below five in number as a substitute for Chi square test in comparing two factors among each other.

3. Results

3.1. Major Ruminant Diseases in the Study Area According to the Farmers' Perception

As complementary to serological analysis, the farmers mentioned that the main prevalent large ruminant diseases in the study area were foot and mouth disease (Anashe), contagious bovine pleauro pneumonia (Samba), pasteurellosis (hidhido) and Black leg (Afefta) as presented in table 1. This study agreed to the finding of Yohhanes (22) and Kuastrose (23) who reported CBPP, CCPP, anthrax, black leg and pasteurellosis as the major infectious disease observed in the study area and other parts of the country.

Table 1. *Major Ruminant diseases according to community response in Southern Zone of Tigray Region.*

Major disease of ruminants			Respondents	
Scientific Name	Local Name	Species	No	%
Foot and Mouth Disease	Anashe	Bovine	79	72.4
Lumpy skin diseases	Dubdubta	Bovine	7	6.4
Anthrax	Tafya	Bovine	69	72.4
Pasteurellosis	Hidhido	Bovine	41	37.6
Contagious bovine pleuro pneumonia	Samba	Bovine	29	26.6
Black leg	Wokie	Bovine	91	83.5
Sheep and goat pox	Enfirir	Caprine	28	26.7
Pastuerellosis	Mieta	Sheep	42	38.5

3.2. Sero-prevalence of Contagious Bovine Pleuro Pneumonia

From the total of 384 sera samples examined,thirty six sera were test positive to CFT giving an overall prevalence of 11.9 as indicated in table 2.The highest sero-prevalence was observed in Alamata district (28%) and lower was 0 (0%) in Ofla and Endamehoni Districts.

Table 2. *The Sero-prevalence of CBPP in the districts of Southern Zone of Tigray Region, Northern Ethiopia.*

District	Number of animal tested	Negative	Positive	District sero-prevalence
R/alamata	105	75	30	28
R/azebo	106	81	16	15.2
Ofla	95	68	0	0
E/mehoni	78	63	0	0
Total	384	338	46	11.9

As shown in Table 3, the sero-prevalence of CBPP in male animals was 11% and 12.5 in female animals and the sero-prevalence between the two sexes were not statistically significant (p>0.05).

Table 3. *Sero-prevalence of CBPPin relation to sex in the four districts of Southern Zone of Tigray region Northern, Ethiopia.*

District	sex	Number of Animals tested	CFT Positive	Sero-prevalence (%)
Alamata	Male	30	9	13.2
	Female	75	21	6.8
Raya azebo	Male	38	6	8
	Female	68	10	33.3
Ofla	Male	45	0	0
	Female	50	0	0
Endamehoni	Male	50	0	0
	Female	28	0	0
Total			46	11.9

Risk factors considered in this study were sex and age of the animals as well as agro-ecology. Sero-prevalence was significantly associated with agro-ecology as indicated in table 4.

Table 4. *Risk factors associated with animal level Sero-prevalence of CBPP.*

Factors		N	CFT positive	Sero-prevalence	Chi-square	P value
Sex of animal					*	0.07
	Female	216	31			
	Male	168	15			
Age of animals	<2 years	97			*	0.28
	> 2 years	287				
Agro-ecology					51	0.001
	Highland	173				
	Midhighland	106				
	Lowland	105				

N= number of animals tested
* Fisher's exact test

4. Discussion

The result of the serological test (11.9 %) is complementary to the community perception that CBPP is common disease in the study area, in which 26.6 % of the respondents mentioned CBPP as one of the major cattle disease. The overall sero-prevalence (11.9 %) in the study area is parallel to other study conducted in different part of Ethiopia under extensive production system; 9.5% in older animals at different export quarantines of Ethiopia Kassaye and Molla (24), 10% in Dassenech district of South Omo Zone, South-Western Ethiopia Molla and Delil (25). Other study out of Ethiopia reported is also comparable to this study; 10.65 in Kwara state-Nigeria, by Olabode *et al.* (26). However, other reports from Ethiopia, 0.4 % by Gezahagn e*t al.*, (12) and Erimiyas *et al.*, (10) are lower compared to this study. The variation of these findings might be due to the variation in temporal and spatial distribution of the disease, animal management difference and the sensitivity of the serological tests used. In this study CFT test was used and others used ELISA though CFT is the recommended test by OIE (14). The sero-positivity of CBPP varies significantly among the study districts and this could be due to slight difference in animal movement though with similar production system. The significant ($P<0.05$) difference in the sero-prevalence may be due to difference in the districts and agro-ecology. The insignificant ($P<0.05$) difference of sero-prevalence among sex and age groups may be due to similar exposure of animals to the disease since the disease is contagious that all animal in the herd can be affected and chronic that a single diseased animal can serve as continuous source of infection to the herd. The disease is mainly transmitted from animal to animal in aerosols. This organism also occurs in saliva, urine, fetal membranes and uterine discharges (18). This could play great role in uniformity of infection in all age groups and sexes).

In conclusion, the sero-prevalence of CBPP in the region needs high attention in implementing the disease control and prevention strategies. The sero-prevalence difference was significantly associated to the agroecology and requires a great attention at the mid highland and lowland. Therefore, there is a need to develop scheme and implement control measures directing at preventing further spread and lowering the prevalence of the disease in the zone through the use of better and coordinated vaccination program especially along the animal movement routes.

Acknowledgment

We would like to express our appreciation to Alamata Agricultural research center in supporting this project both in human power and material. We would like to extend our gratitude to animal health experts of the zone for their unlimited support at the field work.

References

[1] Amanf W., 2009.Contagious bovine pleuropneumonia (lung sickness) in Africa. *Onderstepoort Journal of Veterinary Research, 76:13–17.*

[2] Belay, D., K. Yisehak and G.P.J. Janssens, 2012a. Survey of Major Diseases Affecting Dairy Cattle in Jimma Town, Oromia, Ethiopia. *Global Veterinaria, 8: 62-66.*

[3] Belay, D., K. Yisehak and G.P.J. Janssens, 2012b. Productive and Reproductive Performance of Zebu X Holstein-Friesian Crossbred Dairy Cows in Jimma Town, Oromia, Ethiopia. *Global Veterinaria, 8: 67-72.*

[4] Bureau of African Affairs, 2006. www.state.gov/r/pa/bgn/2859.htm.

[5] CSA, 2007. Population and Housing Census of Ethiopia, Addis Ababa: Central Statistical Agency

[6] CSA, 2008. Central statistics for livestock population in Ethiopia. Addis Abeba, Ethiopia

[7] CSA, 2013. Central statistics for livestock population in Ethiopia. Addis Abeba, Ethiopia

[8] Coopreck, D.L.1994. The Borenaplaute of southern Ethiopia. Synthesis of pastoral research, development and change, 1986-91. System study International Livestock Center for Africa (ILCA), Addis Ababa, Ethiopia.

[9] Dohoo, L., Martin,W., and Stryhn,H., 2003. Veterinary Epidemiologic Research. Prince Edward Island, Canada.

[10] Erimiyas Dele, Berihun Afera, Etsay Kebede, Nesibu Awol and Birhanu Hadush, 2014. Sero-prevalence of Trade Hampering Livestock Diseases in Animals Originated from Borana at Export Quarantine Centers in Adama, Central Ethiopia. *African Journal of Basic & Applied Sciences 6 (2): 30-36.*

[11] Gedlu Mekonnen, 2004. Serological, Clinical and Participatory Epidemiological Survey of Contagious Bovine Pleuropneumonia in Somali Region, Ethiopia (MSC thesis). Addis Ababa University, Faculty of Veterinary Medicine, Debre-zeit, Ethiopia.

[12] Gezahegn Alemayehu, Samson Leta and Berhanu Hailu, 2014. Low sero-prevalence of Contagious Bovine Pleuropneumonia (CBPP) in bulls originated from Borena Pastoral Area of Southern Ethiopia. *Animal and Veterinary Sciences. 2(6): 213-217.*

[13] ILCA Bulletin, 1980. Small ruminant production .Addis Ababa, Ethiopia, pp2-11.

[14] Livestock Data Innovation in Africa, 2012. www.africalivestockdata.org

[15] OIE Terrestrial Manual, 2008. Contagious bovine Pleuropneumonia.

[16] OIE Terrestrial Manual, 2009. Contagious bovine Pleuropneumonia.

[17] OIE Terrestrial Manual, 2014. Contagious bovine Pleuropneumonia.

[18] Radostits, D.M. Blood, D.C. and Gay, C.C., 2008. Veterinary Medicine. A Textbook of diseases of cattle, sheep, pigs, goats and horses. 8th ed. London. Bailliere Tindal. Pp. 748-785.

[19] SPSS, 2007. Statistical package for social science version 16 by Jim Dalrymple, Macworld Software company, USA.

[20] Tambi, N.E., Maina, W.O. and Ndi, C. 2006. An estimation of the economic impact of contagious bovine pleuropneumonia in Africa. Rev. sci. tech. Off. int. Epiz., 25 (3), 999-012.

[21] Thrusfield M., 2008. Sampling in Veterinary Epidemiology. 3rd ed., Black well Science Ltd, London. 46-65, 228-242 Pp.

[22] Yohannes Tekle, 2007. Major animal health problems of market oriented livestock Development in Alamata Woreda. A thesis submitted to the Faculty of Veterinary Medicine, Addis Ababa University, as a partial fulfillment of the requirements for the attainment of Degree, Doctor of Veterinary Medicine (DVM), Debreziet Ethiopia.

[23] Kuastros Mekonnen, Major animal health problems of market oriented livestock development in Alaba woreda, Southern Nations Nationalities and peoples region. A thesis submitted to the Faculty of Veterinary Medicine, Addis Ababa University, as apartial fulfillment of the requirements for the attainment of Degree, Doctor of Veterinary Medicine (DVM), Debreziet Ethiopia.

[24] Kassaye D; Molla W., 2012.Sero-prevalence of contagious bovine pleuropneumonia at export quarantine centers in and around Adama, Ethiopia. *Trop Anim Health Prod*; 45(1): 275-9.

[25] Molla B, Delil F. 2015. Mapping of major diseases and devising prevention and control regimen to common diseases in cattle and shoats in Dassenech district of South Omo Zone, South-Western Ethiopia. *Trop Anim Health Prod.* 47(1):45-5.

[26] Olabode HOK, Mailafia S, Adah BMJ, Nafarnda WD, Ikpa LT, Jambalang AR, and Bello RH, 2013. Serological Evidence of Contagious Bovine Pleuro-Pneumonia antibodies in tradecattle (Bos Indicus) sold in Kwara state-Nigeria. Online *International Journal of Microbiology Research.Volume 1, Issue 1, pp. 14-19.*

[27] FAO-OIE-OAU/IBAR-IAEA Consultative Group on CBPP (Rome, 12–14 November 2003). Rome, Italy. 2004. Towards sustainable CBPP control programmes for Africa.

Assessment of Reproductive Performance and Problems in Crossbred (Holstein Friesian X Zebu) Dairy Cattle in and Around Mekelle, Tigray, Ethiopia

Alemselam Birhanu Mekonnin[1, 2, *], Christopher R. Harlow[1], Goitom Gidey[2], Desalew Tadesse[2], Gidena Desta[2], Tadesse Gugssa[3], Simon C. Riley[1]

[1]MRC Centre for Reproductive Health, CMVM, University of Edinburgh, Edinburgh, UK
[2]College of Veterinary Medicine, Mekelle University, Tigray, Mekelle, Ethiopia
[3]Tigray Bureau of Agriculture and Rural Development, Tigray, Mekelle, Ethiopia

Email address:
A.B.Mekonnin@sms.ed.ac.uk (A. B. Mekonnin)

Abstract: A cross sectional study was conducted in and around Mekelle, Tigray, Ethiopia from November 2013 to May 2014 with the aims to assess reproductive performance and prevalence of reproductive problems in crossbred (Holstein Friesian x Zebu) dairy cattle. A questionnaire survey methodology was used. The study sampled 177 randomly selected dairy farms comprising 1013 crossbred dairy cattle (736 cows and 277 heifers). The mean age at first service, age at first calving, first postpartum estrus and calving interval were 24.8 months, 35.3 months, 114.5 days and 401.5 days, respectively. Prevalence rates of reproductive problems recorded in the study area were anestrus (37.8%), repeat-breeding (21.0%), dystocia (11.6%), retained fetal membranes (11.5%), endometritis (6.6%), abortion (6.4%), prolapsed uterus/vagina (2.9%), stillbirth (2.0%) and freemartin (0.2%). Incidence of abortion did not vary with parity and stages of gestation. Breeding and the possible causes of missing insemination/mating while animals were in estrus are problematic. In conclusion, this study has revealed that the reproductive performance of crossbred dairy cattle was not optimal, and anestrus, repeat-breeding, dystocia, retained fetal membranes, endometritis and abortion were the major reproductive problems. More effective breeding and reproductive health management should be considered to improve the fertility of this crossbred cattle herd. Awareness and training should be provided to the farming community to improve the productivity in the region.

Keywords: Crossbred Dairy Cattle, Reproductive Performance, Reproductive Problems

1. Introduction

Ethiopia owns the largest livestock population in Africa and one of the largest in the world, having 52 million cattle, 33 million sheep, 30 million goats, 2.5 million camels and 38 million poultry [1]. About 85% of the Ethiopian population are engaged in the agricultural sector, which is the backbone of the country's economy, with livestock and its products being important sources of food and income [2]. However, dairying has not been fully exploited and promoted. Cattle play the most important role in the farming economy followed by sheep and goats. This cattle population is primarily of indigenous Zebu type [3]. Barka, Fogera, Boran, Horro, Sheko, Afar and Arsi are also among the Ethiopian local breed cattle which are crossbred with exotic breeds (Holstein Friesian and Jersey). Cattle are well adapted and distributed among diverse ecological conditions and management systems [4].

Dairy cattle production in the country is classified into four major livestock production systems: rural smallholder (mixed crop-livestock) production, pastoral and agro-pastoral production, urban and peri-urban smallholder dairy production, and specialized commercial dairy production systems [2,5]. Infertility is the main problem that affects production in both local and crossbred cows and heifers in Ethiopia [6,7,8]. Consequently, the economic gain for example, calf crops, milk and milk products, from these cows is not satisfactory. Puberty in heifers is usually at 24 months in Zebu X Holstein-Friesian crossbred dairy cattle [7] and, heifers are reported to have an extended later age at first calving. Most cows in smallholder farms do not optimally calve every 12 to 13 months after the first calving [6].

Tigray regional state (northern part of Ethiopia) contributes a significant proportion (3.5 million) to the Ethiopian cattle population [1]. There is also an increased demand for milk and milk products in and around Mekelle city [9], due to increased population growth and urbanization. Consequently, the number of people involved in small scale intensive, large scale intensive and small holder dairy farming has increased dramatically in the vicinity of the city. This growth effort is supported by government extension programs through provision of door-to-door Artificial Insemination (AI) service to improve the genetic potential and increase milk production. Despite the effort by government to enhance the dairy sector, there is limited ongoing livestock research, particularly on assessment of reproductive and productive performance and reproductive problems of dairy cattle. Therefore, the objectives of this study were to assess reproductive performance and to study the prevalence of reproductive problems of crossbred (Zebu x Holstein Friesian) dairy cattle in and around Mekelle, Tigray, Ethiopia.

2. Materials and Methods

2.1. Study Area

The study was conducted from November 2013 to May 2014 in and around Mekelle city, which is the largest city in northern Ethiopia, and the capital city of Tigray. It is located at 39° 29`E and 13° 30` N at an altitude of 2000 metres above sea level. The climate of the study area conforms to that of Ethiopian Highlands. The mean annual rainfall is 619mm, which is bimodal with short rainy seasons occurring from March to May and from mid-September to February. The annual minimum and maximum temperature is 11.8°C and 29.9°C, respectively [10].

2.2. Study Methodology

2.2.1. Study Farms and Animals

The number of farms sampled in the study was determined by $N=0.25/SE^2$, where N= number of sampled farms, SE=Standard error [11]. A list of 210 farms housing crossbred dairy animals were considered as the sampling frame. From this, 173 farms were selected using systematic random sampling. Considering standard error of 0.038 with 95% confidence interval as follows, $N=0.25/ (0.038)^2 = 173$. In total, 177 dairy farms were included in the survey to enhance precision. These farms housed 736 crossbred (Zebu x Holstein Friesian) dairy cows and 277 crossbred dairy heifers aged two years or above. They also housed 55 crossbred dairy bulls and 398 crossbred dairy calves during the study period.

2.2.2. Questionnaire Data Collection and Analysis

The questionnaire (Appendix 1) was translated into local language (Tigrigna) and piloted beforehand. A cross-sectional survey was used to collect information on reproductive performance and assess the common reproductive problems of crossbred dairy cows and heifers. Farm owners, attendants, managers, and veterinary professionals were given a short briefing about the overall aims of the study. They were asked to complete the questionnaire survey information regarding age at first service, age at first calving, calving interval, first post-partum estrus, reproductive health problems, breeding history (AI, natural mating, parity) and other related questions including the year of farm establishment. Data was analysed using two tailed Fisher's exact test where a p value of < 0.05 was considered significant [12].

3. Results

3.1. Reproductive Performance

The average ages at first service and at first calving were 24.8 months (range 10 to 48 months) and 35.3 months (range of 21 to 57 months), respectively. First postpartum estrus and calving interval are indicated in Table 1.

3.2. Common Reproductive Problems

Anestrus, repeat-breeding, dystocia, retained fetal membranes (RFM), endometritis and abortion were the major reproductive problems cited by farmers/attendants or veterinarians in crossbred dairy cattle, with prevalence indicated in Table 2. Among 177 farms, 163 (92.1%) farms were affected by one or multiple reproductive problems. There were similar incidences of abortion in cows and heifers based on stages of pregnancy (Table 3). Overall incidence of abortion in crossbred cattle in first, second and third trimesters were, 17.5%, 42.1% and 40.4%, respectively. There was significantly higher ($p<0.05$) incidence of anestrus in heifers than cows. Conversely, higher incidence ($P<0.05$) of dystocia and retained placenta was recorded in multiparous than in primiparous cattle (Table 2).

The common breeding method in the study area is mixed AI and natural mating by bull (Table 4). Among 177 farms, 68 (38.4%) farms had shown missing insemination/mating due to various factors. Although animals showed typical signs of estrus (including clear vaginal discharge, restlessness, mounting other cows, mounted by other cows), owners failed to get their animals mated or inseminated. Major causes of missed insemination recorded are absence of AI technicians when called to inseminate, or arriving very late (33.8%), poor animal condition (19.1%), inattentiveness (11.8%) and reproductive/other health problems (8.8%).

Table 1. Reproductive performance of crossbred dairy cattle in the study area.

Variable	Range	Mean ± SD
Age at first service (months)	10 to 48	24.8±6.6
Age at first calving (months)	21 to 57	35.3±6.3
First postpartum estrus (days)	9 to 480	114.5±73.7
Calving interval (days)	302.9 to 759.2	401.5±73.0

Table 2. The relative prevalence of major reproductive problems of crossbred dairy cows and heifers in and around Mekelle.

Reproductive problems	Total incidence*	Incidence in multiparous cows*	Incidence in heifers/ primiparous heifers*	P-value (Fisher's exact test)
Anestrus¶	336 (37.8)	225 (31.5)	111 (63.1)	< 0.0001
Repeat-breeding¶	187 (21.0)	153 (21.4)	34 (19.3)	0.6058
Dystocia	103 (11.6)	92 (12.9)	11 (6.2)	0.0122
RFM	102 (11.5)	99 (13.9)	3 (1.7)	< 0.0001
Endometritis	59 (6.6)	52 (7.3)	7 (4.0)	0.1293
Abortion	57 (6.4)	50 (7.0)	7 (4.0)	0.1698
Stillbirth	18 (2.0)	17 (2.4)	1 (0.6)	0.2259
Prolapsed uterus/ vagina	26 (2.9)	26 (3.6)	0	-
Freemartin	2 (2.0)	-	2 (1.1)	-
Total	890	714	176	

Anestrus¶ and repeat-breeding¶ were compared between multiparous cows and heifers; whereas, dystocia, retained fetal membranes (RFM), endometritis, abortion, stillbirth and prolapsed uterus/vagina were compared between multiparous cows and primiparous heifers; freemartin associated with heifers. Animals were reported to have one or multiple exposures to a single or to multiple problems. *Values in parentheses are percentages. P-value of < 0.05 considered significant.

Table 3. Prevalence of abortion based on stages of pregnancy versus parity in crossbred dairy cattle.

Stage of gestation	Total aborted*	Abortion based on parity		P-value (Fisher's exact test)
		Multiparous cows*	Primiparous heifers*	
1st trimester	10 (17.5)	7 (14.0)	3 (42.9)	0.0949
2nd trimester	24 (42.1)	23 (46.0)	1 (14.2)	0.2197
3rd trimester	23 (40.4)	20 (40.0)	3 (42.9)	1.0000
Total	57 (100)	50 (100)	7 (100)	0.1698

*Values in parentheses are percentages. P value of < 0.05 considered significant.

Table 4. Breeding practises with crossbred cattle in the study area.

Breeding methods	Number of farms*
Artificial insemination (AI)	61 (34.5)
Natural mating (bull)	46 (26)
Mixed AI and bull	70 (39.5)
Total	177 (100)

*Figures in parentheses are percentages.

4. Discussion

4.1. Reproductive Performance

4.1.1. Age at First Service and Age at First Calving

In the current study, the age at first service and calving were in accordance with previous studies in small holder dairy farms in Oromia region, Ethiopia [8]. Similar ages were also recorded in crossbred cattle at first service in Gondar town [13] and in Dire Dawa [14], Ethiopia. Ages at first service and first calving were similar to recent studies in small scale farms in and around Mekelle, Ethiopia [15]. Further, comparable ages at first calving were recorded in previous studies in urban and in peri-urban crossbred dairy cattle farms, in central Tigray [16], and in crossbred cattle in Tanzania [17,18]. However, later age at first calving was recorded in the present study than in crossbred (Arsi breed X Jersey, and Arsi breed X Holstein Friesian) cattle in Asella, Ethiopia [19,20]. The current study showed comparatively earlier age in crossbred dairy heifers at first calving than in Zimbabwe [21], other parts of Ethiopia [6] and in Malawi [22]. Heifers can be bred when they attain 60% of their adult body weight [23]. For a dairy farm to be profitable there should be a focus on heifer's timely growth and conception. Age at puberty and calving are highly related to body weight of the heifers [24].

4.1.2. First Postpartum Estrus and Calving Interval

Comparatively longer postpartum estrus was recorded in the present study than in Oromia region, Ethiopia [8]. In contrast, the present study showed shorter postpartum estrus period compared to studies in Abernosa Ranch [25] and in small scale farms in and around Mekelle, Ethiopia [15]. In the present study, the calving interval was similar to previous reports [8,19]. In contrast, the present findings revealed shorter calving intervals compared to previous studies in central part of Ethiopia [6], Abernisa Ranch, Ethiopia [17], small scale dairy farms in and around Mekelle, Ethiopia [15], Malawi [22] and Tanzania [18]. Unlike the present study and other reports in crossbred (Zebu x Holstein Friesian) dairy cattle, pure Zebu (Bos indicus) cattle have a much longer calving interval [26]. Farmers/attendants or farm managers in the present study were asked if they had observed pregnancy overdue. They responded indicating animals bearing male calves tend to have 1 to 2 weeks longer gestation periods compared to female calves, which is in accordance with previous reports [8].

4.2. Prevalence of Reproductive Problems

Anestrus was found to be the most prevalent reproductive problem followed by repeat-breeding. This is in contrast to a previous questionnaire survey [27]. The present study also demonstrated high incidence of anestrus in comparison with a study in crossbred cattle in Bangladesh [28]. Our study indicates that repeat-breeding was a major problem affecting fertility of animals in the study area. High incidence of repeat breeding could be due to lack of nutrition, improper insemination and timing of AI and poor semen quality [29]. Our incidence of repeat breeding is comparatively higher than previous reports from Ethiopia in crossbred cows around Bedelle [27], East Showa [29], in indigenous Boran breed cows in Borena Zone [30], in crossbred cows/heifers in Mekelle city, Ethiopia [31] and in crossbred cows in Bangladesh [28]. Conversely, the present study showed lower incidence of repeat-breeding than incidences in Goa, India [32].

Dystocia is one of the major reproductive problems in crossbred dairy cattle in and around Mekelle, and is comparatively higher than in previous reports from south western [27] and other parts of Ethiopia [29]. Our findings are in contrast to previous studies where incidence of dystocia was higher in multiparous cows compared to primiparous heifers [33]. Incidence of dystocia in primiparous heifers was less than in multiparous cows. The possible causes of dystocia reported by the farmers and veterinarians were failure of cervical dilatation, fetal oversize, twinning, abnormal presentation, position and posture of the fetus, uterine inertia, hypocalcaemia and obesity of the dam.

Prevalence of retained fetal membranes was in agreement with previous studies conducted in south western part of Ethiopia [27]. Contrary to our finding, lower incidence was reported in crossbred dairy cows in other part of Ethiopia [29] and crossbred cows in Bangladesh [28]. The higher incidence of retained fetal membranes in multiparous cows than primiparous heifers were consistent with previous studies in Israel [34]. The reason retained fetal membranes was higher in multiparous cows could be due to previous exposure to reproductive problems or other health problems and nutritional deficiencies.

The prevalence of endometritis in the present study was comparatively lower than previous reports in crossbred cows in other part of Ethiopia [27]. However, it was higher than reports in East Shoa, Ethiopia [29] and Bangladesh [28].

Abortion is one of the major causes of economic losses in the cattle industry. Overall incidence of abortion in the current survey was comparatively higher than in reports by Esheti and Moges [29], although lower than in other studies of crossbred cows elsewhere in Ethiopia [27]. Abortion could be due to metabolic or hormonal abnormalities, nutritional deficiencies, trauma, toxicities, or infectious agents [35,36]. In the present study, although results were not significant, there was comparatively higher prevalence of stillbirth in calves born from multiparous cows to calves born from primiparous heifers. Contrary to our survey, it is speculated that the occurrence of assisted calving is 2.5 times higher in primiparous heifers than multiparous cows and that there is a high incidence of stillbirth [37]. This represents an area for future study.

The exact cause of prolapsed uterus is not clear [38] although high estrogen has been proposed to cause prolapsed vagina [39]. Delayed intervention in cases of uterine prolapse may cause fatal septicaemia [40]. Freemartinism is not a major reproductive problem in crossbred cattle in and around Mekelle, although it is one of the causes of anestrus and sterility in heifers. The occurrence of freemartinism reaches 90-97% in twin pregnancies in cattle [41,42].

This study has noted high incidence of missed insemination or mating. The use of AI is encouraged by government, with a bull rearing and semen collection centre being established in Mekelle, and few farmers have their own crossbred dairy bulls for breeding purposes. When animals are not bred when they come to estrus, this will inevitably result in heifers with a long age at first service and first calving, and cows with a longer calving interval, hence a decreased calf crop or replacement heifers. Strategies to improve breeding management should be developed to achieve one calf per year and therefore improve economic development in dairy production.

In conclusion, this study has noted that the reproductive performance of crossbred cattle was not optimal, and that anestrus, repeat-breeding, dystocia, retained fetal membranes, endometritis and abortion were the major reproductive problems affecting fertility of crossbred dairy cattle in and around Mekelle, Tigray, Ethiopia. Hence, effective breeding and reproductive health management should be considered as a means to improve fertility of crossbred cattle. Furthermore, awareness and training should be given to the farming community to improve productivity for the dairy industry in the region.

Acknowledgments

The authors acknowledge School of Clinical Sciences, College of Medicine and Veterinary Medicine, University of Edinburgh for supporting Alemselam Birhanu Mekonnin and for funding the study. Special thanks would be offered to Mekelle University, College of Veterinary Medicine for the offer of transport and other facilities and support. We also thank the farmers, farm attendants, farm managers, AI technicians and veterinary professionals working in dairy farms who agreed to participate in the survey.

Appendix 1

Pre-screening questionnaire given to livestock owners/ farm managers to study the prevalence of reproductive diseases/ problems in crossbred cows/heifers in and around Mekelle, Tigray, Ethiopia.

1. Name of the farm or farm owner______________________________

2. Address of the farm: ______________________________; phone no. ____________

3. When was the farm established? ☐ 1-5 years ☐ 6-10 years ☐ > 10 years

4. Type of farm: ▭Intensive ▭Semi-intensive ▭ Extensive

5. Number of cattle in the farm (owned)? ____________________

a. No. of Cows___________ c. No. of bulls___________

b. No. of heifers__________ d. No. of calves__________

6. Types of feed cows or heifers are fed:

▭Hay ▭ Straw ▭Concentrate ▭ Concentrate and hay or straw

7. How many times do animals get feed per day? _________________

8. Do animals get water regularly? ______; how many times a day?________________

9. Age of cows and/or heifers and parity (years):

Cow 1._________ (parity________); heifer 1. ____________

Cow 2._________ (parity________); heifer 2. _____________

Cow 3._________ (parity________); heifer 3. _____________

Cow 4._________ (parity________); heifer 4. _____________

Cow 5._________ (parity________); heifer 5. _____________

Cow 6. _________ (parity________); heifer 6. _____________

Cow 7. _________ (parity________); heifer 7. _____________

Cow 8. _________ (parity________); heifer 8. _____________

Cow 9. _________ (parity________); heifer 9. _____________

Cow 10. _________ (parity________); heifer 10 ___________

10. What is the number of pregnant cows/ heifers in the farm?

A) Cows: _______ (trimester:_______ 1st; _____2nd; ____3rd)

B) Heifers: ______ (trimester: _______1st; _____2nd; _____3rd)

11. Method of insemination? Natural AI Both

12. Number of animals in estrous now? A) Cows: ________; B) Heifers: ________

13. How many lactating cows do you have? ________

14. What is the number of anestrus animals in the farm? A) Cows? ______; B) Heifers: ____

15. Were any of your cattle encountered reproductive diseases or problems in the past? ▭Yes ▭No

16. If yes, what reproductive diseases or problems were observed?

____

17. Did any of your cows suffer from abortion? ▭Yes ▭ No

18. If yes, what month of the pregnancy abortion was occurred?

a. before 3 months c. over 6 months

b. 3 to 6 months d. a, b and c

19. Did any of your cows encounter pregnancy overdue in the past? ▭Yes ▭ No

If yes, how many months was the cow pregnant before it was given veterinary assistance?

_________________? Number of cows diagnosed positive? ___________

20. Did any of your cows or heifers give birth to a dead calve at a normal gestation length (9 months) in the past?

▭Yes ▭No

If yes, how many cows? __________

21. Did any of your cows suffer from dystocia in the past? ▭Yes ▭No

If yes, how many of your cows suffered from dystocia? ________

22. Did any of your cows suffer from endometritis in the past? ▭Yes ▭No

If yes, no of cows or heifers suffered from endometritis? ___________

23. Did any of your cows or heifers suffer from vaginal, cervical or uterine prolapse in the past?

▭Yes ▭ No

If yes, number of cows or heifers with vaginal prolapse? ________________; Cervical prolapse?____________ or uterine prolapse?______________

24. Did any of your cows encounter retained fetal membranes in the past? ___________

How did you solve the problem?

____

25. Have any of your cows or heifers been repeater (repeat breeder)?

If yes, what do you think the cause/s for the animal to come back in to estrus again?

What measure did/do you take to get the animal pregnant?

____

26. Did any of your cows suffer from metritis in the past?

If yes, what treatment did the cow get?

What was the effect of the treatment in the reproductive status of the cow after that?

27. Did any of your animals come to estrus, but missed insemination or mating in the past? ▭Yes ▭ No

If yes, why was the animal not inseminated or mated?

a. Lack of bull

b. Lack of AI technician

c. Lack of means of communication to AI technician

d. Called AI technician, but did not come to inseminate or did come very late

e. Reproductive tract problem

f. Size of the animal was very small to breed

g. Lack of nutrition

h. All or some of the above causes

28. Did any of your animals suffer from any health problem other than reproductive health?

If yes, please describe the disease and signs the animals showed.

____

29. What is your future plan to improve the reproductive performance of your animals?

____

30. What do you think the government (agriculture, universities, etc.) and private sectors should do to support improve fertility of your animals? ________________________________

31. Do you have any comment?

____

Thanks!!

References

[1] CSA (2012). (Central Statistics Agency of Ethiopia). http://www.csa.gov.et.

[2] IBC (Institute of Biodiversity Conservation), 2004. The state of Ethiopia's farm animal genetic resources-country report. A contribution to the First Report on the State of the Worlds Animal Genetic Resources. ftp://ftp.fao.org/docrep/fao/010/a1250e/annexes/CountryReports/Ethiopia.pdf.

[3] NABC (2010). Fact Sheet: Livestock Ethiopia; Livestock in Ethiopia and opportunity analyses for Dutch investment September 2010 NABC.

[4] Lobago, F., Bekana, M., Guftafsson, H. and Kindahl, H. (2006). Reproductive performance of dairy cows in smallholder production system in Selalle, Central Ethiopia. Trop. Anim. Health Prod. 38: 333-342.

[5] Lobago, F. (2007). Reproductive and lactation performance of dairy cattle in the Oromia Central Highlands of Ethiopia with special emphasis on pregnancy period. Doctoral thesis Swedish University of Agricultural Sciences, Uppsala.

[6] Shiferaw, Y., Tenhagen, B. A., Bekana, M. and Kassa, T. (2003). Reproductive performance of crossbredd cows in different production systems in the central highlands of Ethiopia. Trop. Anim. Health and Prod. 35: 551-561.

[7] Duguma, B., Kechero, Y. and Janssens, G-P.J. (2012). Productive and Reproductive Performance of Zebu X Holstein-Friesian Crossbred Dairy Cows in Jimma Town, Oromia, Ethiopia. Global Veterinaria 8(1): 67-72.

[8] Dinka H. (2013). Reproductive performance of crossbred dairy cows under smallholder condition in Ethiopia. AJDFMP 1(5): 101-103.

[9] Fisseha, N. E. (2010). Determinants, challenges and prospects of dairy production and marketing in Mekelle city.Master's Thesis.Mekelle University, Mekelle, Ethiopia.

[10] BoPED (2011). (Bureau of Planning and Economic Development), Tigray, Ethiopia.

[11] Arsham, H. (2005). Questionnaire design and surveys sampling, 9th ed. http://home.ubalt.edu/ntsbarsh/stat-data/Surveys.htm (Retrieved July15, 2012).

[12] Prism 6.0 for Windows, GraphPad Inc., La Jolla, California, USA, http://www.graphpad.com. (Accessed online 23 November 2014).

[13] Nuraddis I., Shebir A. and Shiferaw M. (2011). Assessment of Reproductive Performance of Crossbred Cattle (Holstein Friesian X Zebu) in Gondar Town.Global Veterinaria 6(6): 561-566.

[14] Mureda, E. and Mekuriaw, Z. (2007). Reproductive Performance of Crossbred Dairy Cows in Eastern lowlands of Ethiopia. Livestock Research for Rural Development. Volume 19, Article number 161. http://www.lrrd.org/lrrd19/11/mure19161.htm.

[15] Kumar, N. and Tkui, K. (2014). Reproductive performance of crossbred dairy cows in Mekelle, Ethiopia. Sci. J. Anim Sci. 3(2): 35-40.

[16] Weldeslasse, G. T., Zeleke, Z. M. and Gangwar, S. K (2012): Reproductive and productive performance of dairy cattle in Central Zone of Tigray, Northern Ethiopia. I.J.A.B.R. 2(1): 58-63.

[17] Haile-mariam M., Banjaw K., Gebremeskel J., Ketema T. (1993). Productivity of Boran Cattle and their Friesian crosses at Abernossa Ranch, Ethiopia. I. Reproductive performance and prevailing mortality. Trop. Anim. Health Prod. 25: 239-248.

[18] Asimwe, L. and Kifaro, G. C. (2007). Effect of breed, season, year and parity on reproductive performance of dairy cattle under smallholder production system in Bukoba district, Tanzania. Livestock Research for Rural Development 19. http://www.lrrd.org/lrrd19/10/asim19152.htm.

[19] Negussie E., Brannang E., Banjaw, K. and Rottmann, O. U. (1998).Reproductive performance of dairy cattle at Assella livestock farm.Arsi. Ethiopia. I: Indigenous cows versus their F1 crosses. J. Anim. Breed. Genet. 115: 267-280.

[20] Yifat D., Kelay B., Bekana M., Lobago F., Gustafsson H. and Kindahl H. (2009). Study on reproductive performance of crossbred dairy cattle under smallholder conditions in and around Zeway, Ethiopia. Livestock Research for Rural Development. 21(88). Retrieved April 15, 2015, from http://www.lrrd.org/lrrd21/6/yifa21088.htm.

[21] Masama, E., Kusina, K. T., Sibanda, S. and Majoni, C. (2003). Reproduction and lactation performance of cattle in a smallholder dairy system in Zimbabwe. Trop. Anim. Health Prod. 35: 117-129.

[22] Agyemang, K. and Nkhonjera, L. P. (1990). Productivity of Crossbred Cattle on Smallholder Farms in Southern Malawi. Trop. Anim. Health Prod. 22: 9-16.

[23] Hammond, J. (1960), Farm animals their breeding, growth and inheritance. Arnold, London. 49(5): 46-473.

[24] Moore, R. K., Kennedy, B. W., Schaefer, L. H. and Moxley, J. E. (1990). Relationship between reproduction traits, age and body weight at calving and days dry in first lactation Ayrshires and Holsteins. J. Dairy Sci. 73: 835-842.

[25] Bekele T., Kasali O. B. and Alemu T. (1991). Reproductive problems in crossbred cattle in Central Ethiopia. Anim. Prod. Sci. 26: 41-49.

[26] Mukasa-Mugerwa, E. (1989). A review of reproductive performance of female Bos indicus (Zebu) cattle. International Livestock Centre for Africa (ILCA), monograph, Addis Ababa, Ethiopia. http://www.ilri.org/InfoServ/Webpub/Fulldocs/X5442e/x5442e00.htm

[27] Bitew, M. and Prasad, S. (2011). Study on Major Reproductive Health Problems in Indigenous and Cross Breed Cows in and Around Bedelle, South West Ethiopia. J. Anim. Vet. Advan. 10(6): 723-727.

[28] Al-Maruf, A., Paul, A. K., Bonaparte, N., Bhuyian, M. H. and Shamsuddin, M. (2014). Reproductive Disorders that Limits the Reproductive Performances in Dairy Cows of Bangladesh. J. Emb. Trans. 29(2): 189-194.

[29] Esheti, G. and Moges, N. (2014). Major Reproductive Health Disorders in Cross Breed Dairy Cows in Ada'a District, East Shoa, Ethiopia. Global Veterinaria 13(4): 444-449.

[30] Benti, A. D. and Zewdie, W. (2014). Major reproductive health problems of indigenous Borena cows in Ethiopia. J. Adv. Vet. Anim. Res. 1(4): 182-188.

[31] Mandefro, M. and Negash, G. (2014). Repeat Breeder Syndrome in Dairy Cows: Influence of Breed and Age on Its Prevalence. World J. Agric. Sci. 10 (4): 200-203.

[32] Chakurkar, E. B., Barbuddhe, S. B. and Sundaram, R. N. S. (2008). Infertility in farm animals: causes and remedies. Technical Bulletin No: 15, ICAR Research Complex for Goa (Indian Council of Agricultural Research), Ela, Old Goa-403402, Goa, India. pp. 1-14.

[33] Johanson, J. M. and Berger, P. J. (2003). Birth weight as a predictor of calving ease and perinatal mortality in Holstein cattle. J. Dairy Sci. 86: 3745-3755.

[34] Eger, S., Drori, D., Kadoori, I., Miller, N. and Schindler, H. (1985). Effects of Selenium and Vitamin E on Incidence of Retained Placenta. J. Dairy Sci. 68: 2119-2122.

[35] Ortega-Mora, L. M., Gottstein, B., Conraths, F. J. and Buxton, D. (2007). "Ruminants: Guidelines for Diagnosis and Control in Farm Protozoal Abortion. CAB International, UK.

[36] Givens, M. D. (2006). A clinical, evidence-based approach to infectious causes of infertility in beef cattle. Theriogenology 66: 648-654.

[37] Olson, K. M., Cassell, B. G., McAllister, A. J., and Washburn, S. P. (2009). Dystocia, stillbirth, gestation length, and birth weight in Holstein, Jersey, and reciprocal crosses from a planned experiment. J. Dairy Sci. 92: 6167-6175.

[38] Noakes, E. D., Parkinson, T. J. and England, G. C. W. (2001a). Post parturient prolapse of the uterus. Chapter 19. In: Arthur's Veterinary Reproduction and Obstetrics. 8th ed. Harcourt (India) Pvt. Ltd., New Delhi. pp. 333-338.

[39] Roberts, S. J. (1998). Vaginocervical prolapse. In: Veterinary Obstetrics and Genital Diseases (Theriogenology). 2nd ed. [Indian reprint] CBS Publishers and Distributors, New Delhi, India. pp. 196-198.

[40] Bhattacharyya, H. K., Peer, F. U., Buchoo, B. A. and Ansari, M. M. (2007). Management of uterine prolapse in cattle of Kashmir. Indian Vet. J. 84: 744-745.

[41] Esteves, A., Båge, R. and Payan-Carreira, R. (2012). Freemartinism in Cattle, Ruminants: Anatomy, Behavior and Diseases, Chapter: Chapter 7, Nova Science Publishers Inc, pp. 99-120.

[42] SDDP (1999). Calf and heifer rearing. SDDP Extension Manual, Smallholder Dairy Development Project. Ministry of Agriculture. August 1999 Addis Ababa, Ethiopia. 3: 1-15.

Characteristics of Households and Indigenous Chicken Consumption in N'Djamena (Chad)

Issa Youssouf Adoum[1, *], Mopate Logtene Youssouf[2], Vounparet Zeuh[3], Ayssiwede Simplice Bosco[4], Bada Algom Oumar[1], Adam Bakhit Mustapha[1], Ardjoun Khalil Djalal[1], Missohou Ayao[4]

[1]National High Institute of Sciences and Techniques, Abeche (INSTA) Ex University Institute of Sciences and Techniques, Abeche, Chad
[2]Livestock Research Institute for Development (LRID) Ex Zootechnical and Veterinary Research Laboratory, N'Djamena, Chad
[3]Livestock Polytechnic Institute of Moussoro, Moussoro, Chad
[4]Inter-State School of Sciences and Veterinary Medicine, service of Animal Husbandry Food Sciences (EISMV), Dakar-Fann, Sénégal

Email address:
issayou@gmail.com (I. Y. Adoum), mopate.ly@gmail.com (Mopate L. Y.), vounzeuh@yahoo.fr (V. Zeuh), ayissimbos@yahoo.fr (A. S. Bosco), oumar_algo@yahoo.fr (B. A. Oumar), bakhitmusta@yahoo.fr (A. B. Mustapha), djalalardjoun@yahoo.fr (A. K. Djalal), missohou@refer.sn (M. Ayao)

Abstract: The objective of the study was to analyze the home consumption of local chickens in N'Djamena. It was conducted using a crosscutting and retrospective survey of a purposive sample per a quota of 250 households in 10 districts of the city. The heads of household surveyed are in average 41.5±9.4 years old and led families made up of 9.6±4.9 persons. The majority of respondents (94.4%) were married and educated (78.8%) at different levels. Employees were the majority (68%). The majority of households (62%) had an average monthly income ranging from less than 50,000 F CFA[i] to 150,000 F CFA and about 82% of households spend in average 25,000 to 75,000 F CFA for food per month. Indigenous chicken is consumed during parties (32.3%), Christian festivals (38.0%) and visits by VIPs (39.7%). Most respondents (71%) had a monthly consumption frequency ranging from 2 times (45.6%) or 3 times (25.2%). Households headed by women consumed an average 2.01 chickens as against 1.78 heads for households led by men ($p > 0.05$). All respondents (100%) stated having a preference for indigenous chicken. Taste and price are considered as the main determinants of indigenous chicken consumption in households in N'Djamena.

Keywords: Consumption, Indigenous Chicken, Households, N'Djamena, Chad

---

1. Introduction

N'Djamena, the capital city of Chad, with its administrative, economic and political functions, has a population of 993,492 in 2009, representing 41% of the urban population of Chad with a high annual growth rate of about 5% [14].

Urban concentration and city food supply problems are great development concerns in Africa [26]. The contribution of agricultural and pastoral productions in feeding city populations is undeniable [19]. African cities are safe outlets for agricultural products near and distant areas [7].

In Sub-Saharan Africa, over 80% of poultry livestocks are bred in family production systems. Family poultry plays an important role in the fight against poverty in rural areas and an irreplaceable socio-cultural role in African societies [8, 18, 25, 28, 29]. Thus poultry reared are intended for food but also for use in traditional rituals, guest receptions, gifts and used in the barter system [1, 8].

Given the population growth in developing societies and speculation on food prices, consumption of animal products is influenced by various socio-economic factors [21]. Predictions of demographic changes and growth of individual consumption of animal products show that, by 2020, there will be need to produce more than 100 billion tons of meat in developing countries to cope with demand [6].

Village livestock farming provides animal protein readily available to households. Indigenous chicken meat has an organoleptic quality especially appreciated by African consumers in sub-Saharan Africa [2, 16, 27].

In urban areas where consumer habits are changing rapidly, there is not enough information on chicken consumption patterns [27]. N'Djamena does not make exception to this rule and lack of data about local chicken consumption in households.

The objective of this study was to analyze the main determinants of local chicken consumption in households in N'Djamena.

2. Materials and Methods

2.1. Study Framework

The study was carried out between October and December 2010 in 10 districts of N'Djamena city. It focused on the characteristics of households and consumption of indigenous chickens that could be found there. As the Capital city of Chad, N'Djamena borders with Cameroon. Its population was estimated at about one million people in the last census in 2009 [14]. It extends between 12° and 13° North latitude and 15 ° and 16 ° East longitude.

2.2. Data Sampling and Collection Methods

The survey was conducted among a sample of 250 households. This survey is based on a purposive sampling and quota. The number of households to be surveyed in each district was proportional to the population size defined in the district in relation to the total population of the city of N'Djamena. It was conducted in two steps: a questionnaire validation pre-survey in a few households distributed in the different districts and a crosscutting and retrospective survey carried out among heads of households targeting people making family expenses. The information sought included:

- The location and socio-economic characteristics of households;
- The consuming practices of the major meat types, the different species of poultry consumed in their order of preference, the types of meat consumed depending on the circumstances. Moreover, the rank of the consumption frequency of chicken, the consumed quantity, the main dishes and the chicken supply method were analyzed.
- Purchasing practices and expenses on food per month in households, as well as criteria for buying chicken as well as quality attributes were collected.
- Socio-cultural practices of using chicken, including types of selected chickens, ritual sacrifices and offerings in households.

2.3. Statistical Analyses

The raw data were coded and entered into "Excel". Subsequently, these data were imported into SPSS [23] processing software. Descriptive statistical analysis (calculating frequencies, means and standard deviations, chi-two test) and analysis of variance (ANOVA) were performed. The significance level adopted was 5%.

3. Results

3.1. Socio-Economic Characteristics of Households

The heads of households (HH) were in average 41.5±9.44 years old. Men, who were more in number, have an average age (44.7 years) significantly higher ($p < 0.05$) than that of women (33.2 years). Almost all were married with an average of 9.6±4.92 people under their responsibility, of whom 1.3±0.6 wives, 5.41±3.7 children and 2.84±1.4 active. The vast majority (about 79%) of HHs was educated and over half (54%) Islamized (Table I). They are mostly (59.5%) employees (civil servants, police force and private employees) and the rest (40.5%) was made up of traders, workers and others (Table I). Their wives practiced more household and commercial activities than salaried workers. Almost half (49%) of households were indigenous of regions of Chari-Baguirmi and those close to the capital city, such as Mayo-Kebbi, Batha and Tandjile regions.

Table I. *Socio-economic characteristics of household heads surveyed in N'Djamena (Chad).*

Parameter	Status	Number	Percentage (%)
Gender	• Women	70	28
	• Men	180	72
Religion	• Christian	109	43.8
	• Muslim	135	54.2
	• Animist	5	2.0
Region of origin	• Chari-Baguirmi	42	16.8
	• Mayo-Kebbi	32	12.8
	• Batha	25	10.0
	• Tandjile	24	9.6
	• Guera	22	8.8
	• East Logone	16	6.4
	• Others	89	35.6
Education	• University	48	19.2
	• Secondary	83	33.2
	• Primary	66	26.4
	• Illiterate	53	21.2
Marital Status	• Married	236	94.4
	• Divorced	7	2.8
	• Widow	6	2.4
	• Single	1	0.4
Activity of the household head	• Civil servant	79	32.4
	• Trader	43	17.6
	• Private employee	36	14.8
	• Military	30	12.3
	• Worker	21	8.6
	• Other	35	14.3
Activity of wives	• Housewife	116	48.1
	• Trader	73	30.3
	• Private Employee	33	13.7
	• Other	19	7.9

3.2. Monthly Income and Food-Related Expenses

Households had an average monthly income ranging from 50,000 to 150,000 F CFA and those who spent between 25,000 and 75,000 FCFA were in the majority (Table II). Monthly expenses for food were significantly associated ($p<0.05$) with household income.

***Table II.** Categories of income and monthly expenditure of households on food (in F CFA) and number of chickens consumed in N'Djamena (Chad).*

Revenue		Expenditure	
Category	**Rate (%)**	**Category**	**Rate (%)**
50,000 - 150,000	62.0	25,000 – 75,000	81.6
150,000 – 250,000	33.6	75,000 – 150,000	14.0
Over 250,000	4.4	Over 150,000	4.4

In relation to income, monthly numbers of consumed chickens have varied. Households with incomes of more than 150,000 F CFA consumed three (03) chickens. Those with incomes between 100,000 and 150,000 F CFA have eaten two (02) fowls and those whose incomes were below 100,000 F CFA, one (01) chicken.

3.3. Types of Poultry Consumed

The indigenous chicken has ranked at the top of preferences of about 44% of household heads (Table III).

***Table III.** Types of poultry consumed by order of preference in households in the city of N'Djamena (Chad).*

Species consumed	Number	Percentage (%)
• Indigenous Chicken	109	43.6
• Indigenous Chicken, Duck	27	10.8
• Indigenous Chicken, Pigeon	16	6.4
• Indigenous Chicken, Reform chicken	13	5.2
• Indigenous Chicken, Broiler	13	5.2
• Heterogeneous consumption (no special preference)	72	28.8

3.4. Type of Meat Consumed Depending on Circumstances

Meat from small ruminants was mostly consumed during religious (Muslim and Christian) festivals, children's baptisms, on New Year's Day and at weddings (Table IV). As for indigenous chicken meat, it was more consumed during parties and upon receiving a distinguished guest.

***Table IV.** Type of meat consumed depending on circumstances in households in the city of N'Djamena (Chad).*

Event	Type of meat consumed	Number	Percentage (%)
Ordinary Life (n=248)	SR, NC, fish	31	12.5
	Cattle, SR, NC,	29	11.7
	SP, fish	21	8.5
	SR, NC,	20	8.1
	Cattle, SR, NC, fish	20	8.1
	SR	15	6.0
	SR, fish	15	6.0
	Other	97	30.1
Week-end (n=76)	Fish	31	40.8
	NC	17	22.4
	NC, fish	16	23.9
	Other	12	15.8
Party (n=133)	NC	43	32.3
	SR	29	21.8
	SR, fish	17	12.8
	Fish	16	12.0
	SR, NC,	16	12.0
	Other	12	9.00
Moslem Festival (n= 145)	SR	133	91.7
	Cattle, SR	4	2.8
	Other	8	5.5
Christian Festival (n= 50)	SR	25	50.0
	NC	19	38.0
	Other	6	12.0
New Year (n= 99)	SR	52	52.5
	NC	25	25.3
	SR, NC,	7	7.1
	Other	15	15.2
Baptism (n= 156)	SR	88	56.4
	Cattle, SR	54	34.6
	Cattle	11	7.1
	Other	3	1.9
Wedding (n= 145)	SR	69	47.6
	Cattle, SR	54	37.2
	Cattle	19	13.1
	Other		2.1
Funeral (n= 147)	Cattle, SR	59	40.1
	SR	58	39.5
	Cattle	27	18.4
	Other	3	2.0
Distinguished guest (n= 224)	NC	89	39.7
	NC, fish	36	16.1
	Camel, pork	31	13.8
	SR	16	7.1
	SR, NC, camel, pig	16	7.1
	SR, NC,	15	6.7
	Other	21	9.4

SR = small ruminant; NC = indigenous chicken

3.5. Supply, Criteria and Purchase Price, Consumption Frequencies and Cooking Modes

The majority of households (60%) got their supply from markets in N'Djamena focusing, for approximately 44% of them, on price and weight criteria for the purchase of chickens (Table V). The average price of broilers was higher than that of reform hens and indigenous chickens. The majority of households (70.8%) have a consumption frequency of two to three chickens per month. The monthly average was 1.85 ± 1.167 heads, being about two chickens with a variation from 2.01 chickens for households headed by women to 1.78 in those led by men. The sauce is still the most popular practice of cooking in households (26.0%) followed by soup (16.0%).

Table V. Supply, criteria and purchase prices, consumption frequencies and cooking modes of indigenous chickens in households in the city of N'Djamena (Chad).

Character	Status	Number	Percentage (%)
Supply mode	N'Djamena Market	149	59.6
	N'Djamena Market, village market	39	15.6
	N'Djamena Market, own stock	14	5.6
	Own stock	10	4.0
	Other	38	15.2
Rate of consumption	3 times/month	63	25.2
	2 times/month	114	45.6
	Once/month	56	22.4
	Other	17	6.8
Cooking Mode	Sauce	65	26.0
	Soup	40	16.0
	Sauce, soup	28	11.2
	Sauce, fried chicken	26	10.4
	Soup, fried chicken	26	10.4
	Other	65	26.0
Most important purchase criteria (n = 249)	Price	71	28.4
	Weight	38	15.2
	Age, price	38	15.2
	Age	30	12.0
	Size	18	7.2
	Other	55	22.0
Number of chickens consumed / month		1.85 ± 1.167	
Price of village chicken (in F CFA)		2839 ± 414.14	
Price of Reform chicken (in F CFA)		4879 ± 334.6	
Broiler prices(in F CFA)		5055 ± 300.04	

3.6. Meat Type Classification According to Organoleptic Quality

The main organoleptic qualities that motivated the consumption of chicken compared to other meats were the color of the skin, cooking easiness, tenderness, flavor and the natural character of the meat (Table VI).

Table VI. Classification of different meat types of meat in terms of indicators and quality attributes in households in the city of N'Djamena (Chad).

Quality attribute	Type of meat consumed	Number	Percentage (%)
Color of the skin (n=32)	Poultry	20	62.5
	Fish	12	37.5
Cooking facility (n=112)	Poultry	85	75.9
	Fish	25	22.3
	Small ruminants	2	1.8
Tenderness (n=85)	Poultry	80	94.1
	Fish	5	5.9
Taste (n=174)	Poultry	169	97.7
	Fish	4	2.3
Hygienic quality (n=129)	Poultry	114	88.4
	Fish	15	11.6

3.7. Criteria for Choosing the Indigenous Chickens

All of the respondents stated that they had a preference for indigenous chicken. More than half (55.6%) of them justified this preference by its most succulent taste, cheaper price compared to that of reform hens, broilers and other poultry, the natural character of its production and market availability (Table VII).

Table VII. Determining factors for preferring indigenous chicken in households in N'Djamena (Chad).

Characters	Responses	Frequency	%
Reason for preference	Tastier, cheaper	34	13.6
	Tastier	28	11.2
	Tastier, more natural	20	8.0
	Tastier, more natural	18	7.2
	Cheaper	15	6.0
	Tastier, cheaper, more natural,	14	5.6
	Available on market	10	4.0
	Cheaper, preferring one's own	111	44.4
	Other		

3.8. Sociocultural Use of the Indigenous Chicken

More than half (53%) of respondents said they did not use the meat of indigenous chicken in ritual sacrifices as against 47% who made use of it (Table VIII). The chickens used for that purpose were mainly purchased on the market. The frequency of its use was occasional for over half (51.3%) of people or annually (43.7%). The purchase of chicken intended for sacrifice was essentially based on feather color (66.7%), including white, red, multicolored and the male sex (32.7%). As for the ritual practice, chicken is either simply bled (48.6%) or cooked and distributed (35.2%).

Table VIII. Use of indigenous chicken in ritual practices in the households surveyed in N'Djamena (Chad).

Characters	Responses	Number	(%)
Using indigenous chicken for sacrifices	Yes	117	46.8
	No	133	53.2
Chicken Acquisition Mode (n=156)	Purchasing from market	108	69.3
	Choosing from one's stock	26	16.6
	Gift	19	12.2
	Home delivery	3	1.9
Frequency of use (n=119)	Need-based	61	51.3
	Annually	52	43.7
	Other	6	5.0
Criteria for purchasing chicken for sacrifice (n=150)	Feather colour	100	66.7
	Sex	49	32.7
	Other	1	0.6
Practice of ritual sacrifice using local chicken (n=142)	Chicken is bled	69	48.6
	Chicken is cooked and distributed	50	35.2
	Chicken is given to the marabout	23	16.2

4. Discussion

This study establishes for the first time the relationship between the monthly frequency of indigenous chicken consumption and socio-economic characteristics of households in the city of N'Djamena. In addition, it has established the central spot occupied by the meat of local chicken among meats consumed at weekends and during a visit paid at home by a host or a distinguished guest. The same goes for its use in ritual ceremonies. These observations were similar to those made in Cameroon, where urban indigenous chicken consumption is linked to some particular circumstances (traditional ceremonies and religious celebrations) for which the other two types of chicken available on the market (broilers and imported cuts) are not suitable [13]. In Sub-Saharan Africa, the various events and religious celebrations significantly affect the consumption of animal products [2], as does the level of income of household heads. Regarding the use of animal species depending on opportunities, it is consistent with observations made in Burkina Faso [12] and in Sénégal [15]. Indeed, sheep, goats and cattle are sacrificed for ceremonies and events gathering a large number of people while chickens are widely sought to honor guests and friends to strengthen social bonds. During the Ramadan festival period and the New Year, the meat of small ruminants is sought more than chicken meat; unlike some countries such as Sénégal where chicken meat is much sought during these periods [27]. In Chad, sharing meals with family and friends during these celebrations requires a somewhat larger amount of meat, hence the use of small ruminants.

Frequency of consumption is influenced by household income and size. The low-income households do not allow a high frequency of chicken consumption, unlike the middle-income households with fewer dependents. Our frequency of indigenous chicken consumption was lower than those "out homes" in the same city that vary over time; daily (3%), weekly (51%); twice per week (23%); three times a week (5%) and monthly (18%) [11]. The continuous working days and the multiplication of grilling points and street restaurants would explain these high frequencies. The average consumption level per person surveyed was similar to the results obtained in the same city [17]. The annual extrapolations on the basis of average daily sales in the markets and on the total poultry traders indicate an average consumption of 1.80 kg / ht / year in N'Djamena. Note that the data on the average consumption bearing exclusively on indigenous chickens in sub-Saharan African countries are not so much available. In households in N'Djamena, the indigenous chicken is mainly used in cooking stews or sauces and soup. In Dakar in Sénégal [27], the main dishes prepared using indigenous chicken are rice dishes (53.2%), sauces (19.3%), fried chicken (11.1%) and served with some couscous (16.4%). The differences would be put on the account of eating habits. In Sénégal, a variety of chicken dishes is observed.

The main determining factor for choosing the indigenous chicken is the price, due to the fact that the chicken is expensive given the purchasing power of different households [4]. Notwithstanding the survey periods, we see that in N'Djamena, the average price of chicken was higher than that in Niger [3], in Bangui (Central African Republic), in Cotonou (Bénin), in Bamako [10], in Yaoundé [4, 13] and Dakar [27]. At the time of the investigation under consideration, the price of chicken at the market was higher than the national average price of 1,840 F CFA in 2008 [17] and the price recorded during the "out homes "consumer study in 2010 which was 2,160 FCFA [11]. The high cost of indigenous chickens in N'Djamena compared to prices in 2010 and to those in other African cities could be explained by the fact that the studies were conducted in the months of November and December, which corresponds to the period of Christmas and New Year celebrations. Moreover, unlike other African countries, there are very few semi-industrial broiler rearing and egg-laying chicken farms (for reform hens) in Chad. Similar results are obtained in Ethiopia [2] showing that poultry prices are higher during periods of peak sales such as Christmas and New Year (December-January) and Easter (April) and they fall in periods of fasting and Easter (February) which coincide with low sales. Price fluctuations during certain periods of the year are also recognized in the markets of Kampala in Uganda [5]. Besides the price, the weight and age of the chicken are also considered to be criteria that influence the consumers' choice at the time of purchase. Observations made in Ethiopia indicate that Ethiopian consumers preferred young chickens compared to old chickens [2].

The organoleptic quality attributes that led to the consumption of indigenous chicken in N'Djamena compared to other meats in households, were similar to those obtained in Tanzania [16] where local chickens are preferred by consumers because of their pigmentation, the thinness, their taste and the ability to cook special dishes. As for the motivations and factors determining the preference of indigenous chicken in households, our results agree with those obtained in Zimbabwe [20], Ethiopia [2], Sénégal [27] and Uganda [5]. These authors believe that the organoleptic characteristics, including taste and nutritional aspects, are the main characters that drive the consumption of indigenous chicken in households. Consumers in the city of Dakar (Sénégal) believe that the hen, particularly that in time of egg-laying, has a much tastier flesh [27].

Traditionally, poultry is used in mystical practices. Thus, in some local communities, chickens or their products can ward off evil spells targeting the family or a family member [9]. The chicken used in mystical-social practices should meet criteria that differ from the chicken intended for common consumption [27]. In our case, color (66.7%) and gender (32.2%) are the main criteria for the choice of chickens intended for sacrifice. These results are similar to those obtained by some authors [22, 27]. According to these authors, the color of feathers and sex of the chicken can direct its destiny either for sacrifice, or to be used to welcome a guest or to as an offering. As for the mode of the mystical-social use of the local chicken, our results showed that in the majority of cases, the chicken is bled (48.6%), cooked and distributed (35.2%) or given to the marabout. In Sénégal, however, the indigenous chicken can be given alive to a stranger [27]. But in Ethiopia, a rooster with red and white plumage is sacrificed for good rain and harvest, that which has red feathers with black spots is sacrificed to celebrate the New Year, a white and black rooster is sacrificed to prevent evil and disasters, and that with red pullets is sacrificed to the dead ancestors [24].

5. Conclusion

This study made it possible to determine the socio-economic characteristics of household heads, purchasing and consumption practices of indigenous chickens in the households in the city of N'Djamena. The same was done concerning expenditure on food consumption, which remains based on household size and income. In N'Djamena, indigenous chicken is the main poultry meat consumed in households in the form of sauce and soup. In addition, they are widely sought at various festive and ritual ceremonies. Thus, traditional poultry farming plays a major role in favoring animal protein intake and meeting the urban population demand in poultry meat. Price remains the main criterion for choosing the chicken at the time of purchase. The low semi-industrial poultry production highlights the indigenous one to meet chicken meat needs of city dwellers. For the development of traditional poultry farming in Chad and in order to better meet the increasingly growing needs of consumers, it is important to implement a policy of sustainable development of this sector.

References

[1] Agbede G.B., Teguia A. et Manjeli Y., 1995. Enquête sur l'élevage traditionnel des volailles au Cameroun. Tropicultura, 13, (1) : 22 – 24

[2] Aklilu H.A., Almekinders C.J.M, Udo H.M.J., Van Der zijpp A. J., 2007. Village poultry consumption and marketing in relation to gender, religious festivals and market access. Tropical Animal Health and Production. 39:165-177

[3] Assoumane I., Ousseini G., 2010. Revue du secteur avicole du Niger. http://www.fao.org/docup/012/ak770f/ak770f00.pdf. 61 p. (05 Août 2010)

[4] Awono Bessa C., Laroche-Dupraz C., Grongnet J. F., Vermersch D., Havard M., Lhuissier A., 2008. Déterminants de la consommation urbaine de poulet de chair au Cameroun: cas de la ville de Yaoundé. In : Parrot L., Njoya A., Temple L., Assogba-Komlan F., Kahane R., Ba Diao M., Havard M. (éds scientifiques), Parrot L. (coordonnateur), Tome 1 : Gouvernance et approvisionnement des villes, Editions L'Harmattan. 209–218

[5] Emuron N., Magala H., Kyazze F.B., Kugonza D.R., Kyarisiima C.C., 2010. Factors influencing the trade of local chickens in Kampala city markets. Livestock Research for Rural Development, 22 (4), Art. #76. Retrieved May 7, 2011, from http:// www.lrrd.org/lrrd22/4/emur22097.htm

[6] Faye B., Alary V., 2001. Les enjeux des productions animales dans les pays du Sud. Prod. Anim., 14, 3-13.

[7] Guérin H., Faye B., 1999. Spécificité de la problématique périurbaine pour les systèmes d'élevage. In : P. Moustier, A Mbaye, H. De Bon, H. Guerin, J. Pages (éds scientifiques), Actes de l'atelier «Agriculture périurbaine en Afrique subsaharienne ». Cirad-Coraf, 20 – 24 avril 1998, Montpellier, France, p. 43 – 49

[8] Guèye E. F., 2000. The role of family poultry in poverty alleviation, food security and the promotion of gender equality in rural Africa Outlook on Agriculture, 29, 129-136.

[9] Guèye E.F., 2005. Le rôle de la volaille villageoise et des petits ruminants pour la réduction de la pauvreté et la facilitation de la sécurité alimentaire. Rapport de l'atelier mouvements. Du 7 au 8 novembre 2005 Ouagadougou (Burkina Faso).

[10] Horman D., 2004. Le poulet Africain étouffé par l'Europe. http://www.gresea.be. 136p. (25 Octobre 2010)

[11] Issa Y., Mopate L.Y., Louassouabe G., Ayssiwede S.B., Missohou A., 2012. Consommation hors-foyer de poulets traditionnels dans la ville de N'Djaména (Tchad). Revue Scientifique du Tchad Janvier – 2012. Volume 11 - Numéro Spécial 1 (42-52)

[12] Kondombo S.R., Nianogo A.J., Kwakkel R.P., Udo H.M.J., Slingerland M., 2003. Comparative analysis of village chicken production in two farming systems in Burkina Faso. Tropical of Animal Health and Production, 35:563-574.

[13] Laroche Dupraz C, Awono Bessa C., Vermersch D., 2008. Application de la théorie de Lancaster à la consommation de poulet de chair au Cameroun. Revue d'Etudes en Agriculture et Environnement. http://www.raestud.eu/pdf/079_98_laroche.fin.pdf.79-98 p. (05 Août 2010)

[14] Ministère de l'Economie et du Plan (MEP)., 2009. Institut National de la Statistique, des Etudes Economiques et Démographiques (INSEED). Rapport provisoire du 2ème Recensement Général de la Population et de l'Habitat (RGPH2) du Tchad. 88 p.

[15] Missohou A., Dieye P.N., Talaki E., 2002. Rural poultry production and productivity in Southern Sénégal. Livestock Research for Rural Development, 14 (2) http://www.cipav.org.co/lrrd/lrrd14/2/miss142.htm

[16] Mlozi M. R. S., Kakengi A. V. M., Minga U. M., Mtambo A. M., Olsen J. E., 2003. Marketing of free range local chickens in Morogoro and Kilosa urban markets, Tanzania; Livestock Research for Rural Development, 15 (2). Retrieved June 12, 115, from http://www.lrrd.org/lrrd15/2/mloz152.htm

[17] Mopaté L.Y., 2010. La filière volaille locale dans l'approvisionnement en viande des villes : cas de la ville de N'Djaména au Tchad. Atelier pour le Développement de l'Aviculture Professionnelle au Tchad (DAPT), du 09 au 12 juin 2009, à N'Djaména (Tchad). Ministère de l'Elevage et des Ressources Animales (MERA), International Finance Corporation (IFC) of the World Bank Group, FAO, SCAC (Ambassade de France), LRVZ, p. 14-18.

[18] Mopaté L. Y., Awa N. D., 2010. Systèmes avicoles en zone de savanes d'Afrique centrale : performances zootechniques et importance socio-économique. L. SEINY-BOUKAR, P. BOUMARD (éditeurs scientifiques), 2010. Actes du colloque International, avec comité de lecture, intitulé «Savanes africaines en développement : innover pour durer», 20-23 avril 2009, Garoua, Cameroun. PRASAC, N'Djaména, Tchad ; CIRAD, Montpellier, France, Version 1 mise en ligne sur http://hal.cirad.fr/cirad-00472067/fr/, ou Version 2 sans modification sur CD, 11 p.

[19] Moustier P., 1999. Définitions et contraintes de l'agriculture périurbaine en Afrique subsaharienne. In : P. Moustier, A Mbaye, H. De Bon, H. Guerin, J. Pages (éds scientifiques), Actes de l'atelier « Agriculture périurbaine en Afrique subsaharienne ». Cirad-Coraf, 20 – 24 avril 1998, Montpellier, France, p. 29 – 42

[20] Muchadeyi F C, Sibanda S, Kusina N T, Kusina J., Makuza S., 2004. The village chicken production system in Rushinga District of Zimbabwe. Livestock Research for Rural Development, 16 (6), Art. #40. Retrieved July 20, 2011, from http://www.lrrd.org/lrrd16/6/much16040.htm

[21] Salomon A., Workalemahu A., Jabbar M., Ahmed M., Hurnissa B., 2003. Livestock marketing in Ethiopia. A review of structure, performance and development initiatives, (Socio-economic and Policy Research Working Paper 52; International Livestock Research Institute, Nairobi, Kenya).

[22] Savane M., 1996. L'aviculture rurale au Sénégal, contraintes et perspectives zoo-économiques : Cas de la haute Casamance. Thèse Méd. Vét., EISMV, N° 9, Dakar

[23] SPSS, 2009. Statistical Package for Social Sciences. Version 17.0, SPSS Incorporated, Illinois, USA.

[24] Tadelle D., Olge B., 2001. Village poultry production systems in the central highlands of Ethiopia. Tropical Animal Health and Production, 33:521-537

[25] Talaki E., 2000. Aviculture traditionnelle dans la région de Kolda (Sénégal). Thèse : Méd. Vét. EISMV, N° 10, Dakar

[26] Temple L. et Moustier P., 2004. Les fonctions et contraintes de l'agriculture périurbaine de quelques villes africaines (Yaoundé, Cotonou, Dakar). Cahiers Agricultures, 13 (1) : 15 – 22

[27] Teno G., 2009. Etude des déterminants de la consommation du poulet du pays: cas de la région de Dakar (Sénégal). Thèse Méd. Vét., EISMV, N° 36, Dakar

[28] Traoré M., 2005. Evaluation de l'impact d'un transfert de paquet technique (amélioration génétique et des conditions d'élevage) sur la génération de revenus en aviculture traditionnelle dans les Niayes. Thèse Méd. Vét. EISMV, N°23, Dakar

[29] Traoré E. H., 2006. Première évaluation de la structure et de l'importance du secteur avicole commercial et familial en Afrique de l'Ouest. Rome: FAO. 52 p.

---

[i] 1 USD = 500 F CFA

22

Relationship Between the Amount of Subcutaneous Fat, Testicular Morphometry, Epididymis and Some Sperm Parameters in *Leptonycteris yerbabuenae* Bat Before, During and After Mating

Martínez-Coronel Matías[1, *], Munguía-Pérez Alma Alicia[1], Arenas-Ríos Edith[2]

[1]Department of Biology, Autonomous Metropolitan University–Iztapalapa, Iztapalapa, Mexico
[2]Department of Biology of Reproduction, Autonomous Metropolitan University–Iztapalapa, Iztapalapa, Mexico

Email address:
marti17@hotmail.com (Martínez-Coronel M.), alma_chiquitita23@hotmail.com (Munguía-Pérez A. A.), editharenas2000@yahoo.com.mx (Arenas-Ríos E.)

Abstract: Studies in reproductive age mammals show that the increase in fat content is inversely related to sperm quality in response to a decrease in testosterone levels. In turn the decrease in androgen concentration is related to morphophysiological involution in the testis and epididymis. However, the bat *Leptonycteris yerbabuenae* increases the body fat content previous the mating period, contrary to what was reported in most mammals. Therefore the aim of this study was to determine the importance of variation in fat content in *L. yerbabuenae* in relation to testicular and epididymal cycle; and sperm parameters. The results clearly show an increase in the fat content as it approaches the mating season. Also, there is an increase in the size of the testis and epididymis. In the post-mating months, both: fat and testis, decrease and the sperm cells were not presents. *Leptonycteris yerbabuenae* has a different behaviour to most mammals, accumulate fat while producing, transit and sperm storage could be happening. So, in this model, we must do studies that meet these processes emerging from that reported in other mammals.

Keywords: Fat, Testis, Epididymis, Sperm, Bat Reproduction

1. Introduction

Leptonycteris yerbabuenae is a nectarivorous bat, inhabits desert and tropical deciduous forest in the northern hemisphere environments, from southern USA, through México and reaches the Salvador in Central America. In this area the species is composed of two groups or population with different breeding and behavioral period [1-2]. Populations distribution above parallel 21°N behave as a latitudinal migrant and births occur during the spring [1, 3, 4], while populations below that parallel are local residents or regional migrant and births occurs at autumn [12, 5]. Members of the family Phyllostomidae are restricted to the neotropics, except *Macrotus waterhousii*, *Leptonycteris nivalis* and *L. yerbabuenae*, species that reach to the Southern United States, in a subtropical area [6]. So far it is not known that a phylostomid bat hibernates, therefore, it´s interesting that *L. yerbabuenae* has subcutaneous fat accumulation. Originally it was proposed that the accumulation of fat by *L. yerbabuenae* was related to the latitudinal migration that some populations of this species make to breed in Northern Mexico and the southern United States [3, 7] however it was curious that both sexes accumulate fat, even when it know that only females perform the migration journey to northern Mexico and the southern United States for reproductive purposes, while males movements is unknown [3,6]. Another interesting fact registered, at least in populations of Central and Southern of Mexico, is that the males accumulate more fat than females [4, 5]. Martínez-Coronel et al. [6] found that in a resident colony of *L. yerbabuenae* of Chiapas, México, the fat accumulated by males is used for breeding and not for migration [1, 3, 6]. It was also found that compared to other species of bats that accumulate fat, in *L. yerbabuenae*, the increase of fat coincides with the increase in the size of the testis, and considering that increase testicular could be an indicator of spermatogenesis [7], then these observations are contradictory to those reported for most of other species of bats [8] but *Pteropus poliocephalus* and *P. scapulatus* [9, 10].

It has been reported the functions of adipose tissue as energy reserve, but also as endocrine organ, having an influence on hormones and adipokines derived from adipose tissue that relate to the reproductive organs and its hormones [11]. However, the total and intra-abdominal subcutaneous fat, is associated with low testosterone levels and high levels of free and total estradiol [12-13]; altering and reducing the sperm concentration [14], and erectile dysfunction causing an increase in scrotal temperature [15].

For example, in the *Scotophilus heathii* bat has been reported that serum leptin levels are positively correlated with body fat and negatively related to reproductive function [16-17].

Not only that, it is important to note that the testis and epididymis functions in most mammals, is chaired by androgen, since in the absence, a decrease in testicular and epididymal weight is observed, is induces apoptosis in the epididymis starting with the head region and progressively moving up the caudal region of the same [17-18].

Due to the different effects that causes fat accumulation in mammalian reproduction and that in *L. yerbabuenae* has been observed a different behavior than other species analyzed in this aspect, this paper was aimed at evaluating the accumulation of fat, body morphometry, testicular and epididymal sperm parameters of this species during the previous period, during and after mating.

2. Methodology

2.1. Study Area

The cave "Los Laguitos" is located 4 km NW (16° 46′42" N, 93°08′55′′W), Tuxtla Gutierrez, Chiapas, 781m a.s.l. The average temperature of the cave is 32.3°C and relative humidity is 95.4%, which is classified as a "hot cave" [20]. The local climate is warm humid with summer rains, with rainfall less than 60 mm in the driest month, with winter rain less than 5% of annual and annual temperature around 24.7 °C [21]. The vegetation surrounding the cave corresponds to a Tropical Deciduous Forest [22]. During the study period the cave was inhabited by *Mormoops megalophylla*, *Pteronotus davyi*, *P. parnelli*, *P. personatus*, *Artibeus jamaicensis*, *Glossophaga soricina*, *L. yerbabuenae* and *Natalus stramineus*.

2.2. Ethics Statement

L. yerbabuenae is not listed as an endangered species in the Norma Oficial Mexicana NOM-059-ECOL-2010 SEMARNAT-2010 for the protection of native wild species of México (SEMARNAT, 2010). All protocols for the capture and handling of the live animals as well as for the euthanasia procedure used in this study were conducted in strict accordance with the guidelines established by the American Society of Mammologists for the use of wild mammals in research [23] and were approved by the Ethics Committee of our institution. The capture of specimens studied was approved by the scientific collector's license FAUT-0070 issued to Yolanda Hortelano Moncada by the Dirección General de Vida Silvestre de México (an agency of SEMARNAT).

2.3. Fieldwork

Three adult males of *L.yerbabuenae* were captured every month from May to October 2014 using an expand hand-net (Bioquip Tropic net) in a cave. During transport to the laboratory, bats were fed, ad libitum, with fruit puree, brand: "Gerber, Nestlé" apple and tropical fruit diluted in water. The age of the bat was estimated on the fusion of the cartilaginous epiphysis of the metacarpal-phalangeal joint of the 4th digit [24].

2.4. Laboratory Work

Bats were sacrificed by decapitation to obtain serum (under study), the rest of the body was dissected to remove the testis and epididymis. From each organ, wet weight and size, was measured. Subcutaneous fat was also removed and its weight recorded. Under a stereoscopic microscope each epididymis was sectioned in its three principal regions: head, body and tail, and the weight of each region was recorded.

Both epididymal segments of the same region (right and left caput; corpus, and cauda) were pooled and minced with scissors followed by gentle stirring in 1 ml of Ringer solution at 34°C to provoke the output of sperm [25]. Subsequently, the minced material was collected with a Pasteur pipette and filtered by passage through a 20-µl diameter weft lycra mesh (98% Nylon/Polyamide, 2% Lycra/elastane), and the fluid was collected in a 2-ml Eppendorf tube [26]. The sperm suspensions were washed twice by centrifugation at 500 × g for 5 minutes. The supernatant was removed, and the cell pellet was resuspended with 1 ml of Ringer solution. Determinations of sperm number, viability, and morphology were carried out using standard microscopic procedures.

2.5. Statistical Analysis

The Pearson index was applied to determine the correlation between body mass, fat, testicular mass and epididymal mass.

3. Results

3.1. Body Mass and Amount of Fat

The changes that showed the individuals mass over time, were related to the amount of stored fat ($r = 0.90$; $R^2 = 0.82$; $F_{1,\ 17\ d.f.} = 74.78$; $P = 0.0000$). The presence of subcutaneous fat was evident in March and increased at the same time of body mass until late May when start the mating period, during June, fat content and body mass decreased sharply in the following months the two variables continued to decline (Figure 1).

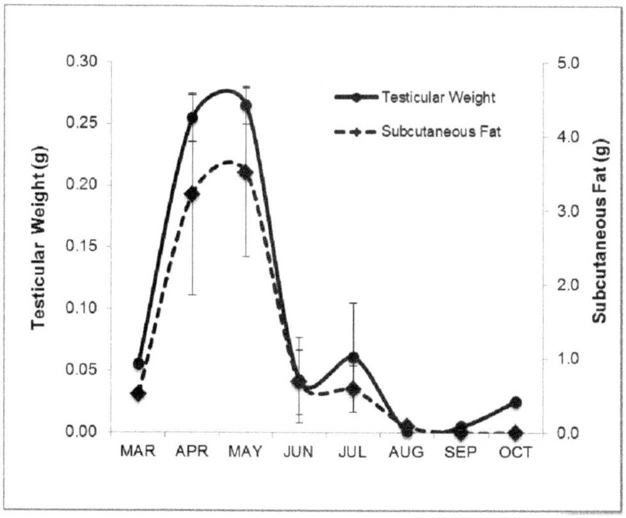

Figure 1. *Temporal variation in body mass and subcutaneous fat accumulation of L. yerbabuenae males in the cave "Los Laguitos", Chiapas, Mexico.*

3.2. Body and Testicular Mass

Like the fat content, the testicular mass showed changes related with the body mass of the individuals ($r = 0.73$; $R^2 = 0.53$; $F_{1,18\ d.f.} = 19.75$; $P = 0.0004$). The testes increase from March to May, when they reached their highest value, then declined sharply in June and continued to decline in the coming months (Figure 2).

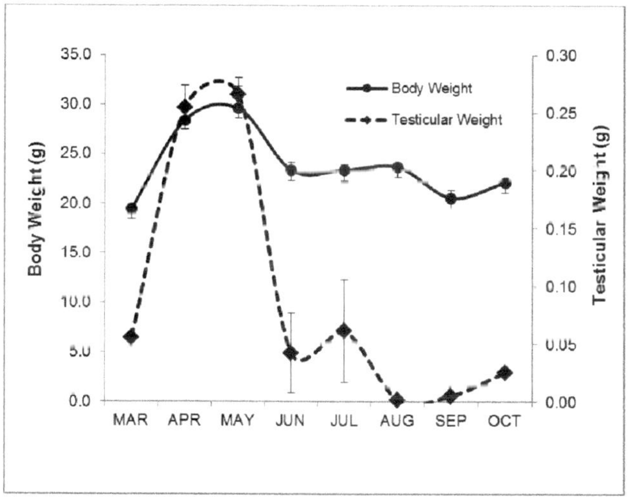

Figure 2. *Temporal variation in body mass and testicular mass of L. yerbabuenae in the cave "Los Laguitos", Chiapas, Mexico.*

3.3. Testicular Mass and Epididymal Mass, and the Subcutaneous Fat Quantity

These three variables showed similar changes over time, prior to mating, the three variables increased their value and peaked in May, when start the mating period. During June, at the time of mating, declined sharply observed this trend until October (Figures 3, 4). The correlation between testicular mass and subcutaneous fat was high ($r = 0.75$; $R^2 = 0.57$; $F_{1,17\ d.f.} = 21.82$; $P = 0.003$) as well as, testicular and epididymal mass ($r = 0.97$; $R^2 = 0.94$; $F_{1,17} = 297.86$; $P = 0.0000$) were high.

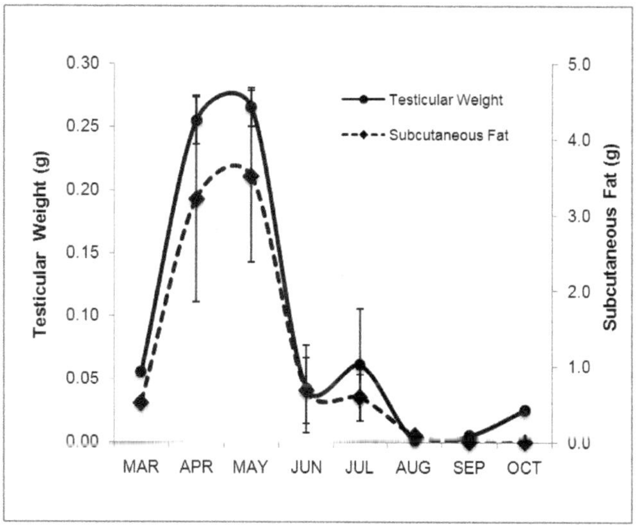

Figure 3. *Temporal variation in testicular mass and subcutaneous fat accumulated by the males of L. yerbabuenae in the cave "Los Laguitos", Chiapas, Mexico.*

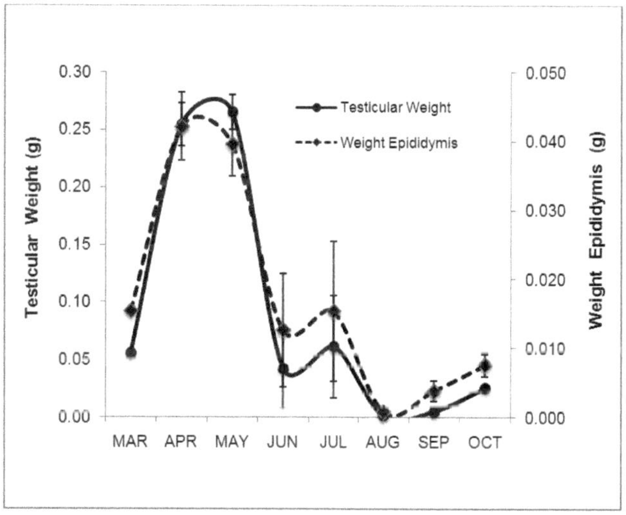

Figure 4. *Temporal variation in testicular mass and epididymis of L. yerbabuenae in the cave "Los Laguitos", Chiapas, Mexico.*

3.4. Sperm Parameters

The presence of sperm in epididymis was only detected in specimens of April and May (Table 1), before and just at the beginning of the breeding season. In some specimens of June 30 and July 30 the presence of sperm was detected, but it was impossible to count because they were isolated, and which were observed degenerates with necrotic appearance. The highest sperm concentration in April and May were found in the tail of the epididymis (108.50 x 106), followed by the body (75.24 x 106) and head (55.73 x 106). Also, the greater amount of alive sperm was found on epididymal cauda (79.83%), while the highest mortality was found to occur in the body (33.33%).

Table 1. Estimated average sperm concentration (x 10^6) stored on different parts of the epididymis, and the percentages of live (V) and dead sperms (M) for each region

	Caput	Body	Cauda	CAPUT		BODY		CAUDA	
				V	M	V	M	V	M
April	81.67	118.75	176.67	67.66	32.33	60.67	39.33	84.67	15.33
May	29.80	31.73	40.33	72.00	28.00	72.67	27.33	75.00	25.00
Average	55.73	75.24	108.5	69.83	30.17	66.67	33.33	79.83	20.17

4. Discussion

Several studies have investigated the relationship of the increased in body fat with conventional sperm parameters according to the WHO, i.e. concentration, motility and sperm morphology [27-29]. Finding a negative effect on these parameters, i.e. sperm count decreased, motility and a DNA fragmentation index increased.

Some of the mechanisms that are involved in male infertility due to a fat quantity increase are: changes in the hormones concentration such as reduction of inhibin-B and androgen levels, accompanied by estrogen elevated levels [15]. This is because the total fat, intra-abdominal and subcutaneous is associated with low levels of free and total testosterone in men. This decrease is explained by overactivity of the enzyme cytochrome P 450 aromatase expressed at high levels in white adipose tissue and it is responsible for being a key in the biosynthesis of estrogens [12].

The integrity and physiology of the testis and epididymis are androgen dependent and is observed that in the absence of these, in testis and epididymis loss weight occurs, affects seriously the gene expression and induce to apoptosis [18-19]. Based on this, it would expect that if a male mammal begins to accumulate fat, the testis would show minimal activity, and the sperm cells would be of poor quality. However, in *L. yerbabuenae* happens that while fat accumulates, it also increases the size of the testis and epididymis, as well as the quantity and quality of sperm stored in the epididymis, prior to the mating period that start in late May and through June [6]. This seasonal phenomenon of fat accumulation and testicular activity increase , in mammals, is not new, was described originally for primates [30], and is known as " fatted male phenomenon", has also been reported in *Pteropus poliocephalus* [10] as well as in large mammals like ungulates [31], pinnipeds [32] and ursids [33], among others. However, here is the first time that the ratio between fat and sperm parameters was studied.

In *L. yerbabuenae*, body mass is reduced in June, and is related to reproductive activity [6], and not with migration as other authors proposed [1, 3], because males and females make up a mating colony inside the cave and individuals do not go out to forage at night, mainly males [6], and in the case of the last point mentioned, energy expenditure can be associated with spermatogenesis, courtship and for defense.

Unlike *P. poliocephalus*, the males of *L. yerbabuenae* are not territorial, and they do not integrate harems, although it was noted that they can spend hours waiting for the opportunity to copulate while showing agonistic behavior with other males [6, 9].

Traditionally, the testis size had taken as a sign of fertility, especially in ecological studies. This criterion is based that for sperm production there should be seminiferous epithelium proliferation, an increase that should be reflected in the overall size of the testis. Different studies such as those conducted in *L. yerbabuenae* [34], Artibeus jamaicensis [35] and *Myotis nigricans* Beguelini et al. [36] provide data, that until more testicular mass, spermatogenesis occurs. In the present study, there was not testis histology, but we found that before the start of the breeding season was increased testicular mass and storing sperm in the epididymis was confirmed in samples of the months April, May and June. After mating we observed the testis regress, while the degenerate sperm were observed in samples of June and July. These results agree with those reported in a histological study in a population of *L. yerbabuenae* of Chamela, Jalisco [34]. Also, in this study we found that the testicular mass varied seasonally similar to body mass, indicating a close relationship between spermatogenesis and the individual condition, as in *P. poliocephalus* [10].

Sperm storage is a strategy that, some bat species have developed, to ensure fertilization, associated with different reproductive strategies, especially in those with different synchrony of gametogenic cycle in females and males, and temperate distribution [37]. But so have some species of tropical distribution as *Lasiurus ega*, *Rhinopoma hardwickei*, *Scotophilus heathi* and *Hipposideros speoris* [37]. The results found in L. Yerbabuenae indicate no sperm storage in the epididymis because, as soon as ends the mating period (May-June), the regression of epididymal and testicular tissue is observed, and sperm cells degenerate. These results agree with those reported for a population of the same specie of Jalisco, Mexico [34] as well as general knowledge that exists for most tropical species [37]. There is also evidence that the sperm storage do not occur in females, because was found female pregnant in the first days of July, indicating that fertilization of ovum occurs immediately after the copula [6].

The concentration and sperm viability found in *L. yerbabuenae*, compared with reports for the cauda epididymis of *Artibeus jamaicensis* ($54.79 \pm 88.14 \times 10^6$) and *Sturnira lilium* ($51.80 \pm 25.93 \times 10^6$) [38] indicate that *L. yerbabuenae* has a higher sperm concentration ($108.50 \pm 93.94 \times 10^6$). These differences in members of the same family may result from the different reproductive strategies that each species have, the first two species are bimodal poliestric, however *L. yerbabuenae* is seasonal monoestric [38].

Another consequence of the body fat increase, wa s the scrotal temperature increase [15], since fat is also deposited in the scrotal region, causing an increase in temperature in this region. A slight increase in scrotal temperature can disrupt spermatogenesis and cause fertility problems [39-42], caused in part by mitochondria degeneration, smooth endoplasmic reticulum dilatation and enlargement of the intercellular spaces between Sertoli cells and spermatids; directly associated with oxidative stress, followed by germ cell apoptosis [43].

However, the results in this study of fat amount, the size of testis, epididymis and presence of sperm in *L. yerbabuenae*, differ from those papers published in another mammals, because in fieldwork we registered higher scrotal temperatures ($x = 38.84 \pm 0.23$, $n = 9$) in June 16th than body temperature ($x = 36.21 \pm 0.09$, $n = 9$ =) during mating period. However, more studies are necessaries, like the register of body and scrotal temperatures, during their annual cycle, and adaptive mechanisms that may be counteracting the scrotal hyperthermia, even in reproductive stages, among which may be acting: the system countercurrent heat exchange between pampiniform plexus and testicular artery; protection mechanisms against hyperthermia as the system "unfolded protein response" [44] and antioxidant mechanisms that protect against oxidative stress.

To achieve a better understanding of what happens in *L. yerbabuenae* in relation with the accumulation of subcutaneous fat and reproductive function, is necessary determine biochemical markers of obesity, and profound studies of testicular and epididymal function and sperm functionality.

5. Conclusions

The results obtained in *L. yerbabuenae* showed that in this species the fat accumulation is positively related with testis increase. These results open a number of questions that actually not been raised in relation to leptin-testosterone metabolic pathways proposed.

References

[1] T.H. Fleming, and J. M. Nassar, "Population biology of the lesser long-nosed bat Leptonycteris curasoae in Mexico and Northern South America", in "Columnar Cacti and their Mutualists: Evolution, Ecology, and Conservation", T. H. Fleming and A. Valiente-Banuet, Eds. University of Arizona Press, Tucson, pp. 283–305, 2002.

[2] A. Rojas-Martínez, A. Valiente-Banuet, M. C. Arizmendi, A. Alcántara-Eguren, and H. T. Arita. "Seasonal distribution of the long-nosed bat (*Leptonycteris curasoae*) in North America: does a generalized migration pattern really exist?", J. Biog. Vol. 26, pp. 1065–1077, 1999.

[3] G. Ceballos, T. H. Fleming, C. Chávez, and J. Nassar, "Population dynamics of *Leptonycteris curasoae* (Chiroptera: Phyllostomidae) in Jalisco, México", J. Mamm. Vol. 78, pp. 1220-1230, 1997.

[4] G. S. Wilkinson, and T. H. Fleming, "Migration routes and evolution of lesser long-nosed bats, *Leptonycteris curasoae*, inferred from mitochondrial DNA", Mol. Ecol., Vol. 5, pp. 329–339, 1996.

[5] C. Galindo G., A. Sánchez Q., R. H. Quijano, and L. G. Herrera-M. "Population dynamics of a resident colony of *Leptonycteris curasoae* (Chiroptera: Phyllostomidae) in central Mexico", Biotropica Vol. 36, pp. 382-391, 2004.

[6] M. Martínez-Coronel, Y. Hortelano-Moncada, V. Corral, and L. Cuevas, "¿Para qué acumula grasa *Leptonycteris yerbabuenae* en la cueva de "Los Laguitos", Chiapas, México?" Submitted to Revista Mexicana de Mastozoología, 2015.

[7] Pfeiffer, B, and Mayer F, "Spermatogenesis, sperm storage and reproductive timing in bats", J. Zool., London, Vol 289, pp. 77-85, 2013.

[8] Roy, VK, Krishna A, "Regulation of leptin systhesis during adipogenesis in males of a vespertilionid bat, *Scotophilus heathi"*, J. Exp. Biol, Vol. 214, pp. 1599-1606, 2011.

[9] M. A. McGuckin, and A. W. Blackshaw, "Seasonal changes in testicular size, plasma testosterone concentration and body weight in captive flying foxes (*Pteropus poliocephalus* and *P. scapulatus*)", J. Reprod. Fert, Vol. 92, pp. 339-346, 1991.

[10] Welbergen, JA, "Fit females and fat polygynous males: seasonal body mass changes in the grey-headed flying fox", Oecologia, Vol. 165, pp. 629-637, 2011.

[11] Wozniak S. E., L. L. Gee, M. S. Wachtel and E. E. Frezaa, "Adipose tissue: The new endocrine organ? A review article", Dig. Dis. Sci, Vol. 54, pp. 1847-1856, 2009.

[12] SS Du Plessis, S Cabler, DA Mc Alister, E Sabanegh, A Agarwal. "The effect of obesity on sperm disorders and male fertility", Nat. Rev. Urol,pp. 1-9, 2010.

[13] Vigueras-Villaseñor RM, Rojas-Castañeda JC, Chavez-Saldaña M, Gutierrez-Perez O, García-Cruz ME, Cuevas-Alpuche O, Reyes Romero MM, Zambrano E. "Alterations in the spermatic function generated by obesity in rats", Acta Histochem, Vol. 113, pp. 214-220, 2010.

[14] Hammound AO, Wilde N, Gibson M, Parks A, Carrell TD, Meikle W. "Male obesity and alteration in sperm parameters", Fertil Steril,Vol. 90, pp. 2222-2225, 2008.

[15] S Cabler, A Agarwal, SS Du Plessis. "Obesity and male fertility" S.J. Parekattil and A. Agarwal. Male Infertility. Contemporary Clinical Approaches, Andrology, ART & Antioxidants, 2012.

[16] A. Banerjee, S. Udin, and A. Krishna, "Regulation of leptin synthesis in White adipose tissue of the female fruit bat, *Cynopterus sphinx*: role of the melatonin with or without insulin", Exp. Physiol, Vol. 96, pp. 216-225, 2010.

[17] R. K. Srivastava, and A. Krishna, "Adiposity associated rise in leptin impairs ovarian activity during Winter dormancy in Vespertilionid bat, *Scotophilus heathi*", Reproduction, Vol. 133, pp. 165-176, 2007.

[18] B. Robaire, S. Seenundun, M. Hamzeh, S.A.Lamour, "Androgenic regulation of novel genes in the epididymis", Asian Journal of Andrology, Vol. 9(4),pp. 545-553, 2007.

[19] Marilia, T.C., Patrão, C., Erick, J.R., Silva, M.C.W., and Avellar.. Androgen and the male reproductive tract: an overview of classical roles and current perspectives. Arquivos Brasileiros de Endocrinologia & Metabologia. 2009; 53 (8):934-945.

[20] Martínez-Coronel, M, García, E, Müdespacher-Zihel, C, and Torres, A, "El microclima de la cueva de Los Laguitos y su relación con los murciélagos", Mundos Subterráneos, Vol. 21, pp. 74-89, 2010, México, D. F.

[21] C. M. D. Cardoso, "El clima de Chiapas y Tabasco". DF, México: Instituto de Geografía, Universidad Nacional Autónoma de México, 1979.

[22] F. Miranda, "La vegetación de Chiapas". Tuxtla Gutiérrez, Chiapas: Consejo Estatal para la Cultura y las Artes de Chiapas, 1998.

[23] R. S. Sikes, W. L. Gannon, "The Animal Care and Use Committee of the American Society of Mammalogists", Guidelines of the American Society of Mammalogists for the use of wild mammals in research, – *J. Mammal* Vol. 92, pp. 235-253, 2011.

[24] T. H. Kunz, and E. L. P. Anthony, "Age estimation and post-natal growth in the bat *Myotis lucifugus*", J. Mamm. Vol 63, pp. 23-32, 1982.

[25] M. Kaabi, P. Pazb, M. Alvareza, E.Anela, J. C. Boixoa, H. Rouissic, P. Herraezband, L. Anela, , "Effect of epididymis handling conditions on the quality of ram spermatozoa recovered post-mortem", – *Theriogenology*, Vol. 60, pp. 1249–1259, 2003.

[26] E. Arenas-Ríos, M. A. León-Galván, E. Mercado, E. Rosado, "Superoxide dismutase, catalase, and glutathione peroxidase during epididymal maturation and prolonged storage of spermatozoa in the mexican big-eared bat (*Corynorhinus mexicanus*)", – *Can. J. Zool. Vol.* 83, pp. 1556-1565, 2005.

[27] E.R. Hofny, M.E. Ali, H.Z. Abdel-Hafez, E.D. Kammal, E. E. Mohamed , H. G. Abd El-Azeem and T. Mostafa, "Semen parameters and hormonal profile in obese fertile and infertile males". Fertil. Steri,. Vol. 94 (2), pp. 581–4, 2010.

[28] J. E. Chavarro, T. L. Toth, D. L. Wright, J. D. Meeker, and R. Hauser, "Body mass index in relation to semen quality, sperm DNA integrity, and serum reproductive hormone levels among men attending an infertility clinic", Fertil. Steril, Vol. 93, pp. 2222–2231, 2010.

[29] R. M. Fariello, J. R. Pariz, D. M. Spaine, F. C. Gozzo, E. J. Pilau, R. Fraietta, R. P. Bertolla, C. Andreoni, and P. Cedenho, "Effect of smoking on the functional aspects of sperm and seminal plasma protein profiles in patients with varicocele", Hum. Reprod, Vol. 27, pp. 3140-3149, 2012.

[30] F. V. Du Mond, and T. C. Hutchinson, "Squirrel monkey reproduction: the "fatted" male phenomenon and seasonal spermatogenesis", Science Vol. 158, pp.1067–1070, 1967

[31] D. M. Forsyth, R. P. Duncan, K. G. Tustin, and J.-M. Gaillard, "A substantial energetic cost to male reproduction in a sexually dimorphic ungulate", Ecology Vol. 86, pp. 2154–2163, 2005.

[32] C. A. Beck CA, Bowen WD, Iverson SJ, "Sex differences in the seasonal patterns of energy storage and expenditure in a phocid seal", J Anim Ecol Vol. 72, pp. 280–291, 2003.

[33] S. A. Atkinson, and M. A. Ramsay, "The effects of prolonged fasting of the body composition and reproductive success of female polar bears (*Ursus maritimus*)", Funct. Ecol. Vol 9, pp. 559–567, 1995.

[34] F. Rincón-Vargas, K. E- Stoner, R. M. Vigueras-Villaseñor, J. M. Nassar, O. M. Chaves, and R. Hundson, "Internal and external indicators of male reproduction in the lesser long-nosed bat *Leptonycteris yerbabuenae*", J. Mamm. Vol. 94, pp. 488-496, 2013.

[35] T. H. Fleming, E. T. Hooper, and D. E. Wilson, "Three Central American bat communities: structure, reproductive cycles, and movement patterns", Ecology Vol. 53, pp. 555–569, 1972.

[36] M. R. Beguelini, R. M. Góes, S. R. Taboga, and36 E. Morielle-Versute, "Two periods of total testicular regression are peculiar events of the annual reproducitive cycle of the black Myotis bat, *Myotis nigricans* (Chiroptera: Vespertilionidae)", Reproduction, Fertility and Development, Vol. 26, pp. 834-846, 2013.

[37] E. G. Crichton, "Sperm storage and fertilization", in "Reproductive Biology of Bats", E. G. Crichton and P. H. Krutsch, Eds, Academic Press, London, pp. 295-320, 2002,

[38] A. L. Álvarez-Guerrero, E. Lira, and N. A: Moreno-Mendoza, "Characterization of gametes in two phyllostomid bats: *Artibeus jamaicensis* and *Sturnira lilium*", unpublished data.

[39] A. Jung, M. Eberl, and W. B. Schill. "Improvement of semen quality by nocturnal scrotal cooling and moderate behavioural change to reduce genital heat stress in men with oligoasthenoteratozoospermia". Reproduction Vol. 121, pp. 595–603, 2001.

[40] A. Jung, W. B. Schill, and H. C. Schuppe , "Genital heat stress in men of barren couples: a prospective evaluation by means of a questionnaire", Andrologia Vol. 34, pp. 349–355, 2002.

[41] Y. H. Lue, B. L. Lasley, L. S. Laughlin, R. S. Swerdloff, A. P. Hikim, A. Leung, J. W. Overstreet, and C. Wang. "Mild testicular hyperthermia induces profound transitional spermatogenic suppression through increased germ cell apoptosis in adult cynomolgus monkeys (*Macaca fascicularis*)", J. Androl. Vol. 23, pp. 799–805, 2002.

[42] C. Paul, A. A. Murray, N. Spears, and P. T. Saunders, "A single, mild, transient scrotal heat stress causes DNA damage, subfertility and impairs formation of blastocysts in mice", Reproduction Vol. 136, pp. 73–84, 2008.

[43] Kanter Mehmet, Aktas Cevat and Erboga Mustafa (2011) Heat stress decreases testicular germ cell proliferation and increases apoptosis in short term: an immunohistochemical and ultrastructural study. Toxicology and Industrial Health 29(2) 99–113

[44] Jung-Hak Kim a,1, Sun-Ji Park a,1, Tae-Shin Kim b, Hyo-Jin Park a, Junghyung Park a, Bo Kyung Kim a, Gyeong-Ryul Kim a, Jin-Man Kim c, Song Mei Huang c, Jung-Il Chae d, Choon Keun Park e, Dong-Seok Lee Testicular hyperthermia induces Unfolded Protein Response signaling activation in spermatocyte. Biochemical and Biophysical Research Communications 434 (2013) 861–866

23

Detection of *Toxoplasma gondii* from Native Cattle in Southwest of Iran

Asghar Arshi, Esmaeil Mahmoudi, Mohammad-Saeid Jami, Abbas Doosti*

Biotechnology Research Center, Islamic Azad University, Shahrekord Branch, Shahrekord, Iran

Email address:

asghararshi@yahoo.com (A. Arshi), esmailmahmoodi72@gmail.com (E. Mahmoudi), sjamimail@yahoo.com (M. S. Jami), bioshk@yahoo.com (A. Doosti)

Abstract: Infections by protozoan parasite *Toxoplasma gondii* are prevalent worldwide in animals and human. *T. gondii* is the causative agent of toxoplasmosis, one of the most prevalent parasitic infections to humans and domestic animals. If first be during pregnancy, *T. gondii* may be transferred vertically by tachyzoites that are passed to the embryo via the placenta. *T. gondii* may be transmitted horizontally in three phases of the life cycle, ingesting infectious oocysts from the environment or tissue cysts or tachyzoites which are contained in gastrointestinal of many different animals. Transmission may also occur via tachyzoites contained in blood products, texture transplants or non-pasteurized milk. Like rest of the world toxoplasmosis is prevalent in Iran. The present study aimed to determine *T. gondii* isolates from native cattle in Chaharmahal Va Bakhtiari province located in south west of Iran by molecular methods. In this study, 155 blood samples were collected from native cattle. Genomic DNA was extracted using DNA extraction Kit (Cinna Gen, Iran) according to the manufacturer protocol and PCR was performed using specific primers (ITS-F and ITS-R). Sixteen (6.95%) cattle were positive to *T. gondii* infection. The positive control samples showed the excepted amplification product specific for *T. gondii* (171 bp). Although the present results showed relatively low prevalence of *T.gondii* infection in Chaharmahal Va Bakhtiari native cattle, control and eradication programs seem to be still necessary to prevent the prevalence of this infection factor and economic losses.

Keywords: *Toxoplasma gondii*, Toxoplasmosis, Native Cattle, PCR, Iran

1. Introduction

Toxoplasma gondii (T. gondii) is a protozoan parasite mandatory which infects all warm-blooded animals such as marine, mammals, humans, animals and birds [1]. This obligate intracellular protozoa was identified in 1908 in a North African rodent. Its intermediate hosts could be humans or other warm-blooded animals [2]. *T. gondii* infection causes mental retardation, loss of vision and other congenital health problems in human newborns [3]. The world prevalence of Toxoplasmosis in human is about 10–30% [4]. In other words up to one-third of the world populations suffer from Toxoplasmosis, an infection caused by *T. gondii* [5,6]. This parasite belongs to apicomplexa, the phylum which also includes main human and domestic animal's pathogens such as Plasmodium (causative agent of malaria), Cryptosporidium (diarrhea), Eimeria (coccidiosis in poultry) and Theileria (East Coast Fever in cattle) [7]. While the infection is asymptomatic in persons with healthy immune system it can be fatal in immune compromised people. Infection during pregnancy can result in feeble offspring, abortion and stillbirth, or birth defects. Moreover, ocular diseases have been reported as toxoplasmosis outcome, that can sometimes be severe in adults resulting in loss of vision and cognitive function and even fatal encephalitis [8,9]. There are three infectious stages of *T. gondii* sporozoites (in oocysts), slow growing bradyzoites (in tissue cysts) and rapidly dividing tachyzoites (in pseudocysts) which can be transmitted through two main routes (sexual and asexual) [8]. The sexual period of the parasite only occurs in the intestine of the definitive host (domestic and wild cat), and results in the excretion of oocytes in stool [10]. Generally *T. gondii* is transmitted through ingestion of partly cooked meat, pork or lamb containing Toxoplasma cysts or unwashed fruits or vegetables that have been in contact with contaminated soil containing infected cat feces [11]. Together with atypical and recombinant species three important clonal lineages of *T. gondii*, specified as Type I, II and III, have been classified according to their genetic multiform. It has been shown that type I and some of the recombinant or atypical species are virulent in mice, whilst genotype II and III are non-virulent [12].

Over the past decade, the use of Polymerase Chain Reaction (PCR) assay has had significant advances for toxoplasmosis detection both in congenital diseases (before birth) and acute toxoplasmosis in immune compromised patients. Among the PCR-based assays, nested-PCR followed by hybridization has been reported as the most sensitive detection technique for the detection of toxoplasmosis [13].

Internal transcribed spacer (ITS) is a fragment of non-functional RNA situated among structural ribosomal RNAs (rRNA) [14]. Read from 5' to 3', the polycistronic rRNA transcript has the 5' ETS (5' external transcribed sequence), 18S rRNA, ITS1, 5.8S rRNA, ITS2, 28S rRNA and the 3' ETS. Since ITSs are easy to amplify even from small quantities of DNA (due to the high copy number of rRNA genes), and they have a high degree of variation even between closely related species, the sequence comparison of the ITS region is widely used in taxonomy and molecular phylogeny [15]. In this work we aimed to investigate the prevalence of *T. gondii* from Iranian native cattle by molecular studies on ITS-1.

2. Materials and Methods

2.1. Samples Collection

One hundred fifty five (155) native cattle blood samples were collected from slaughterhouse in Chaharmahal Va Bakhtiari province and transferred into a sterile tube and stored in 0.05 M EDTA. For ethical approval in this study the protocol and informed consent forms were approved by the Islamic Azad University, Shahrekord Branch, Shahrekord, Iran with 17621105 grant number. Genomic DNA from specimens was extracted using DNA Extraction Kit (Cinna Gen, Iran) according to the manufacturer's protocol. The extracted DNA was quantified by spectrophotometric measurement at a wavelength of 260 nm. The extracted DNA of each specimen was kept frozen at –20°C until used.

2.2. Gene Amplification

Specific primers for ITS-1 of *T. gondii* were used for gene amplification. Forward primer begins at base 97 with the following sequence Toxo-F: 5'-CATTGGAGAGATTTGCATTC -3' and reverse primer begins at base 240 with the sequence Toxo-R: 5'-ATCAGTATCCCAACAGAGACAC -3', therefore a fragment of 171 base pairs was expected. PCR test was performed in final volume of 25 µl PCR reactions containing 100 ng of template DNA, 1.5 mM $MgCl_2$, 200µM dNTPS, 2 mM of each primers and one unit of Taq DNA polymerase enzyme. Thermal PCR conditions consisted of initial 5 min at 95°C and then 32 cycles of denaturing temperature at 94°C for 1 min, annealing temperature at 56°C for 1 min, extension at 72°C for 1 min, and final extension at 72°C for 5 min.

The amplification products were analyzed by 1.5% agarose gel electrophoresis. Electrode buffer was TBE (Tris-base 10.8 g, 89 mM, boric acid 5.5 g, 2 mM EDTA (pH 8.0) 4 ml of 0.5 MEDTA (pH 8.0), with all components joined in enough H_2O and stired to dissolve). Gels were stained with ethidium bromide, aliquots of 10 µl of PCR products were applied to the gel. Constant voltage of 80 V for 30 min was used for products separation. After electrophoresis, generated bands were screened and digitally photographed under UV light.

2.3. Statistical Analyses

Data were analyzed by the chi-square test using the SPSS 17 (SPSS Inc. Chicago, IL, USA) software. P values <0.05 were considered significant.

3. Results

Agarose gel electrophoresis of positive samples revealed a 171 bp fragment. An example of PCR amplification of blood samples is shown in Figure 1. From 155 samples collected, *T. gondii* DNA was detected in 16 cattle blood samples in this study. Our results showed a low frequency (6.95%) of *T. gondii* isolate in native cattle in Chaharmahal Va Bakhtiari province.

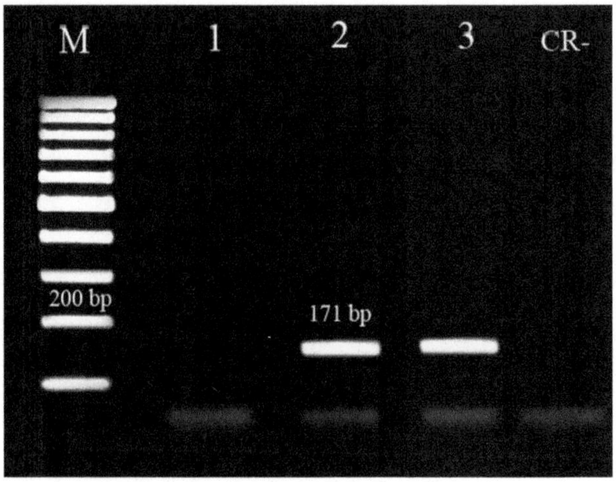

Figure 1. *Gel electrophoresis for detection of T.gondii infection in blood samples. Lane M is 100 bp DNA ladder (Fermentas, Germany); lane 1 is a negative sample, lane 2 and 3 are positive samples, CR- is negative control.*

4. Discussion

Toxoplasmosis is a zoonotic disease caused by *T. gondii* and has been known in many countries since 1908. *T. gondii* infection in cattle is distributed world-wide. There are multitude reports on comparison of different techniques on diagnosis of Toxoplasma infection [16]. PCR used to detect *T. gondii* is very efficient in rapid diagnosis of toxoplasmosis [17]. PCR technique, by which a part of *T. gondii* genome DNA is detectable with high sensitivity and specificity, is preferred to other techniques such as serological tests with variable sensitivity and specificity [18]. Blood samples are the most available sample required to perform PCR for diagnosis proposes in animals, birds and human cases [17]. In a human study Mohammed Yesuf et al. indicated that the prevalence of toxoplasmosis for HIV\AIDS patients in the Ethiopia was 60%. The analysis shows that some health, economic and risk behavior factors influence exposure of patients to toxoplasmosis [19].

In this work we observed a low frequency (6.95%) of native cattle population infected by *T. gondii* in Chaharmahal Va Bakhtiari province in Iran. Some similar studies in different regions of Iran showed the prevalence rate of *T. gondii* up to 15.9% in North-West of Iran [20], 21.6% in coastal region of Caspian Sea [21], 32% in Khuzestan province [22], and 13.8% in Ahvaz city [23].

Comparison of our results with other reports shows that the occurrence of toxoplasmosis varies between countries, influenced by traditions, customs and the life styles of the population. For instances studies have shown the infection rate of 7.8% in France [24], 15.7% in Spain [25], 76.3% in Serbia [26], 5% in north America [27] and 10.5% in Vietnam [28].

In a study in Brazil, the number of *T. gondii* infected animals from farms that had a history of abortion or stillbirth was much higher than in animals from farms without abortion history (P=0.019) [29].

Age seems to be another important factor in toxoplasmosis. It has been reported that younger animals are more likely to become infected than other age groups e.g. cattle under the age of one year were significantly (P>0.05) more infected than the older cattle [23, 30].

5. Conclusion

The results of the present study showed that PCR, as a highly sensitive and specific method can be used for diagnosis, identification and differentiation of *T. gondii* and laboratory support is an important tool in disease diagnosis. Thus, it is essential to screen all regions regularly to prevent the spread of the disease. Although we showed a comparatively low prevalence of *T. gondii* in Iranian cattle, the control and eradication programs still seem to be necessary to prevent and reduce its negative effects on health and economy.

Acknowledgments

The authors would like to express their deep sense of gratitude and sincere thanks to the staff of the Biotechnology Research Center of Islamic Azad University of Shahrekord branch in southwest Iran.

References

[1] Holec-Gąsior, L., Drapała, D., Dominiak-Górski, B. and Kur, J. (2013). Epidemiological study of Toxoplasma gondii infection among cattle in Northern Poland. Ann. Agric. Environ. Med, 20(4): 653-656.

[2] Haeri, M.R., Jalalizadegan, B., Tabatabaie, F. (2014). Recognition of Acute Toxoplasmosis with IgG Avidity ELISA Test in the Pregnant Women (The First Trimester) in Qom Province, Iran, during Two Years (2012-2013). A. J. L. S, 2(6-3): 18-21.

[3] Dubey, J.P., Rajendran, C., Ferreira, L.R., Martins, J., Kwok, O.C., Hill, D.E., Villena, I., Zhou, H., Su, C. and Jones, J.L. (2011). High prevalence and genotypes of Toxoplasma gondii isolated from goats, from a retail meat store, destined for human consumption in the USA. Int. J. Parasitology, 41(8): 827-833.

[4] Lopes, W.D., Rodriguez, J.D., Souza, F.A., dos Santos, T.R., dos Santos, R.S., Rosanese, W.M., Lopes, W.R., Sakamoto, C.A. and da Costa, A.J. (2013). Sexual transmission of Toxoplasma gondii in sheep. Vet Parasitol, 195(1-2): 47-56.

[5] Okada, T., Marmansari, D., Li, Z.M., Adilbish, A., Canko, S., Ueno, A., Shono, H., Furuoka, H. and Igarashi, M. (2013). A novel dense granule protein, GRA22, is involved in regulating parasite egress in Toxoplasma gondii. Mol Biochem Parasitol, 189(1-2): 5-13.

[6] Choi, K.M., Gang, J. and Yun, J. (2008). Anti-Toxoplasma gondii RH strain activity of herbal extracts used in traditional medicine. Int. J. Antimicrob Agents, 32(4): 360-362.

[7] Pratt, S., Wansadhipathi-Kannangara, N.K., Bruce, C.R., Mina, J.G., Shams-Eldin, H., Casas, J., Hanada, K., Schwarz, R.T., Sonda, S. and Denny, P.W. (2013). Sphingolipid synthesis and scavenging in the intracellular apicomplexan parasite, Toxoplasma gondii. Mol Biochem Parasitol, 187(1): 43-51.

[8] Grigg, M.E. and Sundar, N. (2009). Sexual recombination punctuated by outbreaks and clonal expansions predicts Toxoplasma gondii population genetics. Int .J. Parasitol, 39(8): 925-933.

[9] Masatani, T., Matsuo, T., Tanaka, T., Terkawi, M.A., Lee, E.G., Goo, Y.K., Aboge, G.O., Yamagishi, J., Hayashi, K., Kameyama, K., Cao, S., Nishikawa, Y. and Xuan, X. (2013). TgGRA23, a novel Toxoplasma gondii dense granule protein associated with the parasitophorous vacuole membrane and intravacuolar network. Parasitol Int, 62(4): 372-379.

[10] Miller, C.M., Boulter, N.R., Ikin, R.J. and Smith, N.C. (2009). The immunobiology of the innate response to Toxoplasma gondii. Int. J. Parasitol, 39(1): 23-39.

[11] Qu, D., Han, J. and Du, A. (2013). Enhancement of protective immune response to recombinant Toxoplasma gondii ROP18 antigen by ginsenoside Re. Exp Parasitol, 135(2): 234-239.

[12] Döşkaya, M., Caner, A., Ajzenberg D., Değirmenci, A., Dardé, M.L., Can, H., Erdoğan, D.D., Korkmaz, M., Uner, A., Güngör, C., Altıntaş, K. and Gürüz, Y. (2013). Isolation of Toxoplasma gondii strains similar to Africa 1 genotype in Turkey. Parasitol Int, 62(5): 471-474.

[13] Fallahi, S.h., Kazemi, B., Seyyed Tabaei, S.J., Bandehpour, M., Lasjerdi, Z., Taghipour, N., Zebardast, N., Nikmanesh, B., Omrani, V.F. and Ebrahimzadeh, F. (2014). Comparison of the RE and B1 gene for detection of Toxoplasma gondii infection in children with cancer. Parasitol Int, 63(1): 37-41.

[14] Rajaratnam, S. and Thiagarajan, T. (2012). Molecular characterization of wild mushroom. J. Exp. Bio, 2 (2): 369-373.

[15] Kent, T., Lapik, Y.R. and Pestov, D.G. (2009). The 5' external transcribed spacer in mouse ribosomal RNA contains two cleavage sites. RNA, 15(1): 114-120.

[16] Sevinsc, F. (2000). The seroprevalence of Toxoplasma gondii in goats detected by indirect hemagglutination (IHA) and indirect florescent antibody (IFA) tests in the region of Konya. Acta Parasitologica Turnica, 24(1): 57-80.

[17] Tavassoli, M., Ghorbanzadehghan, M. and Esmaeilnejad, B. (2013). Detection of Toxoplasma gondii in sheep and goats blood samples by PCR-RFLP in Urmia. Vet. Res. Forum, 4: 43–47.

[18] James, G.S., Sintchenko, V.G., Dickeson, D.J. and Gilbert, G.L. (1996). Comparison of cell culture, mouse inoculation, and PCR for detection of Toxoplasma gondii: effects of storage conditions on sensitivity. J. Clin. Microbiol, 34: 1572–1575.

[19] Mohammed Yesuf, K., Melese, Z.T. (2015). Prevalence of Toxoplasmosis in HIV/AIDS Patients in Mettu Karl Hospital. A. J. H. R, 3(3): 183-188.

[20] Ghazaei, C. (2006). Serological survey of antibodies to Toxoplasma gondii. Afr J Health Sci, 13(1-2): 131-4.

[21] Sharif, M., Gholami, Sh., Ziaei, H., Daryani, A., Laktarashi, B., Ziapour, S.P., Rafiei, A. and Vahedi, M. (2007). Seroprevalence of Toxoplasma gondii in cattle, sheep and goats slaughtered for food in Mazandaran province, Iran during. Vet. J, 174(2): 422-424.

[22] Nematollahi, A. and Moghadam, G. (2008). Survey on seroprevalence of anti-Toxoplasma gondii antibodies in cattle in Tabriz, Iran by IFAT. American. J. Anim. Vet. Sci, 3(1): 40-42.

[23] Raeghi, S., Akbarei, A. and Sadeghi, S. (2011). Seroprevalence of Toxoplasma gondii in sheep, cattle and horses in Urmia North-West of Iran. Iranian. J. Parasitol, 6(4): 90-94.

[24] Gilot-Fromont, E., Aubert, D., Belkilani, S., Hermitte, P., Gibout, O., Geers, R. and Villena, I. (2009). Villena, Landscape, herd management and within herd seroprevalence of Toxoplasma gondii in beef cattle herds from champagne-Ardenne, France. Vet Parasitol, 161: 36-40.

[25] González-Warleta, M., Castro-Hermida, J.A., Carro-Corral, C., Cortizo-Mella, J. and Mezo, M. (2008). Epidemiology of neosporosis in dairy cattle in Galicia (NW Spain). Parasitol Res 102(2): 243-249.

[26] Klun, I., Djurković-Djaković, O., Katić-Radivojević, S. and Nikolić, A. (2006). Cross-sectional survey on Toxoplasma gondii infection in cattle, sheep and pigs in Serbia: seroprevalence and risk factors. Vet Parasitol, 135(2): 121-131.

[27] Dubey, J.P. (1992). Isolation of Toxoplasma gondii from a naturally infected beef cow. J Parasitol, 78(1): 151-153.

[28] Huong, L.T., Ljungström, B.L., Uggla, A. and Björkman, C. (1998). Prevalence of antibodies to Neospora caninum and Toxoplasma gondii in cattle and water buffaloes in southern Vietnam. Vet Parasitol, 75(1): 53-57

[29] Fajardo, H.V., D'ávila, S., Bastos, R.R., Cyrino, C.D., de Lima Detoni, M., Garcia, J.L., das Neves, L.B., Nicolau, J.L. and Amendoeira, M.R. (2013). Seroprevalence and risk factors of toxoplasmosis in cattle from extensive and semi-intensive rearing systems at Zona da Mata, Minas Gerais state, Southern Brazil. Parasit Vectors, 6, 191.

[30] Dubey, J.P. (2009). Toxoplasmosis in sheep--the last 20 years. Vet Parasitol, 163(1-2): 1-14.

Response of Pullet Chicks to Dietary FumonisinB_1: Growth Indices and Haematological Parameters

Ogunlade Jacob Taiwo

Department of Animal Production and Health Sciences, Faculty of Agricultural Sciences, Ekiti State University, Ado-Ekiti, Nigeria

Email address:
taiwoogunlade2003@yahoo.com

Abstract: Growth indices and heamatological parameters of 180 Isa brownpullet chicks fed graded levels of dietary fumonisin B_1 (an environmental mycotoxin produced by *Fusariumverticillioides*) were studied in a feeding trial that lasted nine weeks. The chicks, having similar initial average weights were randomly assigned to four experimental diets containing 0.2, 5.2, 10.2, and 15.2 mgFB_1/kg constituting diets 1(control), 2, 3, and 4 respectivelyin a completely randomized design. Each dietary treatment had three replicates of 15 chicks each. The feed intake was monitored daily and the chicks weighed weekly. Blood samples were collected at the end of the trial and analyzed. Results revealed a non-significant ($P>0.05$) but FB_1 concentration dependent decrease in daily feed intake, final live weight and daily weight gain of chicks fed diets 2, 3, and 4 when compared with those on diet 1. Crude protein and ether extract digestibility decreased significantly ($P < 0.05$) as the dietary FB_1 levels increased. The dry matter digestibility of chicks on diets 2, 3, and 4 were 94.77, 95.07 and 94.81 % respectively of the control value. Chicks fed diets containing 10.2 and 15.2 mg FB_1/kg suffered significantly ($P < 0.05$) reduced concentration of erythrocytesand mean corpuscular heamoglobin concentration (MCHC). Lymphocytes significantly decline (lymphopenia) while heterophils significantly increased with increase in dietary FB_1 suggesting a condition of immunosuppression and tissue degeneration respectively in chicks fed diets 3 and 4. The study demonstrated that pullets chicks exposed to dietary fumonisin concentration of 10.20mg/kg diet and above would suffer depressed apparent crude protein and ether extract digestibility and decreased synthesis of erythrocyte, MCHC and lymphocytes.

Keywords: Mycotoxin, Poultry, Digestibility, Blood Profile

1.Introduction

Poultry production is an enterprise recognized as a quick means of generating income and improving animal proteins in human diets. The presence of mycotoxin and anti-nutritional factors in most of the ingredients used in formulating rations for this specie of animal is of great concern to the poultry farmersand professionals (12). Fumonisin B_1, a novel mycotoxin produced by the fungus *Fusariumverticillioides,*has been reported to be a major contaminant of maize intended for use in poultry ration formulation and human consumption. The importance of maize, a feed ingredient of high caloric value, in formulation of poultry ration can not be overemphasized.

Fumonisins have been shown to decreased body weight and average daily weight gain of broiler chicks (7), rats (1), rabbits (3) and pigs (4).

Additionally, ingestion of FB_1 contaminated diets has been shown to depress the syntheses of serum parameters and reduce the relative weights of some organs in laying hens (12).

In view of these, and findings from other literatures showing increasing wave of fumonisin contamination of feeds and feedstuffs (4), this study was designed to assess the growth and haematological parameters of pullet chicks fed graded levels of dietary FB_1

2.Materials and Methods

The innocular of toxigenic strain of *F. verticillioides* (MRC 286) obtained from the Mycotoxin laboratory of the International Institute of Tropical Agriculture (IITA), Ibadan, Nigeria were introduced to autoclaved maize grains to produce FB_1 according to the method described by Nelson *et.*

al.,(10).The inoculated maize grains were air-dried, ground and quantified for FB_1 usingCD-ELISA. Four experimental diets containing 0.2, 5.2, 10.2 and 15.2 mg/kg FB_1 were formulated by replacing autoclaved, non-cultured maize with the ground cultured maize at graded levels. The gross composition of the diets are shown in Table 1. 180 day-old pullet chicks having similar initial average weights were randomly assigned to the experimental diets in a completely randomized design such that each experimental diet had 45 chicks replicated thrice with15 chicks per replicate in a feeding trial that lasted for 9 weeks.

Table 1. *Gross composition (%) of the pullet chicks experimental diets.*

Ingredients	Diet 1	Diet 2	Diet 3	Diet 4
	0.2mg/Kg FB_1	**5. 2mg/Kg FB_1**	**10. 2mg/Kg FB_1**	**15. 2mg/Kg FB_1**
Non inoculated Maize	43. 00	41. 26	39. 52	37. 78
Inoculated Maize	-	1 . 74	3 . 48	5 . 22
Soybean meal	23. 00	23. 00	23. 00	23. 00
Wheat offal	28. 00	28. 00	28. 00	28. 00
Fish meal	2 . 00	2 . 00	2 . 00	2 . 00
Bone meal	2 . 00	2 . 00	2 . 00	2 . 00
Oyster shell	1 . 00	1 . 00	1 . 00	1 . 00
Premix	0 .25	0 .25	0 .25	0 .25
Methionine	0 .20	0 .20	0 .20	0 .20
Lysine	0 .30	0 .30	0 .30	0 .30
Salt	0 .25	0 .25	0 .25	0 .25
Total	100. 00	100. 00	100. 00	100. 00
Calculated nutrients	-	-	-	-
Crude protein (%)	20. 02	20. 02	20. 02	20. 02
Crude fibre (%)	4 .90	4 .90	4 .90	4 .90
ME (Kcal/kg)	2678. 42	2678. 42	2678. 42	2678. 42
ME =	Metabolisable energy			

3.Results and Discussion

3.1. Growth Parameters of Pullet Chicks Fed Graded Concentrations of Dietary FB_1

The initial and final live weights, daily fed intakes, daily weights gains and feed conversion ratios (FCR) of the pullets are shown in Table 2. The performance indices of the chicks apparently decreased, except FCR, as the concentration of dietary FB_1 increased, however, the parameters were not significantly ($P > 0.05$) influencedby the dietary treatments. The non –significant reduction in daily feed intake and consequently, the daily weight gains and final live weight of the chicks obtained in this study are consistent with the resultof Voss *et.al.,*(17) and US NTP(16) and could be due to feed refusal effect occasioned by the repellant taste or odour of the contaminated feed as observed by Gelderblom*et. al.,* (6), Ewuola*et. al.,* (3) and Gbore*et. al.,* (5). The reduction in overall feed efficiency over the nine weeks feeding trial suggests the ability of the dietary FB1 to impede nutrient metabolism. However, the findings of Ewuola*et. al.,*(3) and Gelderblom*et.al.,*(6) that dietary fumonisin B_1 significantly reduced body weight gain in rabbits and rats respectively are contrary to the results obtained in this study. This may be due to variations in the sensitivity of different specie of animals to fumonisin(15)

3.2. Nutrient Digestibility of Pullet Chicks Fed Graded Levels of Dietary FB_1

The result of apparent nutrient digestibility of the chicks (Table 3) showed a dietary FB_1 concentration dependent decline in crude protein and ether extract. The dry matter digestibility of chicks on diets 2, 3 and 4 were 94.77, 95.07, and 94.81 % respectively of those on control diet (1). The nutrient digestibility values were an indication of nutrients absorption and utilization. The significant decline in crude protein and ether extract digestibility particularly for chicks on diets 3 and 4 suggests an inhibition of sphingolipid biosynthesis by FB_1 (18) resulting in alteration of epithelial morphology of the chicks and poor digestion, absorption, and utilization of protein and other nutrients (11). Since the pullet chicks were fed *ad-libitum*, and all the experimental diets were iso-nitrogenous and satisfied the protein requirement for pullet chicks(13), the significant decline in crude protein digestibility of the chicks across the dietary treatments is an indication of the ability of fumonisin B_1 to impede protein metabolism. These results may also justify the apparent reduction in the daily feed intake, weight gain and poorer feed conversion ratio obtained for chicks on higher levels of dietary fumonisin.

Table 2. Growth Indices of pullet chicks fed graded levels of dietary Fumonisin.

Parameters	Diet 1	Diet 2	Diet 3	Diet 4	SEM*
	0.2mg/Kg FB_1	5.2mg/Kg FB_1	10.2mg/Kg FB_1	15.2mg /KgFB_1	
Initial Live Weight (g)	179.00	180.67	182.00	181.00	1.25
Daily Feed Intake (g)	32.09	31.92	31.44	30.81	3.09
Final Live Weight (g)	484.67	475.67	447.00	428.00	34.24
Weight Gain (g/day)	5.40	5.27	4.50	4.41	0.90
Feed Conversion Ratio	6.10	6.10	6.89	7.00	0.67

Values shown are means. SEM* =Standard Error of Means.

Table 3.Apparent Nutrient Digestibility (%) of chicks fed graded levels of dietary FB_1.

Nutrient	Diet 1	Diet 2	Diet 3	Diet 4	SEM*
	0.2mg/KgFB_1	5.2mg/Kg FB_1	10.2mg/Kg FB_1	15.2mg/Kg FB_1	
Dry Matter	66.14^a	62.68^b	62.88^b	62.71^b	0.68
Crude Protein	64.07^a	58.07^b	50.11^c	46.82c	0.97
Crude Fibre	58.10	56.18	55.14	55.02	2.49
Ether Extract	72.80^a	66.00^{ab}	61.65^b	50.00	1.80
Ash	47.03	49.05	45.00	45.00	2.19
Nitrogen Free Extract	84.12	83.50	83.29	81.29	1.07

a, b, c. Means differently superscripted across the rows are significantly different ($P < 0.05$) .SEM = Standard Error of Means

3.3. Effect of Graded Levels of Dietary FB_1 on Haematology of Pullet Chicks

The haematological indices of the pullets as shown in Table 4 reveals that the erythrocytes, MCHC and Lymphocyte values decreased significantly ($P < 0.05$) while the heterophils value significantly ($P < 0.05$) increased with increased dietary FB_1 concentration. Other haematological parameters were not significantly influenced by dietary FB1. Although, all the haematological values were within the reported range for normal female chicken (9), pullets exposed to diets 3 and 4 suffered a significant depression in the synthesis of red blood cells (erythrogenesis).The significant reduction in mean corpuscular haemoglobin concentration(MCHC) and red blood cells(RBC) with increasing levels of dietary fumonisin B_1suggested that the red blood cells were hypo chromic. Since the principal function of lymphocytes is in relationship to its immunological activity, it therefore appeared in this study that dietary FB_1 suppressed immune response in pullets fed diets 3 and 4 and induced tissue destruction in the bird as indicated by a significantly higher values of heterophil(2). Similar result of immune suppression in chicken fed maize cultured with *F. verticillioides* was reported by Marijanovic*et.al.*,(8). However, these results are contrary to the reports of Parent-Massin and Parchment(14) and Zomborsky-Kovac*et.al.*,(19) that fumonisin is a non-haematotoxicmycotoxin. This may be due to variations in the sensitivity of different specie of animals to fumonisin(15)

Table 4. Haematological Values of Pullet Chicks Fed graded Levels of Dietary Fumonisin.

Parameters	Diet1	Diet2	Diet3	Diet4	SEM*
	0.2mg/KgFB_1	5.2mg/KgFB_1	10.2mg/KgFB_1	15.2mg/KgFB_1	
Erythrocytes (x 10^6/mm^3)	2.63^a	2.50^{ab}	2.38^b	2.45^b	0.06
Haemoglobin(g/dl)	10.53	10.23	10.07	10.00	0.28
Mean Cell Volume (µ3)	119.33	127.33	123.33	126.67	2.17
MCH (µµg)	40.00	41.00	40.33	41.00	0.63
MCHC (%)	33.00^a	32.33^{ab}	31.00^b	32.33^{ab}	0.49
Packed Cell Volume (%)	31.67	31.67	30.67	31.00	0.58
Platelets (x 10^3/L)	243.67	22.67	238.67	243.33	35.65
Leukocytes(x 10^3/mm^3)	12.90	12.26	11.90	11.30	1.93
Lymphocytes (x 10^3/mm^3)	8.89^a	8.13^a	6.08^b	6.28^b	1.87
Heterophils (x 10^3/mm^3)	3.35^c	3.82	4.76^a	4.69^a	3.01
Monocytes (x 10^3/mm^3)	0.12	0.11	0.22	0.11	0.39
Eosinophils (x 10^3/mm^3)	0.26	0.19	0.26	0.23	0.49

a, b, c: Means differently superscripted across the row are significantly different ($P < 0.05$)
SEM: Standard Error of Means
*MCH: Mean Corpuscular Haemoglobin
*MCHC: Mean Corpuscular Haemoglobin Concentration

4. Conclusion

This study demonstrated that FB_1 of 10.20 mg/kg and above in the diet of pullet chicks will reduce dry matter, crude protein and ether extract digestibility, suppress RBC, MCHC and lymphocytesyntheses and induce liberation of heterophils from the tissues.

Acknowledgements

The author expressed his appreciation to Dr. R. Bandyopadhyhay and Mr. O. Ayinde of Mycotoxin laboratory, International Institute of Tropical Agriculture, (IITA, Ibadan) for their technical assistance.

References

[1] Bondy, G.S., Suzuki, C.A.M., Mueller, R.W., Fernie, S.M., Armstrong, C.L., Hierlihy, S.I., Savard, M.E and Barker, M.G. (1998). Gavage administration of the fungal toxin fumonisin B_1 to female Sprague-Dawley rats. *J. Toxicol. Environ. Health,* 53: 135-151.

[2] Coles, E.H.(1986). Veterinary clinical pathology.4th ed. W.B. Saunders company, Philadelphia, London and Toronto. Pp 99-148

[3] Ewuola, E.O., Ogunlade, J.T., Gbore, F.A., Salako, A. O., Idahor, K.O. and Egbunike, G.N. (2003). Performance evaluation and organ histology of rabbits fed *Fusariumverticillioides* culture material. *Trop. Anim. Prod.* 6 (2): 111-119

[4] Fazekas, B., Bajmocy, E., Glavics, R. and Fenyvesi, A. (1997). Fumonisinmycoticoses in Hungary. Leuco-encephalomalacia in horses, fattening pulmonary oedema in pigs. *Magy. Allartov. Lapja.*, 119 : 137-139

[5] Gbore, F.A, Ogunlade, J.T, Ewuola, E. O. and Egbunike G.N. (2010). Growth indices and haematological parameters of weanling pigs fed dietary fumonisin B_1.*Nig. J. Anim. Prod.* 37 (1) : 123-134.

[6] Gelderblom, W. C. A., Cawood, M. E., Snyman, S. D., and Marasas, W. F. O. (1994). Fumonisin B_1dosimetry in relation to cancer initiation in rat liver. *Carcinogenesis,* 15 : 209-214

[7] Ledoux, D.R., Brown, T. P., Weibking, T.S. and Rottinghaus, G. E. (1992). Fumonisin toxicity in broiler chicks. *J. Vet. Diagn. Invest.* 4: 330-333

[8] Marijanovic, D.R., Holt, P.,Norred, W.P., Bacon, C.W., Voss, K.A., Stancel, P.C. and Ragland, W.L.(1991). Immunosuppressive effects of *F. moniliforme* corn culture in chickens. *Poult. Sci.*, 70: 1895-1901

[9] Mitruka, B. M and Rawnsley, H. M. (1977). Clinical biochemical and haematological reference values in normal experimental animals. Masson Pub. USA Inc., N. Y. pp. 21-84

[10] Nelson, P. E., Juba, J. H., Ross, P. F. and Rice, L. G. (1994). Fumonisin production by Fusarium species on solid substrates. *J. Assoc. Off. Anal. Chem. Int.*, 77: 522-524.

[11] Ogunlade, J. T., Gbore, F. A., Ewuola, E. O., Idahor, K. O., Salako, A. O. and Egbunike, G. N. (2004). Biochemical and Haematological Responses of Rabbits Fed Diets containing micro doses ofFumonisin .*Trop. J. Anim. Sci.* 7 (1) : 169-176

[12] Ogunlade, J. T. and Egbunike, G. N. (2013). FumonisinMycotoxicity in laying hens: Haematology, serum biochemistry and organ characteristics. *Glob. Adv. Res. Jour. Of Env. Sc. and Toxicol.* 2(2) : 47 – 53

[13] Oluyemi, J.A. and Roberts, F.A. (2000). Poultry production in warm wet climates. 2nd ed. Spectrum Book Ltd. (Publ.), Ibadan, Nigeria. pp. 1-7.

[14] Parent-Massin, D. and Parchment, R.E.(1998). Haematotoxicity of mycotoxins. In: Le Bass, J., Galties, P. (eds.). Mycotoxins in the food chain, MYCOTOX '98, Toulouse, July 2-4, pp. 591-598.

[15] US FDA (2000). Background paper in support of fumonisin levels in animal feed. US Food and Drug Administration Center for Veterinary Medicine, June 6, 2000.

[16] US NTP (1999). NTP technical report on the toxicology and carcinogenesis studies of fumonisin B_1(CAS No. 116355-83-0) in F344/N rats and B6C3F1 mice (feed studies). Research Triangle Park, North Carolina, US Department of Health and Human Services National Toxicology Program (NTP TR 496; NIH Publication No.

[17] Voss, K.A., Chamberlain, W.J., Bacon, C.W. and Norred, W.P. (1993). A preliminary investigation on renal and hepatic toxicity in rats fed purifiedfumonisin B_1. *Nat. Toxins.*, 1: 222-228.

[18] Yoo, H. S., Norred, W. P., Wang, E., Merill, A. H. Jr., and Riley, R. T. (1992). Fumonisin inhibition of de novo sphingolipid biosynthesis and cytotoxicity are correlated in LLC-PK_1 cells. *Toxicol. Appl. Pharmacol.*, 114 : 9-15

[19] Zomborszky-Kovacs, M., Kovacs, F., Horn, P., Vetesi, F., Repa, I., Tornyos, G. and Toth, A.(2002). Investigation into the time-and dose-dependent effect of fumonisin B_1 in order to determine tolerable limit values in pigs. *Livestock Production Science*, 76:251-256.

25

Abandoned Mines Used as Roosts for Reproduction by Townsend's Big-Eared Bats (*Corynorhinus townsendii*) in a Protected Area in the Central Highlands of Mexico

León-Galván Miguel Angel[1], Rodríguez-Tobón Ahiezer[2], Cano Espinoza José Sulim[1], Guzman Ledesma Beatriz Samantha[1], Guevara-Chumacero Luis Manuel[1], Leyequien Abarca Lissette[3]

[1]Department of Biology, Autonomous Metropolitan University-Iztapalapa, Mexico
[2]Postgraduate in Experimental Biology, Autonomous Metropolitan University-Iztapalapa, Mexico
[3]Direction of the Sierra La Mojonera Flora and Fauna Protection Area, National Commission of Natural Protected Areas (CONANP), S.L.P. Mexico

Email address:
leon@xanum.uam.mx (León-Galván M. A.), ahiezerrod@yahoo.com.mx (Rodríguez-Tobón A.), sulim.cano@gmail.com (Cano E. J. S.), samantha.guzled@gmail.com (Guzmán L. B. S.), lmgc1@yahoo.com (Guevara-Chumacero L. M.), lleyequien@gmail.com (Leyequien A. L.)

Abstract: In Chihuahuan Desert arid zone, particularly the states of Zacatecas and San Luis Potosi, Mexico, have been distinguished by its large mining activity, however, many of these mines are disuse, becoming potential refuges for various species of cave bats. Monitoring the potential roosts by *Corynorhinus townsendii* was made within the system of mines in the vicinity of the Sierra La Mojonera Flora and Fauna Protection Area, at Mexico's Central Highlands in the states of Zacatecas and San Luis Potosi. Which consisted of visual inspection inside, and mist netting at the entrance of different mines during an annual cycle. The main reproductive roosts for *C. townsendii* were identified. Spermatogenesis takes place during May-September; the mating period in November-December, whereas the sequence of gestation-lactation occurred since March to August of the next year. These data confirm that *C. townsendii* in the area of study follow a seasonally monoestrous reproductive pattern, characterized by an asynchrony between the ovarian and spermatogenic cycles.

Keywords: Bats, Reproduction, *Corynorhinus townsendii*, Central Highlands of Mexico, Conservation

1. Introduction

The diversity of bat species in Mexico is great, including approximately 12.5% of all bat species known worldwide (≈1,150). These animals can use a wide variety of sites as shelters: hollows in trees or beneath their bark, among the leaves of several plant species, and in rocks and fissures, but primarily inside natural caves. Though indirect, the effects of human activity are reflected in the fact that some bats now occupy artificial refuges for their reproductive activity, such as abandoned construction sites, wells, or mines that are no longer exploited to extract minerals.

The arid zone of the Chihuahua Desert –which begins in the southeastern United States and extends southward into the Mexican states of Zacatecas and San Luis Potosi, where the Mexican High Plains is formed, and flanked by the *Sierra Madre Oriental* Mountains– is an area well known for extensive mining activity, as from Colonial times it has been an important producer of such minerals as zinc, silver and copper, among others. Today, many of those mines have fallen into disuse and become potential roosting-sites for various species of cave bats [1, 2]. While the area has a wide variety of vegetation, the most representative types are desert scrubs and temperate coniferous and hardwood forests, which provide abundant food for arthropod populations, especially insects. And these, in turn, constitute the principal food source for insectivore bats. Shelter and food are considered two limiting factors in the biology of bat populations [3], so any place that provides these two key elements may well be adequate for reproduction, since sufficient food is available to ensure the energy supplies necessary to carry out basic reproductive processes. For these reasons, such sites must be considered as of high priority for the conservation of this group of mammals [4-6].

Chiroptera species are notable for the variety of their reproductive modes, which range from "seasonal monoestrous" to "continuous polyestrous" patterns [7, 8]. Seasonal bat species have a single reproductive pattern characterized by asynchrony in the timing of the males' and females' respective reproductive cycles, and in the fundamental processes that make up the sexual cycles of the two sexes. This is the case of several temperate-zone insectivorous bats, including species of the American *Corynorhinus* genus (eg. *C. mexicanus, C. rafinesquii, C. townsendii*). In these bats, spermatogenesis occurs in spring-summer, mating in autumn-winter, and births in the spring of the following year [9-11].

These features are particularly characteristic of Townsend's Big-eared bats, whose habitat stretches from the continental United States into southern Mexico, with five recognized sub-species: *C. t. ingens, C. t. pallescens, C. t. townsendii, C. t. virginianus*, and *C. t. australis*. The distribution of the latter sub-species extends as far south as the state of Oaxaca in Mexico, passing through Mexico's Central Highlands in the states of Zacatecas and San Luis Potosi [12-14].

For several decades, studies have found that *C. townsendii* populations suffer from the accelerated reduction of their habitats and roosting sites [15]. According to the *World Conservation Union's* 2004 IUCN Red List of Threatened Species, all five sub-species of *C. townsendii* are classified as "vulnerable to extinction" (VU) [16]. However, relatively little is known about populations of these bats in Mexico, where they are not listed in any risk category in the Mexican Norm NOM-059-ECOL-2010 [17]. This may be due to the fact that we know so little about their shelters in general and much less about roosts that may serve as active breeding sites. Therefore, the objectives of this study were to: (i) investigate some of the main mines belonging to different mining complexes in the Sierra La Mojonera Flora and Fauna Protection Area region and its hinterland in the Central Highlands of the states of San Luis Potosi and Zacatecas, which can be used as reproduction sites by *C. townsendii* bats; and, (ii) establish the principal reproductive parameters and timing for this species in that area, since reproduction is the main process for perpetuating organisms and species.

2. Material and Methods

2.1. Study Area

The study was conducted in the Potosino-Zacatecano Central Highlands of Mexico, in the so-called "area of influence" surrounding the "Sierra La Mojonera" (SM), a Protected Area of Flora and Fauna (FFPA), located between 23°54' and 24°42' North latitude and 100°42' and 101°30' West longitude, in the municipalities of Vanegas in northern San Luis Potosi, and Concepción del Oro in northern Zacatecas (fig.1).

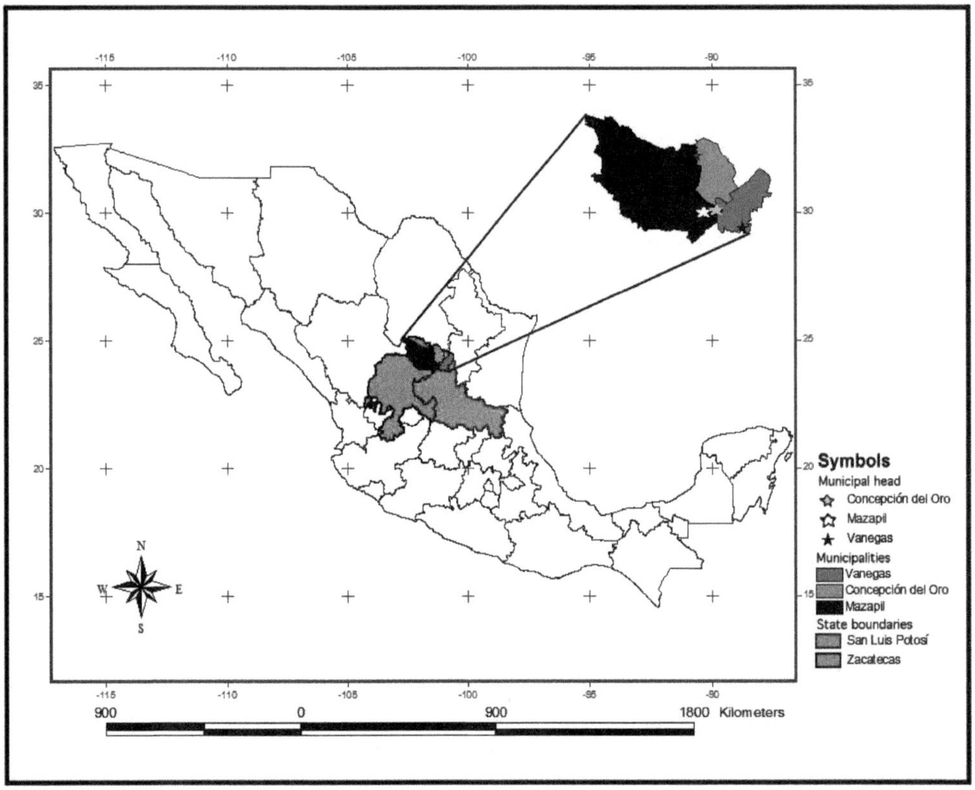

Figure 1. *Study area, the Potosino-Zacatecano highland located at the southern border of the Chihuahuan Desert arid zone of Mexico.*

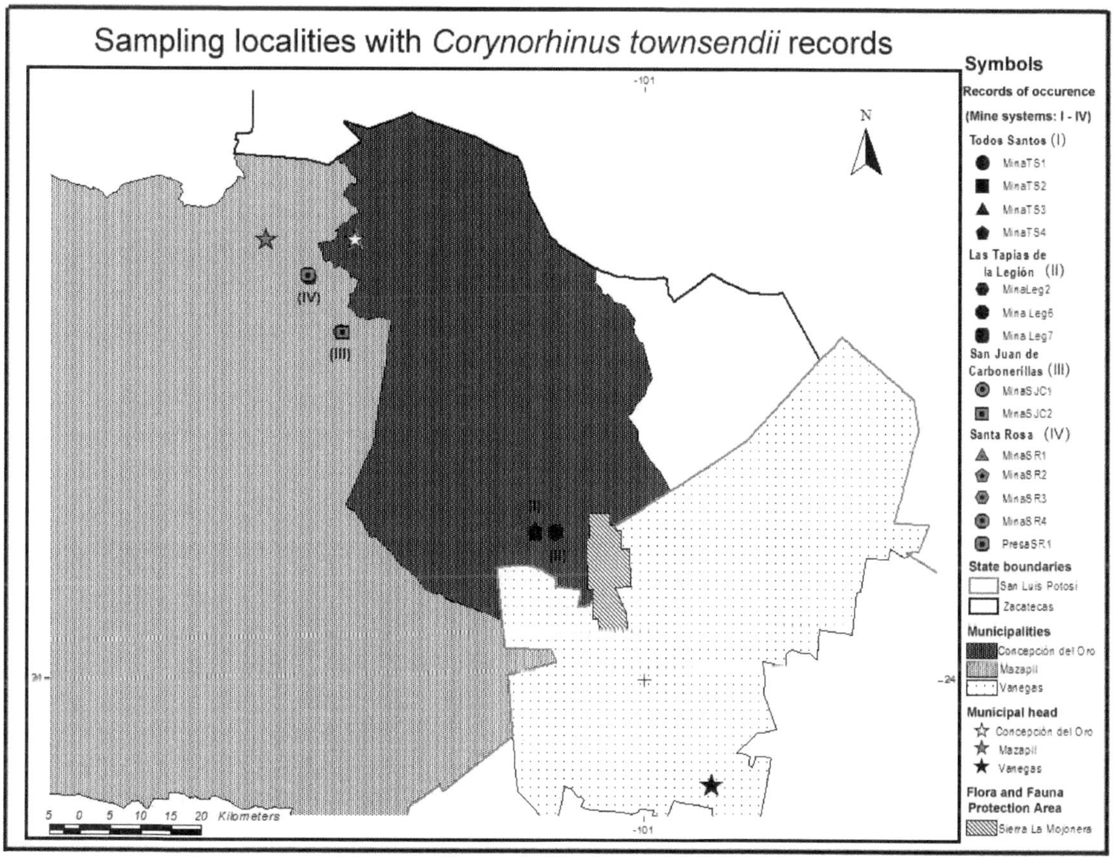

Figure 2. *Map of geographic localization of the Sierra La Mojonera Flora and Fauna Protection Area and the influence zone near it, and the distribution of four abandoned mine systems in which some mines are used as roosts by Townsend's Big-eared bats Corynorhinus townsendii.*

Because this is an ancient mining region, four different systems of mines were located and selected due to they offered potential shelters for Townsend's big-eared bats in some of the hills that intrude into the central plateau from the *Sierra Madre Oriental* mountains. Two of these systems –(I) *Todos Santos* (24°12'31'N; 101°9'31'O, ≈2350 m), and (II) *Las Tapias de la Legion* (24°12'39'N; 101°7'60'O ≈2290 m)– are located in the close vicinity of the SM-FFPA (fig. 2), an area covered primarily by desert scrub vegetation with only a scarce presence of arboreal elements typical of mixed conifer forests. The other two systems are located in the northwest corner of the area of influence of the FFPA, and are called: (III) *San Juan de Carbonerillas* (24°29'46'N; 101°26'28'O, ≈2205 m), and (IV) *Santa Rosa* (24°34'48'N; 101°29'20'O ≈2584 m) (fig. 2). The vegetation around the former is similar to that near *Todos Santos*, while in *Santa Rosa* a mixed conifer forest dominates, with some elements of yucca palms and xeric scrub vegetation.

2.2. Monitoring of Specimens

Sampling was conducted from August 14, 2013 to December 14, 2014. It consisted in 9 visits, each of 3-days' duration, to the different localities and was programmed to cover the key times during which the basic reproductive processes and events of this species take place. During monitoring, visual inspections inside the shelters were performed in daytime, and mist nets were placed at entrances at dusk. They were left open for 3 hours to capture individual bats, which were then examined to obtain somatic and reproductive data. The study was conducted under license from Mexico's National Commission for Natural Protected Areas.

2.3. Identification of the Target Species

Preliminary identification of the target species was conducted in the field by obtaining external morphological data from live animals. However, because sympatric reports exist for *C. townsendii* and *C. mexicanus* in Mexico [13], and because full morphological identification requires measuring skulls, we would have had to sacrifice several specimens, an act that is prohibited by the regulations governing the removal of organisms from Protected Areas or their corresponding zones of influence. Therefore, the decision was taken to determine identification by molecular means. To this end, two bats (one male, one female) were selected from each capture site, and 3-mm diameter biopsies were taken from their wing membrane using a biopsy punch (Fray Products Corp., Buffalo, New York), and then preserved in 70% ethanol. After that, the bats were released alive.

Total DNA extraction was performed using a kit from the Promega Corporation (Madison, Wisconsin) following the manufacturer's instructions. Amplification of about 800 bp of cytochrome b gene via Polymerase chain reaction [18] was performed using primers L14724 [19] and MVZ-16 [20].

Reactions were performed in a volume of 25 ml with approximately 50 ng of DNA, 10 mM of each primer, 200 mM of each deoxynucleoside triphosphate, 2 mM of $MgCl_2$, and 2.5 units of Taq DNA polymerase (QIAGEN, Inc.). The cycles of the polymerase chain reaction were: 94°C followed by 39 cycles of 60s at 94°C, 30s at 45°-50°C and 2 min at 72°C, with a final extension of 10 min at 72°C.

The products of the polymerase chain reaction were purified using the Wizard PCR Prep DNA Purification System (Promega Corporation, Madison, Wisconsin) and utilized to perform sequencing reactions with the Big Dye Terminator Kit (Perkin-Elmer, Norwalk, CT). The sequencing reactions were electrophoresed in an ABI 3100 automated sequencer (Applied Biosystems, Foster City, CA), and sequence alignment was performed with the Clustal W algorithm in the Sequence Navigator 1.0.1 program (Applied Biosystems) and then adjusted manually. Once the sequences were displayed, a basic local alignment –or BLAST [21] – was conducted individually to determine the type of species studied based on the amplified DNA segments and calculations of the percentage of similarity between the sequences obtained in this study and similar sequences deposited in the GenBank database [22].

2.4. Selection of Specimens and Determination of Their Reproductive Status

To determine the reproductive status of the bats only adult males and females were chosen. The selection criteria included somatic measurements (*i.e.*, body weight, forearm length), the general appearance of the fur, and such skeletal features as complete ossification of the metacarpal-phalangeal epiphysis of the 3rd and 4th fingers of the forelimbs, and the degree of tooth wear [10, 23].

Each of the captured male specimens we assigned one of the following reproductive categories: (i) spermatogenesis; (ii) epididymal prolonged sperm storage period; and (iii) mating. This classification was based on the position, appearance and degree of development of the testes and epididymides [9-11, 24]. For the female samples, the categories were: (i) mating; (ii) prolonged sperm storage; (iii) pregnancy; and, (iiii) lactation. Distinctions were based on the degree of development of the mammary glands and nipples, and the presence of fetuses detected by palpation and/or evident bulging of the abdominal-pelvic region [9, 10, 25].

Other conditions that define important stages of the female reproductive cycle (such as oogenesis, ovulation, and parturition) were inferred in light of previously recorded sexual data for this species, so as to avoid the need to sacrifice and dissect any bats. After gathering and recording the required data, all bats were returned to their shelters alive.

3. Results

The sampling procedure produced a total of 121 adult bats (37 males, 84 females) from the main shelters located in the four mining systems chosen in the region (Tables 1, 2).

3.1. Molecular Identification of the Species

Analysis and editing of the sequences obtained from the bats selected for molecular identification confirmed that they were of good quality. Once visualized and edited, fragments of 612 bp of the cytochrome b gene were analyzed. BLAST analysis [21] made it possible to determine that the sequences gathered showed a maximum identity of 99% with the sequence deposited in GenBank that is homologous to *Corynorhinus townsendii* (access number JQ917001), thus confirming that the sequences examined in this study do correspond to the amplified gene for that species. In conclusion: all bats captured at the four sites belonged to the species *C. townsendii.*

3.2. Somatic and Reproductive Characteristics of the Bats

The sex distribution for adult bats of this species from the study area favored females by a ratio of 2.7:1. The average values and ranges of the somatic characteristics recorded for the female specimens were as follows: forearm length, 44.1mm (rank: 39.9-46.3) for all bats caught; and body weight (after excluding the females that were in the different stages of gestation) of 9.7 g (rank: 8.2-13.1). The females of *C. townsendii* have one pair of mammary glands located laterally in the thorax (Fig. 3a). Pregnancy was ascertained by palpation through the month of April until mid-May. Most of the females were in the final stage of pregnancy, as shown by obvious bulging of the abdominal-pelvic region caused by the presence of the product. The changes observed in the region around the breasts of the females, together with the degree of nipple development, allowed us to document the various stages of the cycle of the mammary gland, as shown below (Table 1, Fig. 3):

Table 1. *Somatic data and reproductive conditions of the adult female C. townsendii bats by date of capture, at the roosts of the four mine systems. BW, body weight; FAL, forearm length; nipple size is the relative size of the mammary gland nipple: inconspicuous, small, medium and large; the symbols > and = denote differences or equality in the number of organs with certain size in the sample of bats. NM, variable not measured; body weight of some pregnant and lactating females was not measured to prevent abortion, or to allow them the early foraging. In the number of bats captured by date (n), the number in parenthesis is the total number of specimens in the sample.*

Adult female Corynorhinus townsendii bats				
Capture date	Number of bats (*n*)	Somatic measures (mean and rank)		Reproductive condition
		BW (g)	FAL (mm)	
14/08/13 19/09/14 21/09/13 12/10/13 18/10/14	3 1 6 20	10.1 (8.2 – 13.1)	44.1 (42.3 – 46.0)	Post-lactation inactivity; nipple size: inconspicuous>small>medium

Adult female *Corynorhinus townsendii* bats				
Capture date	Number of bats (*n*)	Somatic measures (mean and rank)		Reproductive condition
		BW (g)	FAL (mm)	
	2 (32)			
15/12/13 12/12/14	3 3 (6)	9.9 (9.5 – 10.4)	43.8 (41.0 – 45.1)	Late mating period, sperm storage; nipple size: medium>small>inconspicuous
05/04/14	7	10.4 (9.0 – 11.0)	44.0 (42.9 – 45.3)	Early gestation; nipple size: small>medium;
05/04/14 16/05/14	4 4 (8)	10.3 (10.0 – 11.0)	44.1 (43.2 – 45.4)	Middle gestation; nipple size: medium>small;
16/05/14	14	NM	44.3 (39.9 – 46.3)	Late gestation; nipple size: medium>large;
16/05/14	15	NM	43.9 (39.9 – 46.3)	Early lactation; nipple size: large, whitish, naked mammary glandular area
15/08/13	2	NM	46.3	Late lactation; nipple size: large, darkened, naked mammary glandular area

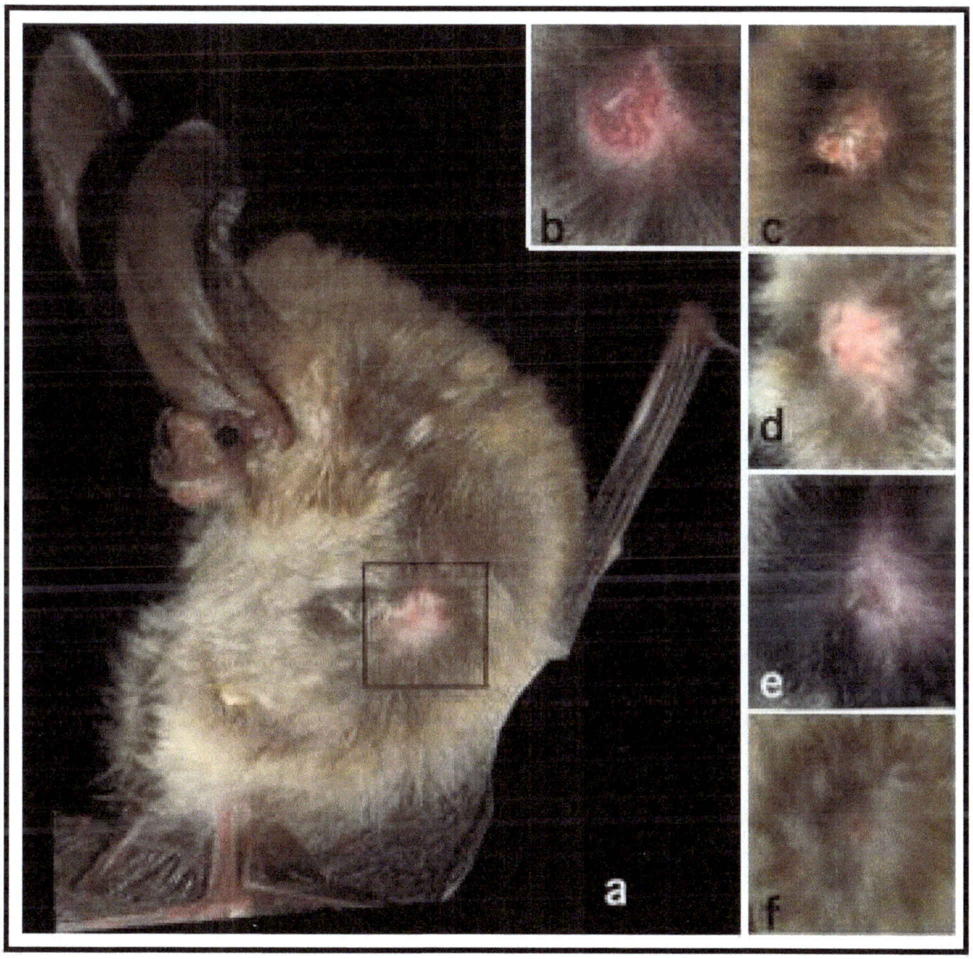

Figure 3. *(a) Photograph of an adult female C. townsendii bat caught in middle May, in late pregnancy; the black square locate the pectoral mammary gland, with a well-developed nipple in a naked skin area. The b-f inserts are photographic magnifications of the same region indicated by the square in (a) but from other specimens that correspond to different development stages of the glandular zone and nipples, and show the main stages of the mammary gland cycle. (b) Early pregnancy; the mammary gland cycle restarts (early April). (c) Late pregnancy, (early May). (d) Lactation (since late May). (e) Retrogression of the mammary gland after the weaning of the young; nipple seen cornified and begins an apparent necrosis. (f) Pos-lactation inactivity (since early October), the skin area around the inconspicuous nipple has been re-covered with hair.*

I- Renewal of the mammary gland cycle in early April, during the first trimester of pregnancy; the nipple is small, translucent in appearance, and located precisely in the center of a circular area of glandular tissue reddish in color due to high blood irrigation, with bare skin caused by hair loss.

II- Pre-lactating condition, in the third trimester of pregnancy, which occurs in early May: the nipple is prominent, while the glandular area is swollen but still reddish.

III- Lactation, beginning in the second half of May; the glandular area is clearly turgid and whitish in color due to the presence of milk; the nipple is highly-developed.

IV- Involution of the mammary gland; once weaning of the young occurs (beginning in August), the nipple shows regression by its dark color and cornified skin; the glandular area has a whitish tone, but is no longer swollen, indicating the cessation of glandular activity.

V- Post-lactation inactivity; beginning in October, the area of glandular tissue and the nipple become very small in size, and the skin is once again coated with fur.

For all the male specimens, the study determined the following somatic values: average forearm length, 43 mm (rank: 41.1-45.0), and mean body weight, 8.8 g (rank: 7.0-10.0) (Table 2). Comparison of these measurements with the corresponding values for the non-pregnant females revealed sexual dimorphism for this species, as females are larger than males.

In adult male *C. townsendii* bats, the testes and epididymides are permanently scrotal and located in the inguinal position (Fig. 4c). Since they undergo dramatic changes in size and appearance according to the different phases of the sexual cycle, it was possible to establish the main stages of the male reproductive cycle for the species in the study area, as shown below (Table 2, Fig. 4):

I- Testicular recrudescence; in the first half of May, males have inconspicuous external testes; the epididymis is small-to-medium in length with a thin and elongated appearance; the caudal end of the tunica vaginalis is black in color.

II- Spermatogenesis, from mid-May to late September; in August, the testes are inguinal and project into the tail membrane because they are fully developed; the cauda of the epididymis takes on a globular appearance; the pigmented area expands and becomes light in color, indicating the onset of the sperm storage period.

III- Mating in November-December; the size of the testes decreases again and they become inconspicuous; spermatogenesis has ceased completely; the epididymis is very elongated with a globular tail likely due to the concentration of sperm.

IV- Inactivity, post-winter; in April, both organs –testis and epididymis– are in a recessed condition; the epididymis is still elongated but the tail is no longer globular, indicating that it has finished storing sperm; the tunic covering them is of dark color due to the presence of pigmentation.

Table 2. *Somatic data and reproductive conditions of the adult male C. townsendii bats by date of capture, at the roosts of the four mine systems. BW, body weight; FAL, forearm length; relative size of the testes and epididymides: inconspicuous, small, medium and large; the symbols > and = denote differences or equality in the number of organs with certain size in the sample of studied bats. NM, variable not measured. In the number of bats captured by date (n), the number in parenthesis is the total number of specimens.*

Adult male Corynorhinus townsendii bats				
Capture date	**Number of bats (*n*)**	**Somatic measures (mean and rank)**		**Reproductive condition**
		BW (g)	**FAL (mm)**	
04/04//14	5	9.0 (7.0 – 10.0)	41.2 (33.6 – 44.6)	Post-winter inactivity; testes: inconspicuous; epididymides: medium>large, globosely, dark cauda
16/05/14	6	NM	42.6 (41.1 – 44.8)	Testicular recrudescence; testes: small; epididymides: medium>large=small, thin, dark
15/08/13	1	NM	41.9	Full spermatogenesis; testes: large; epididymides: large, thin, dark
19/09/14	1	NM	43.0	Late spermatogenesis, epidydimal sperm storage; testes: large; epididymides: medium, globosely, clear cauda
12/10/13	11	8.9 (8.1 – 9.7)	43.4 (41.9 – 45.0)	Testicular involution, epidydimal sperm storage; testes: large>medium; epididymides: large>medium, globosely, clear cauda
24/11/13 13/12/13	1 12 (13)	8.6 (7.4 – 9.6)	43.0 (41.8 – 44.5)	Mating period, epidydimal sperm storage; testes: inconspicuous; epididymides: large>medium, globosely, clear cauda

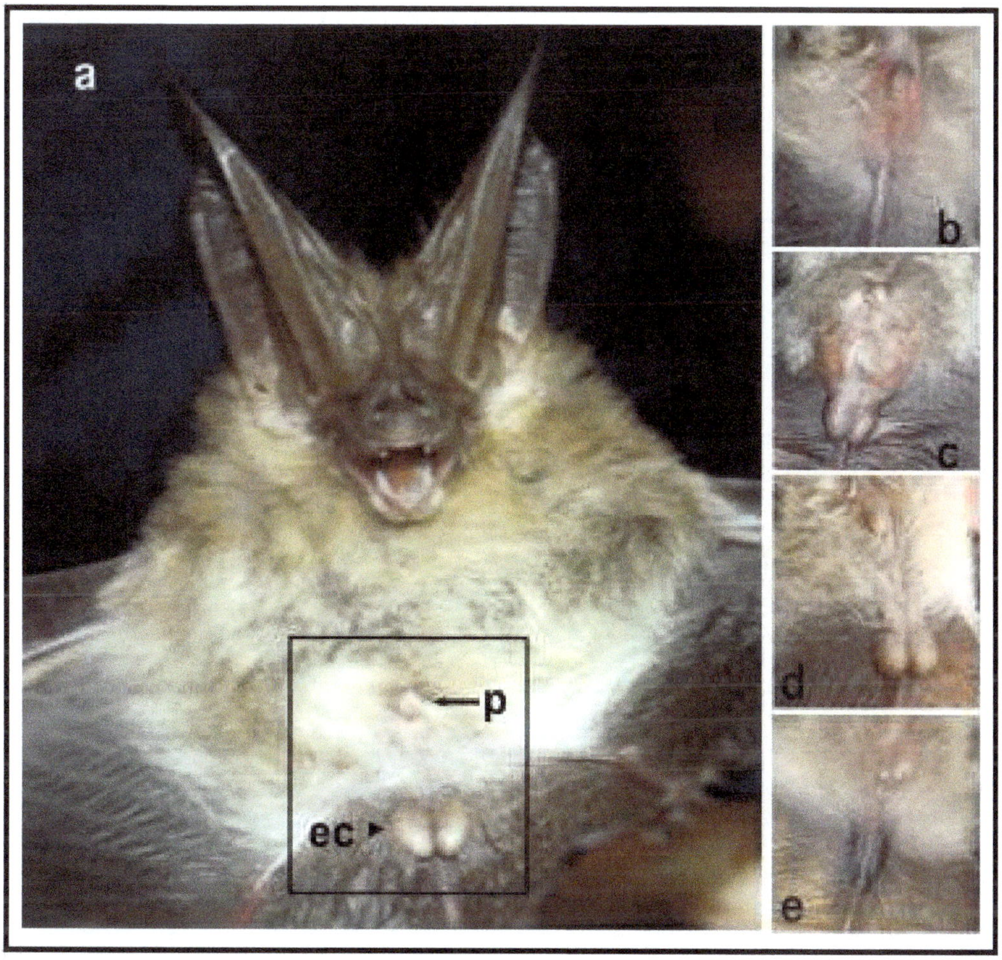

Figure 4. *(a) Photograph in ventral view of an adult male C. townsendii bat caught in the mating period of November; the black square locate the penis (p, arrow) and the cauda of the epididymides (ec, arrow head), this last organs placed on the uropatagium, distal to the groin region, along the vertebral tail. The b-e inserts are photographic magnifications of the same region indicated by the square in (a) but from other specimens that correspond to different development stages of the testes and epididymides, and show the main stages of the sexual cycle. (b) A young specimen about 10 months old caught in April, before its first reproductive season, the testes and epididymides are scrotal but almost conspicuous. (c) Full spermatogenesis (August-September), the testes show maximal size; the prolonged sperm storage has started. (d) Mating period (November-December), spermatogenesis is arrested; the cauda of epididymides is congested with sperm. (e) Post-hibernal reproductive inactivity (March-April), the cauda epididymides are short, thin and surrounded by a dark pigmented tunica albuginea.*

4. Discussion

As mentioned above, the sex distribution of the adult bats in this study favored females by a ratio of 2.7:1, due primarily to the number of females in the gestation-lactation stage, which highlights the importance of the various mining systems monitored that are used as maternal shelters, an aspect that is characteristic of the social organization of the females of this species in U.S. populations [9], and of at least one sister species; namely, *C. mexicanus* found in central Mexico [26].

Based on the reproductive data gathered in this study, together with the information reported in previous works on *C. townsendii* [9, 10], it was possible to establish all the main reproductive stages for both male and female bats (Fig. 5). The stages that were estimated were: oestrus and subsequent intercourse, which begin in autumn and peak in November, though some copulation continues into February. The sperm are first stored in the cauda epididymis of males from mid-August to late October, but after insemination storage continues inside the female genital tract from November to late February, when ovulation, fertilization, and pregnancy should occur.

While this study did not determine whether the specimens of *C. townsendii* from the Mexican Highlands perform true hibernation, the fact that several specimens were captured in the months of November and December as they flew out of their shelters to forage suggests they are characterized by intermittent periods of torpor or, perhaps, that their period of true hibernation occurs in the months of January and February. However, this physiological aspect must be verified through additional studies. As has been reported for several species of vespertilionid bats in temperate zones of America that exhibit delayed fertilization [8] ovulation may occur shortly before, or immediately after, the end of the winter period. In the case of *C. townsendii*, clear evidence of gestation (by palpation) was recorded in early April, after onset of the spring season. In these bats, the gestation period can vary from 56-to-100 days, depending on temperatures in the spring and the degree of torpor experienced by individual females. Births occur in late spring or early summer, followed by a period of anoestrus. Determining when oogenesis and folliculogenesis begin again, the time required for full development of the follicles to ovulation, and the moment of fertilization, will only be possible by performing histological studies that require sacrificing specimens, a procedure that is prohibited for species living in recognized Conservation Areas, such as Sierra La Mojonera Flora and Fauna Protection Area, and its hiterland. One alternative could be to monitor hormone levels –especially of the steroid sex type– using non-invasive quantification methods with urine or feces, but these issues require future studies.

In males of *C. townsendii*, spermatogenesis occurs during the summer and reaches its peak in August-September. In late September-early October the testes regress in a process that coincides with the entry of the sperm into the epididymis (Fig. 5). The accessory sex glands decrease completely in size in late October [9, 10]. One particularly important fact related to the establishment of the full sexual cycle in males is the duration of sperm storage in the epididymis, but determining this would require almost fortnightly monitoring of bats beginning in August when spermatogenesis is complete and continuing until the end of the winter period, when the epididymis regresses [11].

Upon evaluating the data on the seasonality and dynamics of the reproductive processes recognized for Townsend's Big-eared bats in the SM-FFPA and its area of influence, it can be concluded that the reproductive pattern corresponds to that proposed by Pearson et al. [9] for populations of this species in the United States. This pattern that can be characterized as: monoestrous, seasonal, with delayed fertilization and prolonged sperm storage first in the epididymis, and later in the female's reproductive tract. However, because there is no precise correspondence between the dates on which the main reproductive processes of this species occur throughout its area of distribution, it is considered to present an 'emerging' reproductive pattern [4, 5]; with differences in timing most likely due to variations in environmental conditions and variability in the availability of shelters.

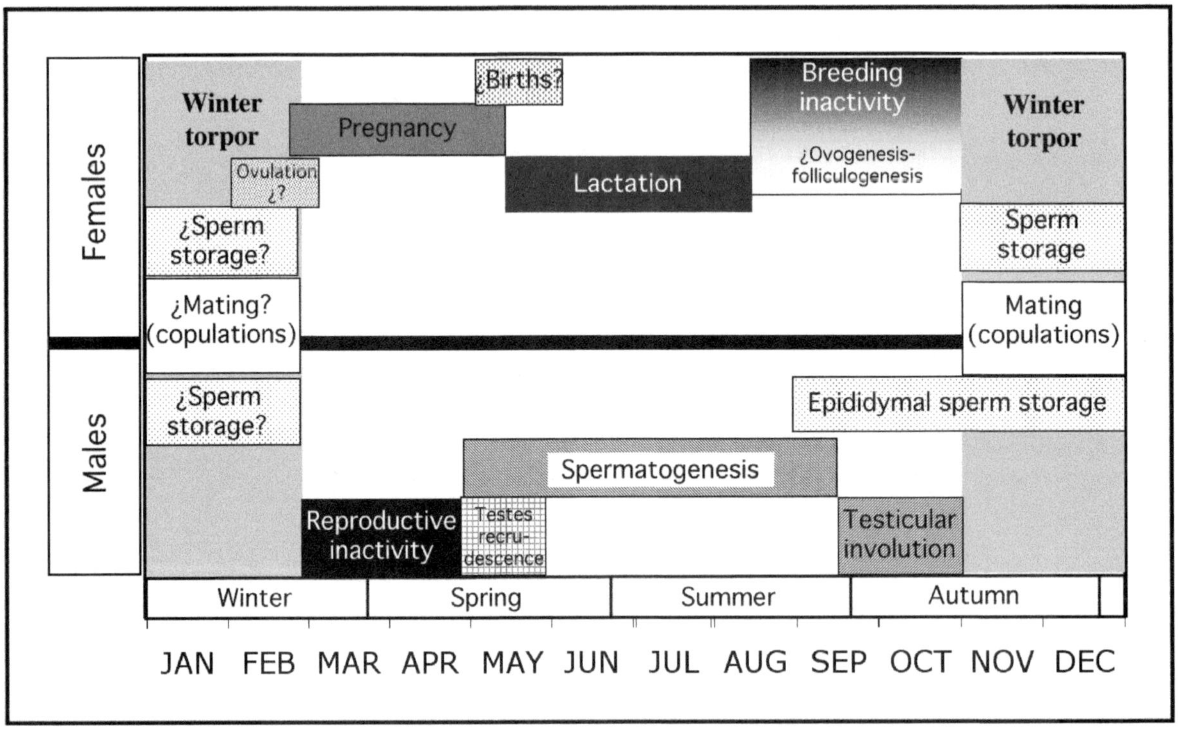

Figure 5. *Annual representation of the timing and duration of the main reproductive processes and events, establishing the full sexual cycle of C. townsendii in the SM-FFPA and its influence zone at the Potosino-Zacatecano Highlands of Mexico. Question forms ¿? of particular reproductive processes or events were estimated by taking into account data about the same species reported in the scientific literature, but also by estimations from our own data in this study*

5. Conclusion

This study clearly suggests that the four mining systems (*Todos Santos*, *Las Tapias de la Legion*, *San Juan de Carbonerillas,* and *Santa Rosa*) studied in the Sierra La Mojonera Flora and Fauna Protection Area ant its hinterland, located at the states of San Luis Potosi and Zacatecas in the Central Highlands of Mexico, have great potential for *Corynorhinus townsendii* bats in relation to the fundamental processes that make up the sexual cycles of males and females. Hence, this zone must be considered as of high priority for conserving this species of Chiroptera.

Acknowledgements

The realization of this work was made possible through funding by CONANP (SEMARNAT, MEXICO), with the

PROMOBI/RNEySMO/sierra-mojonera/04/2014 agreement of its 2014 Biological Monitoring Program; and the full administrative and logistic support of Universidad Autónoma Metropolitana, Iztapalapa. We would like to acknowledge the technical support given by the biologist Aline Méndez Rodríguez, for her advice in the molecular identification of the bat species; and to the MB Osiris Aguilar Romero, for her generous cooperation in the preparation of maps using GIS. Special thanks to Mr. Honorio Pérez Martínez from Huertecillas, Vanegas, SLP, for their great support in the field work.

References

[1] Sherwin, R.E., D. Stricklan, and D.S. Rogers. 2000. Roosting Affinities of Townsend's Big-Eared Bat (*Corynorhinus townsendii*) in Northern Utah. J. Mammal. 81(4): 939-947.

[2] López-González, C. 2005. Use of Abandoned Mines by a Community of Temperate Bats in Durango, Mexico. Acta Chiropterologica. 7(2): 285-292.

[3] Fenton, M.B. 1997. Science and the Conservation of Bats. J. Mammal. 78(1): 1-14.

[4] Clark, B.S., K.C. Bryon, and D.M. Leslie, Jr. 2002. Seasonal Variation in Activity Patterns of the Endangered Ozark Big-Eared Bat (*Corynorhinus townsendii ingens*). J. Mammal. 83(2): 590-598.

[5] Clark, B.S., D.M. Leslie, Jr., and T.S. Carter. 1993. Foraging Activity of Adult Female Ozark Big-eared Bats *(Plecotus townsendii ingens*) in Summer. J. Mammal. 74(2): 422-427.

[6] Comizzoli, P., P. Mermillod, and R. Mauget. 2000. Reproductive Biotechnologies for Endangered Mammalian Species. Reprod. Nutr. Dev. 40(5): 493-504.

[7] Krutzsch, P.H. 2009. The Reproductive Biology of the Cave Myotis (*Myotis velifer*). Acta Chiropterologica, 11(1): 89-104.

[8] Racey, P.A. and A.C. Entwistle. 2000. Life-history and Reproductive Strategies of Bats, *In*: E.G. Crichton and P.H. Krutzsch, Editors. Reproductive Biology of Bats. Academic Press. London. Pp. 364-414.

[9] Pearson, O.P., M.R. Koford, and A.K. Pearson. 1952. Reproduction of the Lump-nosed Bat *(Corynorhinus rafinesquei)* in California. J. Mammal. 33(3): 273-320.

[10] Kunz, T.H. and R.A. Martin. 1982. *Plecotus townsendii* Mammalian Species. 175: 1-6.

[11] León-Galván, M.A., R. López-Wilchis, O. Hernández-Pérez, E. Arenas-Ríos, and A. Rosado. 2005. Male Reproductive Cycle of Mexican Big-eared Bats, *Corynorhinus mexicanus* (Chiroptera: Vespertilionidae). Southwest. Nat. 50(4): 453-460.

[12] Handley, C.O. 1959. A Revision of American Bats of the Genera *Euderma and Plecotus*. Proc. U.S. National Mus. 110.

[13] López-González, C. and L. Torres-Morales. 2004. Use of Abandoned Mines by Long-eared Bats, Genus *Corynorhinus* (Chiroptera: Vespertilionidae) in Durango, Mexico. J. Mammal. 85(5): 989-994.

[14] Smith, S.J., et al. 2008. Subspecific Affinities and Conservation Genetics of Western Big-eared Bats *(Corynorhinus townsendii pallescens*) at the Edge of their Distributional Range. J. Mammal. 89: 799-814.

[15] Pierson, E.D., et al., 1999. Species Conservation Assessment and Strategy for Townsend's Big-eared Bat (*Corynorhinus townsendii townsendii* and *Corynorhinus townsendii pallescens*). ed. I.D.o.F.a. Game. Idaho: Idaho Conservation Effort.

[16] Piaggio, J., K.W. Navo, and C.W. Stihler. 2009. Intraspecific Comparison of Population Structure, Genetic Diversity, and Dispersal Among Three Subspecies of Townsend's Big-eared Bats, *Corynorhinus townsendii townsendii, C. t. pallescens,* and the Endangered *C. t. virginianus*. Conserv. Genet. 10: 143-159.

[17] Secretaría del Medio Ambiente y Recursos Naturales (SEMARNAT). 2010. Norma Oficial Mexicana NOM-059-SEMARNAT-2010, Protección Ambiental -Especies Nativas de México de Flora y Fauna Silvestres-Categorias de Riesgo y Especificaciones para su Inclusión, Exclusión o Cambio- Lista de Especies en Riesgo. Diario Oficial de la Federación, Executive Branch of the United States of México, Mexico City.

[18] Saiki, R.K., *et al.* 1988. Primer-directed Enzymatic Amplification of DNA with a Thermostable DNA Polymerase. Science. 239(4839): 487-91.

[19] Irwin, D., T. Kocher, and A. Wilson. 1991. Evolution of the Cytochrome b Gene of Mammals. J. Mol. Evol. 32(2): 128-144.

[20] Smith, M. and J. Patton. 1999. Phylogenetic Relationships and the Radiation of Sigmodontine Rodents in South America: Evidence from Cytochrome b. J. Mamm. Evol. 6(2): 89-128.

[21] Altschul, S.F., *et al.* 1990. Basic Local Alignment Search Tool. J. Mol. Biol. 215(3): 403-10.

[22] Benson, D.A.M., *et al.* 2012. GenBank. Nucleic Acids Res. D48-D5310.1093/nar/gks1299.

[23] Anthony, E.L.P. 1988. Age Determination in Bats. *In*: T.H. Kunz, Editor. Ecological and Behavioral Methods for the Study of Bats. Smithsonian Institution Press. Washington, DC. Pp. 47-58.

[24] Entwistle, A., P. Racey, and J. Speakman. 1998. The Reproductive Cycle and Determination of Sexual Maturity in Male Brown Long-eared Bats, *Plecotus auritus* (Chiroptera: Vespertilionidae). J. Zool. 244(01): 63-70.

[25] Vela Hinojosa, C., M.A. León-Galván, M. Tapia-Rodríguez, G. López-Ortega, M.A. Cerbón-Cervantes, *et al.* 2013. Differential Expression of Serotonin, Tryptophan Hydroxylase and Monoamine Oxidase A in the Mammary Gland of the *Myotis velifer* Bat. PLoS One. 8(9): e75062.

[26] López-Wilchis, R. 1989. Biología de *Plecotus mexicanus* (Chiroptera: Vespertilionidae) en el Estado de Tlaxcala, México. Doctoral thesis, Universidad Nacional Autónoma de México, México D.F.

26

Anti-coccidial Activity of Moringa Oleifera Plant

El Banna H. A.*, M. Atef, Ghazal Nabil

Department of Pharmacology, Faculty of Veterinary Medicine, Cairo University, Giza, Egypt

Email address:

drelanna3@yahoo.cm (El Banna H. A.), atefshehata@live.com (M. Atef), gazal.nabil@yahoo (G. Nabil)

*Corresponding author

Abstract: *Moringa Oleifera* leaves were screened for its toxicological effect and some pharmacological activities in broiler chicken. Toxicological effect was studied using upgrading oral doses of 75% ethanolic extract in different groups of mice with monitoring the toxicological symptoms and mortality rate. The anti-coccidal activity of *Moringa Oleifera* powdered leaves for prevention and its 75% ethanolic extract for treatment of coccidiosis were studied in broilers. The obtained result proved that there were no toxicological symptoms or mortalities obtained till oral administration of 6000 mg/kg b. wt. Inclusion of Moringa olifera powder (0.5 and 1%) to broiler's feed were very efficacious and equal to diclazuril (1ppm) in preventing symptoms of coccidiosis associated with experimental infection with mixed Eimeria species. The anti-coccidal activity of *Moringa Oleifera* powdered leaves and its 75% ethanolic extract were studied on one-day old chicks. The experimental infected chicks with mixed Eimeria species induced severe coccidiosis in non medicated chicks and led to high mortality reached to (26.76%). Addition of 200 and 400ppm of *Moringa Oleifera* ethanolic extract induced marked curative effect of cocci diosis manifested by reduced mortality percent and improved PM lesion to be 13.3 and 10% respectively compared to 13.3% for group treated with the reference drug (25ppm) toltrazuril.

Keywords: *Moringa Olifera*- prophylactic and treatment - Coccidiosis

1. Introduction

Poultry plays very important role for mankind through food supply, income and employment generation, providing raw materials to some industries. The direct or indirect contribution of poultry industry is very dangerous. Coccidiosis is ubiquitous where chickens are reared (traditional, industrial or organic/bio farms). It is recognized as the parasitic disease that has the greatest economic impact on poultry industries worldwide [1]. Coccidiosis in poultry is still considered as one of the main diseases affecting performance of poultry reared under intensive production systems. Coccidiosis results in intestinal lesions, impaired growth, poor feed utilization, poor flock uniformity and increased mortality. Because it damages the intestinal lining, coccidiosis predisposes birds to the development of necrotic enteritis, another intestinal disease caused by the bacterium Clostridium perfringens.

The intensive use of anticoccidial drugs has led to the development of resistance [2]. Increasing development of drug-resistant coccidial species has stimulated searches for alternative control methods or new drugs. However, this has resulted in the increased cost of poultry products. Furthermore, drug or antibiotic residue in the poultry product is potentially offensive to the consumer. So the finding of natural replacer which improves the growth with prophylactic and curative effect against coccidiosis and without health hazard to human being is worthy.

The use of herbal remedies in the management of coccidiosis is not a new concept. For example, halofuginone, a quinazolinone alkaloid derived from Dichroa febrifuga, has been used as a coccidiostat, and the original extract from D. febrifuga, known as febrifugine, possesses antimalarial and anticoccidial activity [3]. The investigation of herbal materials as anticoccidial remedies therefore holds promise as an alternative in the control of coccidiosis. In addition to possibly lowering the cost of food production in different countries. *Moringa Oleifera* is one of the most important medicinal plants and it is the most widely cultivated species of family Moringaceae. Every part of *Moringa* is said to have beneficial properties that can serve humanity [4]. In addition, various parts of *Moringa Oleifera* contain minerals and area good source of protein, vitamins, β carotene, amino acids and various phenolics. The *Moringa* plant provides a rich and rare combination of zeatin, quercetin, β - sitosterol, caffeoylquinic acid and kaempferol. Various parts of this plant such as the leaves, roots, seed, bark, fruit, flowers and immature pods act as cardiac and circulatory stimulants, antioxidant, antibacterial, antimalarial and antifungal activities, and are being employed for the treatment of different ailments in the indigenous system of medicine, [5]. Furthermore, [6] reported the use of *Moringa Oleifera* acetone leaf extract on broiler chickens naturally infected with Eimeria species while [7], found that different parts of *Moringa Oleifera* were active against Leishmania donovani promastigotes and the flower extract of M. oliefera was found to be the most potent antileishmanial agent when compared to other parts of the plant like leaf, root, bark and stem. Little studies have examined the anticoccidial efficacy of the plant in livestock; thus, this study has provided evidence for the efficacy of Moringa *Oleifer* and its curative and prophylactic anticoccidial activity. In addition its effect on body performance was also investigated

2. Main Body

2.1. Plant Material

The fresh *Moringa Oleifera* (Moringaceae) were collected during November to December, 2012 from private farm in El Sadat city. The plant specimen was authenticated by the Department of Botany, Faculty of Science, and Cairo University, Egypt.

2.2. Plant Preparation

The plant leaves were washed with tap water dried at room temperature then chopped into small fragments and pulverized by using grinder. Cold extraction was done with 75% ethanol for 72 hour at room temperature with intermittent shaking [8]. The extracts were concentrated in a rotatory evaporator at 50°C and refrigerated until use. The plant was used in its powdered form to determine its effect as prophylactic anti-coccidial activity. The plant was used in its ethanolic extract form for determining its curative anti-coccidial activity.

2.3. Animals

Mice: Mature mice weighing (20-25 grams) of both sexes were used for the toxicological study.

Chicks: One day old unsexed chicks weighing (45-55grams) were used for studying the effect on anti-coccidial activity. The birds were kept under good hygienic measures. Chicks were fed on balanced commercial ration and water offered ad libitum. The chicks were floor reared in separate units along the experimental periods.

Coccidia strains: Field strains of sporulated Eimeria oocysts were obtained from Department of Parasitology, Faculty of Veterinary Medicine, Cairo University. These strains include mixed *Eimeria spp (Eimeria acervulina* 19.5 x14.3 (4.5%), *Eimeria maxima* 29 x 23(29.5%), *Eimeria necatrix* 16.7 x14.2 (2.5%), *Eimeria tenella* 22.9 x 19.1(60%) *and Eimeria brunetti* 26.8 x 21.7(3.5%).

2.4. Drugs

Diclazuril obtained from Pharma-Swede Egypt as feed additive (0.2%) under trade name Diclomix ®.

Toultrazuril obtained from Pharma Swede Egypt as oral solution (2.5%) under trade name Tolacox®.

3. Method

3.1. Toxicological Studies

The toxicological pattern of the ethanolic extract of *Moringa Oleifera* leaves was studied by determination of LD50 in mice.

3.2. Determination of LD50

LD50 of the studied extract was carried out in mice according to method described by [9]. For these purpose five groups of 5 mice in each, weighing 20-25 grams one of them served as control group. Other four groups were dosed orally the studied extract on ascending doses (30, 60, 90, and 120 mg/20g b.wt). Animals were put under observation for 24 hours for recording the toxic symptoms, mortality rate and post-mortem findings in each group. LD50 of the tested extract was calculated according to the following formula:

LD50 = "Dm -" "Σ (zxd)" /"n"

Where:

Dm = The largest dose which kill the animals.

z = Mean of dead animals between 2 successive groups.

d = The constant factor between 2 successive doses.

n = Number of animals in each group.

∑ = The sum of (a × b).

3.3. Pharmacological Studies

3.3.1. Anticoccidial Effect

Propagation and isolation of oocytes of mixed *Eimeria spp:* Isolation and propagation of the coccidia was carried according to Long [10] and the experimental design were carried out according to table1.

Preparation of *Eimeria* oocytes: The methods for these procedures are best followed from the description by [11, 12, 13]. The calculated infective dose of culture (74000 oocytes/1ml) was given orally by insulin syringe which introduced intra-crop.

Table 1. Experimental design for the anticoccidial activity.

	Prophylactic capacity	Curative capacity
Groups	Standard (infected & treated with standard drug). • Control +ve (infected & non- treated). • Control –ve (non-infected & non-treated). Treated groups (*Moringa Oleifera* 0.5 & 1%).	• Standard (infected & treated with standard drug). • Control +ve (infected& non- treated). • Control –ve (non- infected & non-treated). • Treated groups(*Moringa Oleifera* 200 & 400 mg/liter)
Standard drug	Diclazuril 1ppm.	Toultrazuril 25ppm.
Onset & form of treatment	Onset: From 1st day on feed Form: Powder.	Onset: After appearance of clinical signs on drinking water Form: Liquid.
Parameter	Clinical signs. Oocyst count. PM lesion. Mortality rate. Fecal score. Histopathological examination. Body weight &FCR.	• Clinical signs. • Oocyst count. • PM lesion. • Mortality rate. • Fecal score. • Histopathological examination.

3.3.2. Post Mortem Examination

It was carried out at 8th for both experiments. Lesion scores were determined according to [14] Lesion score was 0 when no evident lesions were detected while a score was 4 when the lesions were extremely sever.

3.3.3. Parasitological Examination (Oocyst Count)

Fecal samples were collected from freshly evacuated faeces on the litter which spread on the ground for each group from 5th to 11th dpi. The oocysts count was carried out according to the method described by [15] using the McMaster counting chamber.

3.3.4. Fecal Score

A fecal score (1 to 5) was recorded for each group of birds from 5th to 11th day dpi. a score of 1 indicate normal faeces and a score of 5 indicate the presence of severe diarrhea and /or a profuse amount of blood.

4. Result

4.1. Toxicological Studies

LD50: Oral administration of the 75% ethanolic extract on ascending manner 30, 60, 90, and 120 mg/20g body weight showed no toxicological symptoms, mortalities and post-mortem changes. From this observation there is no LD50 recorded till oral administration of 6000 mg/kg body weight which corresponding to 15.5 g of air dried powdered leaves.

4.2. Anticoccidial Effect

4.2.1. Prophylactic Efficacy

Findings pertaining to survival percent, total oocyst count, lesion and fecal scores are presented in table (2). The experimental infected chicks with mixed Eimeria species induced severe coccidiosis in non-medicated chicks and led to high mortality reached to (26.76%). Addition of 0.5 and 1% of *Moringa Oleifera* powdered leaves reduced mortality to be 6.7 and 4.3% respectively. Inclusion of *Moringa Oleifera* powder (0.5 and 1%) to broiler's feed were very efficacious and equal to feed additive in preventing symptoms of coccidiosis associated with experimental infection with mixed Eimeria species and decreased significantly the total oocyst count and lesion score.

The effect of *Moringa Oleifera* as feed supplement on performance of control and coccidia infected chicken was presented in tables (3, 4&5). Use of *Moringa Oleifera* leaves powder in concentration of 0.5 and 1% induced an improvement in body weight with enhancement of the cumulative FCR in both control healthy and coccidia infected broilers.

Table 2. Anticoccidial prophylactic capacity of Moringa Oleifera in experimentally Eimeria-infected broiler chickens (n=15).

Group No.	Used concentration		Survival (%)	Total oocyst No(x 10^3/g)	Lesion score	Fecal score
Control groups	Control non- treated		73.33	629. 75± 23.47^a	3.57 ±0.51 ^{a}	4.8± 0.42^a
	Control non-infected non-treated		100.0	0.0 ± 0.0^d	0.0± 0.0^d	1.0 ± 0.0^b
Treatment	Diclazuril	1 ppm	96.7	36.7± 5.62^c	0.37± 0.042^b	1.3 ±0.1
	Moringa	0.5%	93.3	67.8 ±4.52 ^{b}	0.72 ±0.022^{bc}	1.5 ± 0.23^b
	Oleifera	1%	96.7	44.4 ± 3.38 ^{c}	0.40 ±0.11^{bc}	1.4 ± 0.21^b

Values with different letters (a, b, c, d) within the same column are significantly different at P value ≤ 0.05

Table 3. The effect of Moringa Oleifera as feed additive on performance of control healthy broiler chicken (n=15).

Group		Final body weight g	Feed consumption g	FCR
Control non treated		1850	3348.5	1.81
Diclazuril	1ppm	1900	3002	1.58
M. Oleifera powder	0.5%	1950	3178	1.63
	1%	2100	3130	1.49

***Table 4.** The effect of Moringa Oleifera as feed additive on performance of coccidia infected chicken.*

Group		Final body weight g	Feed consumption g	FCR
Infected non treated		1490	3085	2.1
Diclazuril	1ppm	1885	3092	1.64
M. *Oleifera* powder	0.5%	1818	2910	1.60
	1%	1850	2870	1.55

***Table 5.** Gross P. M and histopathological examination at 8th day of age of the anticoccidial prophylactic capacity.*

Group	Gross P.M examination	Histopathological examination
Standard Diclazuril	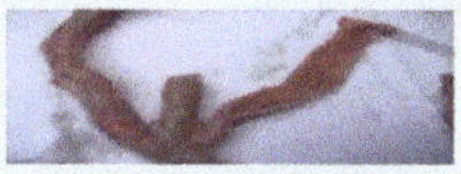	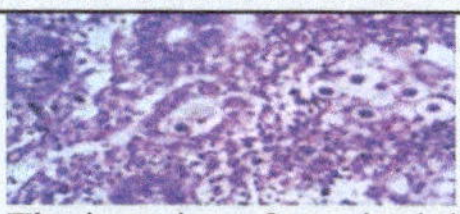 The intestine of standard diclazuril group showed low numbers of Eimeria in the epithelial lining of crypt and necrosis of the villar epithelium. Also Areas of 22haemorrhage were detected in the lamina propria and considerable numbers of inflammatory cells.
0.5%	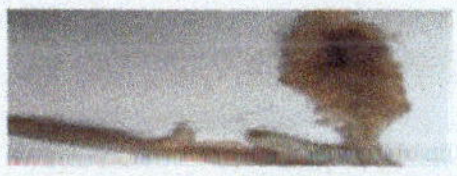	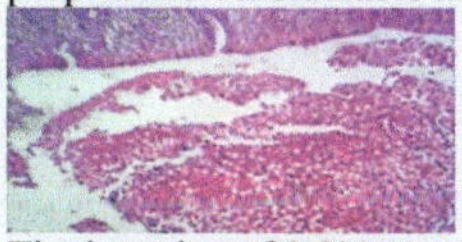 The intestine of 0.5% treated group showed large numbers of Eimeria was detected in lumen
1%	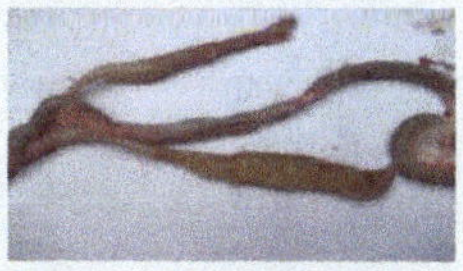	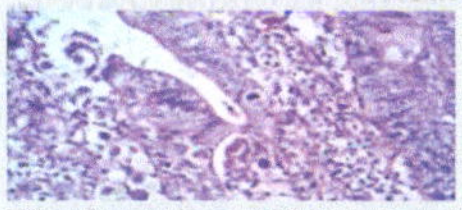 The intestine of 1% treated group showed less pathological changes.
Control negative	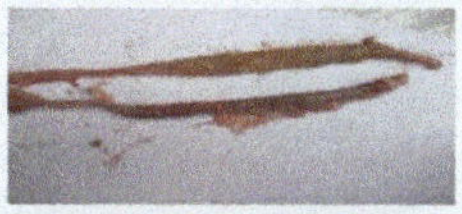	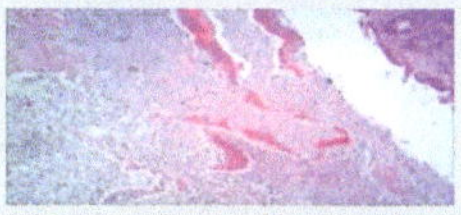 The intestine of control non infected non treated group revealed normal histological appearance of villus epithelium and crypts.
Infected non treated	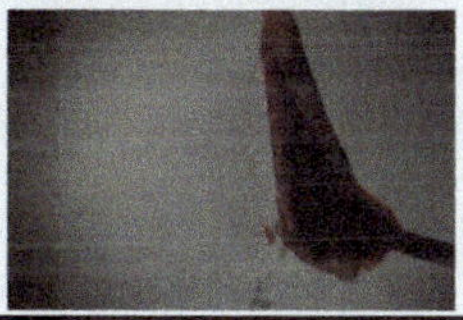	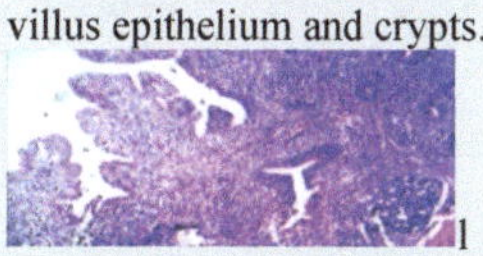 Large numbers of the Eimeria was detected in the lumen and the lamina propria was infiltrated with large numbers of inflammatory cells accompanied with areas of hemorrhages.

4.2.2. Curative Efficacy

Findings pertaining to mortality percent, total oocyst count, lesion and fecal scores, are recorded in table (6&7). The experimental infected chicks with mixed Eimeria species induced severe coccidiosis in non –medicated chicks and led to high mortality reached to (26.76%). Addition of 200 and 400ppm of *Moringa Oleifera* ethanolic extract reduced mortality to be 13.3 and 10% respectively compared to 13.3% for group treated with the reference drug (25 ppm toltrazuril) and decreased significantly the total oocyst count and lesion score.

***Table 6.** Anticoccidial curative capacity of Moringa Oleifera ethanolic extract in experimentally Eimeria infected-broiler chicken.*

Used concentration		Survival (%)	Total oocyst No (x 10^3/g) During two days before treatment	Total oocyst No (x 10^3/g) During 5 days post treatment	Lesion score	Fecal score
Control infected non-treated		73.33	7.5 ± 0.61[a]	6.21.8 ± 17.38[a]	3.57 ±0.51[a]	4.8± 0.42[a]
Control non-infected non-treated		100.0	0.0 ± 0.0[b]	0.0 ± 0.0[d]	0.0± 0.0[d]	1.0 ± 0.0[d]
Toltrazuril	25 ppm	86.67	8.7 ± 1.27[a]	256.75± 21.43[b]	0.97± 0.067[c]	1.4 ± 0.23
Moringa Oleifera	200 ppm	86.67	7.4 ± 0.59[a]	285.2 ±9.45[b]	1.1 ±0.12[b]	1.9 ± 0.44b[c]
	400 ppm	90.0	7.9 ± 0.81[a]	146.6 ± 8.57[c]	0.81 ±0.14[c]	1.5 ± 0.31b[c]

Values with different letters (a, b, c, d) within the same column are significantly different at P value ≤ 0.05

Table 7. *Gross P.M and histopathological examination at 8th day of age of the anticoccidial curative capacity.*

Group	Gross P.M examination	Histopathological examination
Standard Toltrazuril	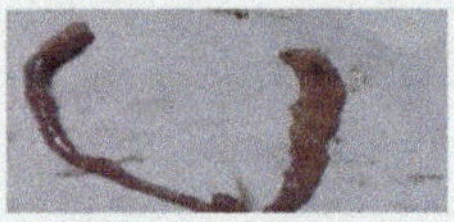	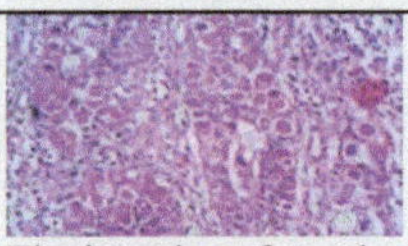 The intestine of standard Toltrazuril treated group showed Eimeriain lamina propria of intestine accompanied with large numbers of inflammatory cells mainly macrophage and lymphocytes.
Moringa Oleifera 200 ppm	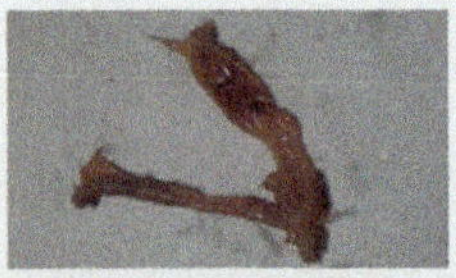	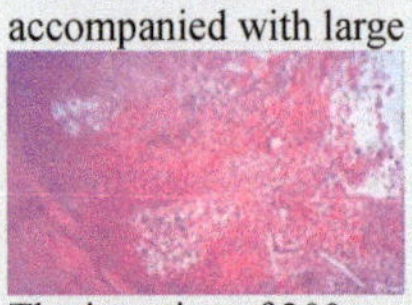 The intestine of 200ppm treated group showed severe pathological changes in which large numbers of Eimeria in the epithelial lining of villi and crypt combined with large areas of hemorrhages.
Moringa Oleifera 400 ppm	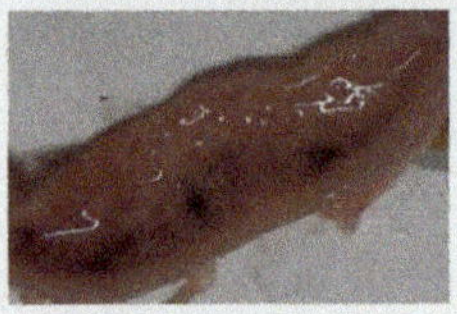	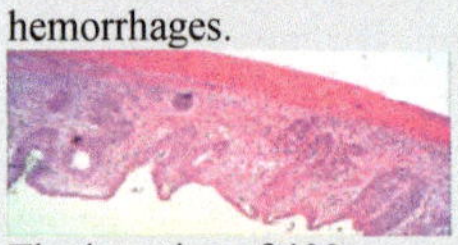 The intestine of 400ppm treated group showed Eimeria with low number and mainly found in the epithelial lining of crypt and areas of hemorrhage were detected in the lamina propria with considerable numbers of inflammatory cells.

5. Discussion

The result of acute oral toxicity (LD50) study of ethanolic leaf extract of *Moringa Oleifera* showed no mortality at the maximum dose of 6000 mg/kg/body weight. In an acute oral toxicity study by [16], *Moringa Oleifera* leaf extract was documented to be non-lethal in animals at 6400 mg/kg body weight. In addition, [17] found that *Moringa Oleifera* leaf extract was documented to be non-lethal in animals at 2000 mg/kg body weight. More so, the report of [18] revealed that the aqueous extract of *Moringa Oleifera leaf* is safe at dosage as high as 5000 mg/kg. These results may indicate safety of ethanolic or aqueous leaf extract of *Moringa Oleifera* when administrated orally as the acute administration of 2 g/kg dose was reported to be the ceiling point for acute oral toxicity of medicinal plants [19].

Eimeria is an intracellular parasite, must adhere to and invade the intestinal epithelial cells in order to replicate. Gut-adapted microorganisms may compete for adhesion and invasion of cells. In the present study and after challenging the chicks with mixed Eimeria especially in the control non treated group, birds showed severe form of coccidiosis represented by a high mortality rate (26.7%), lesion score was 3.57 and fecal score was 4.8 (meaning severe watery diarrhea with obvious amount of voided blood in litter). Addition of 0.5 and 1% of *M. Oleifera* powdered leaves reduced mortality to be 6.7 and 3.3% respectively. In addition, Inclusion of *M. Oleifera* powder (0.5 and 1%) to broiler's feed were very efficacious and equal to diclazuril feed additive in preventing symptoms of coccidiosis associated with experimental infection with mixed Eimeria species. Birds supplemented with *M. Oleifera* (0.5 and 1%) and feed additive form of Diclazuril at a concentration of 1 ppm showed a significant reduction in the cumulative mean oocysts shed (67.8 ±4.52, and 44.4 ± 3.38 & 36.7± 5.62x 10^3/g, respectively) in comparison with the control non-treated birds (629. 75± 23.47x 103/g). Oral supplementation of bird infected with mixed Eimera species by powdered leaves of *M. Oleifera* (0.5 and 1%) showed significant decrease in lesion score (0.72 ±0.022 and 0.40 ±0.011 respectively). These findings were similar or better than those obtained in group treated with standard anticoccidial drug.

Our finding is matched with our histopathological study where the intestine of broilers supplemted with either 0.5 or 1% appeared devoid from Eimeria and the lamina propria was infiltrated with inflammatory cells mainly macrophages and lymphocytes

Birds infected with mixed Eimera species and treated with ethanolic extract of *M. Oleifera* (200 and 400 mg/liter for 5 consecutive days) in drinking water showed a significant anticoccidial activity indicated by decreasing the total ocyst count (285.2 ±9.45 and 146.6 ± 8.57 x 103/ g respectively), decrease in lesion score (1.1 ±0.12 and 0.81 ±0.14 respectively) compared with infected non treated group (Total oocyst of 621.8 ± 17.38 and lesion secore=3.57 ±0. 51) and those treated with reference drug ((Total oocyst of256.75± 21.43 and lesion score of 0.97± 0.067). Concerning the fecal score records, the results of *Moringa.* treated groups were 1.9 ± 0.44and 1.5 ± 0.31 for 200 and 400 mg/liter compared to 4.8± 0.42 for the control non- treated group and 1.4 ± 0.23 for the reference group treated with 25 ppm toltrazuril for 2 consecutive days. The curative anticoccidial activity reported for *M. Oleifera* ethanolic extract in the present study is matched with our histopathological study where the intestine *Moringa* treated group showed presence of low number of Eimeria in the crypt and in the epithelial lining compared with the infected non-treated group and lamina propria was infiltrated by large numbers of inflammatory cells. Bloody colored diarrheal feces indicated by fecal score were seen in all groups following the onset of clinical signs in infected broiler chickens. The bloody diarrhea was milder in all the treatment (toltrazuril and ethanolic extract of *M. Oleifera*) groups as the days progressed. This can be attributed to the reduction of oocyst shed in the feces of the broiler chickens as the day progressed. The reduction of oocyst shed in the feces will result in reduced damage caused on the intestinal lining and as a result the reduction in the level of hemorrhage. On the five day treatment of the present study, the feces of the birds treated with 200 or 400mg/kg body weight of *M. Oleifera* were devoid of diarrhea blood (fecal score, 1.9 ± 0.44 and 1.5 ± 0.31 respectively) compare to values of control non-treated group (4.8 ± 0.42).

The use of *M. Oleifera* is justified on the basis that it possesses anti-malaria properties [5] as well as anti-leishmanial activity [7] and Eimeria belongs to the phylum Apicomplexa as does the Plasmodium parasite. The result of the oocyst inhibition in the fecal matter shows that birds treated with powdered leaves of *M. Oleifera* at prophylactic study or ethanolic extracts at curative one were most promising with marked reduction of the total Eimeria oocyst shed in the feces. The anticoccidial activity of *M. Oleifera* either powdered leaves as prophylactic or ethanolic extract as treatment agents could be attributed to the antioxidant properties possessed by *M. Oleifera* . Antioxidant compounds are also well known to have a cellular protective action against oxidative stress and reduce the severity of *E. tenella* infections by altering the degree of intestinal lipid peroxidation[1]. The antioxidant properties of *M. Oleifera* have been reported previously by [20,21] which are ascorbic acid, flavonoids, phenolics and carotenoid. In different physio-pathological conditions, the systemic amounts of free radicals and reactive oxygen species are higher than normal [22]. Free radical oxidative species are known to be produced during the host's cellular immune response to invasion by *Eimeria* species [23], which play an important role in defending mechanism against parasitic infections. However, their high concentrations may become intolerable to cell causing tissue damage and cytotoxicity and partially contributing to the pathology of infection. In some parasitic infections, decrease in the content of antioxidants like Vitamine A, C and E occur in the host cell [24]. Another free radical oxidative species, nitric oxide enhance vasodilation and hemorrhages in coccidial infections and could be toxic to both parasite as well as to host cells harboring the coccidian parasite [25]. In addition, [26, 27] reported that *E. acervulina* oocysts motivate the lipid peroxidation, increase oxidative damage and imbalance in the antioxidant status in the infected birds by disturbing the oxidative balance. Therefore, to alleviate or reduce the oxidative stress by inclusion of antioxidants as feed supplements either natural as Vitamin E& Se or synthetic as butylated hydroxytoluene are commonly used in the poultry industry.

Inclusion of *M. Oleifera* either powder leaves (0.5 and 1%) to broiler's feed in prophylactic anticoccidial study or the ethanolic extract of *M. Oleifera* leaves (200 and 400mg/kg b.wt.) in curative study had a good dose related response to the improvement of body weight gain in broiler chickens infected with mixed species of Eimeria. Our Findings showed that the infected non- treated group had 19.5% weight loss; this could be as a result of the damaging effect of the Eimeria species on the epithelial lining of the intestines which in turn impairs the absorption of nutrient and water from the intestine. The weight gain observed in the groups treated with *M. Oleifera* leaves could also be due to its nutritional value, having crude protein of 17.01%, carbohydrate (63.11%), crude fat (2.11%) and energy (1440.11 kcal/100 g) according to [28]. However, [29,30] reported that *M. Oleifera* leaf meal has 27.1 and 27.51% crude protein respectively. The improvement of the body weight could as well be attributed to the high levels of vitamins and amino acids in *M. Oleifera* leaves which improve recovery from the disease condition and increase feed intake and feed conversion rate.

6. Conclusion

The present study confirms that *M. Oleifera* possessed a marked anticoccidial activity and could be useful as alternative product for the control of avian coccidiosis in poultry production. It is possible of its use as prophylactic and curative agent for coccidia in addition to its growth promoting effect, safety as well as its antibacterial effect

References

[1] Allen, P. C., Danforth, H. D. & Augustine, P. C. (1998): Dietary modulation of avian coccidiosis. Interenational Journal of Parasitology 28, 1131–1140.

[2] Chapman, H. D. (1997): "Biochemical, genetic and applied aspects of drug resistance in Eimeria parasites of the fowl," Avian Pathology 26, 221–244.

[3] Youn, H. J. and Noh, J. W. 2001. Screening of the anticoccidial effects of herb extracts against Eimeria tenella. Veterinary Parasitology 96, 257–263.

[4] Mishra, G.; Singh, P.; Verma, R.; Kumar, S.; Saurabh, S.; Jha, K. & Khosa, R. L.(2011): Traditional Uses, Phytochemistry and Pharmacological Properties of *Moringa Oleifera* plant: An Overview. Scholars Research Library. *Der Pharmacia Lettre* 3(2), 141-164.

[5] Farooq, A.; Sajid, L.; Muhammad, A. & Anwarul-Hassan, G. (2007): *Moringa Oleifera* : a food plant with multiple medicinal uses. *PhytotherRes*, 21, 17–25.

[6] Ola-Fadunsin, S. D. & Ademola, I. O. (2013): Direct effects of *Moringa Oleifera* Lam (Moringaceae) acetone leaf extract on broiler chickens naturally infected with Eimeria species. *Trop Anim Health Prod.*

[7] Singh M K, Paul J, De T, Chakraborti T. (2015): Bioactivity guided fractionation of *Moringa Oleifera* Lam. flower targeting Leishmania donovani. Indian J Exp Biol.; 53(11): 747-52.

[8] Handa, S. S. (2008): An Overview of Extraction Techniques for Medicinal and Aromatic Plants. In Handa, S. S.; Khanuja, S. P. S.; Longo, G. & Rakesh, D. V., Extraction Technologies for Medicinal and Aromatic Plants, p.p 26. International Centre for Science and High Technology, Italy.

[9] -Kerber, G. (1941): Pharmakologische Methoden Zur Auffindung Von Arzneimitten und Gifter und Analyse ihrer Wirkungsweise Vor. Dr. Med. Leopold Ther.Wissenschaftliche verlage Gerlarge Gesse Gesellschaft. M. B. H.

[10] Long, P. L. (1971): Maintenance of intestinal protozoa in-vivo with particular reference to Eimeria and Histomonas. In Isolation and Maintenance of Parasites in-vivo, 9thSymposium of the British Society for Parasitology, 65–75. Oxford: Blackwell.

[11] Norton, C. C., and L. P. Joyner (1968): The freeze preservation of coccidia. *Res Vet Sci* 9:598–600.

[12] Long, P. L.; Joyner, L. P. & Millard, B. J. (1976): A guide to laboratory techniques used in the study and diagnosis of Av.coccidisis. *Folia Vet. Lat.*, (6), 201-217.

[13] Davis, L. R. (1973): Techniques. In The Coccidia, ed. D. M. Hammond and P. L. Long, 411–58. Baltimore, MD: Univ. Park Press.

[14] Johnson, J. E. & Reid, W. M. (1970): Anticoccidial drugs: Lesion scoring technique in battery and floor pen experiment with chickens. *Exprel.Parasitol.*, 28,30-36.

[15] Hodgson, J. N. (1970): Coccidiosis: Oocysts counting technique for coccidiostat evaluation. *Exprel.parasitol*, 28, 99-102.

[16] Awodele, O.; Oreagba, I. A.; Odoma, S.; da Silva, J. A. & Osunkalu, V. O. (2012): Toxicological evaluation of the aqueous leaf extract of *Moringa Oleifera* Lam. (Moringaceae). *J Ethnopharmacol*, 139(2), 330-336.

[17] Adedapo, A. A.; Mogbojuri, O. M.; Emikpe, B. O. (2009): Safety evaluations of the aqueous extract of the leaves of *Moringa Oleifera* in rats. *J Med. Plants Res.*, 3, 586–591.

[18] Diallo, A.; Eklu-Gadegkeku, K.; Mobio, T.; Moukha, S. & Agbonon, A.; (2009): Protective effect of *Moringa Oleifera* Lam. and Lannea kerstingii extracts against cadmium and ethanol-induced lipid peroxidation. *J Pharmacology and Toxicology*, 4, 160–166.

[19] 1Lu, F. C.; Jessup, D. C. and Lavallée, A. (1965): Toxicity of pesticides in young versus adult rats. *Food Cosmet. Toxicol.*, 3, 591–596.

[20] Siddhuraju, P. & Becker, K. (2003): Antioxidant properities of various solvent extracts of total phenolic constituents from three different agroclimatic origins of drumstick tree (*M. Oleifera* Lam.) Leaves. *J agric. food chem.*, 51, 2144-2155.

[21] Dillard, C. J. & German, J. B. (2000): Phytochemicals: nutraceuticals and human health: A review. *J Sci., Food Agric.*, 80, 1744–1756.

[22] Vladimirov YA, (2004); Reactive oxygen and nitrogen species diagnostic, preventive and therapeutic values. Biochemistry (Moscow), 69: 1-3.

[23] Allen PC, J Lydon and HD Danforth, (1997): Effects of components of *Artemisia annua* on coccidian infections in chickens. Poult Sci, 76: 1156-1163.

[24] Evans P and B Halliwell, (2001): Micronutrients: oxidant/antioxidantstatus. J Nut, 121: 324-338.

[25] Ovington KS and NC Smith, (1992): Cytokines, free radicals and resistance to *Eimeria*. Parasitol. Today, 8: 422-426.

[26] Georgieva NV, M Gabrashanska, V Koinarski and Z Yaneva, (2011). Zinc supplementation against *Eimeria acervulina*-induced oxidative damage in broiler chickens. Vet Med Int, http://dx.doi.org/10.4061/2011/647124

[27] Georgieva NV, M Gabrashanska and V Koinarski, (2011): Ermidou-Pollet S Antioxidant status in *Eimeria acervulina* infected chickens after dietary selenium treatment. Trace Elem Elec, 28: 42-48.

[28] Ogbe, A. O. & John P. A. (2012): Effect of Polyherbal Aqueous Extracts (*Moringa Oleifera* , Gum arabic and wild Ganoderma lucidum) in Comparison with Antibiotic on Growth Performance and Haematological Parameters of Broiler Chickens. *Res. J. Recent Sci.*, 1(7), 10–18.

[29] Booth, F. E. M. & Wickens, G. E. (1988): Non-timber uses of selected arid zone trees and shrubs in Africa. *FAO conservation guide*, Rome, pp 92–101.

[30] Oduro, I.; Ellis, W. O. & Owusu, D. (2008): Nutritional potential of two leafy vegetables: *Moringa Oleifera* and Impomea batatas leaves. *Science Research Essay*, 3(2), 57–60.

Outcome of Gonadotropin Releasing Hormone Treatment 12 Days Post AI and Double Insemination on Conception Rate of Repeat Breeding Cows in Mekelle, Tigray, Ethiopia

Birhanu Hailu[1,*], Berihu Gebrekidan[2], Solmon Raju[2], Alemselam Birhanu[2], Gebrehiwot Tadesse[2], Gezahign Alemayehu[1]

[1]Samara University, College of Veterinary Medicine, Department of Veterinary Epidemiology and Preventive Medicine, Samara, Ethiopia
[2]Mekelle University, College of Veterinary Medicine, Mekelle, Ethiopia

Email address:
birhailu2002@gmail.com (B. Hailu)

Abstract: The aim of the present study was to determine outcome of gonadotropin releasing hormone analogue given 12 days post AI and double inseminations during estrous period of dairy cattle and improvement of conception rate. Field trial was carried out on repeat breeding cross breed dairy cows which are lactating, apparently healthy and exhibits estrus regularly. A total of Sixty three repeat-breeding cows from twenty eight herds were selected and assigned randomly in to three equal groups G (1, 2 and 3); two treated and one control group. Group1 (n=21) cattle were treated intramuscularly with 10 μg buserelin acetate 12 days post AI. Group2 (n=21) cattle were inseminated twice during estrus exhibition with 6-8 hours interval. Group3 (n=21) cattle were receive no treatment, inseminated once as heat was detected and considered as a control group. Dairy cows were examined for pregnancy after three months through rectal palpation. Pregnancy rates recorded were 52%, 38% and 28% in G1, G2 and G3 respectively. Conception rates of treated groups (G1 and G2) exceed control group by 24% and 10% respectively and showed a significant statistical variation ($P<0.05$) as compared to control groups. Comparison between treated groups also indicated that G1 has statistical significant difference from G2. From this experiment, it is recommended that use of GnRH 12 days can improve pregnancy rate as compared to double insemination and single service.

Keywords: Crossbred Cattle, Estrus, Double Insemination, GnRH Analogue, Pregnancy Rates

1. Introduction

Fertility problems in dairy cattle are caused by several factors. Reproductive disorder is most costly problems facing dairy industry and occurs frequently in lactating dairy cows. Repeat breeding is among the most frustrating problems which are defined as cows' failure to conceive from three or more services (Royal *et al.*, 2000; Lucy, 2001 and McDougall, 2006). These are cows that cycle normally and have no clinical abnormalities after a minimum of 3 inseminations (Levine, 1999). The economic losses associated with this problem are highly considerable resulted from increased veterinary expenses, insemination costs, reduced productivity, and losses due to involuntary culling. Reproductive problems have been the primary cause of culling in animal husbandry for many years (Coleman, 1985 and Opsomer *et al.*, 2000).

Several investigations were carried out to find out possible solutions to reduce the number of repeat breeder dairy cows. Some of the possible suggestions that were tried to reduce the incidence of repeat breeding were; strengthening estrus detection, embryo transfer, administration of GnRH at insemination, continued artificial insemination, resynchronization of non-pregnant cows. Double insemination and gonadotropin-releasing hormone treatment twelve days post AI of repeat-breeding dairy cattle were also among the most suggested solutions for this problem by Stevenson *et al.*, 2000. Double insemination increases chances of pregnancy rate due to hidden or error of estrus detection of the dairy men.

Physiologically it is known that gonadotropin releasing hormone (GnRH) is produced by hypothalamus which controls synthesis and release of luteinizing hormone (LH) and follicle stimulating hormone (FSH). These two hormones have combined effects on follicular development, ovulation and corpus lutetium functions (Douglas, 1998). The efficacy of synthetic gonadotropin releasing hormone GnRH analogue mimics the function of this natural hormone in modifying reproductive efficiency of normal as well as repeat breeder dairy cows.

This hormone has improved half life in blood circulation, greater stability to enzymatic degradation, increased receptor affinity, prolonged biological potency and less antigenic than other molecules for repeated use(Cline,2002). The exogenous administration of these hormones at different period of estrus to the cow may lead to treat the disease condition or cysts in the ovary or may rectify hormonal problem or insufficiency to these cows (Morgan, *et al.*, 1993 and Bearden and Fuquay, 1997).

GnRH has generally been used as a therapeutic agent in reproductive management. The GnRH had been used as treatment on rates of fertilization, embryonic mortality and as a therapeutic treatment for the cystic ovaries (Gustafsson *et al.,* 1986). It had been used as treatment along with or 12 days post AI to increase rates of fertilization, reduce embryonic mortality and as a therapeutic treatment for the cystic ovaries, ovarian follicular cysts and for triggering the LH surge to stimulate ovulation (Gustafsson *et al.,* 1986; Thatcher, 1991).

Double insemination with some hours interval reduces incidence of repeat breeding by increasing probability of site and time of semen deposition and estrus detection.

Limited knowledge was available about use of synthetic hormones and double insemination for management of repeat breeding dairy cows in Ethiopia and in Tigray region in particular. Nothing was done to investigate problems of repeat breeding using GnRH analogue on day 12 post AI and double insemination for enhancement of conception rate of cross breed repeat breeding dairy cattle. Therefore, the present study was conducted with the aim of enhancing the fertility rates in cross breed cattle with the specific objectives of: evaluating effects of GnRH analogue (buserellin) 12 days post AI and double insemination with eight hours interval on enhancement of conception rate as compared to control groups.

2. Materials and Methods

2.1. Description of the Study Areas

This controlled trial was conducted in the capital of Tigray regional state, Mekelle. It is one of the seven Administrative Zones and is located at 783 km north of Addis. It is geographically located 39° 29'E and 13° 3'N longitude. Mekelle is surrounded by south east zone in the south and east, Eastern zone from north, central zone from west. It has an average temperature of 20°c and experiences an average annual rain fall of 600 mm. Livelihoods of the people of the city depends on trade, civil servants and agricultural activities. Dairy farming is one of the major farming systems practiced and small holder farmers in vicinity of the city supply moderate amount of milk to the urban dwellers. Some of the farmers in the nearby area practice a mixed crop livestock production system. The area is moderately covered with savanna, bushy and low weed vegetations. Both small holder farmers and commercial dairy farms owners were included the study.

2.2. Study Population and Management Practices

The study was conduct in Mekelle and experiment was conducted in cross breed dairy herds owned by small holder farmers and private commercial dairy farms in the city. The experimental cows were kept in stall facility and feed grass hay, concentrate composed of wheat by products, locally available crop residues, forages and other locally prepared fermented alcohol by products. The cows have good body condition and apparently healthy. They are with history of more than two services and milked twice per day. They were vaccinated regularly against common infectious diseases. Generally, dairy cows were managed in similar agro ecological and climatic conditions. AI was exercised based on visual observation of standing heat and mucosal discharges from vulva by herd keepers.

2.3. Experimental Design and Selection Process

Randomized controlled trial was used to study effects of GnRH analogue given 12 days post AI and double inseminations with 6-8 hours interval on enhancement of pregnancy rates as compared to dairy herds which receive single service. The study period was from December 2009 to February 2010 in and around Mekelle. A total of 63 dairy cows were selected from twenty eight farms. Cows with normal cycling, no clinical abnormalities, failed to conceive after two successive inseminations, not previously assigned for any study and aged from three to ten years were included in the study. Cows that were treated at the first AI and returned to estrus couldn't be reassigned for the study. Sixty three cross breed dairy cows were selected based on this and equally divided in to three groups each consisting of twenty one dairy cows. These repeat breeders were randomly assigned into three protocols of treatment groups.

2.4. Experimental Protocol

This protocol trial consists of three main phases: In the first phase, training was provided for twenty eight herd owners to create awareness about symptom of estrus cycle, behavioral changes observed during estrus exhibition. Some of the signs to be observed by herd owners were mucosal discharges from their vulva, restlessness, frequent urination; allow to be mounted by other animals, raised tails and others. Herd owners were informed that as soon as these symptoms were observed, they would phone to inseminator immediately and these cows were included in the study. The second phase was random assignment of these dairy herds in to three groups; control and treatment groups. The first group G_1 (n=21) was inseminated and 10 µg (2.5ml) buserelin acetate was given intramuscularly 12 days post AI. The second group G_2 (n=21) was inseminated twice with 6-8 hours interval during estrus exhibitions. The last group G_3 (n=21) was given only single service and considered as control group. The last phase of the study was pregnancy diagnosis and was done after 60 days post AI using a rectal palpation in these herds which failed to return to estrus. The cows were considered as pregnant if we were able to palpate or sense fetal membrane, amniotic vesicles, cotyledons and fetus otherwise the cows were classified as negative.

2.5. Data Collections and Statistical Analysis

In addition to recording of data concerning inseminations and owners name, dairy herd owners were asked about breed type, insemination and service history, parity, management condition and milk yield, time and day of estrus exhibition and previous condition of the dairy herds. During study period, pregnancy diagnosis was made through rectal palpation and positive and negative results were recorded. Secondary data was collected from farm records about animals' previous milk yield, clinical cases, origin of the animal and service type. This field trial was of a randomized type in which data was collected from treated and controlled study animals. Collected data was fed to Microsoft Excel spread sheet and process of data cleaning, handling, validating and coding was done on this spread sheet. Difference in pregnancy proportion, age and parity among different treated groups against control one was compared using descriptive statistics and Pearson chi-square tests (SPSS16.0; 2005). The significance level of difference was observed at P value of less than 5%.

3. Results and Discussion

From 63 dairy cows included in the study, 25 cows were found to be pregnant. A total of 11 cows from 21 of G1 were pregnant with conception rate of 52%. In the G2, 8 cows out of 21 (38%) were conceived. The results were indicated in Table 1. G1 treated with buserelin acetate 12 days post AI exceeds in conception rate to G2 by 14% that was given double insemination. In general treated groups recorded higher pregnancy rate as compared to the G3.

Conception rate of G1 (treated) exceeds conception rate of G3 (control) by 24% with statistical significant variation (χ^2=7.636, P=0.006). The pregnancy rates of G2 were greater than group G3 by 10 % with statistical significant variation (χ^2=13.650, P=0.000). Comparison of conception rate between two treated groups: G1 scores more conception rate with statistical significant difference as compared to G2 (χ^2 =11.748, P=0.001).Comparison among the three groups, conception rate in both G1 andG2 were significantly higher thanG3. The overall comparison of treated and controlled group was shown in table 2. Management condition, season and parity variation doesn't show any significant variation in the treated groups as compared to controlled group.

Repeat-breeding dairy cows are sources of frustration and economic loss to dairy producers and the present study was carried out to see effects of double insemination and treatment of GnRH analogue 12 days post AI. G1and G2 scores more 52% and 38% respectively than G3 that scored 28%. These treated groups vary significantly (p<0.05) than control groups. This indicates that incidence of repeat breeding can be reduced through double insemination and GnRH treatment. There is a significance difference between GnRH treatment and double insemination (P<0.05) but numerical difference between double inseminated and controlled group. This may be due to insufficient or defective corpus luetum development (Pursley *et al.*, 1997) and treatment might have produced a healthy CL. This could maintain high progesterone concentration in the serum which reduces embryonic mortality in the early stages.

This result was in agreement with the study by Blowey (1992) that administration of GnRH analogue 12 posts AI improves fertility of cows by 9 % to 12 % and by Drew and Peter (1994) which was already reported. Other study by Beckelr *et al.*, (2006) observed that there was no significant difference between treated and controlled groups which were given 12 days post AI on reproductive performance of dairy cows which is opposite to the present study. Double insemination showed statistical significance variation as compared to control. Time interval at which two inseminations given was six to eight hours. So the observed results may be due to either insemination time is not followed by the owner or by the inseminator, otherwise it may be due to delayed ovulation.

Reduction in incidence of repeat breeding following these treatments results in financial return to farmers as compared to animals with single service. Intramuscular injection of GnRH analogue 12 days post AI exceeds pregnancy rate by 24% from controlled group. Repeat breeding dairy cows with double AI exceed the controlled group by 10%. Still GnRH treated groups overwhelm double inseminated groups by 14% with statistical significance variation. So, all these variations indicated that hormonal treatment will result in a great financial benefit to the farmers.

Table 1. *Results of various protocols with their respective percentages of conception.*

Group	No. animals in each protocol	Type of Protocol followed	Pregnancy rate
1	21	10µg(5ml) buserelin acetate 12 days post AI	11/21(52%)
2	21	Double insemination with 6-8 hours interval	8/21(38%)
3	21	Controlled group(receive no treatment, single service)	6/21(28%)

Table 2. *Cross tabulation of the treated groups with controlled animals.*

Cross tabulated groups			Group 3 Negative	Positive	Total	Significance Level
		Negative	10	0	10	(χ^2=7.636,P=0.006)
G1*G3	Group 1	Positive	5	6	11	
		Total	15	7	21	
			Group 3			
		Negative	13	0	13	(χ^2=13.650,P=0.000)
G2*G3	Group 2	Positive	2	6	8	
		Total	15	6	21	
			Group 2			
		Negative	10	0	10	(χ^2=11.748,P=0.001)
G1*G2	Group 1	Positive	3	8	11	
		Total	13	8	21	

4. Conclusion and Recommendations

The finding our study indicated that double insemination and intramuscular injection can be used as treatment options for repeat breeding dairy cows. Both treated groups; GnRH analogue treated 12 days post AI and double inseminations scores 52% and 38% respectively. There is statistical significance variation between treated and control groups. This experiment provides evidence for continued recommendation of the GnRH treatment to improve conception rates of repeat breeders and farmers could be benefitted financial from these alternative treatment options. Based on these results, the following points are recommended.

- The GnRH analogue administration 12 days post AI could improve the reproductive performance of repeat breeding dairy cows.
- Double insemination can achieve more conception rate for those cows with silent estrus or for the missed detection of heat.
- Farmers should be aware of treatment options to be benefitted from their dairy cows
- Given the cost of GnRH analogue, we continue to recommend the use of this hormone to rectify the problem of repeat breeding crossbred dairy cows to prevent financial losses

Acknowledgements

The authors acknowledge to Ethiopia Ministry of Science and Technology for financial support and Mekelle University for the provision of necessary facilities and administrative work which had remarkable role for the success of research work.

References

[1] Bearden, J. and Fuquay, W. (1992). Applied Animal Reproduction, 3rd edition Mississippi State University.

[2] Beckers, F., Szenci, O., Takacs, E., Sulon, J. and Sousa, N. (2006). Evaluation of GnRH treatment 12 days post A.I in the reproductive performance of dairy cows. Theriogenology.

[3] Blowey, W. (1999). The repeat breeder cow, 3rd edition, A Veterinary Book for Dairy Farmers.

[4] Coleman DA, Thayne WV, Dailey RA. Factors affecting reproductive performance of dairy cows. J Dairy Sci. 1985;68(7):1793–1803.

[5] Dougall, S., Williamson, N. and Macmillan, K. (1995). GnRH induces ovulation of dominant follicle in primiparous dairy cows undergoing anovulatory follicle turn over. *Anim. Reprod. Sci.* 39: 205-214.

[6] Drew, S. and Peters, A. (1994). Veterinary Pharmacology and Therapeutics, Endocrine pharmacology. Vet Rec .134-267.

[7] Goley R and Kadu M. (1995). Efficacy of PGF2 α, GnRH and HCG in treatment of repeat breeder cow. *Indian Veterinary Journal* 72:472-475.

[8] Gustafsson, H, .Larsso, H, Kindah .and A.Madei. (1986) Sequential Endocrine Changes and Behavior during estrus and met estrus in repeat breeder and virgin heifer's *.Anim Repro Sci* 10:261.

[9] Karg, H., Claus, R., Gunzler, O., Rattenberger, E., Pirchner, F. (1980). Hormonal Recognition of cyclicity and infertility in cows under practical conditions. In proceeding of the 11thWorld congress. Disease of cattle Israel, Pp.885-894.

[10] Levine HD. The Repeat Breeder Cow. Bovine Practioner. 1999;33:97–105.

[11] Lucy MC. Reproductive loss in high-producing dairy cattle: Where will it end? J Dairy Sci. 2001;84(6):1277–1293.

[12] Kharche, S. and Srivastava, S. (2007). Dose dependent effect of GnRH analogue on pregnancy rate of repeat breeder cross breed cows. Indian Veterinary Research institute *Anim. Repro. Sci*. India.

[13] Markandeya, N. (2006). Approaches to enhance conception rate and embryo survivability, Department of Gynecology and Obstetrics Veterinary College, Reproductive Techniques to augment Fertility in dairy animals. Karnataka Veterinary Animal and Fisheries Sciences University.

[14] Mauurer, R. and Echternkamp S. (1985). Repeat breeder Females in Beef cattle Influences and causes, J.Anim *Sci*, 61:624.

[15] McDougall S. 2006, Reproduction performance and management of dairy cattle. J Reprod Dev.; 52(1):185–194.

[16] Michael, O, Jeffrey, Stevenson, Brenda, M. and Garth, R. (1993). Administration of GnRH at estrus influences pregnancy rates Serum concentration of LH, FSH estradiol-17 beta, pregnancy specific protein and progesterone, proportion of the luteal cell types and invitro production progesterone in dairy cows. *J Anim Sci 71*:185-198.

[17] Morgan, W .Lean, I. (1993). Gonadotropin Releasing Hormone treatment in cattle a Meta analysis of effects on conception at the time of insemination. *Aust Vet J* 70:205-9.

[18] Opsomer G, Grohn YT, Hertl J, Coryn M, Deluyker H, de Kruif A. Risk factors for post partum ovarian dysfunction in high producing dairy cows in Belgium: A field study.Theriogenology. 2000;53(4):841–857.

[19] Petrie,A. and Watson, P.(2000): Statistics for Veterinary, Revised edition. Blackwel Science Ltd., Osney Mead Oxford OX2 OEL, 25 John Street, London WCIN2 BS.

[20] Royal MD, Darwash AO, Flint APF, Webb R, Wooliams JA, Lamming GE. Declining fertility in dairy cattle: Changes in traditional and endocrine parameters of fertility. Animal Science. 2000;70:487–501.

[21] Schels, H. Mostafawi, D., Morgan, W. (1978). The effect of GnRH on pregnancy rate of artificially inseminated cows. *Vet Rec*; 103: 31-32.

[22] Stevensen, J, Thompson, W. Forbes ,G.Lamb ,D. Gerieger,L,Corah .(2000).Synchronizing estrus and ovulation in beef cows after combination of GnRH, norgestment and prostaglandin with or without timed ovulation .*J Anim sci*,78:1747-1758.

[23] Stevenson J .Caller, Scoby.and .Phatak. (1990).Double insemination and gonadotropin releasing hormone treatment of repeat breeding dairy cattle .*J.DairySc*i 73:1766.

[24] Stojilkovic, S and Catt, K. (1995). *Rec. Prog. Horm. Res 50*: 161-205.

[25] Srivastava, S.K. and Kharche, S.D.(2002). Effect of GnRH on fertility in crossbred cows. *Indian. J.Anim.Sci*. 72:428-430.

[26] Thatcher, W. W., M. Drost, J. D. Savio, K. L. Macmillan, K. L. Entwistle, E. J.-P. Schmitt, R. L. de la Sota, and G. R. Morris.1993. New clinical uses for GnRH and its analogues in cattle. *Anim. Reprod. Sci*. 33:27–49.

[27] Vishwanath R. (2003).Theriogenology, 59:585-598.

Effect of Dietary Yeast (*Saccharomyces cerevisiae*) Supplementation on Performance, Carcass Characteristics and Some Metabolic Responses of Broilers

Mohamed E. Ahmed*, Talha E. Abbas, Mojahid A. Abdlhag, Dafaalla E. Mukhtar

Department of Animal Production, Faculty of Agricultural Technology and Fish Science, University of ALneelain, Khartoum, Sudan

Email address:
moha_555@hotmail.com (M. E. Ahmed)

Abstract: This study was conducted to evaluate the effect of feeding graded levels of yeast on broiler performance, carcass characteristics and some hematological indices. One day old Hubbard broiler chicks (n=160) were randomly allocated to five dietary treatments. Each treatment consisted of 4 replicates of 8 broilers each. The dietary treatments contained 0% yeast (*Saccharomyces cerevisiae*) as a negative control diet, 0% yeast + 30 ppm Oxytetracyline as a positive control, 1%, 2% and 3% yeast in the starter and finisher diets. During the experimental periods of 6 weeks, feed intake, body weight gain and feed conversion ratio values were calculated. At the end of the experimental period (6 weeks of age), some biochemical and hematological indices, carcass characteristics traits and internal organs weights were recorded. Growth performance parameters were significantly ($P \leq 0.05$) affected by experimental diets. Chicks fed either 0 or 3% yeast recorded the highest ($P \leq 0.05$) feed intake, however, the best ($P \leq 0.05$) body weight gain was obtained by birds fed 0 or 1% dietary yeast compared to the positive control diet. The highest ($P \leq 0.05$) feed conversion ratio was reported for birds fed the positive control diet and 3% dietary yeast compared to the negative control diet. The inclusion of different dietary treatments had no significant ($P \geq 0.05$) effects on dressing percentage, hot base and relative weights of heart, gizzard and abdominal fat. Nevertheless, birds fed 3% dietary yeast showed significant ($P \leq 0.05$) decrease in the relative weight of the liver compared to the negative control diet. Relative weights of breast and thigh were significantly ($P \leq 0.05$) higher in birds fed 1% yeast than those fed 3% yeast. There were linear decreases in serum cholesterol and albumin of broilers fed graded levels of dietary yeast. It is concluded that yeast can be included in broiler diet at 1% without detrimental effects on performance, and could therefore serve as a natural substitute for antibiotics.

Keywords: *Saccharomyces cerevisiae*, Broilers, Performance, Carcass, Hematology

1. Introduction

It is well documented that antibiotics benefit animal performance and health. They have long been included as a feed additive to increase broiler's growth performance and control of disease [1]. However, increasing concerns regarding overuse of antibiotics and bacterial resistance has encouraged extensive investigation into alternatives for sub-therapeutic antibiotics in feeds. Furthermore, use of probiotics, prebiotics and organic acids instead of antibiotics has increased in recent times. Probiotics act by competitive exclusion, lower gut pH, produce bacteriocins, lysozyme and peroxides, and stimulate the immune system [2]. Some of the probiotic products contain *Sacharomcyces* spp varieties. *Saccharomyces cerevisiae*, from malted grains fermentation also known as "baker's yeast" is one of the most widely commercialized types of yeast, has long been fed to animals [3]. Moreover, yeast products are important natural growth promoters [4]. Yeast *Saccharomyces cerevisiae* is rich source of protein, vitamin B complex, trace minerals and many other beneficial factors [5].

The mode of action of *Saccharomyces cerevisiae* in enhancing animal performance is not fully understood. Yeasts may beneficially alter the inherent gut microbiota, possibly through controlling pH. The presence of living yeast cells may also act as a reservoir for free oxygen, which could enhance growth of other anaerobes [6]. Effects of yeast products on production and their mode of action in poultry have been reported by [7, 8]. Some studies have confirmed the effects of yeast culture in increasing concentrations of commensal microbes or suppressing pathogenic bacteria [7]. Reference [4] assumed that there may be other mechanisms responsible for effects of yeast culture in monogastrics other than modulation of microbial ecology. Mannan-oligosaccharide and 1,3/1,6 β-glucan are components of the yeast cell wall that have been reported to modulate immunity [9], promote growth of intestinal microflora [10], and increase growth [11]. Yeast culture contains viable cells, cell wall components, metabolites, and the media on which the yeast cells were grown [12]. In in vitro study, [13], postulated that the addition of a soluble fraction of yeast culture showed an anti-inflammatory effect in conjunction with activation of natural killer cells and B lymphocytes. In addition, others have reported that yeast products affect nutrient digestibility [14] and intestinal mucosal development [15, 8].

Reference [16] reported that active dry yeast effectively increases body weight gains without affecting feed/gain ratio in broiler chicks. On the other hand, supplementation of yeast to broiler diets improves feed/gain ratio but not growth rates [17]. In contrast, it has been reported that feeding yeast to chicks improves body weight gain and feed/gain ratio [18]. Recently, [3] indicated that SC supplementation did not affect broiler performance parameters and carcass characteristics. In addition, it has been reported that yeast could be used as an alternative for antibiotic-based drugs in feed in broiler chicks [19, 7].

The present study was therefore conducted to evaluate the effects of feeding graded levels of yeast (*Saccharomyces cerevisiae*) on broiler chicks performance, carcass characteristics and some blood parameters.

2. Materials and Methods

2.1. Chickens and Treatments

The current experiment was conducted in an open-sided poultry house at the premises of Faculty of Agricultural Technology and Fish Sciences, University of Al neelain. The ambient temperature during the experimental period in this location was 23 -39 °C. One day old Hubbard broiler chicks (n=160) were randomly assigned to five dietary treatments, containing 0% yeast (*Saccharomyces cerevisiae*) as a negative control diet, 0%yeast + 30 ppm Oxytetracyline as a positive control, and 3 graded levels of yeast *Saccharomyces cerevisiae* (1%, 2% and 3%). Each treatment was replicated 4 times with 8 birds per replicate. Experimental diets were formulated according to [20], to be fed during starter period (0-3 weeks) (Table 1) and finisher period (4-6 weeks) (Table 2). Each pen was provided with feeder and drinker. Feed and water were offered *ad libitum*.

Table 1. *Composition of experimental broiler starter (1-3 weeks) diets containing graded levels of dietary yeast (Saccharomyces cerevisiae).*

Ingredients%	Dietary Treatments			
	0% yeast	1% yeast	2% yeast	3% yeast
Sorghum	64.00	64.00	64.05	64.83
Ground nut cakes	24.67	23.75	22.79	21.02
Wheat bran	1.00	1.00	1.00	1.00
Super concentrates	5.00	5.00	5.00	5.00
L-Lysine	0.20	0.10	0.10	0.10
DL-Methionine	0.13	0.12	0.11	0.11
Lime stone	1.00	1.10	1.10	1.18
Dicalcium phosphate	0.60	0.53	0.45	0.36
Vegetable oil	3.00	3.00	3.00	3.00
Choline	0.10	0.10	0.10	0.10
Enzymes	0.10	0.10	0.10	0.10
Mycotoxin binder	0.2	0.2	0.2	0.2
Yeast	0.00	1.00	2.00	3.00
Calculated analysis				
ME (kcal/kg)	3171.72	3162.61	3157.81	3155.66
CP%	23.41	23.28	23.23	22.88
Ca%	1.01	1.03	1.01	1.01
Available P%	0.46	0.45	0.45	0.45
Lysine%	1.11	1.06	1.08	1.09
Methionine%	0.52	0.52	0.51	0.51
Methionine+Cystine%	0.74	0.74	0.73	0.73

Table 2. *Composition of experimental broiler finisher (3-6 weeks) diets containing graded levels of dietary yeast (Saccharomyces cerevisiae).*

Ingredients%	Dietary Treatments			
	0% yeast	1% yeast	2% yeast	3% yeast
Sorghum	64.00	64.00	64.05	64.83
Ground nut cakes	24.67	23.75	22.79	21.02
Wheat bran	1.00	1.00	1.00	1.00
Super concentrates	5.00	5.00	5.00	5.00
L-Lysine	0.20	0.10	0.10	0.10
DL-Methionine	0.13	0.12	0.11	0.11
Lime stone	1.00	1.10	1.10	1.18
Dicalcium phosphate	0.60	0.53	0.45	0.36
Vegetable oil	3.00	3.00	3.00	3.00
Choline	0.10	0.10	0.10	0.10
Enzymes	0.10	0.10	0.10	0.10
Mycotoxin binder	0.2	0.2	0.2	0.2
Yeast	0.00	1.00	2.00	3.00
Calculated analysis				
ME (kcal/kg)	3152.28	3157.38	3150.28	3154.68
CP%	19.15	18.98	18.91	18.46
Ca%	0.82	0.82	0.81	0.80
Available P%	0.34	0.35	0.36	0.38
Lysine%	0.85	0.87	0.89	0.90
Methionine%	0.37	0.37	0.37	0.37
Methionine+Cystine%	0.55	0.55	0.55	0.54

2.2. Management

Continuous lighting was provided throughout the experimental period extended from 13/3/2012 to 24/4/2012. Broilers were vaccinated with mix (IB Ma5 + Newcastle clone 30) on day 7, and Gumboro D78 vaccine at 14 days of age, and replicated at 21 days of age. Finally, the birds were vaccinated against Newcastle (live clone 30) at 28 days of age. Feed intake and body weight were measured weekly for starter, finisher and the whole period. Mortality was recorded during the experiment as it occurred. Average feed intake, body weight gain and feed conversion ratio (feed/gain) were calculated for starter, finisher, and overall periods.

2.3. Samples Collection and Analysis

At the end of the feeding trial (6 weeks of age), the birds were fasted overnight and weighed. Two birds from each pen were selected at random and slaughtered following Halal method. This method is in accordance with Islamic rites, which considered as the least painful one. Blood samples were collected from jugular vein during slaughtering process. Hematological indices examined include packed cell volume (PCV), cholesterol, triglycerides, total protein, albumin and globulin. The same samples of birds were used for carcass characteristics analysis. These birds were de-feathered completely using warm water, decapitated, eviscerated and weighed again to obtain the dressed weights. Dressing out percentage was calculated as a percentage of live weight. The weights of liver, heart, gizzard, abdominal fat, breast, thigh and drumstick were expressed as percentage proportion of dressed weights.

2.4. Statistical Analysis

The experiment was arranged in a completely randomized design. Statistical analysis of the data was carried out using the General Linear Models procedure of SAS version 9.0 for Windows [21, 22]. Duncan's Multiple Range Test was used to detect significant differences between treatment means.

3. Results and Discussion

The effects of feeding graded levels of yeast *Saccharomyces cerevisiae* on the growth performance of broiler chicks are shown in Table 3. During the starter period (0-3 wk), dietary treatments did not affect ($P \geq 0.05$) broiler performance parameters. However, during the finisher (4-6 wk) and overall (4-6 wk) periods, supplemental yeast, significantly ($P \leq 0.05$) affected growth performance. During these periods, 3% dietary yeast significantly ($P \leq 0.05$) increased feed intake when compared to the positive control. Similar results were reported by [4]. Moreover, body weight gain at different levels of yeast was not different ($P \geq 0.05$) from either negative or positive controls. Nevertheless, overall body weight gain increased ($P \leq 0.05$) in birds fed on 1% dietary yeast compared with the positive control during the entire period (0 to 6 weeks of age). These findings are in line with the results obtained by [3], who claimed no negative effect of yeast on the growth performance of broiler chickens. The improved body weight gain with yeast supplementation was not due to increased feed intake, and similar results were reported by [4]. On the other hand, a poorer feed conversion ratio was observed in birds fed 3% yeast and positive control compared with negative control. Likewise, [16] demonstrated that active dry yeast increased weight gain without affecting feed conversion ratio in broiler chicks. In contrast with our study, some authors found that the use of yeast cell in broiler diets improved feed conversion ratio [17]. This may be because that in the previous study high-fiber (5.02%) and low-protein (18%) diets were used, and it has been reported that high-fiber diet [23] and low-protein diet [24] reduce feed efficiency.

Table 3. *Effects of graded levels of dietary yeast (Saccharomyces cerevisiae) on broiler performance.*

Parameters	Dietary Treatments					
	0% yeast	0%yeast + Oxytetracyclin	1% yeast	2% yeast	3% yeast	± SEM
0-3 wk						
Feed Intake	1379.7±91.06	1317.5±4.86	1332.9±30.93	1357.3±14.28	1339.7±20.01	22.22
Body W. Gain	729.8±40.80	695.7±50.44	733.6±10.25	690.9±44.31	712.6±24.26	18.53
FCR	1.90±0.20	1.90±0.13	1.82±0.06	1.97±0.12	1.88±0.06	0.06
4-6 wk						
Feed Intake	1951.85[ab]±94.63	1850.21[b]±88.34	1961.94[ab]±37.72	1926.99[ab]±46.33	2016.09[a]±51.32	33.88
Body W. Gain	1132.59[a]±106.17	931.25[b]±70.71	1072.32[ab]±42.07	1068.75[ab]±90.28	1015.40[ab]±43.60	37.48
FCR	1.73[b]±0.08	1.99[a]±0.16	1.83[ab]±0.06	1.81[ab]±0.12	1.99[a]±0.11	0.06
0-6 wk						
Feed Intake	3331.5[a]±172.4	3167.7[b]±91.7	3294.8[ab]±52.5	3284.3[ab]±57.1	3355.8[a]±31.7	47.51
Body W. Gain	1862.4[a]±124.9	1626.9[b]±91.2	1805.9[a]±50.0	1759.6[ab]±79.3	1728.0[ab]±67.0	43.11
FCR	1.79[b]±0.09	1.95[a]±0.1	1.83[ab]±0.05	1.87[ab]±0.06	1.94[a]±0.08	0.04

Values are means of 4 replicates per treatment (8 birds/ replicate).
[ab] Means with different superscripts in the same row were significantly different ($P \leq 0.05$).
SEM: Standard error of the means from ANOVA d.f 15.

The results of the effects of dietary yeast supplementation on carcass weight and relative organs weight are presented in Table 4. Except for dressing % and relative weight of heart, gizzard and abdominal fat, all carcass parameters and internal organs weights were significantly ($P \leq 0.05$) affected by dietary treatments. However, [3,25] revealed that dietary yeast had no effect on carcass characteristics. On the other hand, [26] stated that addition of dietary yeast at all levels improve carcass characteristics of broilers. These different results may be due to dose or kind of yeast used, strain of broilers, basal diet or environmental conditions

Table 4. *Effects of graded levels of dietary yeast (Saccharomyces cerevisiae) on some carcass characteristics and internal organs of broilers.*

Parameters	Dietary Treatments					
	0% yeast	**0%yeast + Oxytetracyclin**	**1% yeast**	**2% yeast**	**3% yeast**	**± SEM**
Dressing%	72.23±5.2	70.10±4.1	69.93±2.5	72.23±1.8	73.08±0.76	1.64
R. W. of heart	0.64±0.06	0.68±0.15	0.65±0.07	0.59±0.03	0.62±0.11	0.05
R. W. of gizzard	2.77±1.54	2.23±0.41	2.18±0.09	2.24±0.17	1.99±0.27	0.36
R. W. of A. Fat	2.58±0.53	2.60±0.24	3.49±0.71	2.61±0.52	3.16±0.80	0.30
R. W. of liver	3.53^{a}±0.51	3.09^{ab}±0.99	2.88^{ab}±0.43	2.63^{ab}±0.56	2.2^{b}±0.15	0.30
R. weight of Br	14.44^{ab}±3.04	16.98^{ab}±2.35	19.05^{a}±2.14	17.16^{ab}±3.85	14.00^{b}±2.57	1.43
M/B Br	5.01^{a}±0.01	3.98^{a}±2.03	4.98^{a}±0.06	2.50^{b}±0.00	4.77^{a}±0.47	0.47
Thig rel	7.54^{ab}±1.13	6.83^{ab}±0.95	8.31^{a}±1.27	7.66^{ab}±1.26	6.07^{b}±0.67	0.54
m/b thigh	5.58^{ab}±0.07	5.87^{a}±0.32	4.74^{bc}±1.24	4.92^{bc}±0.18	4.07^{c}±0.30	0.30
Drum rela	7.27^{b}±0.80	9.21^{a}±2.06	7.93^{ab}±0.49	8.25^{ab}±1.11	9.22^{a}±0.38	0.57
Drum m/b	3.97^{a}±0.06	3.62^{b}±0.11	3.61^{b}±0.00	2.93^{c}±0.16	3.87^{a}±0.26	0.07

Values are means of 4 replicates per treatment.
abc Means with different superscripts in the same row were significantly different (P≤ 0.05).
SEM: Standard error of the means from ANOVA d.f 15.

Table 5. *Effects of graded levels of dietary yeast (Saccharomyces cerevisiae) on some serum metabolites and haematology of broilers*

Parameters	Dietary Treatments					
	0% yeast	**0%yeast + Oxytetracyclin**	**1% yeast**	**2% yeast**	**3% yeast**	**± SEM**
Cholesterol mg/dL	176.00^{a}±7.00	172.33^{a}±3.51	150.00^{ab}±11.00	148.00^{ab}±14.00	141.67^{b}±25.41	8.40
Triglycerides	45.00±10.44	45.00±9.64	46.57±15.23	40.57±14.56	46.57±8.45	5.10
Total Protein g/dL	2.72±1.24	2.81±0.60	2.45±0.72	2.05±0.35	2.13±0.38	0.42
Albumin g/dL	1.50^{ab}±0.51	1.56^{a}±0.22	1.29^{ab}±0.39	0.85^{bc}±0.37	0.79^{c}±0.07	0.19
Globulin g/dL	1.22±0.76	1.25±0.39	1.17±0.46	1.20±0.20	1.33±0.44	0.27
PCV%	31.00^{a}±1.00	29.67^{ab}±5.80	31.33^{a}±0.46	28.00^{ab}±2.00	24.67^{b}±1.15	1.77

Values are means of 3 replicates per treatment.
abc Means with different superscripts in the same row were significantly different (P≤ 0.05).
SEM: Standard error of the means from ANOVA d.f 10.

Table 5 shows the effects of graded levels of dietary yeast on biochemical and haematological indices of broilers. There were no significant (P≥0.05) differences across the different dietary treatments in serum levels of total protein, globulin and triglycerides. These results are in line with the results obtained by [27] who reported that inclusion of yeast into diets of turkey toms doesn't affect serum levels of total protein, globulin and triglycerides. Reference [28] also, found serum levels of protein and triglycerides were unaffected by dietary *S cerevisiae*. In addition, reference [29] declared that there is no significant influence of dietary *S cerevisiae* on serum triglycerides. In reverse to these findings, [26] noticed that dietary yeast decreases serum triglycerides and increases serum concentrations of protein and globulin. Cholesterol, albumin, and PCV were significantly (P≤0.05) affected by dietary treatments. There were linear decreases in serum cholesterol and albumin of broilers fed graded levels of dietary yeast compared to negative and positive control. References [30,31] assured that dietary yeast causes decrease in serum cholesterol when added to broilers diets. Reference [32] confirmed decrease in serum albumin when 2% of yeast culture was added to Japanese quails diets. Opposite to these results [26] mentioned increase in serum albumin as a result of supplementation of yeast to broilers diets. Different results also, obtained by [33] who found supplementation of yeast derived β-glucan has no effect on various concentrations of cholesterol fractions. On the other hand, broilers on 3% dietary yeast expressed significantly (P≤0.05) lowest PCV compared to negative and positive control. This might be due to higher level of yeast used in the experiment. Reference [34] mentioned that increased level of yeast supplementation resulted in increased bacterial load on the bird gut. In reverse to this result [31] reported that dietary yeast has no effects on PCV when introduced into broilers diet. Different results may be due to different dose or kind of yeast used, experimental conditions, basal diet or strain of broilers.

4. Conclusion

It was concluded that yeast can be included in broiler diets at 1% without detrimental effects on performance, and might therefore serve as a natural substitute for antibiotics. More research is however required in both experimental and productive conditions to confirm this conclusion.

References

[1] Chen KL, Kho WL, You SH, Yeh RH, Tang SW, Hsieh CW. Effects of *Bacillus subtilis* var. *natto* and *Saccharomyces cerevisiae* mixed fermented feed on the enhanced growth performance of broilers. Poult Sci. 2009; 88: 309-315.

[2] Grashorn MA. Use of phytobiotics in broiler nutrition– an alternative to infeed antibiotics. J Anim Feed Sci. 2010; 19: 338-347.

[3] Rezaeipour V, Fononi H, Irani M. Effects of dietary L-threonine and Saccharomyces cerevisiae on performance, intestinal morphology and immune response of broiler chickens. SA J Anim Sci. 2012; 42: 266-273.

[4] Gao J, Zhang HJ, Yu SH, Wu SG, Yoon I, Quigley J, Gao YP, Qi GH. Effects of yeast culture in broiler diets on performance and immunomodulatory functions. Poult Sci. 2008; 87:1377–1384.

[5] Reed G, Nagodawithana TW. Yeast Technology. 2nd edition New York: Van Nostrand Reinhold, USA. 1991.

[6] Leeson S, Summers JD. Commercial Poultry Nutrition. 3rd Edition. Nottingham University Press, England. 2008.

[7] Stanley VG, Gray C, Daley M, Krueger WF, Sefton AE. An alternative to antibiotic-based drugs in feed for enhancing performance of broilers grown on *Eimeria* spp.-infected litter. Poult Sci. 2004; 83:39–44.

[8] Zhang AW, Lee BD, Lee SK, Lee KW, An GH, Song KB, Lee CH. Effects of yeast (*Saccharomyces cerevisiae*) cell components on growth performance, meat quality, and ileal mucosa development of broiler chicks. Poult Sci. 2005; 84: 1015–1021.

[9] Shashidhara RG, Devegowda G. Effect of dietary mannan oligosaccharide on broiler breeder production traits and immunity. Poult Sci. 2003; 82: 1319–1325.

[10] Spring P, Wenk C, Dawson KA, Newman KE. The effects of dietary mannanoligosaccharides on cecal parameters and the concentrations of enteric bacteria in the ceca of *Salmonella*-challenged broiler chicks. Poult Sci. 2000; 79: 205–211.

[11] Parks CW, Grimes JL, Ferket PR, Fairchild AS. The effect of mannanoligosaccharides, bambermycins, and virginiamycin on performance of large white male market turkeys. Poult Sci. 2001; 80: 718–723.

[12] Miles RD, Bootwalla SM. Direct-fed microbials in animal production 'avian'. In Direct-Fed Microbials in Animal Production—A Review of the literature. NFIA, West Des Moines, Iowa, US. 1991; 117–146

[13] Jensen GS, Patterson KM, Yoon I. Yeast culture has anti-inflammatory effects and specifically activates NK cells. Comp Immunol Microbiol Infect Dis. 2008; 31: 487-500.

[14] Bradley GL, Savage TF. The effect of autoclaving a yeast culture of *Saccharomyces cerevisiae* on turkey poult performance and the retention of gross energy, and selected minerals. Anim Feed Sci Technol. 1995; 55: 1–7.

[15] Santin E, Maiorka A, Macari M, Grecco M, Sanchez JC, Okada TM, Myasaka AM. Performance and intestinal mucosa development of broiler chickens fed diets containing *Saccharomyces cerevisiae* cell wall. J Appl Poult Res. 2001; 10: 236–244.

[16] Kanat R, Calialar S. A research on the comparison effect on broiler chickens performance of active dried yeast and inactivated and stabilized probiotic yeast supplemented to the rations in different levels. Poult. Sci. 1996; 75 (Suppl. 1):123 (Abstract).

[17] Onifade AA, Odunsi AA, Babatunde GM, Olorede BR, Muma E. Comparison of the supplemental effects of Saccharomyces cerevisiae and antibiotics in low-protein and high-fiber diets fed to broiler chicken. Arch Anim Nutr. 1999; 52: 29–39.

[18] Onifade AA, Babatunde GM, Afonja SA, Ademola SG, Adesina EA. The effect of a yeast culture addition to a low-protein diet on the performance and carcass characteristics of broiler chickens. Poult Sci. 1998; 77 (Suppl. 1): 44. (Abstract).

[19] Hooge DM, Sims MD, Sefton AE, Connolly A, Spring P. Effect of dietary mannan oligosaccharide, with or without bacitracin or virginiamycin, on live performance of broiler chickens at relatively high stocking density on new litter. J Appl Poult Res. 2003; 12: 461–467.

[20] National Research Council. Nutrient Requirement of Poultry. Ninth revised edition, National Academy Press, Washington DC. 1994; 19-26

[21] SAS Institute, Inc. SAS/STAT(R) User's Guide, Version 9, Cary, NC: SAS Institute, Inc. 2003.

[22] Steel RGD, Torrie JH. Principles and Procedures of Statistics. A Biometrical Approach. 2nd ed. McGraw-Hill Book Co, Inc, New York, NY. 1980.

[23] Krás RV, Kessler AM, Ribeiro AML, Henn JDi, Santos Il dos, Halfen DP, Bockor L. Effect of dietary fiber and genetic strain on the performance and energy balance of broiler chickens. Braz J Poult Sci. 2013; 15: 15-20.

[24] Bregendahl K, Sell JL, Zimmerman DR. Effect of low-protein diets on growth performance and body composition of broiler chicks. Poult Sci. 2002; 81: 1156-1167.

[25] Karaoglu M, Durdag H. The influence of dietary probiotic (*Saccharomyces cerevisiae*) supplementation and different slaughter age on the performance, slaughter and carcass properties of broilers. Int J Poult Sci. 2005; 4: 309-316.

[26] Paryad A, Mahmoudi M. Effect of different levels of supplemental yeast (*Saccharomyces cerevisiae*) on performance, blood constituents and carcass characteristics of broiler chicks. Afr J Agr Res. 2008; 12: 835-842.

[27] Konca Y, Kirkpinar F, Mert S, Kayhan B. Performance, intestinal microflora and blood constituents in finishing turkeys fed diets supplemented with dietary mannan oligosaccharide and live yeast. J Anim Feed Sci. 2009; 18: 508-517.

[28] Yalçın S, Eser H, Yalçın S, Cengiz S, Eltan Ö. Effects of dietary yeast autolysate (*Saccharomyces cerevisiae*) on performance, carcass and gut characteristics, blood profile, and antibody production to sheep red blood cells in broilers. J Appl Poult Res. 2013; 22: 55-61.

[29] Pouraziz S, Shahryar HA, Chekani-Azar S. Effects of dietary *Saccharomyces cerevisiae* and butyric acid glycerides on performance and serum lipid level of broiler chickens. Kafkas Univ Vet Fak Derg. 2013; 19: 903-907.

[30] Aluwong T, Raji MA, Hassan BF, Kawu MU, Kobo PI, Ayo JO. Effect of different levels of supplemental yeast on performance indices and serum biochemistry of broiler chickens. The Open Conf Proc J. 2012; 3(Suppl 1-M7): 41-45.

[31] Saied JM, Al-Jabary QH, Thalij KM. Effect of dietary supplement yeast culture on production performance and hematological parameters in broiler chicks. Int J Poult Sci. 2011; 10: 376-380.

[32] Ghally KA, Abd El-Latif SA. Effect of dietary yeast on some productive and physiological aspects on growing Japanese quails. Afr Crop Sci Conf Proc. 2007; 8: 2147-2151.

[33] An BK, Cho BL, You SJ, Paik HD, Chang HI, Kim SW, Yun CW, Kang CW. Growth performance and antibody response of broiler chicks fed yeast derived β-glucan and single-strain probiotics. Asian-Aust J Anim Sci. 2008; 21: 1027-1032.

[34] Onwurah FB, Okejim J, Amaefula KU. Effect of yeast as water additive in the management of litter in the production starter broiler. Asi J Natu Appl Sci. 2013; 2: 27-30.

29

Toxoplasmosis in Small Ruminants from Varied Habitats

Saghir Ahmad*, **ZahidaTasawar**

Institute of Pure and Applied Biology, Bahauddin Zakariya University, Multan, Pakistan

Email address:
saghirahmad@bzu.edu.pk (S. Ahmad), saghir7np@yahoo.com (S. Ahmad)

Abstract: Background: Toxoplasmosis is an infectious disease found all over the world in all the mammalian and avian species. We conceived the hypothesis that the infection might be affected by the various factor differing in various habitats. The present study was conducted to evaluate our hypothesis by investigating the rates if infections different flocks of small ruminants populated in various localities with varied ecological conditions in southernmost part of Punjab, Pakistan. Materials and Method: The blood samples collected from mixed farms of sheep and goats were examined by Latex Agglutination Test to detect rates of seroprevalence of anti-Toxoplasma antibodies. Statistical analyses were applied to ascertain the correlation between habitat variations and rates of toxoplasmosis in three distinct regions of study area including sand dunes of Cholistan desert, Agricultural Region and Marshy areas. Results: The total infection rates collectively found in small ruminants were 31.41%. The incidence rates of Toxoplasma infection in small ruminants were 38.1%, 32.1% and 14.5% in animals reared in Agricultural Region, Riverside region and Sand Dunes region of Cholistan correspondingly. Conclusions: The results showed the varied rates of toxoplasmosis in small ruminants in various habitats in the study area. Furthermore, the overall higher occurrence of toxoplasmosis in small ruminants underlined the threat of zoonotic transmission of infection to human.

Keywords: Toxoplasmosis, Small Ruminants, Habitat Variations

1. Introduction

The Domestic sheep and goats are the vital source of milk, meat, fibers and pelts in almost all the countries of the world. These livestock animals are vulnerable to different parasitic diseases (Gebremedhin et al., 2013) including toxoplasmosis (Othman and Al-Azuheir, 2014) that causes a range of reproductive problems such as prenatal and postnatal mortality, still births or abortions (Edwards and Dubey, 2013) leading to the economic losses and threats to human health via zoonotic transmission (Othman and Al-Azuheir, 2014). The livestock animals in general and small ruminants in particular are exposed to a variety of infectious and noninfectious diseases of parasitic origin (Akhter and Arshad, 2006; Siddiki et al., 2010) leading to the reduction in productivity (Haileleul, 2002). Parasitic infections pose threats to health and limit the productivity due to the associated morbidity and mortality (Nwosuet al., 2007) or due to early death in the embryonic life, mummification, abortion, stillbirth (Panadero et al., 2010), and in some cases the neonatal or postnatal death (Edwards and Dubey, 2013). These infections have become a serious universal threat for livestock (Lashari and Tasawar, 2011).

One of these infections is toxoplasmosis caused by Toxoplasma gondii (hereafter referred as T. gondii or/and Toxoplasma) belonging to class Coccidia of phylum Apicomplexa (Ferguson, 2002; Kopecna et al., 2006). T. gondii is widespread in distribution and can be considered as one of the most successful protozoan parasites (Doskaya et al., 2006) that can inflict serious diseases in all the endothermic animals (Doskaya et al., 2006; Dubey, 2009) such as mammals including small ruminants and humans (Aspinall et al., 2002). Since Toxoplasma is transmitted through zoonosis particularly from sheep and goats (Sevgili et al., 2005), there is dire need to screen the animals whose meat is used by human as food so that the human health is ensured (Hill and Dubey, 2002; Lhafi et al., 2004).

Toxoplasmosis is deleterious in terms of both economy of a country and health of its people (Hill et al., 2005) and approximately thirty three percent of animals and human population of the world has been estimated to be infected with T. gondii at an average (Sensini, 2006) ranging between 1 and 99% rates of infections (Olivier et al., 2007). The open-air meat markets are considered as a potential source of infestation of human by T. gondii. While being transported from slaughter houses, the meat is by far contaminated with oocysts of T. gondii hence resulting as a risk factor of zoonosis to human beings. The incidence of T. gondii seroprevalence in different species of animals has been studied in many countries of the world with results varying from country to country, region to region, herd to herd and season to season. Sometimes even these results vary with variation of methodology utilized on the same herd (Yu et al., 2007). The open-air markets are common in Rahim Yar Khan and Rajan Pur regions of southern Punjab, Pakistan and create a potential source of pathogen contamination as the stray cats and dogs are usually found around the markets which, being a natural reservoir of T. gondii, add many millions of oocysts of parasite through their excreta just within a couple of week after getting infected (Dabritz et al., 2007). Oocysts of T. gondii exhibit a characteristic resistance against a broad spectrum of disinfecting agents due to structural stability principally in warm and humid regions of the world, nevertheless having poor survival in arid and cold climatic conditions (Rorman et al., 2006).

Toxoplasmosis infection has been established as a major economic threat for sheep and goat farming industry particularly due to abortion all over the world (Buxton et al., 2007; Innes et al., 2009). This disease may also cause the monitory losses in terms of the reproductive disorders such as abortions, stillbirth, or weakness of neonates that results in death (Bueno et al., 2004; Soares et al., 2009) or adult mortality, reduced productivity in small ruminants with lower quality of wool and leather (Parthiban et al., 2005). According to the findings of Kijlstra and Jongert (2009), T. gondii is a food hazard as well.

As the survival of T. gondii is affected by environmental factors (Chacin-Bonilla and Sanchez-Chavez, 2000; Hill et al., 2005), we chose to conduct the current study to ascertain the variations in the rates of infections in the animas populated the remote areas of Pakistan. The present study is based on the research conducted to ascertain the association between toxoplasmosis in small ruminants'flocks reared in different habitat of Southern Punjab, Pakistan.

2. Materials and Methods

A total of 1200 blood samples were randomly collected from domestic small ruminants belonging to different localities in Cholistan Sand Dunes region, Agricultural region of district Rahim Yar Khan and Riverside (also called Kacha) Region in district Rajan Pur along the eastern bank of River Indus. Three to five ml of blood was collected from each animal's jugular vein in a vacuum tube. Each sample was allowed for 1 hour time to coagulate and afterwards applied 3000 RPM centrifugation for 10-15 minute so that serum could be decanted from the sample. The serological assay to detect the occurrence of anti-Toxoplasma antibodies (IgG) was carried out by using "Toxoplasmosis Latex" manufactured by "ANTEC DIAGNOSTIC PRODUCTS-UK. The results were analyzed statistically by applying the statistical tests Chi-square test to compute the correlation via Pearson's test through SSPS version 20.

3. Results and Discussion

In the present study, the relationship between habitat variation and occurrence of toxoplasmosis was analyzed and significantly (P=0.000) varied rates of toxoplasmosis infection were found in three different regions of our study area (Table 1). The results revealed that amongst total 556 small ruminants sampled from the agricultural areas region 212 were found positive for anti-Toxoplasma antibodies with the highest rate of toxoplasmosis (38.1%) followed by the animals populated in riverside areas region where, out of 404 total sampled animals 130 were positive for anti-Toxoplasma antibodies showing the infection rate at level of (32.1%)and with least rate of toxoplasmosis infection were found in the small ruminants reared in Cholistan desert region 35/240 (14.5%) as shown in Table 1.

Table 1. *Relationship between toxoplasmosis and habitat variations.*

Region	Animals examined	Animals positive	Prevalence (%)
Desert Areas	240	35	14.58
Agricultural Region	556	212	38.12
Riverside Region	404	130	32.17
Total	1200	377	31.41

Chi-Square = 43.2994 P-Value = 0.000

The results demonstrated the significant (P-Value= 0.000) regional variations in prevalence of Toxoplasma infection consistent with (Yang et al., 2013) who reported same picture in China and (Sechi et al., 2013) whose results demonstrated the association between toxoplasmosis and still water sources contaminated by cats' access to water consumed by small ruminants one of the important determinants in three different regions in the present study area.

These variations in infection rates probably could also be related with the humidity being highest in the habitat of small ruminants' flocks populated in the riverside areas in an agreement with Rorman et al. (2006) that the oocysts of T. gondii exhibit a strong structural stability predominantly in warm and humid regions of the world. It is widely accepted view that the oocysts of Toxoplasma have a poor survival in arid and cold climatic conditions (Van der Puijeet al., 2000; Rorman et al., 2006).

The higher rate of toxoplasmosis (38.1%) (Table 1) in the densely populated Agricultural Region inhabiting animal as compared with the infection rates in the animals reared in desert areas (14.5%) (Table 1) can be attributed to the presence of higher number of cats in the densely populated localities which can boost the number of oocysts in soil (Petersen and Schmidt, 2003) at a rate of many millions just by single defecation (Lopes et al., 2008) thus causing the contamination of the surrounding habitat (Silva et al., 2001) as is evident from the current study area results.

The ecological factors must be taken into account for the variation in the infection rates amongst the small ruminants reared in different habitats of study area (Dubeyet al., 2004; Meerburg and Kijlstra, 2009). The prevalence rates of toxoplasmosis observed in three regions of our study area were in agreement with (Yu et al., 2007) who reported the association between occurrences of T. gondii infection and environmental factors. The similar agreement was found between our findings and (Zewdu et al., 2013).

The rapid sugar industry in Rahim Yar Khan has encouraged the replacement of cotton with Sugarcane and rice crops which increased the humidity in the region suggesting the better chances for the growth of T. gondii in small ruminants and perhaps in the other animal species as well. On the other hand, the animals reared in Cholistan continuously face the stress of the adversely hot summer season along with the scarcity of water and natural vegetation, the mere source of fodder. This is the reason that the nomads of Cholistan desert migrate in the Agricultural areas Region including Sadiqabad, Khan Pur and Liaquet Pur in search of the fodder for their animals particularly on the onset of drought in the dog days of summer season every year. Perhaps during the immigration of the nomad tribes of Cholistan, their small ruminants contract the Toxoplasma infection from the highly infected animals of Agricultural localities.

Furthermore, the Dhands (the seasonal lakes formed by accumulation of rain water) in Cholistan desert, the transient resorts for Siberian migratory birds en route the lakes in the southern limits of Pakistan, are also responsible for the horizontal transmission of T. gondii infection (Cabezon et al., 2011) because, we suspect, the wild cats after feeding on the migratory birds' corps must shed the oocysts in the environment (Amany et al., 2012) which might make their way to the digestive tract of the small ruminants of Cholistan. The stagnant water (Ertug et al., 2005; Sechiet al., 2013) of these Dhands might also be the source of infection as it is shared for drinking by birds as well as small ruminant species simultaneously. This hypothesis is supported by some studies reported in the near past (Taghadosi et al., 2010; Cenci-Goga et al., 2013) providing the evidences of water borne infection of toxoplasmosis.

The Riverside Region showing 32.17% infection in small ruminants exhibits the peculiar picture of humidity due fluctuating floods in the river Indus. In this region of study area, the animals are faced with the scarcity of food in the monsoon season rainfall and some times, for many months displacement also (Ashraf et al., 2013). During the 2010 monsoon, the standing crop of cotton was devastated by flood in the river Indus. The mass migration of human population with their small ruminants occurred due to that flood thus leading to the exchange of variety of infections between animals of Rahim Yar Khan and those migrated from Kacha area region along the river Indus.

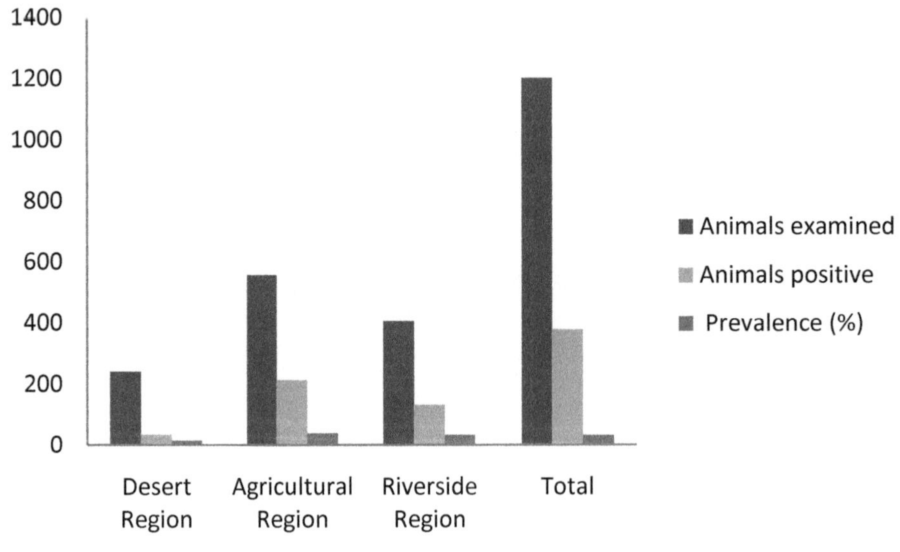

Graph 1. *Prevalence of T. gondii infection in varied habitats*

4. Conclusions

The animals reared in the urban areas with Agri-based population demonstrated the highest rates of seroprevalence of T. gondii (38.1%) suggesting to the hypothesis that canines must be playing a role in the multiplication of parasite. The least incidence of infections (14.5%) was noted in the Sand Dunes dwelling small ruminants perhaps due to harshly high temperature in the Cholistan desert that discouraged the sustenance of T. gondii while the infection rates in small ruminants 32.1% were also influenced by humid environment produced by still water in the region.

Recommendations

- It was noticed throughout the present study that the farmers prefer to mix farming of livestock species including sheep (Ovis aeries), goats (Capra hircus), buffalo (Bos bubalis) and cows (Bos Taurus) particularly where the pasture grazing adapted for feeding the animals. The standing water must be playing the role in exchange of T. gondii infection among different species.

- Therefore, keeping into consideration the horizontal transmission, we suggest the screening of the other livestock species of the study area.
- We also recommend the prompt study to evaluate the infection in humans that might have transmitted by zoonosis.

Author's Contribution

The blood samples collection from sheep, serological and statistical analyses of data were performed by Saghir Ahmad under the supervision of Prof Dr Zahida Tasawar, Institute of Pure and Applied Biology, Bahauddin Zakariya University, Multan.

Acknowledgements

We are grateful to the Higher Education Commission (HEC), Islamabad, Pakistan for providing funds for financial support/scholarship under Indigenous 5000 PhD Fellowship Program, Batch III, PIN: 063-161120-Bm3-093 for completion of present study.

References

[1] Akhter, R. and Arshad, M. 2006. Arid Rangelands in the Cholistan Desert (Pakistan). Secheresse., 17: 210-217.

[2] Amany, M., El-Ghany, A. and Merwad, A. M. A. 2012. Epidemiology and Molecular Detection of Zoonotic Toxoplasma gondii in Cat Feces and Seroprevalence of Anti-Toxoplasma gondii Antibodies in Pregnant Women and Sheep. Life Sci. J.9,133-146.

[3] Ashraf, S., Chuadry, H. R., Farooq, U., Mustafa, Y. S., Fatima, H. and Akhter, S. 2013. Prospective of Dairy Farming in Cholistan. Sci. Int., 25: 345-346.

[4] Aspinall, T. V., Marlee, D., Hyde, J. E. and Sims, P. F. 2002. Prevalence of Toxoplasma gondii in Commercial Meat Products as Monitored by Polymerase Chain Reaction-Food for Thought? Int. J. Parasitol., 32: 1193-1199.

[5] Bueno, J. P., Gozalo, A. Q., Prerez, G. P., Garcia, G. A., Frenandez, E. C. and Mora, L. M. O. 2004. Evolution of ovine abortion associated with Toxoplasma gondii in Spain by different diagnostic techniques. Vet. Parasitol., 121: 33-43.

[6] Buxton, D. S., Maley, W., Wright, S. E., Rodger, S., Bartley, P. and Innes, E. A. 2007. Toxoplasma gondii and ovine toxoplasmosis: New Aspects and Old Story. Vet. Parasitol., 149: 25-28.

[7] Cabezon, O., García-Bocanegra, I., Molina-Lopez, R., Marco, I. and Blanco, J. M. 2011. Seropositivity and Risk Factors Associated with Toxoplasma gondii Infection in Wild Birds from Spain. Plos One., 6: 1371.

[8] Cenci-Goga, B. T., Ciampelli, A., Sechi, P., Veronesi, F., Moretta, I., Cambiotti, V. and Thompson, P. N. 2013. Seroprevalence and risk factors for Toxoplasma gondii in sheep in Grosseto district, Tuscany, Italy. Vet. Res., 9: 25.

[9] Chacın-Bonilla, L. and Sanchez-Chavez, Y. 2000. Intestinal parasiticinfections, with special emphasis on cryptosporidiosis, in Amerindiansfrom western Venezuela. Am. J. Trop. Med. Hyg., 62: 347-352.

[10] Dabritz, H. A., Miller, M. A., Atwill, E. R., Gardner, I. A., Leutenegger, C. M., Melli, A. C. and Conrad, P. A. 2007. Detection of Toxoplasma gondii like Oocysts in Cat Feces and Estimates of The Environmental Oocyst Burden. J. Amer. Vet. Med. Asso., 231:1676-1684.

[11] Doskaya, M., Degirmenci, A., Cicek, C., Ak, M., Korkmaz, M., Guruz, Y. and Uner, A. 2006. Behavior of Toxoplasma gondii RH Ankara strain tachyzoites during continuous production in various cell lines. Parasitol., 132: 315-319.

[12] Dubey, J. P., Navarro, I. T., Sreekumar, C., Dahl, E., Freire, R. L., Kawabata, H. H., Vianna, M. C., Kwok, O. C., Shen, S. K., Thulliez, P. and Lehmann, T. 2004. Toxoplasma gondii infections in cats from Parana, Brazil: seroprevalence, tissue distribution, and biologic and genetic characterization of isolates. J. Parasitol., 90: 721- 726.

[13] Dubey, J. P. 2009. Toxoplasmosis in sheep-The last 20 years. Vet. Parasitol., 163: 1-14.

[14] Edwards, J. F. and Dubey, J. P. 2013. Toxoplasma gondii abortion storm in sheep on a Texas farm and isolation of mouse virulent atypical genotype T. gondii from an aborted lamb from a chronically infected ewe. Vet. Parasitol.192: 129-36.

[15] Ertug, S., Okyay, P., Turkmen, M. and Yuksel, H. 2005. Seroprevalence and risk factors for Toxoplasma infection among pregnant women in Aydin province, Turkey. BMC Pub. Hlth., 5: 66-71.

[16] Ferguson, T. R. 2002. Apicomplexa. J. Parsitol., 18: 355-357.

[17] Gebremedhin, E. Z. and Gizaw, D. 2014. Seroprevalence of Toxoplasma gondii Infection in Sheep and Goats in Three Districts of Southern Nations, Nationalities and Peoples' Region of Ethiopia. W. App. Sci. J., 31: 1891-1896.

[18] Haileleul, N. 2002. Study on Prevalence of GIT Helminthes of Small Ruminants in and Around Wolayta Soddo, Southern Ethiopia. DVM Thesis, Faculty of veterinary medicine, Addis Ababa University, Debre-Zeit, Ethiopia , p. 353.

[19] Hill, D. E. and Dubey, J. P. 2002. Toxoplasma gondii: transmission diagnosis and prevention. Clin. Microbiol. Infect., 8: 634-640.

[20] Innes, E. A., Bartley, P. M., Buxton, D. and Katzer, F. 2009. Ovine Toxoplasmosis. Parasitol., 136: 1884-1891.

[21] Kijlstra, A. and Jongert, E. 2009. Toxoplasma-safe meat: close to reality? Trends Parasitol., 25: 18-22.

[22] Kopecna, J., Jirku, M., Obornik, M., Tokarev, Y. S., Lukes, J. and Modry, D. 2006. Phylogenetic analysis of coccidian parasites from invertebrates: search for missing links. Protist., 157: 173-183.

[23] Lashari, M. H. and Tasawar, Z. 2011. Prevalence of some gastrointestinal parasites in sheep in southern Punjab, Pakistan. Pak. Vet. J., 31: 295-298.

[24] Lhafi, S. K., Mitzscherling, A. T. and Kuhne, M. 2004. Parasitic hazards in meat: a challenge for veterinarians in meat hygiene. Deut. Tierarztl. Woch., 111: 277-281.

[25] Lopes, A., Cardoso, L. and Rodrigues, M. 2008. Serological Survey of Toxoplasma gondiiinfection in domestic cats from northeastern Portugal. J. Parasitol., 155: 184-189.

[26] Meerburg, B. G. and Kijlstra, A. 2009. Changing climate-changing pathogens: Toxoplasma gondii in North-Western Europe. Parasitol. Res.105: 1447-48.

[27] Nwosu, C. O., Madu, P. P. and Richards, W. S. 2007. Prevalence and seasonal changes in the population of gastrointestinal nematodes of small ruminants in the semi-arid zone of north-eastern Nigeria. Vet. Parasitol., 144:118-124.

[28] Olivier, A., Herbert, B., Sava, B., Pierre, C., John, D. C. and Aline, D. K. 2007 Surveillance and monitoring of Toxoplasma in humans, food and animals: a scientific opinion of the panel on biological hazards. The European Food Safety Association J., 583: 1-64.

[29] Othman, R. A. and Al-Azuheir. 2014. Seroprevalence of Toxoplasma gondii in Goats in Two Districts in Northern Palestine. Walailak J. Sci. Technol.11: 63-67.

[30] Panadero, R., Painceira, A., Lopez, C., Vázquez, L., Paz, A., Díaz, P., Dacal, V., Cienfuegos, S., Fernandez, G., Lago, N., Diez-Banos, P. and Morrondo, P. 2010. Seroprevalence of Toxoplasma gondii and Neosporacaninum in wild and domestic ruminants sharing pastures in Galicia (Northwest Spain). Res. Vet. Sci., 88: 111-115.

[31] Parthiban, M., Govindarajan, R., Manoharan, S., Purushothaman, V., Chandran, N. D. J. and Koteeswaran. A. 2005. Comparative sequence analysis of diagnostic PCR amplicons from Indian sheep pox virus. Vet. Arhiv., 75: 203-209.

[32] Petersen, E. and Schmidt, D. R. 2003. Sulfadiazine and Pyrimethamine in the post-natal treatment of congenital toxoplasmosis: What are the options? Exp.Rev. Anti-infect. Ther.1: 175-182.

[33] Rorman, E., Zamir, C. S., Rilkis, I. and Ben-David, H. 2006. Congenital toxoplasmosis--prenatal aspects of Toxoplasma gondii infection. Reprod. Toxicol., 21: 458 - 472.

[34] Sechi, P., Ciampelli, A., Cambiotti, V., Veronesi, F., Beniamino, T. and Cenci-Goga, B.T. 2013. Sero-epidemiological study of toxoplasmosis in sheep in rural areas of the Grosseto district, Tuscany, Italy. Italian J. Anim. Sci., 12: 39.

[35] Sensini, A. 2006. Toxoplasma gondii infection in pregnancy: opportunities and pitfalls ofserological diagnosis. Clncl .Microbiol. Infect., 12: 504-512.

[36] Sevgili, M. C. B., Nalbantoglu, S. and Vatansever, Z. 2005. Determination of Seropositivity for Toxoplasma gondii in sheep in Sanliurfa Province, Turkey. J. Vet. Anim. Sci., 29:107-111.

[37] Siddiki, A. Z., Uddin, M. B., Hasan, M. B., Hossain, M. F., Rahman, M. M., Das, B. C., Sarker, M. S. and Hossain, M. A. 2010. Coproscopic and haematological approaches to determine the prevalence of helminthiasis and protozoan diseases of Red Chittagong Cattle (RCC) breed in Bangladesh. Pak. Vet. J., 30: 1-6.

[38] Silva, J. C., Ogassawara. S., Adania, C. H., Ferreira, F., Gennari, S. M., Dubey, J. P. and Ferreira-Neto, J. S. 2001. Seroprevalence of Toxoplasma gondii in captive neotropical felids from Brazil. Vet. Parasitol., 102: 217-224.

[39] Soares, H. S., Ahid, S. M. M., Bezerra, A. C. D. S., Pena, H. F. J., Dias, R. A. and Gennari, S. M. 2009. Prevalence of anti-Toxoplasma gondii and anti-Neospora caninum antibodies in sheep from Mossoro, Rio Grande do Norte. Brazil. Vet. Parasitol., 160: 211-214.

[40] Taghadosi, C., Kojouri, G. A. and Taheri, M. A. 2010. Detection of Toxoplasma antibodies in sera of Salmonidae by ELISA. Comp. Clin. Pathol., 19: 203-206.

[41] Van der Puije, W., Bosompem, K., Canacoo, E., Wastling, J. and Akanmori, B. 2000. The prevalence of anti-Toxoplasma gondii antibodies in Ghanaian sheep and goats. Acta Trop.76: 21-26.

[42] Yang, N., Li, H., He, J., Mu, M. and Yang, S. 2013. Seroprevalence of Toxoplasma gondii infection in domestic sheep in Liaoning Province, northeastern China. J. Parasitol., 99: 174-175.

[43] Yu, J., Xia, Z., Liu, Q., Liu, J., Ding, J. and Zhang, W. 2007.Sero-epidemiology of Neosporacaninum and Toxoplasma gondii in cattle and water buffaloes (Bubalus bubalis) in the People's Republic of China. J. Parasitol., 143: 79-85.

[44] Zewdu, E., Agonafir, A., Tessema, T. S., Tilahun, G., Medhin, G., Vitale, M., Di Marco. V., Cox, E., Vercruysse, J. and Dorny, P. 2013. Seroepidemiological study of caprine toxoplasmosis in East and West Shewa Zones, Oromia Regional State, Central Ethiopia.Res. Vet. Sci., 94: 43-8.

The Impact of Lead and Nickel Environmental Pollution on Blood Levels of Liver Enzymes in House Sparrow (*Passer domesticus*) in Kosovo

Lulzim Millaku[1, *], Resmije Imeri[2], Jeton Orllati[1], Artan Trebicka[3]

[1]Department of Biology, Mathematics & Natural Science Faculty, University of Prishtina, Prishtina, Kosovo
[2]Department of Biology, Agricultural & Veterinary Faculty, University of Prishtina, Prishtina, Kosovo
[3]Department of Biology, Natural Science Faculty, University of Tirana, Tirana, Albania

Email address:
lulzimmillaku@hotmail.com (L. Millaku)

Abstract: The aim of this study was the evaluation of environmental pollution with heavy metals such as Lead and Nickel on the living organisms in industrial areas, using the blood of House sparrow (*Passer domesticus*) as a bio-indicator of pollution by metals. For this purpose, a blood collection was performed on 32 house sparrows (*Passer domesticus*) males and females, which were captured in Mitrovica town (situated close to smelter "Trepqa", closed in year 2000), Drenas town (near the Ferronickel smelter, pollution area) and in rural area (Ujmir village, not contaminated area). In blood plasma we have analysed: alkaline phosphatase (AP), plasma alanin aminotransferase (ALT), aspartat aminotransferase (AST) and total proteins (TP) in house sparrow (*Passer domesticus*). The results obtained indicate the different values of the enzymes activity (AP, ALT, AST) in blood sparrows between the localities studied. Higher values of AST in significant scale ($p<0.001$) were found in sparrows from Mitrovica and Drenas town compared with the reference site (Ujmirë village). Values of enzymes ALT, AP and total proteins are different between the analyzed groups but the differences are not significant. Further studies are warranted to investigate the mechanism of susceptibility of house sparrow to environmental pollution.

Keywords: Metals, House Sparrow, Biochemical Parameters

1. Introduction

The natural environment has been gradually contaminated by various forms of pollution. A serious group of pollutants are heavy metals that pose a threat to all living organisms, with lead being especially considered as highly toxic [1]. Environmental levels of lead have increased more than 1,000-fold over the past three centuries as a result of human activity. The greatest increase occurred between the years 1950 and 2000, and reflected increasing worldwide use of leaded gasoline. Lead is a heavy, low melting, bluish-gray metal that occurs naturally in the Earth's crust. Most lead used by industry comes from mined ores ("primary") or from recycled scrap metal or batteries ("secondary") [2]. Lead can enter the environment through releases from mining lead and other metals, and from factories that make or use lead, lead alloys, or lead compounds [3]. Nickel normally occurs at very low levels in the environment, so very sensitive methods are needed to detect nickel in most environmental samples. In the environment, it is primarily found combined with oxygen or sulfur as oxides or sulfides. Nickel is released into the atmosphere during nickel mining and by industries that make or use nickel, nickel alloys, or nickel compounds. These industries also might discharge nickel in waste water. Nickel is also released into the atmosphere by oil-burning power plants, coal-burning power plants, and trash incinerators. A lot of nickel released into the environment ends up in soil or sediment where it strongly attaches to particles containing iron or manganese. Under acidic conditions, nickel is more mobile in soil and might seep into groundwater. Nickel does not appear to concentrate in fish. Studies show that some plants can take up and accumulate nickel. However, it has been shown that nickel does not accumulate in small animals living on land that has been treated with nickel-containing sludge [2].

The use of living organisms to monitor heavy metal

pollution provides more promising results than chemical and physical analysis. This results from the fact that we obtain accurate data of bioavailability and bio transference of contaminants as well as observe some physiological and behavioral symptoms of induced toxicity.

Most chemical analyses are conducted on plasma, although testing could also be performed on a serum sample. The reason for this is that collection of serum from birds frequently yields a very small sample size compared to what can be obtained from plasma. Plasma is preferred for routine blood biochemical evaluations of birds. Establishment of normal reference intervals for a given species of bird depends on many factors, including age, state of health, and nutrition. Because of the avian patient's ability to mask illness, it is often difficult to guarantee that a given bird is free of disease for inclusion into a population of normal healthy birds. Factors such as gender, age, temperature, humidity, photo period, season of the year, and time of day may influence the results of a particular analyze [4]. Many studies that are done in avian natural population, the different surroundings of lead and nickel smelters, show a positive correlation between the degree of pollution and accumulation of some heavy metals in different tissues, of different animals, such as urban pigeon - Columba livia [5], the magpies - pica [6], to swallow - hirundo rustica [7].

Alterations in the plasma activity of enzymes used to detect hepatic disease in birds can reflect either hepatocellular injury or increased enzyme production. The liver performs a number of functions and plays an important role in metabolic processes, detoxification of xenobiotics, and hematopoiesis. High aspartate aminotransferase (AST) activity has been reported in the liver of birds. High AST activity has also been found in skeletal muscle, heart muscle, brain, and kidney [8].

In this study, we investigated biochemical parameters as alkaline phosphatase (AP), plasma alanin aminotransferase (ALT), aspartat aminotransferase (AST) and total proteins (TP) in blood plasma of house sparrow (*Passer domesticus*). The purpose of this study was the comparison of biochemical blood parameters of house sparrow (*Passer domesticus*), caught in industrially polluted areas (Mitrovica and Drenas town) and reference areas (Ujmir village) to assess environmental pollution with heavy metals.

2. Materials and Methods

2.1. Study Areas

The pollution of living environment in Mitrovica still presents an ecological problem (the area near foundry "Trepqa" closed since 2000). The main recourses of pollution in Mitrovica, in the past had as starting point different technological departures (metals foundry, refinery, flotation, factory of accumulations and sulfuric acid battery) of "Trepqa" combine and also superphosphates fertilizer factory. The work of these departments has made Mitrovica one of the most polluted cities in Europe. The pollution level can be illustrated from some informations by Popovac [9], who find that the quantity of the emitted lead dust everyday from the Trepça foundry in 1979 was 5 to 6 tons. The concentration of lead in air in Mitrovica from the same period was 20-30 $\mu g/m^3$. Trepça Foundry was closed in August 14th 2000 from the United States Forces. The research that was done from Shehu's [10], analysis of soil taken in the location around Mitrovica had noticed high concentration. More than 13 years have passed by but the pollution left from Trepça's activities, threatens seriously the local environment and people's health.

Drenas town is located 20 kilometres far from Prishtina (capital of Republic of Kosovo) in the West. The smelter (Ferronickel) has operated since 1982. Ferronikeli has three open pit mines: the Dushkaja mine with estimated reserves of 6.2 million tonnes; the Suka mine-0.8 million tonnes and the Gllavica with 6.8 million tones. Ferronikeli smelter is well-known for final production of Ferro- nickel.

In metallurgical processing the mineral base is treated by an oxide mineral of nickel (two sources) with the following average chemical structure: Ni+Co=1.2%; Fe=26.0%; SiO_2=47.0%; CaO=2.5%; Cr_2O_3=1.2%; MgO=11.0%. The produced slag has the chemical structure as follows: Ni-0-08%; SiO_2 55-57 %; MgO 10.0%; Fe total 20%; Ca) 4.0%. The capacity of the smelter in the technological lines (rotating furnace and electrical furnace) is about 12.000 t Ni/year [11]. In recent time, the smelter plant is active and it is known as "New CO Ferronickel".

2.2. Blood Samples and Biochemical Analysis

A blood collection was performed on 32 house sparrows (*Passer domesticus*) males and females, which were captured in Mitrovica town (situated close to smelter "Trepqa", down closed in year 2000), Drenas town (near the Ferronickel smelter, pollution area) and in rural area (Ujmir village, not contaminated area). The blood samples were collected in heparinised tubes by puncturing the alvar vein in the region of the carpal vein joint, after first removing feathers in the area and thoroughly cleaning the skin. We have analyzed: alkaline phosphatase (AP), plasma alanin aminotransferase (ALT), aspartat aminotransferase (AST) and total proteins (TP) in blood plasma of house sparrows (*Passer domesticus*). All biochemical analyses were conducted with an automated analyser (Ciba Express 550).

Statistics: Statistical elaboration of biochemical parameters was done with the method *ANOVA* by determining the average of each indicator, standard deviation. Significant differences were assumed at $p<0.05$. For all statistical analyses, Sigma stat program was used.

3. Results and Discussion

Results of our study on the activity of transaminases (AST, ALT), alkaline phosphatase activity (AP) and total proteins (TP) in blood plasma of the house sparrow (*Passer domesticus*) caught in polluted industrial areas (Mitrovica and Drenas town) and reference area (Ujmir, village) are presented in table 1 and figure 1.

Table 1. *Biochemical values of house sparrow (Passer domesticus) from polluted site (Mitrovica and Drenas town) and reference site (Ujmir village).*

Blood (biochemical parameters)	Reference site	Polluted site	
	Ujmirë (10)	Drenas (12)	Mitrovicë (10)
ALT *(U/L)*	104.8 ± 68.9	205.6 ± 191.4	209.8 ± 199.7
AST *(U/L)*	379.6 ± 284.8	935.3*** ± 654.2	998.3** ± 619.1
AP *(U/L)*	180.8 ± 28.4	251.7 ± 53.4	237.1 ± 119.7
TP *(g/L)*	41.3 ± 10.1	40.1 ± 8.1	35.2 ± 3.5

Note: Values are expressed as means ± SD. In parentheses () number of birds. **P<0.01; ***P<0.001.

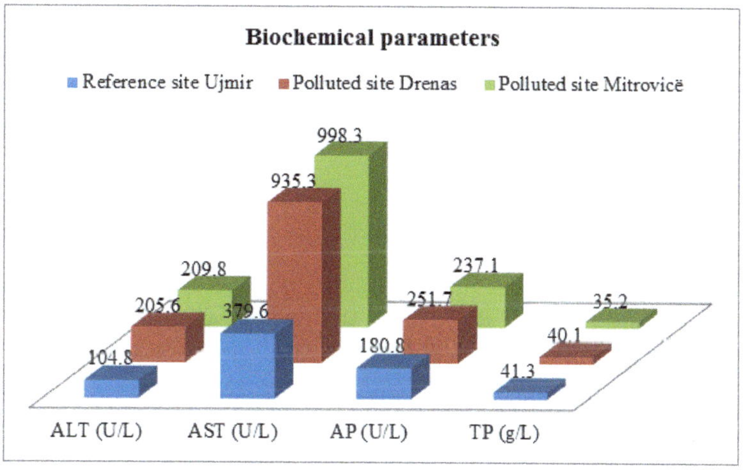

Fig. 1. *Mean concentrations of enzymes ALT, AST, AP (U/L) and TP (g/L).*

In general, increases of plasma AST activity in birds are suggested when such activity is greater than 275 U/L. Increases result from either hepatic or muscle injury, which allow the leakage of intracellular AST into the blood. Plasma AST activity is considered to be markedly increased when the activity is greater than 800 U/L. Activity of this magnitude is suggestive of severe hepatic insult, especially in the presence of biliverdinuria or biliverdinemia. However, increased AST activity does not provide information about hepatic function. It is useful to evaluate Creatine kinase (CK) activity in conjunction with AST activity to differentiate between muscle and liver injury [12, 13]. Increased plasma ALT activity may occur with muscle injury. Plasma ALT appears to have a longer half-life (mean of 11.99 hr from muscle) compared with plasma CK (mean of 3.07 hr from muscle); therefore, activity of ALT remains increased longer than CK does after muscle injury [14, 15]. Alanine aminotransferase (ALT) activity has been reported in the liver, skeletal muscle and many other tissues of birds, and leaks into blood when such tissues are injured.

Plasma ALT activity is considered to be neither a specific nor a sensitive test for hepatocellular injury in birds. Plasma ALT activity in most species of normal birds ranges from 19 to 50 U/L and may be more useful for the detection of hepatic disease in carnivorous birds. Plasma ALT activity increases with significant liver or muscle injury in birds (especially carnivores) and has no advantage compared with AST as a test for hepatocellular disease [12, 13]..

Alkaline phosphatase activity occurs in multiple tissues including bone and intestine, and increased plasma AP activity results not from leakage of the enzyme but from increased cellular production. Plasma AP activity in birds results primarily from osteoblastic activity. Therefore, increases in the plasma AP activity are suggestive of skeletal growth, nutritional secondary hyperparathyroidism, healing fractures, and the preovulation condition of medullary calcification in hens. Plasma AP activity is not useful in the detection of hepatobiliary disease in birds. Aflatoxin B1-induced liver necrosis and bile duct hyperplasia have not significantly increased the serum AP activity in the pigeon, cockatiel (*Nymphicus hollandicus*), great horned owl (*Bubo virginianus*), and red-tailed hawk (*Buteo jamaicensis*). Plasma AP activity appears to be a sensitive indicator of intestinal diseases, such as coccidial infections in the duodenum, jejunum, and cecum [14].

The normal plasma protein concentration in birds is less than that in mammals, generally ranging from 2.5 to 4.5 g/dL (25–45 g/L). Albumin, which represents 40–50% of the total plasma protein in birds, is produced in the liver. Other plasma proteins also produced in the liver include transport proteins, proteins of coagulation, fibrinogen, enzymes, and hormones. Immunoglobulin's produced by B lymphocytes and plasma cells represent a significant component of the total plasma protein concentration.

The normal plasma protein concentration is essential to the maintenance of the normal colloidal osmotic pressure, which preserves normal blood volume and pH. Hens demonstrate a marked increase in plasma total protein concentration just before egg production [15, 16]. This estrogen-induced hyperproteinemia is associated with an increase in vitellogenin and lipoproteins, which are necessary for yolk production. These proteins are produced in the liver, transported in the blood, and incorporated into the oocytes of the ovary.

Capture myopathy in Sandhill cranes (*Grus Canadensis tabida*) was associated with increased plasma activity of CK, AST, and LDH within 1 hour of capture [17]. The peak activity of these enzymes occurred 3 days following capture and by 10–17 days, CK and LDH activities had returned to normal; however, plasma AST activities were still 2–5 times higher than normal reference values.

The increase level of transaminases (ALT, AST) in the blood plasma of sparrows from Mitrovica and Drenas are in accordance with results of Rozhaja [18], in case of treatment with lead in laboratory mice and in cases of environmental pollution with this metal. In cases of acute liver damage, enzyme ALT values are higher than the values of AST [19].`

4. Conclusions

The changes in the biochemical parameters show that the house sparrow (*Passer domesticus*) can be used as a bioindikator of environmental pollution with lead and nickel. The results obtained are correlative but further studies are warranted to investigate the mechanism of susceptibility of thc house sparrow (*Passer domesticus*) to environmental pollution.

References

[1] Roux, E., Marra, P. 2007 "The presence and impact of environmental lead in Passerine birds along an urban to rural land use gradient". Arch Environ Contam Toxicol 53:261–268.

[2] Agency for Toxic Substances and Disease Registry. 1989. Agency for Toxic Substances and Disease Registry. Decision guideline for identifying substance-specific data needs related to toxicological profiles. Part V. Fed Regist 54:37619-37633.

[3] Miranda, M., Benedito, L., Blanco, I., Lopez, C., Merino, A., Lopez, M. 2009 "Metal accumulation in cattle raised in a serpentine - soil area: Relationship between metal concentrations in soil, forage and animal tissues". J. Trace Elem. Med. Biol., 23: 231- 238.

[4] Scope, A., Frommlet, F., Schwendenwein, I. 2004 "Circadian and seasonal variability and influence of sex and race on eight clinical chemistry parameters in budgerigars (*Melopsittacus undulatus*, Shaw, 1805)". *Res Vet Sci* 78: 85–91.

[5] Elezaj, R. I., Selimi I. Q., Letaj Rr. K., Kurteshi, H.K.(2001): The effects of air pollution by heavy metals on biochemical and hematological parameters of the feral pigeons *(Columba livia)* from Mitrovica and Prishtina area. Federation of American Societies for Experimental Biology (The FASEB Journal). Abstract Number: Volume 15, Number 4, A 54. 50.5. March 7.

[6] Hahn, E., Optapczuk, P., Ellenberg, H., Stoeppler, M. (1985): Environmetal monitoring of heavy metals with birds as pollution integrating biomonitors II. Cadmium, Lead and Copper in Magpie (Pica Pica) Feathers from heavy polluted and control area. Proceedings of International Conference "Heavy Metals in the Environment". Vol.1, pp. 721-723, Athens- September.

[7] Grue, C. E., O'Shea, O.J. (1984): Lead concentrations and reproduction in Highway-nestin Barn Swallows. The Condor, 86: 383-389.

[8] Franson, J.C., Murray, H.C., Bunck, C. 1985 "Enzyme activities in plasma, kidney, liver, and muscle of five avian species". *J Wildlife Dis.* 21: 33–9.

[9] Popovac, D., Colakovic, B., Popovac, R., Saljic, L., Rodorovic, P. 1981 "Environmental poll-ution in the industrial region of Mitrovica e Kosoves and possible effects on human health". Acta. Biol. Med. Exp., 6, 61-65.

[10] Shehu, I., Demaku S., Arbneshi, T., Jusufi, S., Shala, F., Dobra, B. 2011 "Heavy Metals in Landfill Waste of Trepça, after Flotation Process as Pollutants of Water and Soil". J. Int. Environmental Application and Science. 6 (3): 429 – 433.

[11] Rizaj, M., Beqiri, E., McBow, Z., Kongoli, F. 2008 "The mineral base and productive capacities of metals and non-metals of Kosovo". JOM. vol.60 No.8, 18-22.

[12] Lumeij, J.T. 1987. "A Contribution to Clinical Investigative Methods for Birds, with Special Reference to the Racing Pigeon (*Columbia livia domestica*)" [thesis]. Utrecht, Proefschrift.

[13] Lumeij, J.T. 1994 "Avian clinical enzymology". *Semin Avian Exotic Pet Med* 3: 14–24.

[14] Lumeij, J.T., De Bruijne, J.J., Slob, A. 1998. "Enzyme activities in tissues and elimination half-lives of homologous muscle and liver enzymes in the racing pigeon (*Columbia livia domestica*)". *Avian Pathol* 17: 851–64.

[15] Kogut, M.H., Powell, K.C. 1993 "Preliminary findings of alterations in serum alkaline phosphatase activity in chickens during coccidial infections". *J Comp Path* 108: 113–19.

[16] Johnson, A.L. 1986 "Reproduction in the female. In: Stukie PD (ed.)", *Avian Physiology*. New York: Springer-Verlag, pp. 403–31.

[17] Businga, N.K., Langenberg, J., Carlson, L. 2007 "Successful treatment of capture myopathy in three wild greater sandhill cranes [*Grus Canadensis tabida*]". *J Avian Med Surg* 21: 294–8.

[18] Rozhaja, D.A., Jablanoviq, M. 1983 "Ndotja dhe mbrojtja e ambientit të njeriut". Enti i teksteve dhe mjeteve mësimore, Prishtinë.

[19] Wolf, P.L., Williams, D., Von Der Muehll, E. 1973 "Practical clinical enzymology: Techniques and interpretations and biochemical profiling" pp. 215-226. John Wiley and Sons, Inc., New York.

31

Growth of different infectious bursal disease virus strains in cell lines from origin of lymphoid leukosis tumors

Ahmed Hassan[1, 2, *], Mostafa Shahata[2], Elrefaie Refaie[2], Ragab Ibrahim[2], Jun Sasaki[1], Masanubu Goryo[1]

[1]Department of Veterinary Pathology, Faculty of Agriculture, Iwate University, 3-18-8, Ueda, Morioka, 020-8550, Japan
[2]Department of Poultry diseases, Faculty of Veterinary Medicine, Assiut University, Assiut, 71526, Egypt

Email address:
khalaf_poultry@yahoo.com (A. Hassan)

Abstrac: Growth and propagation of infectious bursal disease virus (IBDV) in chicken embryo is time consuming and costly, and an appropriate serological test is required to detect and identify IBDV strains, therefore, a suitable cell lines in which different IBDV strains can grow well has been needed. The aim of the present work was to study the growth of different IBDV strains in cell lines from lymphoid leukosis tumors using histopathological staining, indirect immunofluorescence, immunohistochemistry and transmission electron microscopic examination. In conclusion, cell lines from origin of lymphoid leukosis tumors; LSCC-BK3 and LSCC-CU10 are suitable for growth and propagation of different IBDV strains. IBDV strains resulted into histopathological lesions of variable severity differ according to the patho-type of IBDV and time after virus inoculation. Indirect immunofluorescent test could be used for detection and differentiation of IBDV strains inoculated into cell lines from origin of lymphoid leukosis tumors. Trials of immunohistochemistry technique for detection of different IBDV strains in cell lines, were unsuccessful. Using transmission electron microscopy, IBDV particles could be detected in all infected cell lines.

Keywords: Infectious Bursal Disease Virus, Cell Lines, Histopathological Staining, Immunohistochemistry, Immunofluorescence

1. Introduction

Infectious bursal disease (IBD) was first described in 1962 [2]. IBD is one of the most economically important diseases that affect chickens and it possesses a great threat to the poultry industry worldwide [9].The economic importance of the disease is manifested in two ways. Firstly, some virus strains may cause mortalities up to 30% or more in three to six weeks old birds [9]. Secondly, and very importantly, the manifestation of severe, prolonged immunosuppression in chickens infected at early age and which have recovered [29].The immunosuppression increases the risk of secondary infection and reduces antibody response to vaccinations [21].The etiological agent of IBD is a double stranded RNA virus which is nonenveloped and icosahedral in symmetry [13]. The virus is resistant to ether and chloroform, to extremes of PH, high temperatures and some disinfectants, which is why the viral particles persist in poultry farms [16]. The disease is seen mostly in chickens between 3 to 6 weeks old, and common signs will include rapid drop in feed and water consumption, whitish to greenish-white diarrhea with soiled vent, ruffled feathers and listlessness with unsteady gait or sitting in hunched position, vent picking and sleeping with beak touching the floor. IBD virus primarily affects the bursa of Fabricius, resulting in inflammation and swelling and leading to damage of the organ with consequent immunosuppression [26]. Biosecurity measures and proper vaccinations are used in the control of IBD [30].

***Table (1).** Results of histopathological changes in different cell lines at different intervals after infection with different four IBDV strains.*

DPI[a]	Cell lines/Strains									
	993		JI		BDA		Ni		control	
	Lscc-cu10	Lscc-bk3	Lscc-cu10	Lscc-bk3	Lscc-cu10	Lscc-bk3	Lscc-cu10	Lscc-bk3	Lscc-cu10	Lscc-bk3
1 day	+	+	+	+	-	-	-	-	-	-
2 days	++	++	++	++	+	+	+	+	-	-
3 days	+++	+++	+++	+++	++	++	++	++	-	-

[a] Days post-inoculation
(-) Non visible, (+) mild, (++)moderate, (+++) sever.
BDA: IBDV- BDA strain (Vaccine I strain), Ni: Nisseiken strain (Vaccine I strain)

Detection and identification of IBDV strains have been performed in chick embryos [8] because IBDV does not grow well in cell cultures originating from chickens or other animals [15, 23]. Examination of IBDV in chicken embryo is time consuming and costly, and an appropriate serological test is required to detect and identify IBDV strains, so it is impossible to examine many viral samples at once when using chicken embryo [31]. Therefore, a suitable cell lines in which different IBDV strains can grow well has been needed.

It was reported that LSCC-CU 10 line cells derived from a lymphoid leukosis tumor was susceptible to IBDV [6]. It was concluded that LSCC-BK3 line was more susceptible to IBDV and could be used for detection and identification of the virus [31].

The aim of the present work was to study the growth of different IBDV strains in cell lines from lymphoid leukosis tumors using histopathological staining, indirect immunofluorescence, immunohistochemistry and transmission electron microscopic examination.

2. Materials and Methods

2.1. Cell lines and IBDV Strains

Established cell lines; LSCC-BK3, which originated from lymphoid leukosis lymphomatous bursa [5] and LSCC-CU10, which originated from lymphoid leukosis transplant TLT [1], were used for growth and propagation of IBDV strains; Very virulent IBDV 993 strain [4], moderately virulent IBDV J1 strain [31], Vaccine strain I: IBDV-BDA vaccine strain (Embrex Inc., Japan) and Vaccine strain II: Nisseiken vaccine strain (Nisseiken Co. Ltd, Japan). The growth medium for cell lines consisted of nutrient mixtures RPMI-1640 (Nisssuri) supplemented with 10% fetal bovine serum, 0.15% dehydrated tryptose phosphate broth (Difco), 100 units of penicillin, and 0.1 mg of streptomycine per ml.

2.2. IBD Virus Inoculation into Cell Lines and Samples Collection

1 ml from each IBDV strains was centerifugated at 104 RPM for 5 minutes and 0.5 ml of supernatant was mixed with 4.5 ml of growth mixture and then filtered using cellulose filter in petri dishes. 1 ml from each cell line containing 5 x 105 was added to each petri dish. Control cell lines without virus inoculation were prepared. All cell lines were incubated at 37 °C with 5% CO2 for 3 days. 1 ml from each petri dish, including IBDV inoculated and control cell lines, was collected at 1, 2, and 3 days post inoculation, then centerifugated at 1.24 RPM for 5 minutes and discard supernatant then the washed 3 successive times with phosphate buffer saline (PBS). Slides were prepared from collected cell line samples then used for histopathology, indirect immunoflurocsence, and immunohistochemistry.

2.3. Histopathology

Slides which prepared from collected cell line samples at 1, 2, and 3 days post inoculation were fixed using acetone then deparaffinized in xylene, rehydrated by passing through descending grades of ethyl alcohol to distilled water, and stained by hematoxylin and esosin, mounted with neutral balsam. The stained sections were observed under microscope for assessing histopathological changes. The severity of histological lesions was scored as non visible (-), mild (+), moderate (++) or sever (+++).

2.4. Indirect Immunoflurocsence

Slides which prepared from collected cell line samples at 1, 2, and 3 days post inoculation were fixed using acetone then deparaffinized and hydrated. Cell line sections were covered with 0.1% trypsin Ca (antigen retrieval) for one hour at 37 °C. Sections were incubated with polyclonal chicken anti serum to IBD virus (1/10) overnight at 4 °C in a humidified chamber. After being rinsed three times for 5 min each with TBS, the sections were incubated with Fluorescein isothiocyanate (FITC)-labeled secondary antibody (1/200) for 30 minutes at 37 °C. After a rinse with TPS, the sections were mounted. The procedure for negative control sections was the same as described above except the primary antibodies were substituted with PBS. The immunofluorescence results was scored as none visible (-), mild (+), moderate (++) or sever (+++).

2.5. Immunohistochemistry

Slides which prepared from collected cell line samples at 1, 2, and 3 days post inoculation were fixed using acetone then deparaffinized and hydrated. Cell line sections were covered with 0.1% trypsin Ca (antigen retrieval) for one hour at 37 °C. The endogenous peroxidase activities were removed with 1% (v/v) hydrogen peroxide (H2O2), and the non-specific binding sites were blocked by 10% normal goat serum for 20 minutes at room temperature. Sections were incubated with polyclonal chicken anti serum to IBD virus (1/10) overnight at 4 °C in a humidified chamber. After being rinsed three times for 5 min each with TBS, the sections were incubated with peroxidase-labeled rabbit anti-chicken IgG (1/200) for 30 minutes at 37 °C. After a rinse with TPS, the sections were reacted for 4 minutes with 0.02% (w/v) 3,3-diaminobenzidine (DAB)-4HCL and 0.001% (v/v) H2O2 in 100 mM distilled water, Subsequently, the sections were counterstained with hematoxylin and dehydrated and mounted. The procedure for negative control sections was the same as described above except the primary antibodies were substituted with PBS. The immunohistochemical lesions was scored as none visible (-), mild (+), moderate (++) or sever (+++).

2.6. Transmission Electron Microscopic Examination

Cell line samples which collected at 1, 2, and 3 days post inoculation were fixed using 25% glutaraldehyde for 1 day then washed 3 times with PBS and incubated at 4 °C for 1 day. Cell line samples were post-fixed using 1% osmic acid for 2 hours and then dehydrated and replaced using ascending grades of ethyl alcohol, butyl-glycidyl ether (QY-1), QY-1 + Epon, and Epon. Cell line samples were embedded in Epon at 60 °C for 3 days. Epon embedded blocks were trimmed to expose cell line samples then roughly sectioned using glass knife and stained by toluidine blue. Thin sections (0.5 µm) were cut using platinum knife and then sliced and mounted on sheet mesh. Samples were stained with both uranium acetate and lead salt aqueous solution. The stained cell line sections were observed under transition electron microscope for detection virus particles.

3. Results

3.1. Histopathology

Results of histopathologic staining are shown as lesion scores in table (2).

Table (2). *Results of indirect immunofluroscence technique of various cell lines at different intervals following inculation with different IBDV strains.*

DPI[a]	Cell lines/Strains									
	993		JI		BDA		Ni		control	
	Lscc-cu10	Lscc-bk3	Lscc-cu10	Lscc-bk3	Lscc-cu10	Lscc-bk3	Lscc-cu10	Lscc-bk3	Lscc-cu10	Lscc-bk3
1 day	+	+	-	-	-	-	-	-	-	-
2 days	++	+	+	+	-	-	-	-	-	-
3 days	++	++	+	+	+	+	+	+	-	-

[a] Days post-inoculation
(-) Non visible, (+) mild, (++) moderate, (+++) sever.
BDA: IBDV- BDA strain (Vaccine I strain), Ni: Nisseiken strain (Vaccine I strain)

No histological changes were observed in control cell lines, whereas other infected cell lines with each of the four strain of IBDV showed degeneration and necrosis of lymphocytes as shown in figure (1).

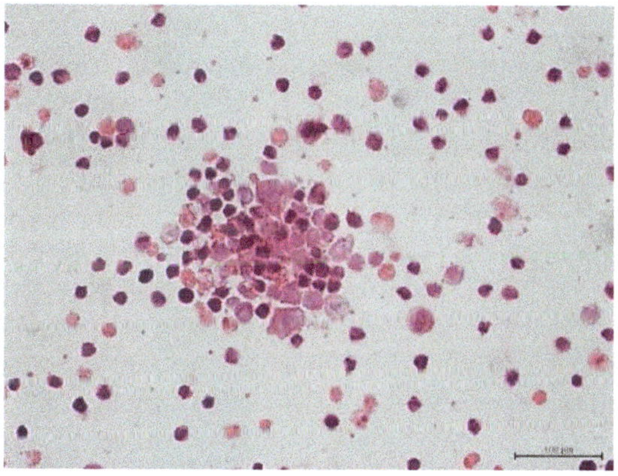

Figure (1). *Histopathology, LSCC-CU10 cell line infected with vvIBDV 993 strain 3 days post infection, showing degeneration and necrosis of lymphocytes, (magnification 40X).*

It was observed that histological changes in cell lines increased in severity with the time post inoculation. It was recorded that vvIBDV (993) strain resulted in lesion scores similar to virulent (J1) strain, while both vaccine strains resulted into similar lesion scores which are less in severity than vvIBDV and virulent strains.

3.2. Indirect Immunofluorescence

Indirect immunofluorescence technique was used to detect viral antigen of IBDV in LSCC-CU10 and LSCC-BK3 cell lines infected with 993 (vvIBDV), J1 (moderately virulent IBDV) and vaccine strains of IBDV. Results revealed that IBDV antigen could be detected abundantly, moderately and rarely in cell lines infected with 993, J1 and vaccine strains of IBDV, respectively at 1, 2 and 3 days post inoculation as shown in table (2). The positive reaction for immunofluorescense in cell lines appears as immunofluoresent green color [Figure (2)].

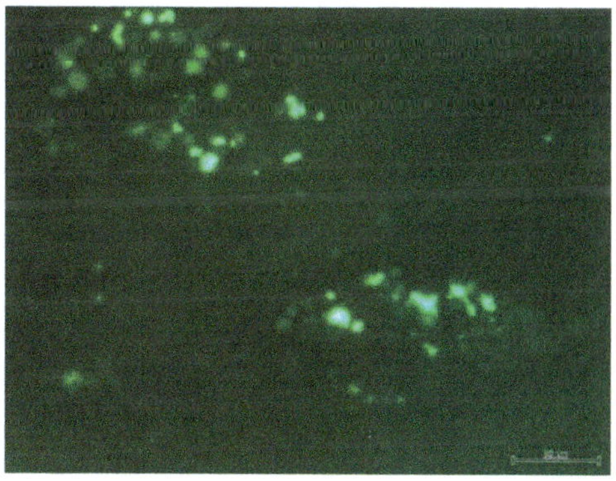

Figure (2). *Immunofluorescence, fluoresent antigens in cytoplasm of the LSCC-BK3 cell line infected with vvIBDV 993 strain 3 days post infection (magnification 40X), the viral antigen appears as immunofluoresent green color.*

Control cell lines showed negative results for immunofluorescence technique.

3.3. Immunohistochemistry

Immunohistochemistry technique was used to detect viral antigen of IBDV in LSCC-CU10 and LSCC-BK3 cell lines infected with 993 (vvIBDV), J1 (moderately virulent IBDV) and vaccine strains of IBDV. Results revealed that trials of immunohistochemistry technique for detection of different IBDV strains in cell lines, were unsuccessful.

3.4. Transmission Electron Microscopic Examination

Transmission Electron Microscopic examination was used to detect viral antigen of IBDV in LSCC-CU10 and LSCC-BK3 cell lines infected with 993 (vvIBDV), J1 (moderately virulent IBDV) and vaccine strains of IBDV. Results revealed that IBDV particles could be detected in all infected cell lines at 2 days post infection. IBDV particles 62 nm in diameter were recognized in the cytoplasm of infected cells by electron microscopy as shown in figure (3).

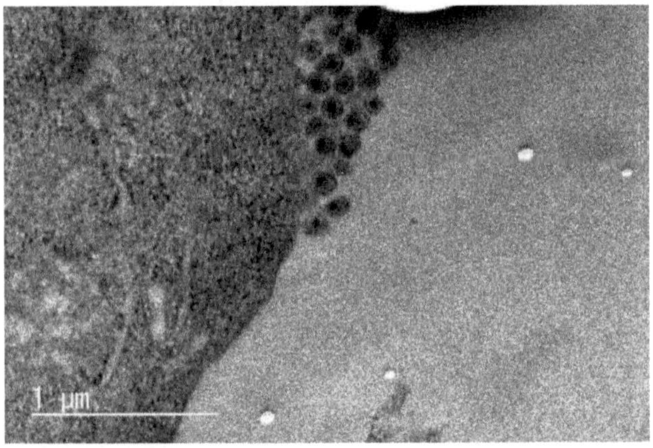

Figure (3). *Transmission Electron Microscopy, electron micrograph of LSCC-CU10 cell line infected with moderately virulent J1 strain 2 days post infection, clusters of virus particles are seen in cytoplasm (magnification 100,000 X).*

No virus particles were detected in control cell lines.

4. Discussion

IBDV has been successfully adapted to cell lines originated from chicken embryo, including chicken embryo bursal cells, kidney cells, and fibroblast cells [3, 15, 20, 25, 27]. IBDV also has been propagated on cell cultures including turkey and duck embryo cells [20], mammalian cell lines derived from rabbit kidneys [24], Vero cells [7, 10, 17], derived from African green monkey kidneys; BGM-70 cells [10], derived from givet monkey kidneys; and MA-104 cells [10] from fetal rhesus monkey kidneys. IBDV may be adapted to cell line, but isolation and propagation of some IBDV strains may be difficult with this technique [14, 19, 22, 25, 28]. Results of our study indicated that cell lines from origin of lymphoid leukosis tumors including LSCC-BK3 and LSCC-CU10 are suitable for growth and propagation of different IBDV strains. Our research scored the severity of histological lesions in these cell lines 1,2 and 3 days post inoculation with different IBDV strains and results revealed that cell lines showed degeneration and necrosis of cells with variable severity differ according to the patho-type of IBDV and time after virus inoculation. It was observed that histological changes in cell lines increased in severity with the time post inoculation. It was recorded that vvIBDV (993) strain resulted in lesion scores similar to virulent (J1) strain, while both vaccine strains resulted into similar lesion scores which are less in severity than vvIBDV and virulent strains.

Indirect mmunoflorescence technique [18] and electron microscopic examination [20] of the infected cell line or embryonating eggs are suitable methods for observation the growth and propagation of IBDV. It is possible to grow IBDV in transformed cell lines [6, 11, 12, 13, 15, 31]. In the present study, indirect immunofluorescence technique was used to detect viral antigen of IBDV in LSCC-CU10 and LSCC-BK3 cell lines infected with 993 (vvIBDV), J1 (moderately virulent IBDV) and vaccine strains of IBDV. Results revealed that IBDV antigen could be detected abundantly, moderately and rarely in cell lines infected with 993, J1 and vaccine strains of IBDV, respectively at 1, 2 and 3 days post inoculation. In our study, transmission electron microscopic examination was used to detect viral antigen of different IBDV in the same cell lines and results indicated that IBDV particles could be detected in all infected cell lines at 2 days post infection. IBDV particles 62 nm in diameter were recognized in the cytoplasm of infected cells by electron microscopy.

Trials of immunohistochemistry technique were used to detect viral antigen of IBDV in LSCC-CU10 and LSCC-BK3 cell lines infected with 993, J1 and vaccine strains of IBDV, but results reported that all these trials, were unsuccessful. Further studies are required to understand why immunohistochemistry is unable to detect IBDV in infected cell lines.

In conclusion, Cell lines from origin of lymphoid leukosis tumors; LSCC-BK3 and LSCC-CU10 are suitable for growth and propagation of different IBDV strains. IBDV strains resulted into histopathological lesions of variable severity differ according to the patho-type of IBDV and time after virus inoculation. Indirect immunofluorescent test could be used for detection and differentiation of IBDV strians inoculated into cell lines from origin of lymphoid leukosis tumors. Trials of immunohistochemistry technique for detection of different IBDV strains in cell lines, were unsuccessful. Using transmission electron microscopy, IBDV particles could be detected in all infected cell lines.

Acknowledgments

The authors would like to thank the stuff members of laboratory of Veterinary Pathology, Iwate university for their help to finish this work. The authors acknowledge the financial support of Egyptian government represented by Ministry of higher education scholarship.

References

[1] Calnek, BW, Murthy, KK and Schat, KA. Establishment of Marek's disease lymphoblastoid cell lines from transplantable versus primary lymphomas. Int J Cancer 1978; 21: 100-107.

[2] Cosgrove, AS. An apparently new disease of chickens – avian nephrosis. Avian Dis 1962; 6: 385-389.

[3] Eterradossi, N and Saif, YM. Infectious Bursal Disease. In Saif, YM, Fadly, AM , Glisson, JR, McDougald, LR, Nolan, LK and Swayne, DE, editors. Diseases of Poultry, 12th ed, Ames, Iowa, USA: Blackwell Publishing Professional; 2008, p. 185-208.

[4] Goryo, M. Experimental study of very virulent infectious bursal disease virus (vvIBDV). Avian Dis 1992; 36: 13-22.

[5] Hihara, H, Yamamato, H, Arai, K, Okazaki, W and Shimizu, T. Conditions for successful cultivation of tumor cells from chickens with avian lymphoid leukosis. Avian Dis 1980; 24: 971:979.

[6] Hirai, K and Calnek, BW. In vitro replication of infectious bursal disease virus in established lymphoid cell lines and chicken B lymphocytes. Infect Immun 1979; 25: 964 970.

[7] Hirai, K. and Shimakura, S. Structure of infectious bursal disease virus. J Virol 1974; 14: 957-964.

[8] Hitchner, SB. Infectivity of infectious bursal disease virus for embryonating eggs. Poult Sci 1970; 49: 511-516.

[9] Hussain, I, Rasool, MH and Mahmood, MS. Production of hyperimmune serum against infectious bursal disease virus in rabbits. Pak Vet J 2004; 24: 179-183.

[10] Jackwood, DH, Saif, YM and Hughes, JH. Replication of infectious bursal disease virus in continuous cell lines. Avian Dis 1987; 31: 370-375.

[11] Kibenge, FSB, Dhillon, AS and Russell, RG. Growth of serotypes I and II and variant strains of infectious bursal disease virus in vero cells. Avian Dis 1988; 17: 298-303.

[12] Kibenge, FSB, Dhillon, AS and Russell, RG. Biochemistry and immunology of infectious bursal disease virus. J Gen Virol 1988; 69: 1757-1775.

[13] Kibenge, FSB, McKenna, PK and Dybing, JK. Genome cloning and analysis of the large RNA segment (segment A) of a naturally avirulent serotype 2 infectious bursal disease virus. Virology 1991; 184: 437-40.

[14] Lee, LH and Lukert, PD. Adaptation and antigenic variation of infectious bursal disease virus. J Chin Soci Vet Sci 1986; 12: 297-304.

[15] Lukert, PD. and Davis, RB. Infectious bursal disease virus: growth and characterization in cell cultures. Avian Dis 1974; 18: 243-250.

[16] Lukert, PD and Saif, YM. Infectious bursal disease virus. In: Calnek, BW, Barnes, HJ, Beard, CW, Mc Dougald, LR and Saif, YM, editors. Diseases of Poultry, 10th ed. Ames, Iowa, USA: Iowa State University Press; 1997, p.721-738.

[17] Lukert, PD, Leonard, J and Davis, RB. Infectious bursal disease virus: Antigen production and immunity. Am J Vet Res 1975; 36: 539-540.

[18] MacDonald, RD. Immunofluorescent detection of double-stranded RNA in cells infected with reovirus, infectious pancreatic necrosis virus, and infectious bursal disease virus. Can J Microbiol 1980; 26: 256-261.

[19] McFerran, JB, McNutly, M, McKilliop, ER, Conner, TJ, McCracken, RM, Collins, DS and Allan, GM. Isolation and serological studies with infectious bursal disease virus from fowl, turkeys and ducks: demonstration of a second serotype. Avian Pathol 1980; 9: 395-404.

[20] McNulty, MS, Allan, GM and Mc Ferran, JB. Isolation of infectious bursal disease virus from turkeys. Avian Pathol 1979; 8: 205-212.

[21] Muller, H, Islam, MR and Raue, R. Research on infectious bursal disease – The past, the present, and the future. Vet Microbiol 2003; 97:153-165.

[22] Muller, H, Lange, H and Becht, H. Formation, characterization and interfering capacity of a small plaque mutant and of incomplete virus particles of infectious bursal disease virus. Virus Res 1986; 4: 297-309.

[23] Petek, M, D'Aprile, PN and Cancellotti, F. Biological and physicochemical properties of the infectious bursal disease virus (IBDV). Avian Pathol 1973; 2: 135-152.

[24] Rinaldi, A, Lodetti, E, Cessi, D, Lodrini, E, Cervio, G and Nardelli, L. Coltura del virus de Gumboro (IBA) su fibroblast de embrioni di pollo. Nuova Vet 1972; 48: 195-201.

[25] Rosenberger, JK, Saif, YM and Jackwood, DJ. Infectious Bursal Disease. In: Dufour-Zavala, L, Swayne, DE, Glisson, J. RJ, Pearson, E, Reed, WM, Jackwood, MW and Woolcock, PR, editors. A laboratory manual for the isolation and identification of avian pathogens 5th ed, American Association of Avian Pathologists; 2008 p. 188-190.

[26] Roy, P, Raja, A and Dhillon, AS. Counterimmunoelectrophoresis for diagnosis of infectious bursal disease: comparative efficacy of three different electrophoresis buffers. J. Appl Poult Res 2008; 17: 116-120.

[27] Skeeles, JK and Lukert, PD. Studies with an attenuated cell-culture-adapted infectious bursal disease virus: Replication sites and persistence of the virus in specific-pathogen-free chickens. Avian Dis 1980; 24: 43-47.

[28] Tsukamoto, K, Matsumura, T, Mase, M. and Imai, K. A highly sensitive, broad spectrum infectivity assay for infectious bursal disease virus. Avian Dis 1995; 39: 575-586.

[29] Van den Berg, TP. Acute infectious bursal disease in poultry: a review. Avian Pathol 2000; 29: 175-194.

[30] Vieltiz, E. Aspects of Protection against Gumboro virus. Zoo International 1993; 16: 42-49.

[31] Yamaguchi, S, Imada, I and Kawamura, H. Growth and infectivity titration of virulent infectious bursal disease virus in established cell lines from lymphoid leukosis. Avian Dis 1981; 25: 927-935.

32

Investigation of Biometric Sexual Differences on Humeral Articular Surfaces of New Zealand Rabbits via Photogrammetric Techniques

Abdullah Varlik[1], Sema Ozkadif[2, *], Emrullah Eken[3], Ibrahim Kalayci[1]

[1]Department of Geodesy and Photogrammetry, Faculty of Architecture and Engineering, Necmettin Erbakan University, Konya, Turkey
[2]Department of Nursing, School of Health, Batman University, Batman, Turkey
[3]Department of Anatomy, Faculty of Veterinary Medicine, Selcuk University, Konya, Turkey

Email address:
avarlik@konya.edu.tr (A. Varlık), semaerten80@gmail.com (S. Ozkadif), eeken@selcuk.edu.tr (E. Eken), ikalaycı@konya.edu.tr (I. Kalayci)

Abstract: The glenohumeral joint is a one of the joints most of which frequently dislocate. Moreover, in this joint various developmental disorders and pathological situations can be seen. The fact that it can perform the widest and the most diverse movements of our body makes the joint surfaces constituting the joint important. Therefore, in this study, surface areas of humeral head and glenoid cavity which form glenohumeral joint of 12 New Zealand rabbits of both sexes were measured, and their proportions to each other were determined on a three dimensional (3D) model obtained via photogrammetric methods. In conclusion, a statistically significant difference was identified between male and female rabbits regarding the joint surfaces constituting glenohumeral joint. Moreover, it was observed that the surface of humeral head was 3 times as large as the surface area of glenoid cavity. It has been suggested that the photogrammetric method that was used and the data that were obtained will shed light on forensic medicine applications and contribute to the information pool in the field of anatomy in veterinary medicine.

Keywords: Glenohumeral Joint, Photogrammetry, Rabbit, Surface Area, Three Dimensional Reconstruction

1. Introduction

Various cases such as developmental anomalies, fractures, dislocations, arthritis, different inflammatory and tumoral phenomena can be encountered in shoulder (glenohumeral) joint. Due to this critical significance of the area, morphometric studies in this regard gain importance at the stages of both diagnosis and treatment [1]. Before some simple surgical interventions, simulations of the shoulder joint can be used after making a 3D model of it [2]. The morphology of glenoid cavity and definition of various parameters were conducted on a reconstructed 3D model formed from computed tomography (CT) images [3]. 3D models are useful in shoulder arthroplasty especially in cases where pre-surgical planning is necessary [4].

Analysis and morphometry of human or animal bones, especially of their uneven surfaces is quite difficult. Various approaches exist to create 3D models of objects that have different shapes and characteristics. Among them are 3D coordinate measurement machines (CMM), laser scanning, photogrammetry and robotic methods. The most suitable method to create a 3D model in terms of both precision and cost, photogrammetry is regarded as a reliable method that deserves to be preferred in the examination and evaluation of bones [5]. Photogrammetric methods are quite advantageous in that they cost little, patients are not exposed to radiation and desired measurement values can be taken via the model formed [6]. Photogrammetry is a technology and branch of science where reliable information is obtained about objects and environment by recording, measuring and interpreting the photographic images formed by rays radiating from objects and the environment created by them. This method is used with high precision to identify measure and interpret the formal and characteristic properties of animate and inanimate beings. The greatest advantage of photogrammetry over the other methods of measurement is that measurements are taken on the photographic projection of the object rather than directly on the object. This property of indirect measurement allows photogrammetry to be used in different fields [7].

A photogrammetric system was formed to identify deformation that occurred in the vertebrae due to scoliosis and to monitor its progress, a 3D body model was created and measurements were taken on it [6].

Photogrammetric studies are also used in dentistry. In an orthodontic study, a 3D skull model created by making a photogrammetric evaluation of the images taken from 5 different angles and positions instead of X-ray images [8].

In addition, deformation analyses are also made using photogrammetric methods in veterinary surgery. Method was developed to measure deformation in horse hooves in different weight conditions and the hooves were evaluated photogrammetrically after their photographs were taken [9]. Photogrammetric technique was assessed for the characterization of equine foot volume changes associated with foot trimming [10].

Photogrammetric methods began to be used in veterinary anatomy studies, too. Different measurements were taken on a 3D model of the joint surfaces of the bones forming the shoulder joints of sheep, cats and rabbits created through photogrammetric methods, and differences among the species were revealed irrespective of gender [11]. Glenoid cavity which constitutes the shoulder joint, exhibits differences between the genders [12].

3D photogrammetry technique was developed to estimate morphometrics and body mass of Steller sea lions (*Eumetopias jubatus*) [13]. And also researches applied photogrammetric techniques to photographs taken by bird over 70 years ago, before the trackway was removed to digitally reconstruct the site as it was prior to excavation [14].

A review of literature that was conducted revealed that there were no studies explaining the morphometric properties in males and females of humeral head and glenoid cavity, which form the shoulder joint of the New Zealand rabbit. In order to meet this shortcoming in the relevant literature, measurements were taken on a 3D model created through photogrammetric methods, and a study was conducted to see the proportions of joint surfaces in terms of area and to determine whether the morphometric measurement values were statistically significant between the sexes.

2. Materials and Methods

The bones used in the study were obtained from New Zealand rabbits used in a project completed in early 2011 and supported by Coordination Office of Selcuk University Scientific Research Projects. Also it was accepted by the ethics committee of the Veterinary Faculty of Selçuk University on 24 June 2009 (decision number: 2009/056).

2.1. Age and Weight

In this study, a total of 12 New Zealand rabbits, 6 male and 6 female, aged 1-1.5 years and weighing between 3 and 3.5 kg, were used.

2.2. Dissection

Rabbits were duly slaughtered and then the upper extremities were taken from the animals' bodies after dissecting them. The upper extremities, which were taken together with muscles and fat, were boiled in potassium hydroxide solution in order to rid them of these tissues. Scapula and humerus, which constitute glenohumeral joint, were thoroughly cleaned.

2.3. Photogrammetric Assessment

As a basis for photogrammetric assessment, objects need to be defined within a known coordinate system or coordinates need to be assigned to some points on the object during the taking of photographs (Fig.1). Since it is virtually impossible to measure the 3D coordinates of the points on the object via traditional methods, a new device was designed and coded targets were used for the control points.

Coded targets can be used to define a local coordinate system and model scale or to make accurate matching in picture alignment. The identification and matching of the coded targets in pictures is performed automatically by the software. The automatic marking of the targets saves time compared with the manual marking and alignment of the targets and produces more precise results than manual marking.

The measurements of the target points were also measured using this device. These points, which were measured and taken as known during the evaluation process, were measured two dimensional (2D) using a compass having a precision of 1/20 mm.

Before photographs were taken, marks whose coordinates were known but had a size of 1.5mm so as to yield clear images in the pictures taken were made on the bones surfaces randomly and in a way to be seen in all pictures.

The geometry of taking photographs has a significant place in the field of photogrammetric picture taking. In the study, a photograph scale was determined depending on the size of the object and taking into account the digital camera used, as well as a B/H (base height) rate in accordance with this photograph scale and a shooting angle (plan). Pictures belonging to the object surfaces were taken using a 16-megapixel Sony DSC-W570 digital camera by raising the camera at an angle of about 30° at an equal distance to the object, at a rate of 70 % overlapping with one another and with a Base/Height ratio of 1/3 (Fig. 2)

Photoscan software was used in our study for photogrammetric evaluation. First, the internal routing elements of the camera used were calculated. The internal routing procedure requires reconstruction of the perspective rays of the setup in the camera in similar conditions. With this procedure, the focal length of the camera (f), coordinates of the projection center (x_p, y_p), radial distortion (k_1,k_2,k_3) and tangential distortion (p_1,p_2) values were calculated. The camera used in the study had been calibrated in previous studies and its calibration values were given in Table 1.

The photogrammetric evaluation procedural steps of the

Photoscan software consist of photograph alignment, formation of dense point clouds, formation of 3D model grid network, model tissue coating and location-referencing.

During the photograph alignment procedure, the software perceives the coded target points on the pictures automatically, performs automatic matching between the pictures and creates connection points by finding common points outside these coded target points. The position and routings of the camera during a photograph shooting are calculated by the help of these points. After this procedure, a point cloud model is created by making intensive point matching procedure between the stereo photograph couples (Fig. 3).

The georeferencing of the model is performed by conducting a 7-parameter (3- shifts, 3- rotation, 1 scale) transformation with at least three points whose real world coordinates are known. Since only the real dimensions of the model were needed in our study, transformation was implemented by scaling the model using the lengths between the coded target points. After the transformation, the differences between the real lengths of the control points and their calculated lengths were calculated by the software. Table 2 shows the results of a model belonging to the left humerus of a female New Zealand rabbit.

After conducting the georeferencing of the model, a digital surface model was formed by creating a 3D grid network from the dense point cloud (Fig. 4), and then the real 3D model of the object was obtained by coating (covering) the picture texture (Fig. 5). These procedures were performed for each bone and thus real 3D models were obtained for all the bones. The overall mean errors of the models that were obtained remained at about 0.00007 m (0.07 mm). In other words, measurements can be taken on our models at a precision rate of 0.1 mm.

The joint surface of the bones were selected manually on the real 3D models that were formed and thus their surface areas were measured (Fig. 6).

2.4. Statistical Analysis

The statistical analisis was performed by using SPSS 16.00 for Windows. The independent samples t-test was carried out and the mean values, standart deviations and P-values of surface area belonging to glenohumeral joint in the right and left side for males and females were calculated.

Nomina Anatomica Veterinaria [15] was used in terminology.

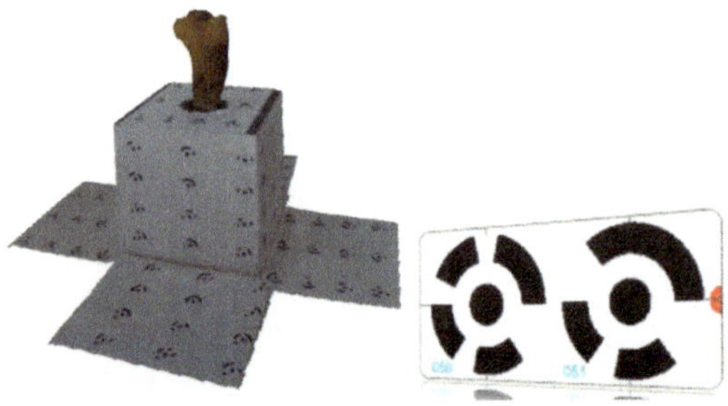

(a) (b)

Figure 1. *The device used to take photographs and coded target points (a, b).*

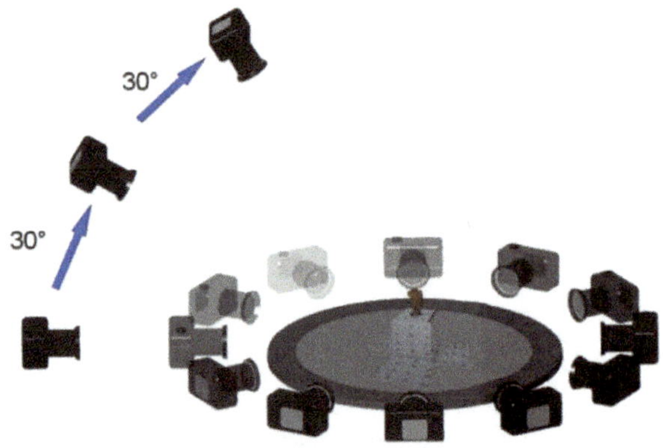

Figure 2. *The simulated picture-taking procedure.*

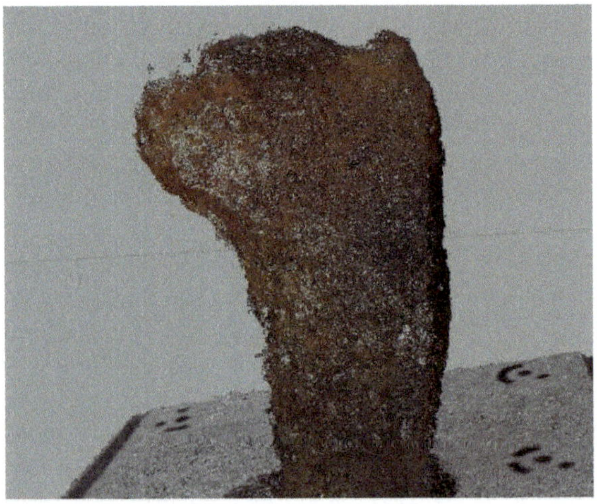

Figure 3. *The point cloud model created as a result of intensive point matching.*

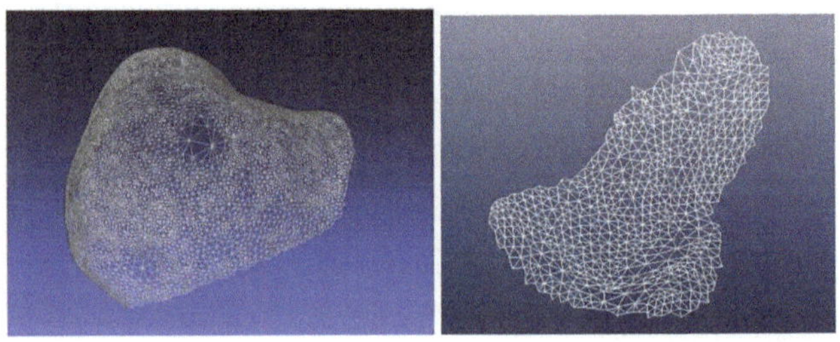

(a) (b)

Figure 4. *Creation of a digital surface model of a: humeral head and b: glenoid cavity by forming a 3D grid network.*

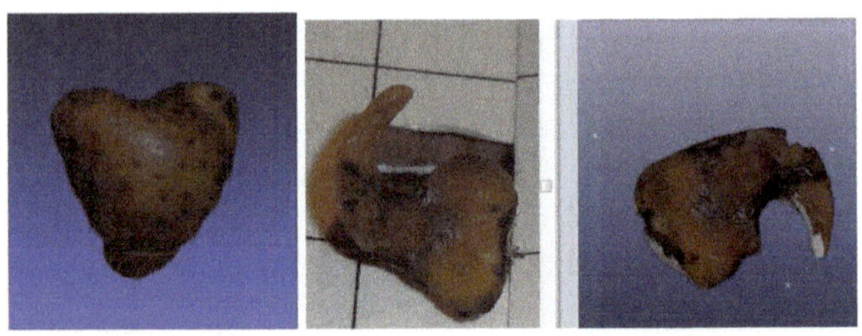

(a) (b)

Figure 5. *3D modeling of the joint surface of a: humeral head and b: glenoid cavity.*

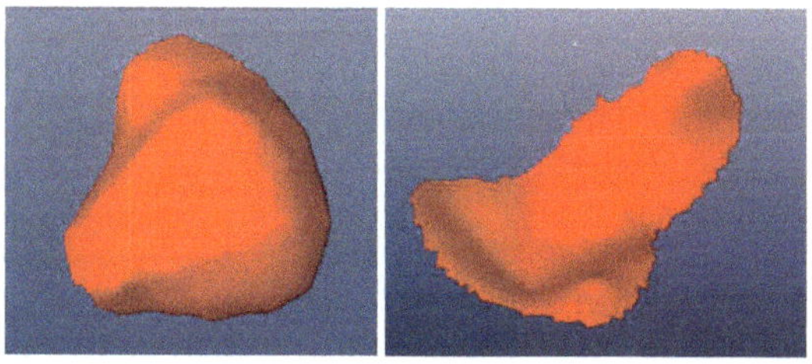

(a) (b)

Figure 6. Calculation of surface areas of a: humeral head and b: glenoid cavity, which constitute glenohumeral joint.

Table 1. The calibration values of the camera (Sony DSC-W570) had been used in the study.

Focal Length- Shutter	4.5mm- 1/250(sn)
K1,k2,k3	4608x3456
P1,p2	0,0524 mm/pix
xo	1.31527 pix
yo	0,104 mm

Table 2. The transformation results of a model belonging to the left humerus of a female New Zealand rabbit.

Points Id	Length (m)	Error (m)
1-3	0.0092	0.000014
1-5	0.0159	0.000017
3-7	0.0159	0.000059
5-7	0.0092	0.000054
5-9	0.0159	0.000002
7-11	0.0159	0.000018
9-11	0.0092	0.000046
13-15	0.0092	0.000032
11-15	0.0159	0.000021
13-17	0.0092	0.000079

Table 3. Statistical results of biometric measurements belonging to glenohumeral joint obtained as a result of 3D reconstruction (mean± SD).

	Photogrammetric Analysis	Right (n=6)	Left (n=6)
Male	Humeral head (cm^2)	1.539±0.187	1.547±0.182
	Glenoid cavity (cm^2)	0.492±0.060	0.498±0.060
	Humeral head / Glenoid cavity	3.128±0.096	3.108±0.076
Female	Humeral head (cm^2)	1.937±0.194	1.972±0.207
	Glenoid cavity (cm^2)	0.655±0.053	0.651±0.058
	Humeral head / Glenoid cavity	2.953±0.093	3.026±0.103

$P > 0.05$; there was no statistically significant difference in the same line.

Table 4. Statistical comparison of biometric measurements belonging to left and right sides of glenohumeral joint obtained as a result of 3D reconstruction (mean± SD)

	Photogrammetric Analysis	Male (n=6)	Female (n=6)
Right	Humeral head (cm^2)	1.539±0.187^a	1.937±0.194^b
	Glenoid cavity (cm^2)	0.492±0.060^a	0.655±0.053^b
	Humeral head / Glenoid cavity	3.128±0.096^a	2.953±0.093^b
Left	Humeral head (cm^2)	1.547±0.182^a	1.972±0.207^b
	Glenoid cavity (cm^2)	0.498±0.060^a	0.651±0.058^b
	Humeral head / Glenoid cavity	3.108±0.076	3.026±0.103

^{a,b}: Different letters in the same line are statistically significant ($P < 0.05$).

3. Results

3D coordinates and 3D digital terrain models of the required points in scapula and humerus, which form glenohumeral joint in the New Zealand rabbits, were obtained through the close-up picture photogrammetry method. Joint surface areas were calculated by the help of 3D digital terrain model, their proportions were identified and it was found that there was no statistically significant difference between the right and left sides in both males and females (Table 3.) that there was a statistical difference between the genders (Table 4).

According to Table 3, there were no statistically significant differences between the right and left sides in both sexes in the surface areas of humeral head and glenoid cavity and in the proportion of the surface area of humeral head to the surface area of glenoid cavity.

It was seen that in both sexes and in both sides, the surface area of humeral head was almost 3 times as large as the surface area of glenoid cavity.

According to Table 4, a difference at the level of $P < 0.05$ was found in the surface areas of male and female New Zealand rabbits constituting glenohumeral joint and their proportions to each other.

4. Discussion

Surface area measurements through photogrammetric methods of humeral head and glenoid cavity, which constitute glenohumeral joint in male and female New Zealand rabbits and their proportions to each other, were evaluated statistically. According to this, no statistically significant differences were observed between the joint surfaces in the right and left sides of both male and female rabbits whereas differences were found between the sexes. There weren't any statistically significant differences observed in glenoid cavity measurements of south Indian population [16] and Egyptian population [17] in the right and left sides as in New Zealand rabbit.

As a result of metamorphic measurements they conducted on male and female scapula, Taşer and Başaloğlu [1] found a statistical difference between the sexes. Moreover, it was shown through studies conducted that both the height and width measurements of glenoid cavity exhibited a statistically significant difference between the sexes [18]. Prescher and Klümpen [12] argued that glenoid cavity displayed sexual dimorphism but this alone was not sufficient in distinguishing the sexes and that other characteristic features belonging to the bone should be used to confirm this.

The shape of the glenoid cavity in New Zealand rabbits was look like to ellips and extended in one side, but in feral pigs (*Sus scrofa*) it was circular [19]. In Turkish adult population there were some variations of glenoid cavity according to the types of gleoid notch [20].

It was found in this study that the surface area of humeral head in New Zealand rabbits was about three times that of the surface area of glenoid cavity. Karabork [11] measured humeral head in rabbits as 161 mm^2, and glenoid cavity as 64.7 mm^2 which yielded a proportion of 2.5 times. In humans, on the other hand, humeral head was found to be 4 cm^2, whereas glenoid cavity was measured to be 1.6 cm^2 and the proportion was calculated to be 2.5 times [21].

In conclusion, according to the surface area measurements of the glenohumeral joint of New Zealand rabbits obtained through photogrammetric methods on 3D models, it was found that humeral head and glenoid cavity were important in sex assignment. It is believed that the photogrammetric method used and the data obtained could shed light on forensic medicine practices and contribute to the wealth of knowledge in the field of veterinary anatomy. In addition, it can be said that 3D data that were obtained in this study, which brought together the medical and photogrammetric disciplines/methods harmoniously, made a significant contribution to the medical field.

References

[1] Taşer FA, Başaloğlu H (2003) Morphometric dimensons of the scapula. Ege Journal of Medicine 42: 73-80.

[2] Atmani H, Merienne F, Fofi D, Troulloud P (2008) From medical data to simple virtual mock-up of scapulo-humeral joint. ELCVIA 7: 115-128.

[3] Moineau G, Levigne C, Boileau P, Young A, Walch G (2012) Three-dimensional measurement method of arthritic glenoid cavity morphology: Feasibility and reproducibility. Orthop Traumatol Surg Res 98: 139-145.

[4] Bryce CD, Pennypacker JL, Kulkarni N, Paul EM, Hollenbeak CS, Mosher TJ, Armstrong AD (2008) Validation of three-dimensional models of in situ scapulae. J Shoulder Elbow Surg 17: 825-832.

[5] Şeker DZ, Duran Z, Ege A (2002) Digital fotogrametrinin tıp alanında uygulanmasına bir örnek. 30. Yıl Sempozyumu, Konya, PP: 382-388.

[6] Chang YC (2008) A Photogrammetric system for 3D reconstruction of a scoliotic torso. Thesis of master program of biomedical engineering, university of Calgary, Alberta.

[7] Ege A, Şeker DZ, Tuncay İ, Duran Z (2002) Radius distal eklem yüzünün digital fotogrametrik yöntemle ölçme değerlendirmesi, VIII. Congress Book of the Turkish Society for Surgery of the Hand and Upper Extremity, Adana, 21/10: 128- 132.

[8] Schewe H, Ifert F (2000) Soft tissue analysis and cast measurement in orthodontics using digital photogrammetry. ISPRS 33: 699-706.

[9] Jordan P, Willneff J, D'Apuzzo N, Weishaupt M (2001) Photogrammetric measurement of deformations of horse hoof horn capsules. Videometrics and Optical Methods for 3D Shape Measurement, Proceeding of SPIE, San Jose, California, 4309: 204-211.

[10] Labens R, Redding WR, Desai KK, Orde KV, Mansmann RA, Blikslager AT (2013) Validation of a photogrammetric technique for computing equine hoof volume. Vet J 197: 625–630.

[11] Karabork H (2009) Three- dimensional measurements of glenohumeral joint surfaces in sheep, cat and rabbit by photogrammetry. J Anim Vet Adv 8: 1248-1251.

[12] Prescher A, Klümpen TH (1995) Does the area of the glenoid cavity of the scapula show sexual dimorphism? J Anat 186: 223-226.

[13] Waite JN, Schrader WJ, Mellish JAE, Horning M (2007) Three- dimensional photogrammetry as a tool for estimating morphometrics and body mass of Steller sea lions (*Eumetopias jubatus*). Can J Fish Aquat Sci 64: 296–303.

[14] Falkingham PL, Bates KT, Farlow JO (2014) Historical photogrammetry: Bird's Paluxy river dinosaur chase sequence digitally reconstructed as it was prior to excavation 70 years ago. Plos One 9(4): 1–5.

[15] International Committee on Veterinary Gross Anatomical Nomenclature (2012) Nomina Anatomica Veterinaria. 5th ed., Hannover, Columbia, Ghent, Sapporo: World Association of Veterinary Anatomists.

[16] Mamatha T, Shakuntala R, Murlimanju BV, Kaltur SG, Mangala M, Kumar B (2011) Morphometry of glenoid cavity. OJHAS 10: 1–4.

[17] El-Din WAN, Ali MHM (2015) A morphometric study of the patterns and variations of the acromion and glenoid cavity of the scapulae in Egyptian population. J Clin Diagn Res 9: 8–11.

[18] Churchill RS, Brems JJ, Kotschi H (2001) Glenoid size, inclination, and version: An anatomic study. J Shoulder Elbow Surg 10: 327- 332.

[19] Karan M (2012) Macro-anatomical study of ossa membri thoracici in the feral pigs (*Sus scrofa*). Fırat Univ Vet J Health Sci 26: 17–20.

[20] Coskun N, Karaali K, Cevikkol C, Demirel BM, Sindel M (2006) Anatomical basics and variations of the scapula in Turkish adults. Suudi Med J 27: 1320–1325.

[21] Sager M, Herten M, Ruchay S, Assheuer J, Kramer M, Jager M (2009) The anatomy of the glenoid labrum: A comparison between human and dog. Comp Med 59: 465–475.

Epidemiology, Economic Importance and Control Techniques of Lumpy Skin Diseases

Birhanu Hailu*, **Gezahign Alemayehu, Nuru Seid**

Samara University, College of Veterinary Medicine, Department of Veterinary Epidemiology and Preventive Medicine, Samara, Ethiopia

Email address:
birhailu2002@gmail.com (B. Hailu)

Abstract: Lumpy skin disease (LSD) is an acute infectious disease of cattle endemic in most Sub-Saharan African countries. It is economically devastating viral diseases which cause several financial problems in livestock industries as a result of significant milk yield loss, infertility, abortion and death. It is caused by lumpy skin diseases virus of capripoxvirus. The disease is characterized by fever, enlarged lymph nodes, firm, and circumscribed nodules in the skin and ulcerative lesions particularly in the mucous membrane of the mouth. It occurs in all agro climatic conditions and has the potential to extend its boundaries. It is transmitted by insect vectors among the cattle sharing similar grazing and watering areas and those congregate in the same barn. Good understanding of epidemiology, economic significance and control mechanisms of the disease enabled to design suitable control measures. LSD could be diagnosed using appropriate serological and molecular techniques. Effective control measure of the disease is achieved through mass vaccination though separation and culling of infected animals are optional methods.

Keywords: Lumpy Skin Disease, OIE, Epidemiology, Control, Transmission

1. Introduction

Lumpy skin disease is one of the most economically significant transborder, emerging viral diseases. It is currently endemic in most Africa countries and expanded to Middle East region (Tuppurinen and Oura, 2011). It is a disease with a high morbidity and low mortality rate and affects cattle of all ages and breeds. It causes significant economic problems as a result of reduced milk production, beef loss and draft animals, abortion, infertility, loss of condition and damage to the hide (CFSPH, 2008). It becomes an important threat to livestock and dairy industry in the Middle East and Africa (Kumar, 2011).

Lumpy skin disease is an acute infectious disease characterized by fever, nodules on the skin, mucous membranes and internal organs, emaciation, enlarged lymph nodes, edema of the skin, and sometimes death Radostitis *et al.* (2006).It is caused by the virus classified in capripoxvirusof family poxviridae. Various strains of capripoxvirus are responsible for the disease and these are antigenically and serologically indistinguishable from strains causing sheep pox and goat pox but distinct at the genetic level (Babiuk*et al*, 2008). LSD has a partially different geographical distribution from sheep and goat pox, suggesting that cattle strains of capripoxvirus do not infect and transmit between sheep and goats (OIE, 2010). The disease occurs in different ecological and climatic zones and extends its boundaries to different areas (Davies, 1991).

The lumpy skin disease virus in combination with sheep and goat pox viruses severely affects ruminants. Consequently it brought high economic pressure on subsistence of the poor farmers particularly pastoralists at which their central economy relay on the production of livestock and mixed farming system (Buller *et al.*, 2005). As a transborder disease, causes international ban on the trade of livestock and their products (Merck Veterinary manual, 2011). LSD was spread to East Africa in 1957 in Kenya and disease was extensively expanded to rest of region in subsequent years (Davies, 1991).Determination of seroprevalence of LSD has a time limitation for the presence of detectable antibodies in the serum for more than seven months of post infection. Serological tests such as virus neutralization are less sensitivity and time consuming to detect the low level antibody titres following the infection of the animals (Vorster, 2008; OIE, 2010). In Ethiopia limited works has been done on this disease so far and few works have been reported on risk factors assessments, epidemiological aspects, seroprevalence and financial impacts in selected areas of the country (Getachew *et al.*, 2010,2011; Alemayehu *et al*,2013 and Hailu *et al*,2014). Recently, a report on seroprevalence of disease using virus neutralization and indirect fluorescents antibody test indicated that the disease is widely distributed across the country and increases its impacts (Getachew *et al.*, 2012).There were frequent outbreak reports of the disease though information available on the prevalence of the disease and its financial impacts in North Eastern part of Ethiopia is scarce. Therefore; the aim of this review is to present epidemiological findings, economic impacts and control mechanisms of the disease.

2. Historical Perspectives

For the first time in 1929, skin disease with new clinical symptoms was occurred in Zambia. At that time it was considered as it was caused by either plant poisoning or an allergic response of insect bite (Weise, 1968; Bagla, 2005). After fourteen years, in October 1943, another outbreak of the disease was occurred in Botswana and named it provisionally as "Ngamiland cattle disease" as the case was occurred for the first time in Ngamiland. After two years, 1945 the disease spreads to Zimbabwe and South Africa where the disease named as the lumpy skin disease and demonstration of transmission of the infectious agent by inoculation of cattle with suspension of the skin nodules was determined (Davies, 1991).

The disease was diagnosed in Kenya in 1957; Sudan in 1971; Chad and Niger in 1973; Nigeria in 1974 and Somalia in 1983 (Tuppuraninen, 2005). In 1988, the first outbreak was occurred in Egypt in Ismailia and although control and eradication measures had been taken place the disease remains endemic in these areas (Ali *et al.*, 1990). It was also observed clinically in Israel in herds of dairy farms in 1989 which was suggested as it was spread from Egyptian outbreaks by insect vectors carried by wind (Yeruham*et al.*, 1995). The disease was primarily considered as an endemic disease to Africa and Middle East and other areas. According to annual disease information released by OIE, outbreak cases have reported from Bahrain in 1993/94,2002 Iran in 1996,2001 and other similar cases has been reported in United Arab Emerate, Kuwait and Oman (OIE, 2010).

3. Pathogenesis and Clinical Signs

3.1. Pathogenesis

LSDis developed by infectious LSDV and accompanied with febrile reaction (Vorster, 2008). Mechanism by which the virus observed to cause skin lesions was dueto replication of the virusin specific cells such as pericytes and endothelial cells of lymphatic and blood vessels walls. LSD is generalized and epitheliotrophicdisease that cause localized and systemic reaction and results in vasculitis and lymphadenitis. In some severe cases thrombosis and other symptoms were observed (Radostitis *et al.*, 2006; Merck Veterinary manual, 2011).Incubation period of LSD can vary under field condition and experimental conditionsvary from 5 days in experimentally inoculated animals and 2–4 weeks in naturally infected animals, gives a maximum incubation period, for regulatory purposes, of 28 days (Wood, 1990; Barnard *et al.*, 1994; OIE, 2010).

Nodules of LSD may be found on subcutaneous tissues, muscle fascia and musculature, which are grey-pink with caseous necrotic cores. Gross lesions of LSD were according to description by Haig (1957) and Barnard (1994) which are congested, haemorrghic, edematous and necrotic and involves all layers of skin, epidermis, and dermis, subcutaneous and underlying musculature. Circumscribed necrotic lesions may appear in muzzle, mucous membrane of mouth, respiratory tract, trachea, vulva and prepuce which may ulcerate (Bagla, 2005,Radostitis *et al.*, 2006). Histopathological sections of early skin lesions of epidermis show an epitheloid cells, lymphocytes, macrophages, plasma cells and fibroblast proliferation appear in later stages and if secondary infection occurs ,necrosis, polymorph nuclear and red cells seen. Typical eosinophilic, intracytoplasmic pox inclusion bodies may be seen in cells of epithelioid, hair follicles and cells of muscles and skin glands (Bagla, 2005; AUSVETPLAN, 2009).

3.2. Clinical Signs

Lumpy skin disease is infectious, eruptive and occasionally fatal disease of cattle. It is an acute to chronic viral disease characterized by skin nodules in the skin and other body parts. It might be exacerbated by secondary bacterial complication (Merck Veterinary Manual, 2011). It is an acute to in apparent cattle disease caused by LSDV. It is characterized by fever, nodule in the skin, mucous membrane and internal organs and swelling of superficial lymph nodes (OIE, 2010; Tuppurinen and Oura, 2011).

Course of lumpy skin disease may be acute, sub acute and chronic and infection of LSDV may occur both experimentally and under natural condition. The virus causes from in apparent infection to severe clinical symptoms and those animals which develop clinical disease may have a biphasic febrile reaction. Some of the visible clinical signs are; fever of 40-41.5°C which may last 6-72 hours, lachyrimation , increased nasal and pharyngeal secretion ,loss of appetite, reduced milk production ,some depression and movement reluctance. Severity of clinical signs depends on strain of capripoxvirus and breed of the host cattle and in case of experimental infection route of transmission and dose of the virus also has determinant factor (Carn and Kitching, 1995; LSD contingency plan for the Netherland, 2002; OIE, 2010).

According to Davies (1991) infection of cattle under field condition may develop generalized skin lesions after one to two days of febrile, nodular cutaneous lesions appear which may cover whole body ranging from a few to multiple nodules but in majority of the cases, initial evidences of symptoms are lachyrimation and fever but some cases are non-febrile. Prescapular and precrural lymph nodes are some of the superficial lymph nodes which commonly seen during clinical manifestation of the disease (Tuppurinen and Oura, 2011). The most common sites are head and neck, perineum, genitalia, limb and udder; involve skin, cutaneous tissues and some time underlying part of the muscle.

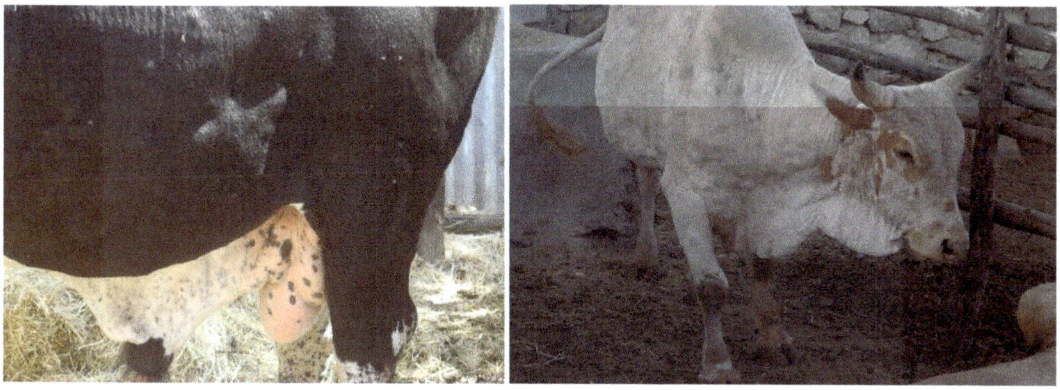

Figure. *Appearance of lumpy skin disease nodules in feedlot cattle taken by the second author*

Diameter of nodular lesion may be up to 1-7 cm diameter appears as round, circumscribed areas of erected hair. In severe cases, ulcerative lesions may develop in mucous membrane of mouth, trachea, and larynx and esophagus(Radostitis*et al.*, 2006). Such ulcerative lesion also develops in conjunctiva, muzzle, nostrils and small nodules may resolve spontaneously without any consequence. Secondary bacterial complication and infestation of fly worms may be occurred (CFSPH, 2008). As stated by Barnard (1994), nasal discharge and salivation may be developed in to mucoid or mucopurulent,lachyrimation to conjunctivitis, superficial lymph nodes markedly enlarged and inflammatory and edematous lesions in limbs, brisket and genitalia may develop and skin lesion may be necrotic and ulcerative lesions may become fibrotic.

Some of the scabbed lesion remains there and other sloughed leaving a hole full of skin thickness which becomes infected by pus-forming bacteria and large areas of skin may slough. Lesions in skin, subcutaneous tissue, and muscles of limbs, together with severe skin inflammation caused by secondary infection of lesions, greatly reduce mobility as indicated by Murphy *et al.* (1999). Rapid deterioration in body condition results and animals that recover may remain in extremely poor condition for up to 6 months. Pneumonia is a common bacterial complication and usually fatal disease and absence of estrus cycle and abortion are common consequences observed in female animals and painful genitalia may prevent bulls from serving (AUSVETPLAN, 2009).

4. Epidemiology

Lumpy skin disease is an important, economically devastating, notifiable disease which brought production loss in cattle due to generalized malaises and chronic debility (Tuppurainen and Oura, 2011). Good understanding of epidemiological aspects LSD related to pathogen, host and environment might aid for prevention mechanisms. Particular emphasis was given to exposure of hosts and pathogen in suitable environment that was facilitating transmission and distribution of the disease (Dohoo*et al.*, 2003). The frequency of morbidity and mortality of the disease, its geographic distribution and mode of transmission in large herds of cattle were observed to cause severe economic losses (Salib and Osman, 2006; Tuppurainen and Oura, 2011).

4.1. Risk Factors

4.1.1. Pathogen Risk Factors

LSDV is one of the species of capripoxviruses affecting cattle of different breeds and this virus is resistant to different chemical and physical agents (Murphy *et al.*, 1999). The virus can persist for about 33 days in necrotic skins and remain viable for at least 18 days in lesions in air-dried hides at ambient temperature. It can survive in a wet environment which can protect them from rays of sun light (Weiss, 1968). LSDV is very resistant in environment and can remain viable for long periods on or off animal hosts. They may persist for up to six months in a suitable environment, such as shaded animal pens. Capripoxviruses have lipid-containing envelopes and susceptible to a range of disinfectants containing detergents. They are susceptible to sunlight, but survive well at cold temperatures (Davies, 1981). The virus is inactivated by heating for 1 hour at 55°C.

The virus is present in nasal, lachrymal and pharyngeal secretions, semen, milk and blood and it may remain in saliva for up to 11 days and in semen for 22 days (Barnard *et al.*, 1994). It can also persist for up to 33 days in necrotic tissue remaining at the site of a skin lesion. Material from skin lesions also contains infective virus when shed (Barnard *et al.*, 1994; Annandale, 2006).There is no evidence of the virus persisting in meat of infected animals, but it might be isolated from milk in early stages of fever (Davies, 1991). The virus may persist for months in lesions in cattle hides. LSD virus may persist for 6 months on fomites, including clothing and equipment but there is no evidence that virus can survive more than four days in insect vectors.

Prototype strain of LSDV is Nettling virus as reported by Alexander (1957). This is one of most strain mainly affects cattle. The virus can't be distinguished by routine neutralization or conventional molecular tests from other species of capripoxviruses(Mathews, 1982). LSD virus is essentially identical with each other and with a Kenyan strain (O 240/KSGP) of sheep and goat pox virus (SGPV). Kenyan group of SGPV strains showed differences when compared with ones from India, Iraq, and Nigeria. Strain variation and persistence of virus for surviving in the environment is among the pathogen risk factors of LSDV(Kitching, 1989).

4.1.2. Host Susceptibility

Lumpy skin disease is a disease of cattle and causes several disorders. Though all breeds and age group are susceptible, Bos*taurus*are particularly more susceptible to clinical disease than zebu cattle. Among *Bostaurus,* fine-skinned Channel Island breeds develop more severe disease (OIE, 2010). Lactating cows appearing to be severely affected and result in a sharp drop in milk production because of high fever caused by viral infection itself and secondary bacterial mastitis (Tuppurainen and Oura, 2011). Young animals are severely affected and clinical symptoms are rapid to appear. Apart from these animals, few cases have been reported in Asian water buffalo (*Bubalusbubalis*). Clinical cases or antibodies have been reported in other species such as oryx, but may have been caused by closely related poxviruses.Generally clinical severity of disease depends on susceptibility and immunological status of the host population (CFSPH, 2008).

4.1.3. Environmental Factors

Environmental determinants play a great role in the epidemiology of lumpy skin disease. It had major impact on the agent, host and vectors as well as interaction between them. These predisposing factors have a great role in maintenance of arthropod vector and transmission of the virus to susceptible animals (Thomas, 2002). These are herd risk factors that have an influence on the outbreak of the disease. Animals share the same grazing and watering points and unrestricted movement of animals across different borders following rainfall were some of the factors(Tuppurainen and Oura, 2011). Distribution of the disease in various agro climatic conditions, introduction of new animals to the herd and the presence water bodies are among the other risk factors that would facilitate the spread of outbreaks in various localities (Getachew*et al.*, 2011; Tuppurainen and Oura, 2011, Hailu*et al*, 2014). The vectors which play a great role in the transmission of the virus are maintained in such environment associated with the coming of the wet season followed by autumn (Ali *et al*, 2006).

4.2. Geographical Distribution

Geographic distributions of LSDV, GPV and SPV is distinctly different and both SPV and GPV geographically ranged and restricted to Africa and Asia for the last fifty years extending from Africa to the north of equator (Kitching, 1989). LSD was originated from Sub Sahara Africa countries in 1929 and spread to the north and south during the last seventy years. The geographic coverage of LSD has extended its range to include all countries in sub-Saharan Africa as well as Madagascar and it is endemic to every African countries and occurs in various ecological zones from temperate areas to dry semi arid and arid areas (Davies, 1991; Kitching and Carn, 2000).

4.3. Transmission

Though there was no clearly defined method of transmission of LSD, circumstantial evidences suggestions that disease might be transmitted by biting insects (Weise, 1968). Later on, the virus was isolated from arthropod vectors and the role of vectors in transmission of the virus was experimentally confirmed. According to Carn and Kitching (1994), lumpy skin disease is endemic to most Sub-Saharan countries and natural infection of cattle by the virus may be brought by different routes of infections.

Epidemiological evidence suggests that, outbreaks of LSD were highly associated with prevalence of high insect vectors population and with upcoming of rainy season. As Magori-cohen (2012) reported that biting insects play major role in transmission of LSDV. Epidemics ofLSD are associated with rainy seasons, river basins and ponds during which cattle grazed in and humid areas conducive to insect multiplication. These biting insects transmit the virus mechanically during their blood meals Chihota *et al.* (2001).

Currently it is widely accepted that LSDV is transmitted mainly by arthropod vectors. This vector-related transmission is apparently mechanical, rather than biological. This distinction is important because infectious organisms do not generally survive in vectors for long periods for multiplication or over-wintering in these insects. Study by Chihota*et al.* (2001) indicated that the virus can survive 2-6 days post feeding from infected cattle and transfers this to susceptible cattle by female mosquito,*Aedesegypti* during experimental infection.The virus can survive only for about average four days and this can't permit for recurrence of disease in the coming season. It was thought that infected vectors can transmit the disease some distance kilometers from the foci of infection as the occurrence of outbreak in 1989 in Israel following aerial movement of infected insect vectors from Egypt (Yeruham*et al.*, 1995).

Mosquitoes and other flies such tabanids, Culicoides, biting midges and *Glossina*species like tsetse fly are among the other arthropod vectors that play a great role in the transmission of the virus. The participation of these flies in the spread of LSDV have been confirmed by isolation of the virus from the stable flies feed on infected cattle and this indicated that these flies are efficient vectors of capripoxviruses (Bruce *et al.*, 2004). Flies, including housefly, bush fly and blowflies are also very commonly associated with infected cattle possible to siphon off infected lachrymal, nasal or other secretions and transfer the virus to another susceptible animal. Vermin, predators and wild birds might also act as mechanical carriers of the virus (Kitching and Mellor, 1986; AUSVETPLAN, 2009).

Outbreaks of LSD are highly associated with seasonal

peak of mechanical vectors in wet and warm weather conditions in Ethiopia (Getachewet *al.*, 2010). Recently Tuppurinenet *al.* (2010) showed the molecular evidence of the potential viral transmission by hard ticks. The virus could be transmitted through transstadial and transovarian in *Boophilus.decoloratus* and mechanical transmission by *Repicephalusappendiculatus* and *Ambylomahebraeum.* Transmission of LSD is also possible by sharing of the same feeding and watering troughs which may be contaminated by the viruses in the saliva of the infected animals or ingestion of the already contaminated food or by iatrogenic agents (Haig, 1957) and suckling calves may be infected through infected milk (Thomas,2002).

Transmission by contact in the absence of the arthropod vectors was not efficient (Carn and Kitching, 1995). A study in Ethiopia also showed that communal grazing and watering points were found to be associated with the occurrence of LSD (Getachew *et al.*, 2010); introduction of new animals to a herd had a strong association with an increased risk of disease in the herd. Excretion of LSDV in semen was detecting using PCR from experimentally challenged bulls by Osuagwuh (2006). Great risks are imposed that semen or movement of semen from countries where the disease is endemic can transmit the disease (Irons *et al.*, 2005) but no standard procedures were present to detect the presence of LSDV in semen. Information was unavailable on transmission of LSD virus via semen or embryos. The virus excretes in the semen for up to 22 days in clinically affected bulls and about 12 days in sub clinically affected bulls (Weiss, 1968). There were also assumptions that virus also secreted in vaginal secretions. The extremely resistant nature of the virus to the environment would therefore make venereal transmission very likely (Committee on Managing Global Genetic Resources, 1993). Due to insufficient information, the International Embryo Transfer Society has not classified LSD virus regarding likelihood of its transmission via embryos.

Experimentally, virus inoculation can cause generalized infection following parental inoculation but it was observed to cause mild local lesions by intra dermal inoculations. Generally transmission of the virus by contact is inefficient and field evidence reported that the disease is not contagious as reported by Tuppurainen in (2005). Experimentally, transmission has occurred between cattle in adjacent insect proof enclosures that share the same water trough. Nasal and laryngeal secretions, semen and blood could potentially play some part in the transmission of the virus, but virtually in all outbreaks the virus appears to be propagated continuously from infected cattle to arthropod and then to cattle that forms cycle.

Virus can be transmitted by animal productssuch as milk, fomites such as equipments and clothing as well as personnel. Though most infection is thought to be the result of insect transmission, field observations have demonstrated that the spread of the virus from farm to farm and district to district might be due to the absence of complete restriction of all animal movements (Tuppurainen, 2005; AUSVETPLAN, 2009). The main factors that could influence transmission of the disease was, prevalence of insect vectors which affect rate of transmission of the virus and would be sharply reduced in the transmission of LSD after cold weather and frosts, which are associated with reduced insect vector populations.

The movement of infected stock, road and rail transport could play an important role in rapidly spreading LSD over larger areas (Kitching and Mellor, 1986). As indicated in the Australian veterinary emergency plan for lumpy skin disease (2009), risk of introduction of disease virus to one country or new areas may be through movement of infected animals or infected premises. Presence of wild life reservoirs has potential for spread of the virus. Though the virus has narrow host rang, limited information are available about natural infection of the virus to the wild buffalos but according to Ali *et al.* (1990), there were five water buffalos during outbreak in Egypt 1988 outbreak in Egypt.

Later in the second outbreak in 2006, the virus was detected by PCR from tissue samples and their milk and confirmed their susceptibility to the virus. Circumstantial evidence indicated that the virus can also observed infecting the Arabian female Oryx and the disease was clinically observed in experimentally inoculated giraffe and impala (Young *et al.*, 1970; Grethet *al.*, 1992).Capripoxvirus was detected using electron microscopy from skin nodules oforyx, and raised antibody levels against capripoxvirus were detected in paired serum samples tested using a neutralization test.

5. Economic Impact

Capri pox viruses are becoming an emerging worldwide threat to sheep, goats and cattle (Babiuket *al.*, 2008). Lumpy skin disease is one of the economically significant diseases in Africa and the Middle East countries that cause severe production loss in cattle. The world organization for animal health (OIE) categorizes the disease as notifiable diseases because of its severe economic losses. The economic importance of the disease was mainly due to having high morbidity rate rather than mortality (Tuppurainen and Oura, 2011). The financial implication of these losses is greatly significant to the herd owners, consumers and the industrial sectors which can process the livestock products and by products.

In intensive farming of cattle, the direct and indirect production losses caused by LSD were estimated to be as high as 45-60% (Tuppurainen and Oura, 2011). It was reflected that the severity of the disease was much more in developing countries where the poorest small scale farmers was found. Reports from Ethiopia indicated that the financial loss estimated based on milk , beef, draught power, mortality, treatment and vaccination costs in individual head of local zebu were lost 6.43 USD and for the Holstein Friesian 58 USD (Getachewet *al.*, 2010).

The disease was mainly affects cattle with subsequent effects on production through the morbidity and reduced productivity (CFSPH, 2008). Major consequences of the disease are retarded genetic improvement, limits the ability of the animal to work, draught power and traction loss, abortion in pregnant cows, marked reduction of milk yield during the active case of the disease, sterility and infertility in both sexes of cattle, permanent damage to hide and chronic debility in beef cattle (Tuppurainen, 2005; OIE, 2010). Control of the disease with special emphasis to endemic areas is an important way to reduce the losses and increase the incomes of cattle owners.

Control costs associated with disease might depend on the type of program to carry out. Israel and Egypt was tried to eradicate the disease by slaughter and mass vaccination. The compensation for the compulsory slaughter of infected and dangerous contact animals would impose some hardship, for loss of valuable genetic potentials and lack of finance for compensation. Prevention of restocking until after a possibly lengthy prescribed period had elapsed would exacerbate serious cash flow problems on infected premises and dangerous contact premises (Thomas, 2002).

Movement restrictions within restricted area and area control would cause loss of market opportunities and associated financial losses to unaffected properties and to support industries such as stock transport (Tuppuraine, 2005). Therefore, the disease must be major foci of activity for its control and economic implication of the disease must be established and return to the investment for its control. Impact of the disease is beyond a single farm unlike to some of the parasitic diseases. Outbreaks of the disease in one herd impose risk to the neighbors in production system where there is poor control of cattle movement. This significant economic impact of the disease is mainly due to the morbidity and to lesser extent because of mortality.

The morbidity and mortality rates for LSD vary greatly in different endemic areas depending on the severity of strain, prevalence of insect vectors and susceptibility of the host (Getachew*et al.*, 2010). An outbreak in a previously free country could be expected to result in a high morbidity rate. If LSD became endemic, continuing economic loss and poor productivity would occur due to stock losses, reduced production in cattle industries and cost of preventative vaccination. Permanent loss of some markets would also be expected, with associated downturn in rural economy and increased rural unemployment (Tuppurainen and Oura, 2011).

Overall, LSD is considered as a disease of high economic pressure because of its ability to compromise food security through protein loss, draft power, reduced output of animal production, increase production costs due to increased costs of disease control, disrupt livestock and their product trade, result of reduced milk yield, weight loss, abortion, infertility in cows, mastitis and infertility in lactating cows, infertility in bulls (Weiss, 1968; Kumar, 2009). Permanent damage to the skin and hide greatly affect leather industry. It causes ban on international trade of livestock and causes prolonged economic loss as it became endemic and brought serious stock loss (AUSVETPLAN, 2009; Getachew*et al.*, 2010).

6. Diagnosis

According to Carn (1995) LSD would be presumptively diagnosed based on case history and apparent clinical (OIE, 2010). Rapid laboratory tests are needed to confirm the disease. Laboratory test of LSD can be made by identification of the agent, routine histopathological examination and immune histological staining (Tuppurainen, 2005). Isolation of virus can be made from collected biopsy or at post-mortem from skin nodules, lung lesions or lymph nodes within the first week of the occurrence of clinical signs, before the development of neutralizing antibodies (House, 1990; OIE, 2010; Davies, 1991; CFSPH, 2008). Primary cell cultures are bovine skin dermis and equine lung cells, but growth of such viruses is slow and requires several passages (Tuppurainen, 2005).

Serological tests are used for retrospective confirmation of lumpy skin disease but they are much more time consuming to be used as primary diagnostic methods and limited presence of detectable antibodies in serum (Vorster, 2008; AUSVET PLAN, 2009; OIE, 2010). Polymerase Chain Reaction (PCR) is the other recently developed molecular technique that changes biological science as it revolutionized detection and characterization of microorganisms, enables minute DNA of the organism to replicate very rapidly and makes easy to detect, study and use for any medical purpose. Conventional gel based PCR is more time and labor consuming and could not differentiate between species of capripox viruses but real- time PCR was faster than the former one (Valonese*t al.*, 2009 ; Tuppurinen and Oura,2011; Ireland and Binepal, 1998). PCR for the diagnosis of LSD is with a greater sensitivity and good specificity and it is most appropriate technique (Kholy*et al.*, 2008; OIE, 2010).

7. Prevention and Control

7.1. Vaccination in Endemic Areas

Immunity acquired from natural infection of the disease might be lifelong and vaccination has been successfully used. LSD could be kept under control by vaccination of cattle every year (Thomas, 2002). All strains of capripoxvirus examined so far, whether of bovine, ovine or caprine origin, share a major neutralizing site, so that animals that have recovered from infection with one of the strains are resistant to infection with any other strain. Consequently, it is possible to protect cattle against LSD using strains of capripoxvirus derived from either of the sheep or goats as used in Egypt by Romanian sheep pox strain (OIE, 2010).

Live, attenuated vaccines against LSD are commercially available. These have antigenic homology and there is cross protection among them. Local strain of Kenyan sheep and goat pox virus has been shown to effectively immunize sheep, goats and cattle against infection with capripoxvirus with a remarkable success. The next one is attenuated South African LSD virus (Neethling strain) vaccine derived from cattle, freeze dried product is also available (OIE, 2010). In countries where LSD is endemic, vaccination against this infection was successfully used by vaccinating animals every year. LSDV has been used as a recombinant capri poxvirus, combined with rinderpest or rabies virus and cappripox virus is an excellent vector for recombinant vaccines because of its narrow host range even it is a novel candidate vector for HIV-1 which is the serious public health, based on the replication deficient, as it will not complete its cycle in non-ruminant hosts (Shen *et al.*, 2011).

7.2. Vaccination in New Areas

Risks of introduction of the disease in to the new areas are by the introduction of infected animals and contaminated materials (Davies, 1991;Kitching, 1995).If the occurrence of LSD is reported or confirmed in new areas, before the spread of the disease to other areas extensively, quarantine of the area, slaughtering of the diseased and in contact animals and contacted equipments must be cleaned and disinfected (Davies, 1991; Netherland contingency plan of LSD, 2002; AUSVETPLAN, 2009). Ring vaccination of cattle within the foci of infection with a radius of 25-50 Km , quarantine and animal movement should be restricted to eradicate the disease from the area, but if the area coverage of the disease is large, the most convenient techniques for the control of the disease is mass vaccination of the cattle. These two techniques, slaughter and vaccination were practiced in Israel and Egypt since the first outbreak of the disease occurred and it was effective for the time being (Yeruham*et al.*, 1995).

7.3. Other Control Techniques

For countries free of the disease, the introduction of the disease can be prevented by restriction of the importation of the animals and their products but in those nations which experience the infection can limit the spread of the lumpy skin disease by restriction of the animal movement from one place to another, quarantine, keeping of sick animals well apart from the rest of the herd and must not share drinking or feeding troughs by making awareness creation of the farmers (Thomas, 2002).

Animals older than six months must be vaccinated against lumpy skin disease during spring. It is safe to vaccinate pregnant cows. All animals must be vaccinated once a year. When vaccinating the animals during a disease outbreak, it is important to use one needle per animal so that the virus is not spread from sick to healthy animals. Professional help and recommendation on vaccines must be carefully followed and practiced. Antibiotics also given to prevent the secondary bacterial complication as the defense mechanism of the body weakened which can prolong the complete recovery of the diseased animals (CSFPH, 2008).

References

[1] Alexander, R. A., Plowright, W., and Haig, D. A., (1957). Cytopathogenic agents associated with lumpy-skin disease of cattle. *Bull. Epiz. Dis. Afr., 5:489-492.*

[2] Ali, A. A., Esmat, M., Attia, H. Selim, A. and Abdel-hamid, Y. M., (1990). Clinical and Pathological Studies of on the lumpy skin disease in Egypt. *The veterinary record, 127:549-550.*

[3] AUSVETPLAN., (2009). Australian Veterinary Emergency Plan, Disease Strategy, Lumpy skin disease.

[4] Babiuk, S., Bowden. T. R., Boyle. D. B., Wallace D. B. and Kitching R. P., (2008). Capripoxviruses: An Emerging Worldwide Threat to Sheep, Goats and Cattle. *TransboundaryEmergeging Disease. 55(7):263-72.*

[5] Bagla, P. V., (2005). The demonstration of the lumpy skin disease virus in semen of the experimentally infected bulls using different diagnostic techniques, MSc thesis.

[6] Barnard, B. H. J., Munz, E., Dumbell, K. and Prozyesky, L., (1994). Lumpy skin disease. In: *Infectous disease of livestock* with special reference to South Africa. 1:604-612.

[7] Brenner, J., Haimovitz, M., Orone E., Stram Y., Fridgut O., Bumbarov V., Kuznetzova, L., Oved Z., Waerrman A., Garazzi S., Perl S., Lahav D., Edery N. &Yadin H., (2006). Lumpy skin disease (LSD) in a large dairy herd in Israel. *Isr. J. Vet. Med., 61:73–77.*

[8] Bruce F., Eldridge, Edman J. D., (2004). Medical Entomology: A Textbook on Public Health and Veterinary Problems Caused by Arthropods. Capripox viruses Lumpy skin disease. 488p.

[9] Buller, R. M., Arif B. M., Black D. N., Dumbell K. R., Esposito J. J., (2005). Virus Taxonomy: Classification and Nomenclature of Viruses. Eighth Report of the International Committee on Taxonomy of Viruses, pp. 117–133. Elsevier Academic Press, San Diego.

[10] Carn, V. M., (1993). Control of capripoxvirus infections. *Vaccine*, 11:1275–1279.

[11] Carn, V. M. and Kitching, R. P., (1995). An investigation of the possible route of the transmission of lumpy skin disease virus. *Epidemiology and infection. 114:219-226.*

[12] Carn, V. M., (2002). Control of Capripoxvirusinfections11(13):1275–1279.

[13] Carter, G. R., Wise, D. J. and Flores, E. F., (2005). A Concise Review of Veterinary Virology, G. R. Carter, D. J. Wise and E. Furtado Flores (Eds.) International Veterinary Information Service, Ithaca, New York, USA.

[14] CFSPH ., (2008) . The Center for Food Security and Public Health, Iowa State University, College of Veterinary Medicine and Institution of International cooperation in Animal Biologics, an OIE collaborating center.

[15] Chihota, C. M., Rennie, L. F., Kitching, R. P. and Mello, R P. S., (2003). Attempted mechanical transmission of lumpy skin disease virus by biting insects, *Medical and Veterinary Entomology 17:294–300.*

[16] Committee on Managing Global Genetic Resources, 1993

[17] Coetzer, J. A. W. and Venter., E. H., (2010). A Potential Role for Ixodid (Hard) Tick Vectors in the Transmission of Lumpy Skin Disease Virus in Cattle. *Transboundry and Emerging Disease. 58:93-104.*

[18] Davies, F. G., Kraussh., Lund, L. J. and Taylor M., (1971). The laboratory diagnosis of lumpy skin disease. *Res. Vet. Sci.*, 12:123–127.

[19] Davies, F. G., (1981). Lumpy skin disease. In: Virus Diseases of Food Animals, Gibbs EPJ (ed), *Academic Press, London, 2 :751–764.*

[20] Davies, F. G., (1991a). Lumpy skin disease of cattle: A growing problem in Africa and Near East. *world Animal Review*; 68:37-42.

[21] Davies, F. G., (1991b). Lumpy skin disease, an African capripoxvirus disease of cattle. Br. Vet. J. 147:489–503.

[22] Diesel, A. M., (1949). The Epizootiology of Lumpy Skin Disease in South Africa. In Proceedings of the 14th International Veterinary Congress, London, U. K., pp. 492-500.

[23] Dohoo, I., Martin, W., Stryhn, H., (2003). Measures of Associations, Veterinary Epidemiological Research, 2ndedition, Canada. pp121-137 and pp65-82.

[24] Getachew, G., Bonnet, P., Roger, F. and Waret-Szkuta, A., (2011). Epidemiological aspects and Financial Impacts of the Lumpy Skin Disease in Ethiopia, PhD thesis. pp87-110.

[25] Getachew, G., Waret-Szkuta, A., Grosbois, V., andJacquite, P., (2010). Risk Factors Associated with observed clinical lumpy skin disease in Ethiopia. PhD thesis. PP68-84.

[26] Getachew, G., Grosbois, V., Waret-Szkuta, A., Babiuk S, Jacquiet P, Roger F., (2012). Lumpy skin disease in Ethiopia: Seroprevalence study across different agro-climate zones. p1

[27] Green, H., (1959). Lumpy skin disease; its effect on skin and hide and a comparison in this respect with some other skin diseases. *Bulletin of the epizootic disease of Africa, 7:63-79.*

[28] Greth., A, Gourreau, J. M., Vassart, M., Nguyen-Ba-Vy, Wyers, M., Lefevre. P. C., 1992. Capripoxvirus disease in an Arabian oryx (Oryx leucoryx) from Saudi Arabia. *J Wildl Dis. 28(2):295-300.*

[29] Haig, D. H., (1957). Lumpy skin disease. *Bulletin of Epizootic disease of Africa 5:421-430.*

[30] House, J. A., 1990. Lumpy Skin Disease. In Proceedings of the 93rd Annual Meeting of the United States Animal Health Association, Las Vegas, Nevada, . Pp. 305-314.

[31] House, J. A., Wilson, T. M., Elnakashly, S., Karim, I. A., Ismail, I., ELDanaf, N., Moussa, A. M., and Ayoub, N. N., (1990). The isolation of lumpy skin Disease virus and bovine herpesvirus-4 from cattle in Egypt. *J. Vet. Diagn. Invest. 2: 111-115.*

[32] ICTV (2002), International Committee on Taxonomy of Viruses, Taxonomy of Pox virus

[33] Ireland, D. C., and Binepal, Y. S., (1998). Improved detection of capripoxvirus in biopsy samples by PCR, *Journal of Virological methods*, 74:1-7.

[34] Irons, P. C., Tuppurainen, E. S. M., and Venter, E. H., (2005). Excretion of the lumpy skin disease virus in bull semen. MSc dissertation.

[35] Kholy, A. A. E., Soliman, H. M. T. and Abdelrahman, K. A., (2008). Polymerase chain reaction for rapid diagnosis of a recent lumpy skin disease virus incursion to Egypt, Veterinary Serum & Vaccine Research Institute. *Arab J. Biotech., 11 (2): 293-302.*

[36] Kitching, R. P. and Mellor, P. S., (1986a). Insect transmission of capripoxvirus. *Research in Veterinary Science 40:255–258.*

[37] Kitching, R. P. &Smale, C., (1986b). Comparison of the external dimensions of capripoxvirus isolates. *Res. Vet. Sci.* 41:425–427.

[38] Kitching, R. P., Bhat, P. P., and Black, D. N., (1989). Characterization of the African Strain of Capri pox virus, AFRC Institute for animal Health Pirbright laboratory, *Epidemic. Inf. 102:335-343.*

[39] Kitching, P., and Carn, V., (2000). The involvement of wild life and insect vectors in the epidemiology of Lumpy skin disease in South Africa.

[40] Kumar, S. M., (2009). An outbreak of Lumpy Skin Disease in a Holstein Dairy Herd in Oman: A Clinical report, Asian Journal of Animal and Veterinary Advances 6(8):851-859.

[41] Lumpy skin disease contingency plan for the Netherlands(2002). Veterinary Services, Ministry of Agriculture and Fisheries. pp1-22.

[42] Mac Owen, K. D. S., (1959). n the epizootiology of lumpy skin disease during the first year of its occurrence in Kenya. *Bull. Epiz. Dis. Afr., 7:7-20.*

[43] Magoricohen, R., Louzoun, Y., Herziger, Y., Oron, E., Arazi, A., Tuppurainen, E., Shipgel, Y. N., Klement, E., (2012). Mathematical modeling and evaluation of the different routes of transmission of lumpy skin disease virus, *Veterinary Research 43:1.*

[44] Mathews, R. E. F., (1982). Classification and nomenclature of viruses. Intervirol. 17:1-99.

[45] McFadden, G., (2005). Poxvirus tropism. *Nat. Rev. Microbiol.* 3:201–213.

[46] Merk Veterinary Manual, (2011)., Integumentary System : Pox Diseases : Lumpy Skin Disease, Economic impact of lumpy skin disease.

[47] Mlangwa, J. E. D., and Samui, K. L., (1996). The nature of Animal health Economics and Veterinary Epidemiology, *Rev. sci. tech. Off. int. Epiz., 15 (3) :797-812.*

[48] Murphy, F. A., Gibbs, E. P. J., Horzinek, M. C., Studdert, M. J., (1999). Veterinary Virology. Poxviridae, pp277-292

[49] OIE . 2010. OIE Manual of Diagnostic Tests and Vaccines for Terrestrial Animals . Lumpy skin disease. Chapter2. 4. 14. pp768-778.

[50] Osuagwuh, U. I., (2006). Semen Quality and the Excretion of Lumpy skin disease Virus in Semen Following Vaccination and Experimental Challenge of Vaccinated Bulls, MSc thesis, Pretoria University, pp3-28.

[51] Otte, M. J. and Chilondda, P., (1996). An Introduction to animal health economics, Livestock information, Sector analysis and policy branch, Animal production and health division.

[52] Preeze, J. D., (2006). Control of Lumpy Skin Disease, Vaccinate Every year for Lumpy skin disease.

[53] Pyride, . J and Coakley, M., (1959). Lumpy skin disease: Tissue culurestudies, Bulletin of Epizootic disease of Africa 7:37-50.

[54] Radostitis, MO., Gay, C., Hinchcliff., and Constable, PD., (2006). Veterinary Medicine, Text book of the disease of Cattle, Sheep, Goat, pig and horses, 10th edition.

[55] Regassa, C., (2003). Preliminary study of the Major skin diseases of cattle coming to Nekemit Veterinary Clinic, Faculity of veterinary Medicine, Addis AbebaUnivesity, Debrezite. DVM Thesis

[56] Salib, F. A., and Osman, A . H., (2011). Incidence of lumpy skin disease among Egyptian cattle in Giza Governorate, Egypt, Veterinary World, Vol. 4 (4):162-167.

[57] Shen, J. Y., Shephard, E., Douglass1, N, Johnston, N., Adams, C., Williamson, C., and Anna-LiseWilliamson, A. L., (2011). A novel candidate HIV vaccine vector based on the replication deficient Capri poxvirus, Lumpy skin disease virus.

[58] Thomas, L., (2002). Lumpy-skin disease, a disease of socio-economic importance.

[59] Traktman, P., (1996). Pox virus DNA replication, DNA replication in Eukaryotic cells, Department of cell biology and microbiology, Cornell University Medical College, New York.

[60] Tuppurainen, E. S. M and Oura. C. A. L., (2011). Review: Lumpy Skin Disease: An Emerging Threat to Europe, the Middle East and Asia, Institute for Animal Health, Pirbright, Surrey, UK.

[61] Tuppurainen, S. M., (2005). Detection of the lumpy skin disease virus in samples of the experimentally infected cattle using different diagnostic techniques, MSc thesis.

[62] Valones, A. A., Guimarães, L. R., Brandão. LA. C., de, Souza. P. R. E., Carvalho. A. D. T., Crovela, S., 2009. Principles and Applications of polymerase chain reaction in medical diagnostic fields: a review Brazilian Journal of Microbiology 40:1-11.

[63] Vorster, J. H., Mapham, P. H., (2008). Lumpy skin disease, Livestock health and Production review.

[64] Weiss, W. E., (1968). Lumpy Skin disease. In Emerging Diseases of Animals.

[65] Woods, J. A., (1988), Lumpy Skin Disease, *Review. Tropical AnimalHealthproduction. 20:11-17*

[66] Wood, J. A., (1990). Lumpy skin disease. In: Virus Infections of Ruminants, Dinter Z and Morein B (eds), Elsevier, Amsterdam, pp 53–67.

[67] Yeruham, I., Nir, O., Braverman, Y., Davidson, M., Grinstein, H., Haymovitch, M. andZamir, O., 1995. Spread of Lumpy skin disease in Israel dairy herds. *The Veterinary record 137: 91-93.*

[68] Young, E., BassonP. A., and K. E. Weiss., 1970: Experimental infection of game animals with lumpy skin disease virus prototype strain Neethling. Onderstepoort*J. Vet. Res. 37: 79–87.*

Effects of Sorting on Cannibalism in Catfish (*Clarias gariepinus*) Rose in Concrete Tanks in Maiduguri, North-Eastern Nigeria

Abubakar Abdullahi Biu[1], Gwana Adamu Mohammed[2, *], Bukar-Kolo M. Yachilla[3], Bako M. Modu[4], Umaru Buba Wakil[4], Abdullahi M. Mai[5], Ali Abba Gana Benisheikh[5, 6], Adarju M. B.[7]

[1]Department of Veterinary Microbiology, Parasitology and Virology, Faculty of Veterinary Medicine, University of Maiduguri, Nigeria
[2]Laboratory Unit, A.H.P Department, Mohamet Lawan College Agriculture, Maiduguri, Nigeria
[3]Department of Medicine, Faculty of Veterinary Medicine, Unimaid, Nigeria
[4]Department of Fisheries, Faculty of Agriculture, Unimaid, Nigeria
[5]Department of Basic Science, Mohamet Lawan College of Agriculture, Maiduguri, Nigeria
[6]Biotechnology Centre, University of Maiduguri, Maiduguri, Nigeria
[7]Chad Basin Development Authority, Gambaru-Ngala Road, Maiduguri, Nigeria

Email address:
biuvet@yahoo.com (A. A. Biu), admuwana@yahoo.com (A. M. Gwana), yachillabukar@yahoo.com (Y. M. Bukar–Kolo), mammadu09@gmail.com (M. M. Bako), ubwakilgza@yahoo.com (Umaru. B. W), mumin_abdullahi@yahoo.com (Abdullahi M. M.), alibenisheikh@yahoo.com (A. A. G. Benisheikh)

Abstract: This research study was carried out on the effects of cannibalism in catfish (*Clarias gariepinus*; commonly called "*Tarwada*" in Hausa language), rose in indoor aquaculture, at the hatchery complex, NIFFRI, Maiduguri. The experiments were designed into three treatments; 'A' no sorting (control), 'B' daily sorting and 'C' weekly sorting, performed after stocking with two replications. Randomly sourced, sampled brood stocks (2 males and 2 females). Standard method was used to induce breeding of *Clarias gariepinus* by using Ova-prim and fry were obtained. The Juveniles catfish were sorted, counted and stocked into tanks. Their average weight were taken (2.45kg) and density of 100 fish / m^2 was tested in each treatment, water parameters, survival rate, growth performance, rates and effects of cannibalism in *Clarias gariepinus* were determined. Treatment A had the highest mean weight (11.45g ± 2.4), cannibalism rate (40%), with lowest survival rate (60%). Highest survival rate was observed in C (86%), while optimum growth performance was observed in B (4.2g, 5cm, and 8cm). Results revealed that cannibalism is high in treatment A, less in C (2%), same with shooters. High cannibalism in *Clarias gariepinus* juveniles has been established, this could be controlled by frequent sorting (daily). Further studies are to be conducted on the cost implication of controlling cannibalism in outdoor aquaculture.

Keywords: Aquaculture, Cannibalism, *Clarias gariepinus*, Concrete Tank, Fry, Hatchery, Indoor, Ova-Prim

1. Introduction

Catfishes of the family Clariidae, known as "*Tarwada*" in Hausa language, "*Kumudu*" in Kanuri and "*Gbotongo*" in Fulfulde languages, comprise the most commonly cultivated in Nigeria. The growth of Aquacultures rising in Nigeria at the expense of catfish now is largely being boosted. Fishes, especially, catfish (*Clarias gariepinus*) are sources of food for human beings. It is very rich in proteins and vitamins, especially, vitamin A (Retinol). They are source of animal protein. Fishes such as those in the class Clariidae are highly, used and commercialized [31]. Every fish require energy for living, for growth maintenance, migration and reproduction, which is must to obtain food for its survival [22, 26, 29, 34]. Understanding diet and feeding habits (behavior) of fish is useful to all fisheries Scientists who were concerned with the aspect of fisheries [13, 7]. Royle (2001) reported that food of fish consist of all materials present in its environment. Fishes have been known to food on wide variety of things ranging from Sandy particles, phytoplankton, zooplanktons, leaves, roots, insects, insect larvae, warms, fishes e.t.c. [10, 30, 28, 32]. *Clarias gariepinus* is a benthopelagic fish which is known to have wide range of diet [1, 8, 11, 32, 33]. According to Yalcin *et. al.,* (2002), this specie is economically exploited for food and ornamentals purpose [5]. Catfishes (*Clarias* species) are some of the important fish species for aquaculture due to its high growth rate, significant tolerance to environment stress; reproduction in captivity, resistance to high density culture and its market demand [16]; especially *Clarias gariepinus* is widely accepted by Nigerian consumers and was acknowledged that, these bigger fish are sold for about twice the price of 30 days old fish [16, 24]. *Clarias gariepinus* has an average adult length of more than 1 metre long. These fish have slender bodies, a flat bony head, and a broad, terminal mouth with 4 pairs of barbells. They also have a large accessory breathing organ. They can weigh up to 29 kg or more [4]. Cannibalism is the act of killing and consuming the whole or major part of an individual belonging to the same species, irrespective of its stage or development. It is a common and widespread phenomenon throughout the animal kingdom [18, 27]. Young fish exhibit allometric growth patterns, high growth potentials than the older ones, the intensity of cannibalism would reach a maximum in the early weeks or months of the history when the variability of individual growth would be maximum [10]. Heterogeneous size distributions often lead to social dominance, which in turn results in aggressive behaviour and cannibalism [17]. Cannibalism is thus facilitated by size heterogeneity. But it also affects size heterogeneity, since the smallest fish are consumed by the larger ones, and thus be view as a cause or consequence of heterogeneity [6, 16]. Cannibalism among *Clarias gariepinus*, *Tilapia*, *Heterobranchus longifilis* fry and fingerlings have been identified as one of the major problems by small – scale hatchery operators [26]. Despite the increasing interest in this species, cannibalism among cultured *Clarias gariepinus* has received little attention and the factors underlying it have not much been investigated in details [2]. Therefore, Aquaculture remains the viable alternative for increasing fish production in order to meet the protein need of the people [2, 3, 19, 25]. It was observed that of the over 3,000,000 million tonnes of various freshwater and brackish water fish species in the years 2000, catfish were more abundant next to tilapia [12, 24]. It was reported by Food and Agricultural Organization [12] that 27, 488 million tonnes of catfish produced in 1990 were consumed locally. There is still great need for higher production for both local and international markets which would create labour opportunity. The objectives of this study are to ascertain and assess the effects of cannibalism in *Clarias gariepinus* rose in concrete tanks, the number of juveniles and shooters, determine the optimum sorting frequency for raising and the growth rate of *Clarias gariepinus* juveniles in concrete tanks.

2. Methodology

2.1. Study Area and Location

The study was conducted in Maiduguri, North – Eastern Nigeria. Majority of the local people are small scale business men, farmers, fishermen and herdsmen, Islamic and Western scholars [14]. The major languages are Kanuri, Shuwa-Arab, Hausa and English. It has an area land-mark of 300 square kilometres (300 km^2), lies between latitude 12^0 North to 13^0 North and longitude 13^0 East to 15^0 East. With an estimated population of 629,486 people, out of which 340,809 are males and 288,977 are females [23]. The climatic condition in this area is of a hot dry season (27^0C to 42^0C), and an annual rainfall of 500 to 600 mm has been recorded [14].

2.2. Materials

2.2.1. Apparatus Used

Constructed concrete tanks structure size of 4 m^2 (2 m x 2 m x 1 m), galvanized pipe connected to bore hole, hatchery metre rule, counting table, pH meter, thermometer, Koi air pump (50 KA), Analytical balance, glass container, syringes and needles, Petri-dishes, bowl and siphon, kankabans (Sponge).

2.2.2. Reagents Used

Hormone (Ova-prim), Normal saline solution (0.85% of NaCl salt), salt (NaCl), Artemia feed and 2mm Copens feed, detergent and bore-hole water.

2.3. Methods

2.3.1. Preparation and Sanitation of Experimental Tanks or Ponds

Six concrete tanks were constructed, having the sizes of $4m^2$ (2m x 2m x 1m) each. They were then supplied with water from the Institute bore-hole through galvanized pipe to each. Each tank has independent inlet and outlet ports as part of drainage system. These tanks were first thoroughly washed with water, later with detergent, salt solutions, and rinsed with water finally. They were later filled with water for the experiment. The temperature and the pH of the water were taken and recorded by using the thermometer and the Ph meter respectively.

2.3.2. Sampling of Sample Brood Stocking of Catfish (Clarias Gariepinus)

Four sampled brood stocks (2 males and 2 females), each weighed between 1.2 kg and 1.5 kg, and were randomly sourced from a commercial farm in Maiduguri metropolis, for the purpose of breeding fingerlings for the experimental research study. These brood stocks were stocked in to 2 tanks with high water levels flow for five days for acclimatization as described by [21].

2.3.3. Experimental Stage of Induced Breeding of Clarias gariepinus

The breeding of *Clarias gariepinus* were induced by using the standard method, Ova-prim (hormone) was used to carry out and to obtain fry for the experiment that is research study.

The gravid females were weighed individually and injected intramuscularly with Ova-prim (hormone) at a dosage of female, 0.5ml / kg of body weight. The injected breeding stocks were kept in a glass container with little water and well covered to avoid the breeding stocks from escaping. The stripping of the female was carried out after a latency period of 8 hours at 28°C water temperature, by means of gentle hand stripping into clean Bowls. The males were sacrificed, testes were removed into clean Petri-dish and milt were collected by maceration of the testes and mixed 0.85% saline solution as described by [20]. This was added to the eggs and mixed by gently shaking the Bowl. The eggs were allowed to fertilize by adding small volume of clean water. The fertilized eggs were then spread on kankabans inside the breeding tanks already prepared with water level of 0.2m respectively.

2.3.4. Experimental Observation of Hatching Fertilized Eggs

The eggs were observed to hatch after 22 hours at 28°C water temperature; hatchings were noticed swimming around the spawning mats, carrying their yolk. The spawning mats were removed on the second day after hatching took place, the tanks were cleaned and the dead eggs were siphoned out. The feeding commenced on the third day after absorption of the yolk. The early fry were fed six times a day between 6:00 AM and12:00 mid-nights with artemia. Aeration through powered aerator and flow through was ensured for five hours daily. Feeding with artemia had being continued, until lasted for two weeks as described by [29].

2.3.5. Experimental Design and Observation

(i) The experimental designed were completely randomized designed, which was consisted of three (3) treatments with two (2) replications; Treatment A, no sorting was done, that is, Control treatment. Treatment B, sorting was done on daily basis after stocking. Treatment C, sorting was done on weekly basis after stocking.

(ii) Prior to the start of the experiment, juveniles were sorted and counted before stocking into experimental tanks. The average weight of the juveniles catfish were taken (2.45g), and the density of 100 fish per metre square (100 fish / m^2) was tested in each treatment. The fish (juveniles catfish) were fed three (3) times daily at 7:00 am, 12:00 pm and 5:00 pm with 2mm Copens feed at 5% body weight respectively. Each tank was supplied with compressed air from Koi-Air Pump (50KA) via air stone. Dead fish were removed and recorded daily, juveniles fish were cropped and counted in the last observation day at the 8th weeks respectively. Data were obtained and recorded accordingly.

2.4. Data Analysis

Data obtained from this research study were subjected to statistical analysis by using means for the measurement of central tendency, and standard deviations for measurement of dispersion and or discrepancy within the variables (determined in triplicates) reported in percentage as described by [30] and as performed by [15].

3. Results and Discussion

3.1. Results

The Data obtained from this research study conducted on the effects of cannibalism in the catfish (*Clarias gariepinus*) rose in the indoor concrete tanks, hatchery complex of the National Institute of Freshwater Fisheries Research, along Gamboro – Ngala Road, Eastern part of Maiduguri, Borno state, Nigeria. Observed to yield the following results in tabulated:

Table 1 shows the stocking density (800 Juveniles Catfish), number of tanks used (6), 2 tanks per treatment which contained 400 Juveniles in each, mean water temperature of the tanks in treatments were; A (28.2^{O}C), B (28.0 ^{O}C) and C (27.9 ^{O}C), the pH in each of the treatment was; A (pH 7.15), B (pH 7.14) and C (pH 7.17) respectively.

Table 2 shows the growth performance of the Catfish (*Clarias gariepinus)* in each treatment A, B, and C to their weight in grams, standard length and the total length in centimetres per the sampling period of eight (8) weeks per each week, and the values obtained were expressed as mean of 2 tanks in each treatment.

Table 3 shows the number and the percentage of fish mortality (natural dead rate) per treatment during the experiments, thus; treatment A had 5 (1%), B had 32 (4%) and C had 102 (13%), which varies significantly with the treatments.

Table 4 shows the mean values of shooters in relation to number, weight, standard length and total length within the experiment conducted, thus; treatment A had 112 shooters, 19.02g, 11.8cm and 13.6cm; treatment B had 48 shooters, 11.41g, 9.4cm, and 10.5cm, then treatment C had 27 shooters, 6.06g, 8.0cm and 9.0cm respectively.

Table 5 shows the survival rate in percentage out of the total number of fish (800 Juveniles Catfish) in each treatment been stocked, thus; treatment A had 478 fish been harvested and the percentage of survival is 59.75%, treatment B had 562 fish been harvested with survival rate of 70.75%, while treatment C had 685 fish been harvested and the percentage of survival is 85.63%.

Table 6 shows the rate of Cannibalism in *Clarias gariepinus* Juveniles under the trial which occurred in the three (3) treatments of the experiments, thus; treatment A recorded 39.62%, and treatment B had 25.75%, while treatment C had been recorded1.62% respectively.

Table 7 shows the summarized rates of fish mortality, survival rate and the cannibalism rate occurred in the three treatments, thus; treatment A had the fish mortality rate of 0.63%, survival rate of 59.75% and the cannibalism rate of 39.62%. Treatment B had the fish mortality rate of 4%, survival rate of 70.25% and the cannibalism rate of 25.75%, while Treatment C had the fish mortality rate of 12.75%, survival rate of 85.63% and the cannibalism rate of 1.62% only.

Table 1. *Values of Density, Number of Tanks Used, Mean Water Temperature and pH.*

Treatment.	Sorting Times.	Density.	Number of Tanks Used.	Mean Water Temperature (°C).	Mean Water pH.
A	no sorting	800	2	28.2	7.15
B	Twice weekly	800	2	28.0	7.14
C	weekly	800	2	27.9	7.17
Total (Mean ± SD).		2400 (800 ± 0).	6 (2 ± 0).	84 (28 ± 0.2).	21.5 (7.2 ± 0.02).

Table 2. *Growth Performance of Clarias gariepinus Juveniles under Trials*

Sampling Periods. (Week).	Treatment A. W (g).	SL (cm).	TL (cm).	Treatment B. W (g).	SL (cm).	TL (cm).	Treatment C. W (g).	SL (cm).	TL (cm).
1	2.16	3.1	3.7	2.15	3.0	3.6	2.16	3.1	3.7
2	2.68	3.8	4.5	2.39	3.6	4.1	2.4	3.8	4.1
3	3.2	4.6	5.3	2.94	4.0	4.6	2.4	4.0	4.5
4	4.14	6.5	6.4	3.51	4.6	5.4	3.19	4.6	5.3
5	5.83	6.5	7.5	4.13	5.5	6.4	3.41	5.1	5.8
6	7.3	7.7	8.8	4.99	6.1	7.0	3.86	5.7	6.4
7	8.76	9.0	10.4	6.12	6.9	7.9	4.11	6.2	6.8
8	11.45	10.8	12.0	7.20	8.0	9.0	4.57	6.5	7.2
(M±SD).	46(6±3.3).	52(7±2.6).	59(7±3).	33(4.2±2).	42(5±2).	48(8±2).	26(3.3±0.9).	39(4.9±1).	44(5.5±1.3).

Note: Values are expressed as Mean of two (2) tanks in each Treatment.

Table 3. *Catfish Mortality Rate In The Experiment.*

Treatment.	Number of Death.	Percentage of Mortality.
A	5	0.63
B	32	4.00
C	102	12.75
Total (Mean ± SD).	139(46.33 ± 50.06).	17.4 (5.8 ± 6.3).

Table 4. *Mean Values of Shooters in Relation to Number, Weight and Length*

Treatment.	Number of	Weight Shooters (g).	Standard Length	Total Length
A	112	19.02	11.8	13.6
B	48	11.41	9.4	10.5
C	27	6.06	8.0	9.0
(Mean±SD).	18 (62.33 ± 44.3).	37 (12.2 ± 7).	29 (10 ± 2).	33 (11 ± 2.4).

Table 5. *Survival Rate of Clarias gariepinus Under Trials.*

Treatment.	Number of Fish Stocked.	Number of Fish Harvested.	Percentage of Survival of Fish.
A	800	478	59.75
B	800	562	70.75
C	800	685	85.63
Total (Mean±SD).	2400 (800 ± 0).	1725 (575 ± 104).	216 (72 ± 13).

Table 6. *Rate of Cannibalism on the Clarias gariepinus Under Trials*

Treatment.	Number of Fish Stocked.	Number of Fish Lost.	Percentage of Cannibalism.
A	800	322	39.62
B	800	238	25.75
C	800	115	1.62
Total (Mean±SD).	2400 (800 ± 0).	675 (225 ± 104).	67 (22 ±19).

Table 7. *Rate of Fish Mortality, Survival and Cannibalism Occurred in the Three Treatment*

Treatment.	Fish Mortality Percentage.	Survival Rate Percentage.	Percentage of Cannibalism.
A	0.63	59.75	39.62
B	4.00	70.25	25.75
C	12.75	85.63	1.62
Total (M±SD).	17.4 (6 ± 6).	216 (72 ± 13).	67(22 ± 19).

4. Discussion

The research study on the assessment of cannibalism rate in the growth of *Clarias gariepinus* juveniles in indoor concrete tanks which was conducted in Maiduguri, was designed into three experimental treatments; A (no sorting), B (twice sorting weekly), and C (weekly sorting), with two tanks each, which were stocked 400 juveniles catfish each, and gave a total of 2400 juveniles catfish. The mean temperature and pH of the water used in experiments were 27.9°C and pH 7.17 recorded.

These results revealed that the growth performances of the Catfish in the 3 treatments are expressed as mean value of the two tanks in each treatment. In treatment A, the weight, standard length and the total length were found to be 6g, 7cm, and 7cm. In treatment B, are c, while that of treatment C, are 3.3g, 4.9cm, and 5.5cm respectively. It implies that, in terms of weight treatment A is the highest, seconded by B and the lowest is treatment C. Likewise, with regard to the total length and standard length, treatment C had the highest values, and then followed by treatment B and the lowest is treatment A. This could be as a result of the cannibalism rate amongst the Juvenile catfish. This is due to the cannibalism by shooters which feed on the younger ones. Shooters are those juvenile catfish which grow faster than their counter of the same age.

In another observation made, the results revealed that, number of Catfish mortality in each of the treatments were observed to be in treatment A, B and C are 0.63%, 4% and 13%. This shows that, treatment C has the highest loses, followed by treatment B and the least is treatment A respectively. In another findings, the mean values of shooters in relation to their numbers, weights and lengths in the experimental treatments revealed that, treatment A had the highest number of shooters (112), followed by treatment B (48) and the least was treatment C (27) only. The mean weight of shooters in the 3 treatments A, B and C are that A had the highest values than B, while the least was observed C. i.e. treatment A has the highest, seconded by treatment B and the lest is treatment C. Likewise, the highest mean values of the standard length of the shooters in the 3 treatments A, B and C were 12cm, 9cm and 8cm, and that of the total length are 14cm, 11cm and 9cm respectively. That means, with regard to both lengths, treatment A possessed the highest, treatment B followed and the least is treatment C.

The results revealed that, the survival rates of the Catfish (*Clarias gariepinus*) juveniles under the experimental trials, which were stocked with 800 juveniles each, treatment C had the highest with 685 (86%), followed by treatment B with 562 (71%) and the least is treatment A with 478 (60%). Within the same research study, it revealed that the rates of cannibalism in Catfish under the experimental trials in the 3 treatments A, B and C are found to be 40%, 26% and 2% approximately, of which the highest is treatment A, seconded by treatment B and the least is treatment C and this support the work of most authors such as Hecht, T. & Pienaar, 1993; Dadebo E, 2009.

Finally, the total rate of Catfish mortality is 17%, the total Catfish survival rate is 26% and the total Catfish cannibalism rate is 67% approximately and also the growth performance were high when compared with, there was no sorting. Cannibalism is facilitated by size heterogeneity. But it also affects size heterogeneity, since the smallest fish are consumed by the larger ones, and thus be view as a cause or consequence of heterogeneity. The results obtained from this study supports the works of most authors amongst others are; Hecht and Appelbaum, (1988); Pantastico *et. al*, (1988); Hecht & Pienaar, 1993; Baras, (1999); Dadebo, 2009; Yalcin et al, 2002. Cannibalism among cultured *Clarias gariepinus, Tilapia, Heterobranchus longifilis* fry and fingerlings have been identified as one of the major problems by small – scale hatchery operators, despite the increasing interest in this species, cannibalism among cultured *Clarias gariepinus* especially, has received little attention and the factors underlying it have not totally been investigated in details. From the findings of this study, it revealed that frequent sorting could reduce the cost of fish lost due to cannibalism, and if that is the case, it will encourage farmers and unemployed persons to take part in the fish production, processing and entrepreneurship as means of job creation.

With the recent plan of the Federal Government of Nigeria's programme on the structured ban on fish importation, according to the Agricultural and Rural Development Minister, statement on the programme [9], "the Government decision to gradually stop the importation of fish is understandable, spends a whopping Ninety seven billion Nigerian Naira (NGN 97 billion) on the importation of 700,000 metric tonnes of fish every year" he made this known at the 27th ANC of Fisheries Society of Nigeria held at Yenago, Delta state. He reiterated that, "there is no debating the wisdom in reducing Nigeria's over-dependence on imported fish, it is important that we develop the capacity to produce the adequate food that we need in adequate quantities. The ban will boast local fish production; create jobs for unemployed Nigerians and some foreign exchange". This study provides the solutions to the problems of catfish cannibalism (by frequent sorting of the shooter which reduces the cannibalism) and the programme on the ban on fish importation is an opportunity to aquaculture farmers and it is a challenge to all fish farmers and fish entrepreneurs at large.

5. Conclusion and Recommendations

5.1. Conclusion

The findings obtained from the research study conducted on the effects of sorting on cannibalism among juveniles catfish growth, had been experimentally designed into three treatments A, B and C, and observed to revealed this results. The total rate of cannibalism is much higher. The rate of cannibalism in treatment A, when compared to other treatments (B and C) revealed that there could be high loss of juveniles' catfish where no sorting was applied when raising *Clarias gariepinus* in indoor rearing system. Also the optimum performance of treatment B in terms of cannibalism rate and survival rate gave a clear indication that sorting is been required (on daily bases) when raising *Clarias gariepinus* juveniles, which was observed in this research study by the used of optimum sorting in the treatment B, when considered its optimum growth performance, survival rate is high and mortality rate is low and the growth performance is high. The rate of cannibalism is highly noticed in treatment A and less in treatment C, and likewise, same with the number of shooter obtained, this gave a clear indication that there is a high cannibalism rate in *Clarias gariepinus* juveniles and this could be influence by sorting frequencies. The problem of cannibalism in juvenile fish production should be considered. This is because many farmers are being discouraged already from stocking their ponds with fingerlings. The need to encourage and sustain fish in Arid-zone, Nigeria, so as to make aquaculture more reliable and resilient prompted this study with a view of recommending strategies to fish farmers, most particularly in Maiduguri, Borno state, north – eastern Nigeria.

5.2. Recommendations

We recommends that further studies are to be carried out on the cost implication, to evaluate cannibalism rates in *Clarias gariepinus* juveniles in outdoor rearing operations and within a large scope, and same research studies are to be carried out both in indoor and outdoor to ascertain and evaluate the effects of sorting on cannibalism in the same Catfish species raising.

Acknowledgement

It is a great pleasure to acknowledge with most honoured and duly respected; we owe particular thanks to all those researchers cited in this piece of work and most grateful to all persons who have helped or assisted in one way or the other in the course of carrying out this study.

Reference

[1] Abdel-Aziz, N.E and Gharib, S.M. "Food for feeding habits of rund sardinella (sardInellaaurıta) in El- mex Bay, Alexandria, Egypt" Egypt: *J. Aquat Res*.33:202-221. 2007.

[2] Ahmed, E. "Sustainability Aquaculture Grows in Importance as Demand for Fish Increase", http //: www. Fao.org. Pp. 1 – 3. 2006.

[3] Aminu, R & Omoyeni, A. B "Integrating Culture, Economics and Environmental Requirements for Fish Production in Borno State", In: Eyo, A.A. and Ajao, E.A. (Eds), Proceeding of the 16th Annual Conference of Fisheries Society of Nigeria, (FISON), Maiduguri, Held on 4th – 9th November, 2001; Pp. 58 – 62. 2001.

[4] Anoop, K.R; Sunday, K.S.G; Khan, B.A. & Las, S. "Common Moorhen *Gallinuba chlorus* in the Diet of the African Catfish *Clarias gariepinus* in Keolado, Ghana National Park, India Birds", 5 (2); Pp. 22- 23. 2009.

[5] Babatunde, D.O., and Aminu, R. "Field guide to Nigeria freshwater Fisheries", second edition; 47-49. 2004.

[6] Baras, E. "Sibling Cannibalism among Juvenile Vundu under Controlled Condition, In: Cannibalistic behaviours, Prey Selection, Prey Selectivity, *Journal of Fish Biology*, 54 (5); Pp. 82 – 105.1999.

[7] Dadebo E. "Filter feeding habits of the African catfish *Clarias gariepinus*" Burchell, 1822 (pises: Clariidae) in Lake Chamo, Ethiopia. Ethiopia. J. Biol. Sci. 8(1):15-30. 2009.

[8] Dadebo E. "Reproductive Biology and feeding habits of the catfish *Clarias gariepinus* Burchell (pices: clariidae) in lake Awassa, Ethiopia" SINET. Ethopia. J.Sci.23:231-246. 2000.

[9] Dailysun. "The Structured Ban on Fish Importation", In: Editorial, DailySun, www.sunnewsonline.com Monday, January 20th, 2014, Volume 10, Number 2800; Pp. 19. 2014.

[10] David, D.L; Edward, A; Adass, PA and Jesse C. "Some aspect of water quality and the Biology of *Clarias gariepinus* in Vimtim Stream, Mubi Adamawa state, Nigeria." World J. fish mar. Sci. 2(2):129-133. 2010.

[11] EL Gamal Ael-R Ismail NM. "Food composition and feeding habit of some fresh water of fishes in various water systems at Abbassa, Egypt, with special reference to snail transmitting diseases." *J. Egypt. Soc. Paracitol*. 35(2):637-52. 2005.

[12] F.A.O. Fisheries Statistic, In: Aquaculture Production, FAO Fisheries Series, Number 58, FAO, Rome, 1999.

[13] Getabu A. "A comparative study on the feeding habits of *Oreochromis niloticus* in Nyanza Gulf, Lake Victoria and sewage ponds," In: proceeding of the second EEC Regional seminar on Recant Trend of Research on Lake Victoria Fisheries, Kisumu, Kenya, 25-27 September 1992 (Eds. Okemwa E. Wakwabi E and GETABU A). ICIPE, press, Nairobi, Kenya. 1994.

[14] Gwana, A.M; Auwal, M.S; Bagudu, B.Y. & Gazali, Y.A "Study Area and Location, In: Comparative of Parasitological Diagnostic Techniques in the Survey of Haemoparasites of Camel Slaughtered in Maiduguri Central Abattoir, North – eastern Nigeria", *Journal of Laboratory Science*, Volume 1, number 2; Pp. 57 – 65. 2013.

[15] Gwana, A.M; Mshelia, Ngita Hassan; Abdullahi, Mumin Mai; Auwal, Mohammed Shu'aibu; Bagudu, Buhari Yawuri; Mala, B. Mohammed, Abdullahi, Hala Mal; Sadiq, Aji Bukar. "Effects of Domestic Wastes on Water from Shallow – Wells in Moduganari, Nigeria." *International Journal of Environmental Monitoring and Analysis*. Vol. 2, No. 4, 2014, pp. 185-190. doi: 10.11648/ijema. 20140204.11

[16] Haylor, G.S. "The Case for African Catfish, *Clarias gariepinus* (Burchell, 1882), A Comparison of Relative of Tilapia, Especially *Oreochromis niloticus* (L) and *Clarias gariepinus* (Burchell, 1882) for African Aquaculture", *Aquaculture and Fisheries Management*, Volume 20, Pp. 279 – 285. 1989.

[17] Hecht, T. & Appelbaum, S. "Observation on Intra-specific Aggression and Coeval Sibling Cannibalism by Leave and Juvenile *Clarias gariepinus*, (Clarias: Pisces), Under Controlled Condition," *Journal of Zoo*, London, 214; Pp. 21 – 44. 1988.

[18] Hecht, T. & Pienaar, A. "A Review of Cannibalism and its Implication in Fish Larviculture," *Journal of World Aquaculture Society*, 24 (2); Pp. 246 – 261. 1993.

[19] International Labour Organization. "Meeting the Challenges of Unemployment", Report Submitted by the ILO Employment Policy Strategy Formulation Mission in Nigeria; Pp. 2 – 5. 2006.

[20] Lue, M.Y & Chou, Y.C."Induced Spawning and Larva of Captive Yellow Fin Porgy *Aconthopagus latus* (Honttuyn), Aquaculture," 143; Pp. 155 – 166.1996. [21]Luis Anthonio, K.A.I; Jose, A.S & Evoy, Z.F. "Growth of Pace Juveniles in Nightly Aerate System", Acta Scientarium, Aminu Sciences, Maringa, Vol. 25, Number 1; Pp.4 – 48. 2000.

[21] Munro. "African Inland water fisheries and environmental processing of fishes" *Fisheries Society of Nigeria*, Pp. 74. 2001.

[22] National Population Commission (2006): Census De Facto, In: Census Report; Vital statistical Unit, Gidan Madara, Maiduguri, Borno State Nigeria. 2006.

[23] Omitoyin, B.O. "Introduction to Fish Farming in Nigeria", Ibadan University Press, ISBN 978-121-427-9, 1st Ed; Pp. 87. 2007.

[24] Oresegun, A; Oguntade, O.A & Ayinla, A. "A Review of Catfish Culture in Nigeria", *Nigerian Journal of Fisheries*, 4 (1); Pp. 27 – 52. 2007.

[25] Pantastico, J.B; Dangilan, M.M.A & Eugia, R.V. "Cannibalism Among Different Sizes of Tilapia (*Oreochromis niloticus*) Fry and Fingerling, and the Effect of Natural Food", In: The Second International Symposium on Tilapia in Aquaculture, ICLARM Conf. Proceeding, 15, 623P, Bangkok, Thailand; Pp. 465 – 468. 1988.

[26] Royle, W. "Observation on feeding habits of Clarias barrage experimental pond found in food scheme Technology." No.5, Vol. 2. 76 - 79. 2001.

[27] Smith, C. & Reay, P. "Cannibalism in Teleost Fish, Reviews in Fish Biology and Fisheries", 1st Ed; Pp. 41 – 64. 1991.

[28] Sorgeloos, P. "The Use of Brine Shrimp Artemia in Aquaculture", In: Persons, G.P, Sorgeloos, O.A & Roels, E.J (eds.), University Press Wetteren, (Belgium), 3; Pp.23 – 27. 1980.

[29] Stroud, K.A & Booth, D.J." Statistical Package", In: *Engineering Mathematics.* WWW. Palgrave.Com / Stroud, Pal grave, GB, London, 5th Edition; 1130 – 1139. 2001.

[30] Yalcin, S; Solak, U & Solak K. "Stomach Contents of the catfish (*Clarias gariepinus* Burchell, 1822) in the River Asi, Turkey". *Turk.J. zool.*25: 461-468. 2001.

[31] Yalcin, S; Solak, K & A. Kyurt, I. "Growth of catfish, *Clarias gariepinus* (Claridea) in River Asi (Orontes), Turkey." Cybium 26(3): 163-172. 2002.

[32] Zaret, T.M. "Predation of freshwater communities" Yale University press. New Haven. P.187.1980.

Optimum Dietary Crude Protein Level for Fattening Yearling Arsi-Bale Lambs

Getahun Kebede Yadete

Ruminant Livestock Research, Debre Zeit Agricultural Research Center, Debre Zeit, Ethiopia

Email address:
getkeb2000@yahoo.com

Abstract: This study was aimed to determine the optimum dietary crude protein for fattening yearling Arsi-Bale sheep. Thirty-two intact male lambs (live weight=17.53±1.57 kg) were randomly assigned to five iso-caloric (2.12 Mcal/kg DM) dietary treatments (T), varying in crude protein: 9.4% CP (T1), 10.2% CP (T2), 11% CP (T3), 12% CP (T4) and 13.1% CP (T5). Intake and growth trial lasted for 87 days, followed by digestibility trial and carcass analysis. Treatments did not differ (P>0.05) in DM intake, ranging from 918.29 (T1) to 928.09 g DM/day (T3). Crude protein intake increased ($P<0.001$) with increase in dietary CP (T1, 86.71 g/day; 120g/day - T5). Intake of fiber fractions was highest (P<0.001) with 12% CP diet. Treatments varied in apparent digestibility of DM (P<0.05), CP (P<0.05), NDF (P<0.001) and ADF (P<0.001). Average final live weight, total gain and daily gain of lambs were increased non-significantly (P>0.05) from 22.71 to 23.96 kg; 5.37 to 6.35kg; 61.78-73.00 g/day, respectively. Feed conversion ratios were higher (P<0.001) in lambs fed 12%CP diet (12.61) and 13% CP diet (12.76). Urinary nitrogen and total nitrogen excretion were highest for 13% CP diet (5.02 and 9.19 g/day; P<0.001). Nitrogen balance was peaked (12.70 g/day, P<0.001) with 12% CP diet. There was no significant differences (P>0.05) among treatments in slaughter weight, hot carcass weight, DP, fat and bone proportions. However, hot carcass weight increased from 8.8 to 9.8kg and DP from 39.4 to 42.15, with feed CP increase to 12%. The results of this study indicated that optimum dietary CP for improved growth and feed utilization of yearling Arsi-Bale lambs, growing from 17 to 25 kg is 12% at the specified dietary energy. Suggested, detail study, applying "comparative slaughter technique" is warranted to support the present findings.

Keywords: Yearling Lambs, Weight Gain, Dietary Protein

1. Introduction

Sheep production plays a crucial role in Ethiopia, majorly serving as a family food (meat) and income source from sale of live sheep. There exist 29.33 million sheep population in Ethiopia [5] that entirely raised under traditional production system- characterized by low input-output. The productivity of sheep is very low as explained by annual off-take rate of 33% and average carcass weight of 10 kg/head [7]. The productivity is hindered by feed deficit (inadequate amount and quality), low genetic potential of sheep and prevalence of disease and parasites. Sheep are raised entirely on grazing pasture and rarely supplemented with concentrates. Feed deficit is aggravated with dry season and drought occurrence, when dry roughages remain major available feed and protein is the most limiting macronutrient. Most sheep are sold to local markets at around yearling age (live weight below 20 kg) often without supplementation (body conditioning) before marketing. However, some farmers traditionally fatten their sheep before marketing, with little concentrate supplementation on top of grazing.However, there is uncertainty that the supplementation could support the nutrient requirement for maximum growth of sheep. Moreover, this system of feeding would sometimes lead to over or under utilization of available feed nutrient that may lead to its wastage and uneconomic feeding.

Feeding sheep based on their nutrient requirement at different production phases is not common practice in Ethiopia. On the other hand, most of the developed feeding standards initially based temperate wool breed sheep [17] and some tropical sheep breeds [12, 19] have been used in improved sheep production systems. According to Andrew and Orskov [3], the maximum live weight gain and nitrogen retention of temperate breed lambs on high plane of nutrition, growing from 15 to 40 kg were achieved at 17% dietary CP. In addition, National Research Council (NRC) [17] recommended a diet containing 14.5% CP for maximum growth of early weaned lambs. Unlike that for temperate breeds, Kearl [12] and Paul et al [19] recommended a lower levels of dietary CP and energy for growing tropical sheep at different growth rates and live weights.

Although nutrient requirement tables developed for tropical sheep are believed to meet the requirements of indigenous sheep breeds of Ethiopia, it has been rarely accepted and applied, as the recommendations based estimates obtained from a specific breed, which may not necessarily represent local sheep. Also, differences in the quality of feed and utilization efficiency by animal may contribute to this uncertainty. The differences in nutrient requirement of animals lie on breed, age, physiological status, growth potential, feed quality and environmental factors, such as temperature, air humidity, solar radiation and wind speed [17]. However, there is no/little information on nutrient requirements specific to indigenous sheep breeds of Ethiopia. Therefore, this study was aimed to determine the optimum dietary crude protein for maximum growth and feed utilization of yearling Arsi-Bale lambs in feedlot.

2. Materials and Methods

2.1. Study Area

The experiment was conducted at sheep research station of Debre Zeit Agricultural Research Centre, located at 45 km South East of Addis Ababa (08°44'N 38°,58'E; average altitude of 1900 m a.s.l), Ethiopia. The area is known for bimodal rainfall pattern with average annual rainfall of 845 mm and annual minimum and maximum temperature of 10 and 22 °C, respectively. The area is characterized by mixed-crop-livestock production system, with major crops grown include tef (*Eragrostis tef*), wheat, chick pea and lentil.

2.2. Treatments and Feed Composition

Table 1. Feed ingredients and chemical composition (%DM).

	T1	T2	T3	T4	T5
% Diet composition					
Straw	Straw	Straw	Straw	Straw	Straw
*Noug cake	-	6.0	19.9	35.0	47.2
*Wheat bran	82.3	80.8	62.9	49.9	6.0
*Maize grain	15.6	3.0	7.0	12.9	16.1
*Wheat middling	-	8.1	8.1	-	28.6
*Limestone	1.1	1.1	1.1	1.1	1.1
salt	1.0	1.0	1.0	1.0	1.0
Total	100	100	100	100	100
Chemical composition:(% DM)					
DM	91.46	91.55	91.53	91.84	92.30
CP	9.43	10.26	11.06	12.06	13.10
Ash	12.25	12.69	12.91	10.67	9.71
NDF	48.66	52.86	55.79	56.77	54.80
ADF	26.71	26.43	28.15	31.65	29.18
ADL	5.65	5.75	6.33	7.61	7.20
ME (Mcal kg-1)	2.14	2.13	2.12	2.11	2.11

ME =Metaboliszable energy; calculated according to Kearl [11]. * % DM of concentrate mix. Ratio of straw to concentrate offered was 65: 35, on as fed basis.

The diets were similar in composition, with the exception of noug seed cake and wheat middling (diet1) and wheat middling (diet4) exclusion for the purpose of balancing (Table 1). Maize grain, wheat bran, noug seed cake, wheat middling, salt and limestone constituted concentrate part that contained 14, 16, 18, 20 and 22% CP in the respective treatments, leading to differences in dietary CP (9.43% CP in T1, 10.26% CP in T2, 11.06% CP in T3; 12.06 % CP in T4 and 13.1% CP in T5). The diets were formulated to be nearly iso-caloric (2.12 Mcal ME/Kg DM) and meet the energy requirement for growing tropical sheep [12]. The diet containing 9.4% CP was used as negative control, while 13% CP diet was positive control. All diets were similar in DM content, but differed in NDF, ADF and ADL.

2.3. Animals and Feeding Management

Thirty-two yearling male Arsi-Bale sheep with mean initial live weight of 17.53 ±1.57 kg were purchased from local markets and treated against endo-and ecto-parasites and vaccinated for common viral diseases. All animals were individually penned in a house with concrete floor and adapted to indoor feeding management for two weeks, before commencing the experiment. Then, they were randomly assigned to five dietary treatments in completely randomised design.

Feed was provided twice daily at 8:30 a.m and 2:00 p.m ensuring 15% refusal for each animal. The amount of straw and concentrate offered were adjusted daily based on previous day intake, where straw to concentrate ratio was 65:35, on as fed basis. Water was provided in a bucket free of choice. Feed offered and refusals were measured daily and feed intake was calculated as the difference between the two measurements. Representative feed samples were taken daily and sub-sampled every 15 days. All animals were weighed biweekly after overnight (~16 hours) deprivation of feeds and water.

At the end of the feeding period (87 days), three lambs were selected per treatment and transferred to metabolic crate with slotted floor, individually. The animals were adapted to the attached fecal bags and urine funnels for three days followed by collection of fecal and urine for seven days. All animals were with unlimited access to water. Urine was directly poured into a glass bottle containing drops of sulfuric acid to prevent ammonia loss. The amount of feces and urine produced per animal/day was measured and recorded. About 10% of the daily fecal and urine outputs were sampled per animal and stored in a deep freezer (-20°C) until sub-sampled for laboratory analysis. Moreover, three animals were randomly selected per treatment and slaughtered for carcass analysis. The animals were slaughtered after 24 hour of feed deprivation. Measurements were taken for slaughter weight, hot carcass weight (HCW) and carcass components (bone, fat and lean, trimmings). Dressing percentage (DP) was calculated as: (HCW/SW)*100.

2.4. Sample Chemical Analysis

Feed and fecal dry matter (DM), crude protein (CP) and Ash were determined according to the procedures of AOAC [4], while neutral detergent fiber (NDF), acid detergent fiber (ADF) and acid detergent lignin (ADL) were determined according to Van Soest et al [22].

2.5. Statistical Analysis

Data was analyzed using the General Linear Model (GLM) procedure of SAS [20]. Treatment means of the parameters were separated using Duncan Multiple Range Test. The statistical model used for feed intake, live weight change, digestibility, feed conversion ratio, carcass parameters and nitrogen utilization was: $Y_{ij} = \mu + \alpha_i + \epsilon_{ij}$, Where, μ = Grand mean; α_i = Effect of treatment feeds; and ϵ_{ij}=Experimental error. Data on average daily gain (ADG) for each lamb was computed by regressing the live weight incurred in two weeks interval over the number of days elapsed.

3. Results and Discussion

3.1. Nutrient Intake and Digestibility

The effect of treatments was not significant on dry matter intake (P>0.05), ranging from 918.3 (T1) to 928.1 g/day per lamb (T3). The magnitude of DM intake observed in the present study is comparable with previous studies for Arsi-Bale lambs maintained on roughage and concentrate [6, 8], but higher than that reported for Afar and Black head Ogaden lambs [9]. Studies have shown that a non-significant feed intake with sheep fed diets containing 9% to 13% CP [2], in Saanen kids fed 14% to16% CP diets [15] and Korean black goats consumed 14-20% CP diet [11]. In the present study, intake of crude protein linearly increased (P<0.001) with increase in dietary CP, where lambs on 13% CP diet consumed 120g CP/day. Also, intake of fiber fractions increased with increase in dietary CP, the highest value obtained with 12% CP diet. Although change in the apparent digestibility of nutrients was non-linear with change in dietary CP, there was variation in digestibility of DM (P<0.05), CP (P<0.05), NDF (P<0.001) and ADF (P<0.001). The apparent digestibility of nutrients was greater with T2 and T4 diets, and lowest with T3 diet.

Table 2. *Effect of dietary crude protein level on intake and apparent digestibility of nutrients.*

Parameter		Treatments T1 (n=6)	T2 (n=6)	T3 (n=6)	T4 (n=7)	T5 (n=7)	SEM	P value
Intake	DM	920.26ba	918.29b	928.09ab	920.33ab	922.23ab	3.17	0.2262
(g/day)	CP	86.71e	94.13d	102.61c	110.87b	120.63a	0.37	<.001
	ME	1.97a	1.95ab	1.96ab	1.94b	1.95ab	0.01	<.001
	Ash	112.71c	116.61b	119.81a	98.22d	89.51e	0.39	<.001
	NDF	447.81e	485.39d	517.68b	522.41a	505.52c	1.74	<.001
	ADF	245.86d	242.83d	261.25c	290.93a	269.31b	0.94	<.001
	ADL	52.05e	52.85d	58.72c	70.05a	66.41b	0.22	<.001
Digestibility	DM	55.59b	61.56a	54.66b	64.30a	60.92ab	2.18	0.0393
(%)	CP	59.91ab	59.55ab	58.55b	65.49ab	66.54a	2.32	0.0477
	NDF	64.88bc	74.79a	63.0bc	67.11b	60.41c	2.07	<.001
	ADF	62.24b	71.75a	49.58c	66.60ab	53.4c	2.65	<.001

a,b,c,d,e Values with different superscripts within same row are significantly different; DM=dry matter intake; CPI=crude protein intake; AshI= ash intake; NDFI= neutral detergent fiber intake; ADFI= acid detergent fiber intake; ADLI= acid detergent intake, SEM= standard error of mean; n= number of lambs

3.2. Live Weight Change and Feed Conversion Ratio (FCR)

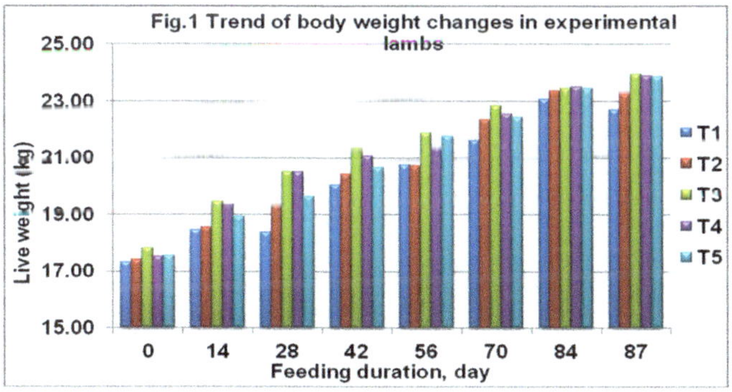

Although non-significant (P>0.05), an improve in the average final live weight (22.71 vs. 23.96 kg), total gain (5.37 vs 6.35kg) and average daily gain (61.78 vs 73.00 g/day) were observed with increase in dietary CP. The observed changes in growth performance with higher CP diet probably resulted from increase in feed intake. In agreement with the present results, Paul et al [19] recommended 9.7%CP to 12.1% CP) diet for tropical sheep, growing from 15 kg to 25 kg. However, improved growth performances were reported at higher (16 to 18%) than lower (10-14%) dietary crude protein for Awassi lambs [10, 21] and Kivircik lambs [13]. Similarly, Hwangbo et al [11] reported the highest gain for growing Korean black goats at higher (18%CP) than lower level of dietary CP. The present study has also shown that changes in live weights of lambs were incremental throughout feeding period (Fig 1). There was differences in FCR (P<0.001): the highest FCR were observed in lambs fed 12% CP diet (12.61 DMI/g gain) and 13% CP diet (12.76 g DMI/g gain),while the lowest value (14.9) was in lambs fed 9.4% CP diet, suggesting a higher nutrient availability at given feed protein and energy contents. Previous studies by Abebe et al [1] and Ermias [6] have indicated an improve in feed utilization and growth performances of Arsi-Bale lambs at higher than lower level of protein source concentrates.

Table 3. *Effect of dietary crude protein on live weight change and feed conversion ratio (FCR).*

	T1 (n=6)	T2 (n=6)	T3 (n=6)	T4 (n=7)	T5 (n=7)	SEM	P value
Initial wt, kg	17.33	17.41	17.83	17.53	17.57	0.68	0.9886
Final wt, kg	22.71	23.25	23.96	23.88	23.86	0.81	0.7814
Total gain, kg	5.37	5.83	6.12	6.35	6.28	0.70	0.8673
ADG, g	61.78	67.05	70.40	73.00	72.25	8.12	0.8673
FCR	14.90c	13.70b	13.18b	12.61a	12.76a	0.24	<0.001

a,b,c Values with different superscripts within same rows are significantly different; FCR= feed conversion ratio(g DMI/g gain); ADG=average daily gain; SEM= standard error of mean; n=number of animals.

3.3. Nitrogen Utilization

Table 4. *Nitrogen utilization (g/day) in lambs fed the experimental diets.*

Treatments	NI	UN	FN	TN	NB
1	15.03e	1.52c	3.76	5.29d	9.74d
2	16.21d	4.12ab	4.20	8.32c	7.89e
3	17.72c	2.43c	4.68	7.11c	10.61cd
4	19.57b	3.06bc	3.81	6.87dc	12.70ab
5	21.08a	5.02a	4.18	9.19a	11.89cb
SEM	0.103	0.431	0.417	0.623	0.646
P- value	<0.001	<0.001	0.5358	0.0005	<0.001

a,b,c,d,e values with different superscripts within same column are significantly different; UN=urine nitrogen, g/d; FN=fecal N; NI= N intake; TN= total N excreted; NB= nitrogen balance; SEM= standard error of mean

Nitrogen intake (NI), urinary nitrogen(UN) and total nitrogen excretion (TN) increased ($P<0.001$) with increase in dietary CP (Table 4). The highest NI(21.08), UN(5.02), and TN excretion (9.19 g/day) were observed in 13% CP diet. Treatments did not vary ($P>0.05$) in the level of fecal nitrogen excretion. An increase ($P<0.001$) in nitrogen balance (NB) was seen with increased dietary CP, being the highest (12.70 g/day) in12% CP diet. Osuagwuh and Akinsoyinu [18] reported an increase in NI, UN, FN and N retention for West African dwarf goats, as the level of crude protein in the supplement increased from 5% to 25% DM. However, there was no significant difference ($P>0.05$) in nitrogen balance between lambs fed 12% and 13% CP diets. The result shows that the higher nitrogen balance, the better the growth performances of lambs.

3.4. Carcass Analysis

There was no real difference ($P>0.05$) among treatments in SW, HCW, DP, fat and bone yields (Table 5). However, the magnitude of HCW increased by about 10% (8.88 vs. 9.8kg) and that of DP increased by 6.5% (39.38 vs. 42.15kg), as feed CP increased from 9.4% to 12%. Studies have shown that DP increases as SW increases [14, 16]. However, the fact that no remarkable change in DP in the present study might have resulted from the lower SW of sample animals. In this study, lean meat yield increased ($P<0.05$) with increase in feed CP%, where the highest value (6.52kg) was observed with 13% CP diet. Similarly, lean to bone and lean to fat ratios were highest for 13% CP diet compared to 9.4% CP diet. There was no significant change in the proportion of fat, bone and meat for Korean Black goat kept on 14% to 20% CP diet [11].

Table 5. *Effect of dietary crude protein level on carcass parameters of experimental lambs.*

Parameter	T1 (n=3)	T2 (n=3)	T3 (n=3)	T4 (n=3)	T5 (n=3)	SEM	P-value
SW (kg)	22.50	23.75	23.83	23.33	23.83	1.46	0.9580
HCW(kg)	8.87	9.07	9.73	9.80	9.83	0.63	0.7177
DP (%)	39.39	38.21	40.77	42.15	41.34	1.60	0.4684
Lean(kg)	4.95b	5.18b	5.58ab	5.96ab	6.52a	0.45	0.0148
Fat(kg)	1.26	0.90	1.35	1.14	1.01	0.19	0.4987
Bone(kg)	2.26	2.65	2.43	2.24	2.10	0.18	0.2980
Trimming, g	393.3a	339.1ab	365.0ab	460.3a	201.5b	56.18	0.0794
LBR	2.19b	1.98b	2.35b	2.68ab	3.12a	0.24	0.0524
LFR	3.96b	6.05ab	4.41ab	5.47ab	6.89a	0.87	0.1868

a,b,c,d,e Values with different superscripts within same row are significantly different; SW = slaughter weight; HCW= hot carcass weight; DP= dressing percent (HCW/SW*100); LBR= lean to bone ratio; LFR=lean to fat ratio; SEM= standard error of mean; n= no. of slaughtered animals

4. Conclusion

Based on the results of this experiment, the optimum dietary CP for improved performance and feed utilization of yearling Arsi-Bale lambs, growing from 17 to 25 kg, is about 12%,which synchronizes with 2.11 Mj/kg DM feed energy. However, detail studies using "comparative slaughter techniques", is suggested to support the present findings. Moreover, applying the same work for other indigenous sheep breeds is equally important.

Acknowledgement

The author acknowledged Ethiopian Institute of Agricultural Research for funding this research and availing research inputs. The efforts of technical assistance- Mr Solomon Abiy and animal attendants: Mrs Workiye Shibru; Mrs Asrat Endale and Mrs Topiya Muhiye is well appreciated. Also, a useful help given by veterinary technician - Mrs Kasech Melese is acknowledged.

References

[1] Abebe Tafa & Solomon Melaku & Kurt J. Peters. 201Supplementation with linseed (*Linum usitatissimum*) cake and/or wheat bran on feed utilization and carcass characteristics of Arsi - Bale sheep. Trop Anim Health Prod (2010) 42:677–68.

[2] Ahn BH, Moon YH (1985). Effect of dietary protein and calcium levels on nutrition in sheep I. Effect of dietary protein and calcium levels on digestibility, nitrogen balance and some mineral retention in sheep. Kor. J. Anim. Sci. 27:507-51.

[3] Andrews, R. P., Orskov, E. R., 1970. The nutrition of early weaned lamb. I. The influence of protein concentration and feeding level on rate of gain in body weight. J. Agric. Sci. (Camb.) 75, 11-1.

[4] AOAC (Association of Official Analytical Chemists), 1990. Official method of analysis.15th ed. AOAC Inc., Arlington, Virginia, USA. pp. 12-9.

[5] CSA (Central Statistic Authority) of Ethiopia, 201Agricultural sample survey 2014.Vol.II. Report on livestock and livestock characteristics (Private peasant holdings). 194p.

[6] Ermias Tekletsadik. 2008. The Effect of Supplementation with barely bran, linseed meal and their mixtures on the performance of Arsi-Bale sheep fed a basal diet of faba bean haulms. MSc Thesis. Haramaya University, Ethiopia.

[7] FAO (Food and Agricultural Organization of the United Nations), 2004. FAOSTAT data. http://www.faostat.fao.org/faostat/collections?subset=agriculture.

[8] Getahun Kebede and Kassahun Melese, 2010. Evaluation of poultry litter as substitute of urea in urea molasses block on growth and carcass characteristics of finished lamb. Ethiopian Journal of Animal Production (EJAP). Vol.10;No.,201Pp: 19-3.

[9] Getahun Kebede Yadete. Effect of Concentrate Supplementation on Performances of Ethiopian Lowland Afar and Blackhead Ogaden Lambs. Animal and Veterinary Sciences. Vol. 2, No. 2, 2014, pp. 36-41. doi: 10.11648/j.avs.20140202.14.

[10] Haddad, S. G., R. E. Nasr & M. M. Muwalla, 2001.Optimum dietary crude protein level for finishing Awassi lambs. Small Ruminant Research, 39, 41–4.

[11] Hwangbo Soon, Sun Ho Choi, Sang Woo Kim, Dong Soo Son, Ho Sung Park1Sung Hoon Lee2 and Ik Hwan Jo. 2009. Effects of Crude Protein Levels in Total Mixed Rations on Growth. Performance and Meat Quality in Growing Korean Black Goats. Asian-Aust. J. Anim. Sci. Vol. 22, No. 8: 1133 – 113.

[12] Kearl, L. C., 1982. Nutrient Requirements of Ruminants in Developing countries. International Feedstuffs Institute, Utah State University, Logan, Utah 84322, USA.

[13] Keser, O., T. Bilal and H. Cankutay, 2008. The effect of different dietary crude protein level on performance and serum immunoglobulin g in male Kivircik lambs. Bulgarian Journal of Veterinary Medicine (2008), 11, No 1, 49–5.

[14] Marinova, P., Y. Banskalieva, S. Alexandrov, V. Tzvetkova and H. Stanchev. 2001. Carcass composition and meat quality of kids fed sunflower oil supplemented diet. Small Ruminant. Res. 42:217-22.

[15] Mohammad Sharifi, Moslem Bashtani, Abbas Ali Naserian, Hamid Khorasani, 2013. Effect of dietary crude protein level on the performance and apparent digestibility of Iranian Saanen kids. African Journal of Biotechnology Vol. 12(26), pp. 4202-420.

[16] Mourad, M., G. Gbanamou and L. B. Balde. 2001. Carcass characteristics of West African dwarf goats under extensive system. Small Ruminant. Res. 42:81-8.

[17] NRC (National Research Council), 1985. Nutrient Requirements of Sheep. Sixth Revised Edition. Washington, D.C; National Academic Press.

[18] Osuagwuh, A. I. A., and A. O. Akinsoyinu, 1990. Efficiency of nitrogen utilization by pregnant West African dwarf goats fed various leveles of crude protein in the diet. Small Ruminant Research, volume 3, Issue 4, July 199Pages 363-37.

[19] Paul, S. S., A.B. Mandal, G. P. Mandal, A. Kannan and N. N. Pathak., 2003. Deriving nutrient requirements of growing Indian sheep under tropical conditions usin performance and intake data emanated from feeding trials conducted in different research institutes. Small Rumin. Res. 50: 97-10.

[20] SAS (Statistical Analysis System).2003. SAS Institute. Inc., Cary, NC, USA.

[21] Titi, H. H., M. J. Tabbaa, M. G. Amasheh, F. Barakeh & B. Daqamseh, 2000. Comparative performance of Awassi lambs and black goat kids on different crude protein levels in Jordan. Small Ruminant Research, 37, 131–13.

[22] Van Soest. P. J., Robertson, J. B., Lewis, B. A, 1991. Methods for dietary fiber, neutral detergent fiber and non starch polysaccharides in relation to animal nutrition. J. Dairy Sci, 74, 3583-359.

Quality Constraints in the Market Chains for Export of Small Ruminants from Afar Pastoral and Agro-Pastoral Areas

Gezahegn Alemayehu*, Birhanu Hailu, Nuru Seid

College of Veterinary Medicine, Samara University, Samara, Ethiopia

Email address:
gezahegnayalew@yahoo.com (G. Alemayehu)

Abstract: The study was conducted in four districts of Afar Pastoral and Agro-pastoral Area to determine quality constraints in the market chains for export of Afar's small ruminants. A total of 291 producers, 8 traders and 4 exporters were interviewed with separate semi-structured questionnaires. The result of study indicated that small ruminant made by far the greatest contribution to livestock-based livelihoods in all study districts. About 72.2% of pastoralist offers shoat for sale to meet their urgent needs at any time during the year. Majority (51.9%) of the producers have no specific target to sale their shoat. Quality and other criteria required by importers were known only by 7.6% of the producers, while majority of them (92.4%) did not know quality and other criteria required by importer. Even though sheep were most demanded by exporters, sheep accounts only 20% from total shoat presented for sale. Only 14.4% of the producers offer adult male for sale which were fit for export. Along the market chain pre-purchase inspection and selection for quality assurance and certification for live shoat were none existent. In all Afar's livestock markets there is no objective standard for selling and buying animals. The result of this study showed that small ruminants supplied to the markets by pastoralist do not meet the quality attributes required by export markets. Appropriate extension service that will respond to the peculiar needs of export markets, especially on the aspect of providing information and knowledge on the desired shoat characteristics and quality requirements of importing countries should be provided for the producers.

Keywords: Afar, Export, Market, Small Ruminants, Quality

1. Introduction

Ethiopia is a resourceful country bestowed with the largest livestock resource in the Africa continent with about 54 million cattle, 25.5 million sheep and 24.06 million goats. From the total small ruminant population 99.8% of the sheep and nearly all goat population of the country are local breeds [1].

The livestock subsector has an enormous contribution to Ethiopia's national economy and livelihoods of many Ethiopians, and still promising to rally round the economic development of the country [2, 3]. Livestock and livestock products export are among the major earners of foreign exchange for the Ethiopian economy. Of the total number of live animals exported 19% was sheep. In shoat marketing system, 95% of the exported animals were sheep [4].

Of the total small ruminant population of the country, pastoralists own about 26 percent of sheep (about 6.5 million heads of sheep) and nearly two-third of the goats' population (about 15.2 million heads of goats) [5]. Sheep and goat are valued for a variety of important contributions in lives of pastoral households. Thus, pastoralists raise them with several objectives to meet the socio-economic and cultural need [6, 7]. Small ruminants play an important role in financial security, women's empowerment and insurance. Pastoral areas output underpins almost all of Ethiopia's live animal and meat exports [8]. A large percentage of the live shoat and meat exported from Ethiopia originates from Afar pastoral area [4, 9].

Despite the reported high livestock population of the country, the major meat and live animal exporters are complaining of shortage of supply and inferior quality of animals (especially shoats). As the country has the largest number of livestock in Africa, Ethiopia has much to gain from the growing global market for livestock products. The problem faced by Ethiopia is thus one of enhancing its competitiveness in the international markets for live shoat and shoat meat in order to increase and maintain its market share. Nearly all Ethiopian live sheep and goat are exported to Saudi Arabia. This indicates live animals export from the country lack diversified export destinations. Additionally, Ethiopian market share and absolute exports to the Saudi market have declined in recent years while the share of the competitors increasing. Ethiopia's current share in the global market is very limited. In 2004, the share of Ethiopia was only 0.23% of global figure [10].

For small ruminant production to contribute its full potential to national economic growth and to support livelihood of the pastoral community require improving the efficiency of internal marketing systems and livestock export procedures, and improving product quality. With regard to quality, serious attention needs to be given to grades, standards and SPS measures, in compliance with international agreements of world trade organization (WTO). Ensuring product quality and reducing trade barriers, particularly in the rapidly integrating market of Europe will ensuring the profit of the livestock sectors and product business. Moreover, the country also benefits from the influx of foreign currency through revenue gained by exporting animals and meat. This is achieved mainly by improving quality of small ruminants supplied for exporters. Information on quality of small ruminants for export from Ethiopia in general and from Afar's in particular is highly scanty. Hence, there is a need for assessment of quality constraints in Afar's small ruminant market chain for export. The aim of this study was therefore to assess quality constraints in the market chains for export of small ruminants from Afar Pastoral and Agro-pastoral areas.

2. Material and Methods

2.1. Study Areas

The study was conducted in two zones of Afar Regional State namely in zone 1 and 3. Afar is one of nine regional states situated in the North-Eastern part of Ethiopia. The altitude of the region ranges from 1500 m.a.s.l. in the western highlands to -120 meters below sea level in the Danakil/Dallol depression. The regional capital, Samara is located in zone 1 (Dubti Woreda) some 588 Kms North-east of Addis Ababa on the main Addis–Djibouti road. Afar is characterized by an arid and semi-arid climate with low and erratic rainfall. Temperature varies from 20°C in higher elevations to 48°C in lower elevations. Rainfall is bi-modal throughout the region with a mean annual rainfall below 500 mm in the semi-arid western escarpments decreasing to 150 mm in the arid zones to the east (Figure 1). There are 16 livestock markets in Afar regional state in which only 75 % (14) of them are functional. The most important livestock markets in the region used for live shoat marketing are Adiatu, Ayisaita, Awash 7, Elewha, Chifra, Mille, Gedamayetu, Endufo, and Logia.

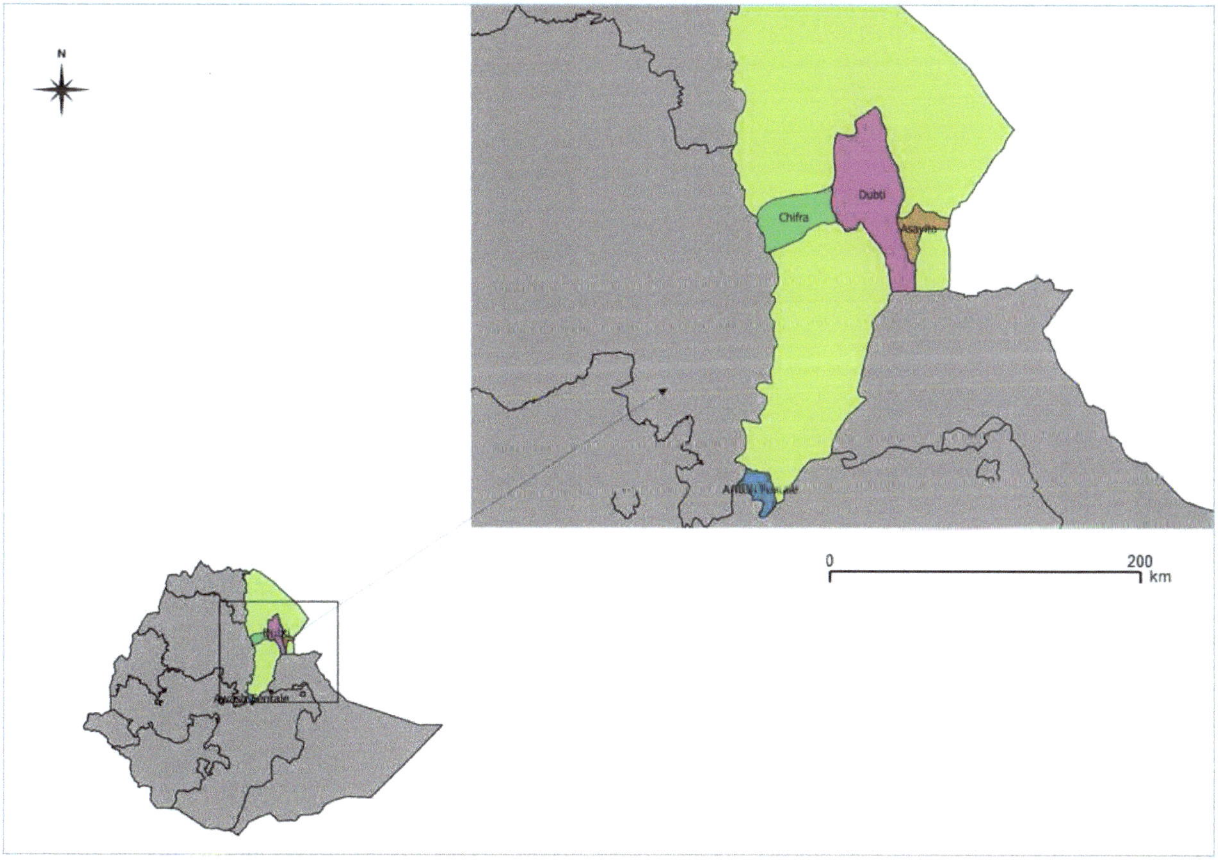

Figure 1. Study areas

2.2. Source of Information and Sampling Procedure

At producers' level, four districts of Afar pastoral region namely Aysaita, Dubti, Chifra and Awash Fentale were selected purposely from the Afar regional states based on their relative importance of export quality shoat, relative importance of domestic vs. export market outlets, their geographical location and socioeconomic characteristics. A total of 291 producers, 8 traders and 4 exporters were interviewed with separate semi-structured questionnaires to collect information on quality constraints of traded shoat along export market chain.

2.3. Data Collection and Analysis Technique

A field surveys were conducted by means of three sets of semi-structured personal interview. The first set was designed for the producers to obtain information on shoat production, marketing, and their awareness on quality requirements for export. The other set was designed for traders to collect shoat supply pattern, shoat quality problems in the market, buying and selling system, their criteria to buy shoat and their awareness on quality requirements for export. The third set was design for exporters to collect shoat supply pattern, shoat quality problems in the market, buying and selling system, their criteria to buy, reason for shoat rejection and quality assurance system along the chain. Data from producers and traders were collected in each month in one of main market day found in each selected districts a period of one year during June 2013- October 2014. The data was subjected to statistical analysis using Statistical Package for Social Sciences (SPSS) software, version 20.0 (SPSS Inc., Chicago, Illinois, USA). Descriptive statistics such as frequency distribution and percentages were used.

3. Results

3.1. Characteristics of Producers

Table 1. *Main source of livelihood for Afar's pastoral and Agro-pastoral community.*

Livelihood dependence	Frequency	Percentage (%)
Only Livestock	199	68.4
Mainly livestock, minor crop	42	14.4
Mainly crop, minor livestock	4	1.4
Livestock and crop equally important	12	4.1
Livestock and other non agricultural activities	34	11.7

The study showed that in Afar pastoral and agro-pastoral areas, livelihoods depend, at least in part, on livestock (Table 1). Small ruminant made by far the greatest contribution to livestock-based livelihoods in all study districts. The main benefit derived from small ruminants in the area was reported to be food, which include meat, milk and fat. The second most important benefit was income from sales of surplus animals. Other lesser benefits include various socio-cultural roles. Majority, 97.3% of the respondents practiced the free range (extensive) production system and only 2.7% of them practiced tethering (subsistence) system, while none of them practiced intensive livestock production system. Interview result indicated that 82.5 % of males involved in shoat selling while only 17.5% of females involved in shoat selling.

3.2. Quality Indicators at Producers' Level

According interview result, 72.2% of pastoralist offers shoat for sale to meet their urgent needs at any time during the year. About 19.2% of the producers sale during drought due to feed shortage, while only 8.6% of the producers indicated that they supply shoat according to seasonal variation in demand and select the appropriate type of shoat according to function (Hajj, Ramadan or other holiday) (Table 2).

Table 2. *Major reasons of pastoralist and Agro pastoralist to sale their shoat.*

Reason to sale	Frequency	Percentage (%)
Immediate cash need	210	72.2
During high demand	25	8.6
During Drought	56	19.2
Total	291	100

Furthermore, the survey result indicated that 12.4% producers targeted primarily restaurants to sell their shoat, while 23.3% and 4.5% targeted primarily household consumers and butchers respectively. While, majority (51.9%) of the producers have no specific target to sale their shoat. Only 7.9% of producers targeted traders who supply shoat for export market (Table 3). The prices received by pastoralist were lower when they sold for traders compared to other costumers. Pastoralist indicated that they receive higher price when they sold during Hajj, Ramadan or other holiday (during high demand) compared to sale immediate cash need as well as drought. The lower price was paid for pastoralist when sold due to drought compared to sales for cash shortage and holiday.

Table 3. *Target of the pastoralist and agro-pastoralist to sale their shoat.*

Target customers	Frequency	Percentage (%)
Household consumers in urban area	68	23.3
Traders	23	7.9
Restaurants	36	12.4
Butchers	13	4.5
No specific target	151	51.9
Total	291	100

Quality and other criteria required by importers were known only by 7.6% of the producers, while majority of them (92.4%) did not know quality and other criteria required by importer. Furthermore, only 18.2% of pastoralists informed about Afars' shoat are demanded by Middle East consumers. Majority of Afar's shoat were exported to Saudi Arabia markets. Quality requirements of shoat in Saudi market is presented in Table 4. The Saudi markets have a preference for Afar's sheep above 26 kg live weight. The animals should be no more than four years of age (three pairs of permanent incisor teeth). Large numbers of shoat are demanded mainly during Hajj and for religious purposes. During Hajj, live weight requirement of Saudi market of sheep is lower to 20-22 Kg. Compared to live goat; live sheep are more preferred by importers. In terms of breed, Afars' sheep are the most demanded by importers next to Somali black head.

Table 4. *Quality requirements of live shoat for Saudi's markets from Ethiopia.*

Products	Quality requirements
Live sheep	Afar's and Somali black head breed
	1. Above 28 Kg live weight for Somali black head , above 26 KG live weight for Afar breed
	2. Below 3 years age
	3. Disease free
	4.None castrated male
Live goat	1. Desert local breed (Afar, Short eared Somali, Long eared Somali
	2. Above 35kg for Afar, Above 40kg for Short eared Somali, Long eared Somali
	3. Below 3 years age
	4. Disease free
	5.None castrated male

Against the above requirements and preferences in the Saudi market, from total shoat presented for sale, sheep accounts only 20%. Majority of producers (40.9%) indicated that they presented young male for sale and 28.2% of producers presented culled female shoat for sale. Only 14.4% of the producers offer adult male for sale which are fit for export. Characteristics of traded shoat in Afar region livestock markets are indicated in Table 5.

Table 5. *Characteristics of traded shoat in Afar region livestock markets as reported by producers.*

Characteristics	Frequency	Percentage (%)
Matured male	9	3.1
Adult male	42	14.4
Young male	119	40.9
Culled female	82	28.2
Breeding female	10	3.4
Male kid	23	8
Young female	6	2
Total	291	100

3.3. Quality Indicators at Market Level

Of four markets surveyed, all markets were fenced and all markets had loading and unloading facilities. None of these markets have water and feed trough and holding facilities. Except the market at Logia which meets 5 day per week, the rest of the markets meet 1 day per week.

Market survey indicated that at various points in market chain from primary market up to quarantine center, there was no veterinarian performing pre-purchase inspection and selection for quality assurance and certification for live shoat. The traded animals were not subjected to any tests before they were moved into quarantine. Per-purchase selections along the market chain have been conducted by traders or purchaser groups without necessary animal health knowledge.

In the markets, purchased decision was reached based on traders' physical evaluation of the animals while moving freely in the market by palpation of the shoat at points for fatness; tail, chest, back. Purchasers knew the age of the shoat using teeth eruption. The traders tried to select shoat with good general health and not emaciated, clean smooth glistening hair not rough coat, good appearance condition (active) and tried fulfill export quality criteria. The traders tried to avoid diseased animals (such as these having emaciation, diarrhoea, pneumonia and severe cases of mange).

Animals are not weighed in Afars' primary and secondary markets but the animals are weighed at export terminal markets. In all livestock markets there is no objective standard for selling and buying animals. Trader may buy a particular type of shoat, e.g. adult male, young male etc or a combination of types in a mob or batch as a unit or as single animals. Sales for exporters occurred in the same manner. Average price per animal from these combinations (or mix) differs greatly. The traders mix shoat different type and making a batch consisting of animals within a range of weight, e.g. underweight, medium or heavy weight to make a balanced batch to maximize net return form shoat. The price of the batch was fixed using shoat which was bought with high prices as bench mark.

3.4. Quality Indicators at Quarantine Level

Exporters exported live shoat to Saudi Arabia, Dubai, Oman and Beirut. Majority of them are exporting only Afra's sheep because of their adaptation to harsh environments and importers preference for sheep sourced from these areas. According to the discussion with exporters exporting live goat is very risky because of high mortality rate during 21 days confinement at quarantine station. Some exporters export immediately after they finished collection of goats without 21 days quarantine. Exporters collect sheep from either from the main source markets through their agents or from secondary markets found Bati and Methara. As part of SPS requirements and according to the rules and regulations of animal quarantine, shoats are exported after providing the shoat with necessary vaccines and medication. The exporter held sheep for 21 days in their own/rented quarantine center found in Methara, Awash 7 killo and Mile.

The facility receives only uncastrated male animals intended for export as live animals; they originate mainly from Afar and oromia region. All animals were bought as batch and arrived by truck. Previous health statuses of the admitted animals were not known. Those animals were not subjected to any tests before they were moved into facilities. There was no primary inspection at the point of entry before the animals are accepted for quarantine. Therefore, the sheep and goat were admitted into quarantine facilities with all their problems. After collections of the animals were completed, animals are examined individually and identified with ear tags before vaccination. Reasons for culling included sub-optimum body condition and signs of clinical disease.

3.5. Quality Assurance System along Export Market Chain

At market level there are no government veterinarians to perform inspection and selection for quality assurance and certification. Screaming of animals at the time of purchase was performed by purchase team on the basis of a number of criteria. The purchase team observe and inspect animals individually by visual assessment to avoid the following: inferior quality, over aged (full permanent teeth > 4 years) or castrated, enlarged lymph nodes and abscesses, generalized mange, infected wounds, scratches, diarrhoea, or any disease which cannot respond to fast treatment, or will leave a scar on the body, phenotypical abnormalities on shoat body or its limbs.

At quarantine centers level, inspection and selection for quality assurance of export sheep is performed both by centers veterinarian and form Adama Quarantine Station. Before the animals were admitted to quarantine facilities, the veterinary authority from federal quarantine service through Adama quarantine station inspects the premises whether the facilities meet the required quarantine standards or not. To ensure completion of quarantine period, veterinary inspectors with technicians perform inspection and checking at entrance, vaccination and departure of quarantine premises.

During departure, the veterinary inspectors screen unfit animals using visual inspection. The leading causes of rejection at terminal export markets were underweight and sheep and goat pox. Other conditions leading to rejection during departure inspection include orf (contagious pustular dermatitis), mange, diarrhea, pneumonia and foot rot. Finally, after they reject unfit animals for export they issued certification for exported animals.

4. Discussions

Afar pastoral community is one of major pastoral groups in Ethiopia occupied northeast of the country. Afar pastoral areas are generally characterized by unpredictable and unstable climatic features where the potential for crop cultivation is limited. Therefore, livestock are centre of pastoral lives and livelihoods. Abdulahi [11] indicated that an estimated minimum of 93% of the population in pastoral areas is directly dependent on livestock for subsistence. The reported greatest contribution of small ruminant in livestock-based livelihoods in this study was also reported by Jost et al. [12] in North Eastern Province of Kenya in which small ruminant especially goats made the greatest contribution to livelihoods Kenyan pastoralist. The main benefits derived from small ruminants in the study areas was reported to be food, income, socio-cultural. Schwartz and Schwartz [13] indicated that the main functions of livestock production in pastoral households are to provide subsistence products (milk, blood and meat), to meet social obligations (bride price, stock alliances and stock patronages) and to insure against disaster (drought, epidemics, raids). Goats and sheep are valued as a source of meat, as well as a resource that can be sold for cash [14,15]. The reported extensive production practice in this study is one of the features of Ethiopian sheep and goat production system. Sheep and goats production in pastoral and agropastoral systems is of subsistence nature. Market-oriented or commercial production is almost non-existent [16].

This study indicated that selling of shoat was done mainly by men. Ayele et al. [17] also reported higher percentages (92%) male sellers in Ethiopia. Even though, women play a significant role in pastoral communities and are key agents in livelihood development, the great majority of pastoral societies continue to be dominated by men, and women's participation in decision-making processes is limited or totally absent. Decisions regarding herd mobility, planning, conflict resolution, and relations with neighboring groups are usually made by older men. With some exceptions, men own the animals and have sole rights to dispose of them through sale and slaughter [18].

The result of this study also showed that majority (72.2%) of pastoralist offers shoat for sale to meet their urgent needs at any time during the year. This might be due to the fact that the small ruminant production system in the study areas is only for subsistence rather than market orientation. The extensive production systems that dominate small ruminant production in area not only inhibit producer access to market information, but limit the learning process on production changes required to meet the quality demands of the export market [19]. The study furthermore indicated that majority (51.9%) of the producers have no specific target to sale their shoat. This indicated that the producers in study area did not offered quality shoat which responding export market demands but to satisfy their immediate cash need. In such a situation, the purchase price of an animal will reflect not only the bargaining skills of both buyers and sellers but also the buyer's preference for the characteristics of the animal and the seller's willingness to sell, sometimes leading to transaction failure [20].

In this study majority of producers (92.4%) did not know quality and other criteria required by importer. Even though Afar sheep and goat breeds most preferred in the Middle East market [4,19, 21], only 18.2% of pastoralists informed about this. However, this information is well known to traders and exporters. Therefore, vertical linkage between traders and producers in terms of both forwards and backwards information would improve the pastoralist capacity to share information and learn strategies for responding to the market. Strengthened agribusiness linkages would improve the efficiency to respond to market demands [19].

The Saudi markets have a preference for uncastrated male Afar's sheep below 4 years and above 26 kg live weight. However, against these requirements and preferences in the Saudi market, sheep accounts only 20% total shoat presented for sale and only 14.4% of the producers offer adult male for sale which are fit for export. The preferences Afra's sheep may have been due to the breed's adaptation to harsh environments and importers preference for sheep sourced from these areas. Hailemariam et al. [4] indicated that in shoat marketing system, 95% of the exported live animals were sheep. This might be due to fact that exporting goat is much risky due to they fail to adapt 21 days of confinement at quarantine centers.

Along the market chain pre-purchase inspection and selection for quality assurance and certification for live shoat were none existant. Purchased decision was reached based on traders' physical evaluation of the animals while moving freely in the market by palpation of the shoat at points for fatness; tail, chest, back. Since there is no disease free zone in Ethiopia including Afar pastoral area [22, 23, 24, 25], some diseases, especially trade related (transboundary) diseases might pass undetected along the market chain. This could limit market supply of export quality animals by compromising most important quality criteria related to health and diseases.

In all Afar's livestock markets there is no objective standard for selling and buying animals. The traders buy shoat with visual estimation of live weight at both primary and secondary markets. This might increase the culling rate of shoat due to underweight at export terminal market since selling of shoat at export terminal conducted on per kg live weight basis of individual animal. Furthermore, buying animals as batch from traders (collectors) could increase the probability of inferior quality shoat inter the quarantine facilities.

Sheep and goat which were collected from producers were admitted to quarantine facilities which were found in Awash 7, Methara and Mile for 21 days. The existing quarantine stations in Ethiopia are small in size and without adequate facilities and owned and run by private entrepreneurs but certification is only made by a "competent authority" [26]. This quarantine is not recognized by the Gulf Cooperation Council (GCC) countries, and animals must be re-quarantined at the port of export. For animals that go through the Djibouti quarantine the Ethiopian certification is neither required nor seen by the final recipient, as all animals are re-certified as Djibouti origin [21]. This practice is potentially leading to duplication of tests, doubling of quarantine waiting requirements, feed costs and the like. However, in order to bring the existing practice to an end and secure the country's proprietary rights, the government of Ethiopia on the way to finalized the constriction of large quarantine facilities at Mile area.

This study indicated biosecurity practice of the quarantine centers are none existent. This poor biosecurity measures in quarantine centers increase risk of the introduction and spread of disease agents within and between facilities. Introduction and spread of diseases in quarantine centers reduce the efficiency of production and thus it makes economic sense. Most stringent biosecurity requirements are concentrated on the people in the high-risk category, such as those who have direct contact with animals or manure on the farm, as well as other farms [27, 28]. Therefore, improving biosecurity practices is the most cost-effective in protection of animal diseases in quarantine facilities [29, 30].

There is also a need to emphasise issues of animal welfare in the in Ethiopian livestock trade, particularly in animal transport [9, 31, 32]. The trucks used for transport are not designed for the purpose and lack many biosafety measures.

Introducing traded animal into quarantine facilities without health certificate and any test along market chain resulting in high rates of rejection within quarantine facilities and between the export and import ports. Such high rejection rates cause severe financial hardship for the business owners by increasing the costs and reduce the competitiveness of the country. Importing countries such as Saudi Arabia are strict in screening unfit animals intermes of health and quality. Such action provides a good signal and an incentive to undertake inspection and screening in a serious manner.

5. Conclusion

The finding of this study indicated that livelihoods depend on livestock and small ruminant made by far the greatest contribution to livestock-based livelihoods in all study districts. The result further showed that small ruminant supplied to the market by pastoralist do not meet the quality attributes required by export markets. There was no government body which assures quality of traded animals along the export market chain. Appropriate extension service that will respond to the peculiar needs of export markets, especially on the aspect of providing information and knowledge on the desired shoat characteristics and quality requirements of importing countries should be provided for producers.

Acknowledgment

We would like to express our gratitude to all those who gave us the possibility to complete this research. We are very grateful to Adama quarantine station, live animal exporters and producers for his provision of valuable information for the research. Finally, and most importantly, we would like to express our deepest gratitude to Samara University research and community service vice president office for financial support for the research.

References

[1] CSA 2013. Agricultural Sample Survey, 2012/13 (2005 E.C.), Volume II: Report on Livestock and livestock characteristics (Private peasant holdings). Statistical Bulletin 570. Addis Ababa. Central Statistical Agency (CSA), Federal Democratic Republic of Ethiopia.

[2] Metaferia, F., Cherenet, T., Gelan, A., Abnet, F., Tesfay, A., Ali, J.A., Gulilat, W. 2011. A Review to Improve Estimation of Livestock Contribution to the National GDP. Ministry of Finance and Economic Development and Ministry of Agriculture, Addia Ababa, Ethiopia.

[3] Behnke, R. 2010. The Contribution of Livestock to the Economies of IGAD Member States: Study Findings, Application of the Methodology in Ethiopia and Recommendations for Further Work. IGAD LPI Working Paper 02-10. Great Wolford, UK: Odessa Centre, IGAD Livestock Policy Initiative. In.

[4] Hailemariam, T., Legese, G., Alemu, D.,and Negassa, A. 2009. Market Structure and Function for Live Animal and Meat Exports in Some Selected Areas of Ethiopia. Research Report 79. EIAR, Addis Ababa, Ethiopia.

[5] SOS 2013. Pastoralism In Ethiopia: Its Total Economic Values and Development Challenges. SOS SAHEL ETHIOPIA, Addis Ababa, Ethiopia.

[6] Devendra, C. 2001. Small ruminants: imperative for productivity enhancement improved livelihood and rural growth. *A review. Asian-Aust. J.Anim.sci.* 14(10)1483-1496.

[7] Jahnke, H.E. 1982. Livestock Production Systems and Livestock Development in Tropical Africa. Kieler Wissenschaftsverlag Vauk.

[8] IGAD 2013. The Contribution of Livestock to the Ethiopian Economy. IGAD Center for Pastoral Areas & Livestock Development (ICPALD). Policy Brief No: ICPALD 5/CLE/8/2013

[9] Legese, G., Hailemariam, T., Alemu, D.,and Negassa, A. 2008. Live animal and meat export value chains in prioritized areas of Ethiopia: Constraints and opportunities for enhancing meat exports. ILRI Discussion Paper 12. ILRI (International Livestock Research Institute), Nairobi, Kenya.

[10] FAO 2005. Addressing marketing and processing constraints that inhibit agri-food export. *AGS* bulletin 160, FAO, Rome.

[11] Abdulahi, M. 2003. Pastoral Development Strategies/ Policies in Ethiopia: A Critical Analysis and Evaluation," Proceedings of the Third National Conference on Pastoral Development in Ethiopia, December 23-24, 2003, Addis Ababa. Pastoral Form Ethiopia: Addis Ababa

[12] Jost C.C, Nzietchueng S. , Kihu S. Bett, B. , Njogu G , Swai Emmanuel, and Mariner J. C. 2010. Epidemiological Assessment of the Rift Valley Fever Outbreak in Kenya and Tanzania in 2006 and 2007. *Am. J. Trop. Med. Hyg.,* 83(Suppl 2) 65–72.

[13] Schwartz, S. and Schwartz, H.J. 1985. Nomadic pastoralism in Kenya: still a viable production system? *Quarterly Journal of International Agriculture,* 24 (1): 5-21.

[14] Abdullahi, A.M. 1990. Pastoral Production Systems in Africa: A Study of Nomadic Household Economy and Livestock Marketing in Central Somalia. Farming Systems and Resource Economics in the Tropics, No.8. Kiel, Germany.

[15] Sieff, D.F. 1999. The effects of wealth on livestock dynamics among the Datoga pastoralists of Tanzania. Agricultural Systems, 59: 1-25.

[16] Gizaw S., Tegegne A., Gebremedhin B. and Hoekstra D. 2010. Sheep and goat production and marketing systems in Ethiopia: Characteristics and strategies for improvement. Improving Productivity and Market Success (IPMS) of Ethiopian Farmers Project, International Livestock Research Institute (ILRI), Addis Ababa, Ethiopia . Working Paper No. 23

[17] Ayele G, A. Jabbar M., Teklewold H., Mulugeta E. and Kebed G. 2006. Seasonal and inter-market differences in prices of small ruminants in Ethiopia. *Journal of Food Products Marketing (USA), 12(4): 59-77.*

[18] Rota A. and Sperandini S. 2009. Livestock and pastoralists. Livestock Thematic Papers Tools for project design. International Fund for Agricultural Development, Rome, Italy.

[19] Sebsibe A. 2011. Export requirements for meat and live small ruminants. How can development agents assist producers to improve small ruminant export? Technical Bulletin No.47

[20] Williams T.O., Spycher B. and Okike I. 2006. Improving livestock marketing and intra-regional trade in West Africa: Determining appropriate economic incentives and policy framework. ILRI (International Livestock Research Institute), Nairobi, Kenya. 122 pp.

[21] Farmer, E. 2010. End Market Analysis of Ethiopian Livestock and Meat. A Desk Study Micro report 164

[22] Delil F., Asfaw Y. and Gebreegziabher B. 2012. Prevalence of antibodies to peste des petits ruminants virus before and during outbreaks of the disease in Awash Fentale district, Afar, Ethiopia. Trop Anim Health Prod, 44:1329–1330

[23] Regassa F. Netsere M., Tsertse T. 2010. Sero-Prevalence of Contagious Caprine Pleuropneumonia in Goat at Selected Woredas of Afar Region. Ethiop. Vet. J., 14(1), 83-89

[24] Zewdie S., 2009. Peste des Petits Ruminants (PPR). Ethiopia Sheep and Goat Productivity Improvement Program (ESGPIP). Technical Bulletin No.20

[25] Dawit, T. 2006. Seroprevalence study of peste des petits ruminants in Gewane district, Afar Regional State, Ethiopia. Unpublished DVM thesis, Addis Ababa University

[26] Aklilu, Y. 2008. Livestock Marketing in Kenya and Ethiopia: A Review of Policies and Practice. Feinstein International Center, Addis Ababa

[27] Gekara O, Leite-Browning ML, (2012). Biosecurity Practices for Small Beef Cattle Producers. A Series for Small-Scale Producers and Hobby Owners.

[28] Anderson David E. 2010. Survey of Biosecurity Practices Utilized by Veterinarians Working with Farm Animal Species. The Online Journal of Rural Research and Policy 5.7: 1-13.

[29] Van Schaik G, Dijkhuizen AA, Benedictus G, Barkema HW, Koole JL 1998. Exploratory study on the economic value of a closed farming system on Dutch dairy farms. Veterinary Record 142: 240–242.

[30] Van Schaik G., Nielen M., Dijkhuizen, A.A. 2001. An economic model for on-farm decision support of management to prevent infectious disease introduction into dairy farms. Preventive Veterinary Medicine 51: 289–305.

[31] Lawrence M., Riccardo C., Ibrahim O.O., Samuel O.O., Jabbar M., Negassa A. and Amos O. 2008. – A rapid appraisal of institutions supporting Somali livestock export. Improvement and Diversification of Somali Livestock Trade and Marketing Project. Discussion Paper No. 14. Improving market opportunities. International Livestock Research Institute, Nairobi.

[32] Negassa A., Costagli R., Matete G., Jabbar M., Oyieke S.O., Abdulle M.H. and Omore A. 2008. Towards improving livestock export marketing support services in the Somali context: survey findings and implications. Improvement And Diversification Of Somali Livestock Trade And Marketing Project. Discussion Paper No. 13. Improving market opportunities. International Livestock Research Institute, Nairobi.

Incidence of Major Clinical Reproductive Health Problems of Dairy Cows at Bako Livestock Research Farm over a Two-Year Period (September 2008-December 2010)

Temesgen Ayana[1, *], Tegegn Gudeta[2]

[1]Department of Veterinary Laboratory Technology, Ambo University, Ambo, Ethiopia
[2]Max Planck Institute for Developmental Biology, Tuebingen, Germany

Email address:
tadefa2005@yahoo.co.uk (T. Ayana)

Abstract: A prospective follow up study was carried out on 372 dairy cows at Bako Agricultural research center between September 2008 and December 2010 to determine the incidence of reproductive problems and associated risk factors in the cows. The animals were continuously followed from insemination/mating until 45 days postpartum for occurrence of clinical reproductive problems. Data were collected during farm visits by observation and clinical examination of animals. The cumulative incidence of clinically observed major reproductive problems was 35.2% (131/372). No statistically detectable effect ($p>0.05$) of breed was shown on the occurrence of clinical reproductive problems evaluated. In addition, number of parities, body condition score (BCS), age of dams, calf sex and service type were not found to have a significant influence on the occurrence of reproductive problems in the study farm ($p>0.05$). The most common reproductive problems recorded in the present study were retained fetal membrane (8.3%), dystocia (6.7%), abortion (5.9%), uterine infections (5.6%) and stillbirths (4.8%). In this study, the incidence of dystocia, uterine infections, stillbirths and repeat breeding were more common in crossbred cows whereas abortion was more common in local cows but the effect of these factors was not significant ($p>0.05$). This study revealed that nearly one cow out of every three cows encountered at least one type of clinical reproductive problems indicating the widespread occurrence of the problems among dairy cows at Bako Agricultural Research Center. However, considered plausible factors such as breed, parity number, body condition score (BCS), age of dams, calf sex and service type had no significant influence on the occurrence of reproductive problems in the study farm indicating that some other factors are responsible for precipitating the conditions. It is, therefore, recommended that other factors that precipitate the occurrence of the problems in the farm should be investigated and appropriate interventions implemented in order to minimize the occurrence of these problems and associated losses in the farm.

Keywords: Bako, Dairy Cows, Incidence, Follow Up, Reproductive Problems, Risk Factors

1. Introduction

Reproductive efficiency is a critical component of a successful dairy operation and acts as an important component of a profitable dairy farm, whereas reproductive inefficiency is one of the most costly problems facing the dairy industry today. Reproductive problems occur frequently in dairy cows and can dramatically affect reproductive efficiency in a dairy herd [1]. Reproductive problems have been implicated to cause considerable economic loss to the dairy industry due to slower uterine involution, reduced reproductive rate, prolonged inter-conception period and calving interval, high cost of medication, drop in milk production, reduced calf-crop and early depreciation of potentially useful cows [2, 3]. Low reproductive efficiency also hinders genetic improvement in Zebu (Bos indicus) cattle and causes a direct economic loss [4]. In addition, several studies have shown that reproductive disorders are the most frequent culling reasons [5, 6, 7].

Among the most common reproductive disorders that have direct impact on reproductive performance of dairy cows include, twinning, dystocia, abortion, retained fetal membrane, stillbirth and metritis. These are diverse disorders that are similar in that they all can result in impaired reproductive function. Deciding whether to breed, treat, or cull dairy cows exhibiting one or more of these reproductive problems is a challenge for both veterinarians and dairy producers [1].

Bako Agricultural Research center is one of the leading public dairy research centers in Ethiopia that is engaged in dairy development research endeavor for more than five decades. The center has played a significant role in adopting and generating appropriate technologies and promoting the transfer of improved dairy technologies to smallholder farmers for dairy development in the country [8, 9]. However, limited effort has been made to assess the conditions of reproductive problems of dairy cows under on-station condition [10]. In addition, the effect of reproductive disorders on reproductive performance of dairy cattle has not been sufficiently studied. This study was, therefore, designed to determine the incidence of periparturient reproductive conditions and associated factors in both local Zebu and crossbred dairy cows under on-station condition.

2. Materials and Methods

2.1. Study Area

The study was carried out at Bako Agricultural Research Center between September 2008 and December 2010. The center is located at 260 km west of Addis Ababa in East Wollega Zone of Oromia National Regional State, Ethiopia. It lies between $9^0$6'N latitude and $37^0$09' E longitude and has an altitude of 1650 meter above sea level (masl). The long-term weather information collected at the center reveals that the area gets a bimodal pattern of rainfall with the main rainy season extending from June to September and a short rainy season that extends from March to May with an average annual rainfall of 1300 mm. The area has sub-humid agro-ecology. The mean minimum, mean maximum and average air temperatures were 14.1, 27.9 and 20.6 ^{0}C, respectively [11]. Majority of soil in western Oromia (Ethiopia) in general and the study site in particular are Nitosols or Alifisols according to USDA soil classification systems [12]. The topography of the area ranges from gently undulating to dissected hills and its geology is characterized by Tertiary and Quaternary age rhyolite and basalt volcanics [13]. The soil is deep and highly weathered, well drained, clay texture and slightly acidic in reaction [14]. Semi-deciduous primary natural vegetation and grassland surround the research center. Maize (*Zea mays*), sorghum (*Sorghum bicolor*), teff (*Eragrostis tef*), hot pepper (*Capsicum frutescence*), sweet potato (*Ipomoea batatas*), haricot bean (*Phaseolus vulgaris*), mango (*Mangifera indica*), banana (*Musa* spp.) and sugar cane (*Saccharum officinarum*) are the major annual and perennial crops grown in the study area. Dominant grasses species include Hyperhenia and Sporobolus [15].

2.2. Animals and Their Management

The livestock farm of the center is mandated to evaluate the growth, productive and reproductive performances of the indigenous Horro cattle breed and their crosses with various exotic bloods [15]. The study animals, aged between 3 to 16 years, were of varying parities, body condition scores, and breeds. Breeds of the animals were identified from the existing records. The proportion of exotic blood in crossbred animals ranged from 50% to 62.5%. Horro cattle (zebu that are reared in the area) has traditionally been used for draft power, milk and meat production in low-input production systems. The breed is classified as an intermediate (Sanga-Zebu) with fine skin and uniform brown color which is lighter around the muzzle and on the flanks, abdominal floor and perineum and in between the hind legs [16].

The study animals were managed by semi-intensive production system. The animals were housed (in herds) in a barn with concrete floor and corrugated iron roof. Pregnant cows and heifers were separated into maternity pens during night. The feeding system of heifers and cows of all breeds were similar. All animals above 6 months of age were let in a group to graze natural pasture (8 am to 5 pm). Concentrate supplement was restricted to calves, milking cows and pregnant cows (mainly during the last trimester of pregnancy). The concentrate mixture included maize (49.5%), Noug seed cake (49.5%), and salt (1%). Supplementation with hay (Rhodes grass/*Chloris gayana* and natural pasture) or silage (Rhodes grass and maize silage) at night was practiced depending on the availability of hay and silage and the condition of the grazing paddocks. All animals were routinely monitored for any health problem and those above six months of age were annually vaccinated against Black leg, Anthrax, Bovine Pasteurellosis, Lumpy Skin Disease (LSD) and Foot and Mouth disease (FMD). All the animals were de-wormed with anthelmintics twice a year; during the beginning of the main rainy season and end of the main rainy season. The animals were sprayed with acaricide (Diazinon 60% EC) against external parasites; the frequency of spray varies depending on the degree of infestation and season of the year [17].

Heat detection was based on daily visual observation (6-8 am and 5-6 pm) by a trained inseminator and throughout the grazing time by the herdsmen. Cows and heifers observed in heat were bred either naturally (local or crossbred bull) or inseminated either with frozen Friesian, or Jersey semen obtained from National Artificial Insemination Center. Those animals that were bred and hence, not returned to estrus were checked for pregnancy using rectal palpation after two months. Postpartum breeding took place after 45 days of voluntary waiting period [15].

2.3. Study Design

A longitudinal study design was used to estimate incidence of reproductive health problems in dairy cows kept at Bako livestock research farm. A total of 372 pregnant dairy cows were continuously followed for occurrence of major reproductive health problems for two consecutive years. Individual cows were followed from insemination/mating until 45 days postpartum. Clinical examination of the reproductive system was regularly carried out to determine the nature of vaginal discharge during the postpartum period. The vulva and perineal area were inspected for the presence of any afterbirth (RFM) if not expelled out with in the first 12 hours [2] and for the presence of any discharge.

2.4. Data Collection

Baseline herd data were collected through direct observation and administration of self administered semi-structured questionnaire. During the initial and subsequent visits, detailed data about the individual cow/heifer participating in the study were collected using a clinical record form. Farm record books were used to collect data on animal identification, age, parity, breed, and others. Monthly visits were carried out for pregnant animals that had not entered the peri-parturient period (more than three weeks prior to parturition) and weekly visits were carried out as soon as the animals entered the peri-parturient period (3 weeks before and after parturition). Data on service type, date of insemination, sex of offspring, reproductive health problems, including but not limited to dystocia (difficult calving requiring considerable assistance), stillbirth (calf born dead at term), abortion (expulsion of the fetus before the end of pregnancy), retained fetal membrane (retained longer than 12 hours after calving), prolapse (vaginal and/or uterine), uterine infections (metritis, endometritis, pyometra or uterine discharge), repeat breeder (cows requiring three or more services before conception or culling) [18, 19] were recorded from the study cows followed during the study period. Body condition of the study animals was scored based on the criteria set by Richard [20] with minor modifications to condense body conditions scores into three groups (poor, medium and good).

2.5. Data Management and Analysis

The collected data were entered and stored in Microsoft Office Excel 2007 (Microsoft Corporation, USA) and EpiData (EpiData version 3.1, The EpiData Association, Odense, Denmark). Reproductive conditions were recorded as binary variables (1=presence; 0=absence), screened for errors and exported into SPSS for Windows (Version 20.0; Statistical Package for Social Sciences Inc, Chicago, Illinois, USA) for analysis. Descriptive statistics such as mean and proportions were used to express the characteristics of different independent variables. Incidence rate was used as a measure of occurrence of reproductive problems per 100 cows calved [21]. Proportional morbidity rates (PMR) were calculated by dividing the number of cases of each reproductive problem by the total number of cases. For the purpose of analysis, crosses of local Horro with Friesian or Jersey, were combined to a single group and described as 'crossbred.' The chi-square (χ^2) statistic was used to determine the associations between predictor variables and incidence of reproductive problems [22]. Logistic regression was employed to check the influence of the independent variables on the dependent variable. In all the analysis, $p>0.05$ was considered to have a significant effect.

3. Results

The mean and standard error of the mean age and parity of the study animals were 7.30±0.17 (mean±SE, 7.30±0.17) and 4.87± 0.16 (mean±SE, 4.87± 0.16), respectively. In the present study, the cumulative incidence of clinically observed major reproductive problems related to the 372 cows (Local zebu=313 crossbred=59) was 35.2% (131/372). The cumulative incidence of major reproductive problems among the two genotypes were 34.2% (107/313) and 40.7% (24/59), respectively for local Horro and crossbred animals and the incidence between the two genotypes did not differ significantly (χ^2=0.65, $p>0.05$) (Table 1).

Despite lack of effect of parity on incidence of reproductive disorders (χ^2=0.74, $p>0.05$), the problems were more common among single parities (38.5%) than multiple parities (33.8%) (Table 1). In addition, the incidence of reproductive problems were also assessed in relation to body condition score of the study cows and statistically insignificant associations (χ^2=1.76, p=0.41) were found. However, incidence was high in animals with poor conditions (44.7%) than good ones (35.4%). On the other hand, the incidence of clinical reproductive problems were higher in cows that were bred by artificial insemination than those that were bred by natural service and those that gave birth to male calves relative to those that gave birth to female calves though the differences were insignificant in both cases. Moreover, factors such as calf sex, dam age and service type did not significantly influence ($p>0.05$) the occurrence of reproductive problems (Table 1).

Table 1. *Bivariate associations of potential host risk factors with incidence of major clinical reproductive problems in local and crossbred dairy cows at Bako, Western Oromia, Ethiopia.*

Factors	Factor categories	No. of observations	No. affected (%)	χ^2	p-value
Breed	Local Horro	313	107 (34.2)	0.655	0.418*
	Crossbred	59	24 (40.7)		
Parity	Primiparous	109	42(38.5)	0.552	0.457*
	Pluriparous	263	89(33.8)		
Body condition score	Good	79	28(35.4)	1.760	0.415*
	Medium	255	86(33.7)		
	Poor	38	17(44.7)		
Age of dam (years)	3-5	127	49(38.6)	2.479	0.290*

Factors	Factor categories	No. of observations	No. affected (%)	χ^2	p-value
	6-10	171	53(31.0)		
	>10	74	29(39.2)		
Calf sex	Male	165	66(40.0)	2.719	0.099*
	Female	202	63(31.2)		
Service type	AI	314	113(36.0)	0.332	0.565*
	Bull service	58	18(31.0%)		

*: Not significant; AI: artificial insemination

The major types of reproductive problems recorded in the present study were retained fetal membranes (8.3%, n=31), dystocia (6.7%, n=25), abortions (5.9%, n=22), uterine infections (5.6%, n=21) and stillbirths (4.8%, n=18) (Fig. 1).

The incidence of major reproductive problems among local Horro and crossbred cows are given in Figure 2. The incidence of the problems didn't differ significantly between the genotypes (p>0.05). In this study, the incidence of dystocia, uterine infections, stillbirths and repeat breeding were more common in crossbred cows while abortion was more frequent in local cows.

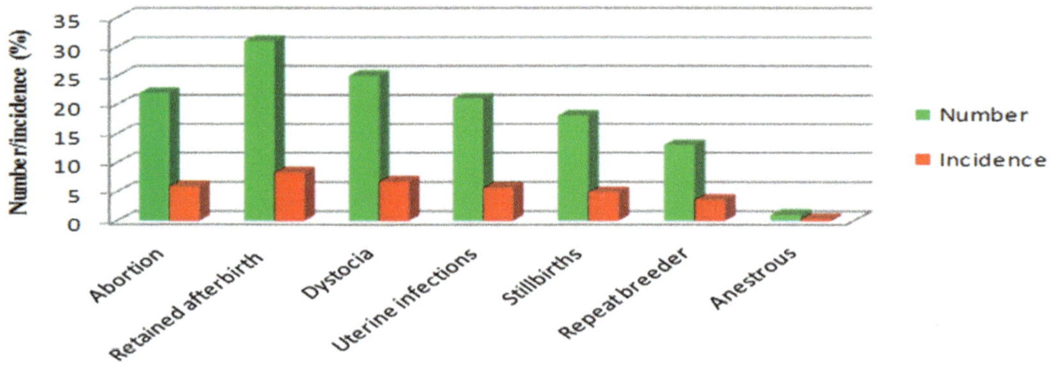

Figure 1. *Number, incidence and types of clinical reproductive problems of dairy cows at Bako livestock research farm, Western Oromia, Ethiopia.*

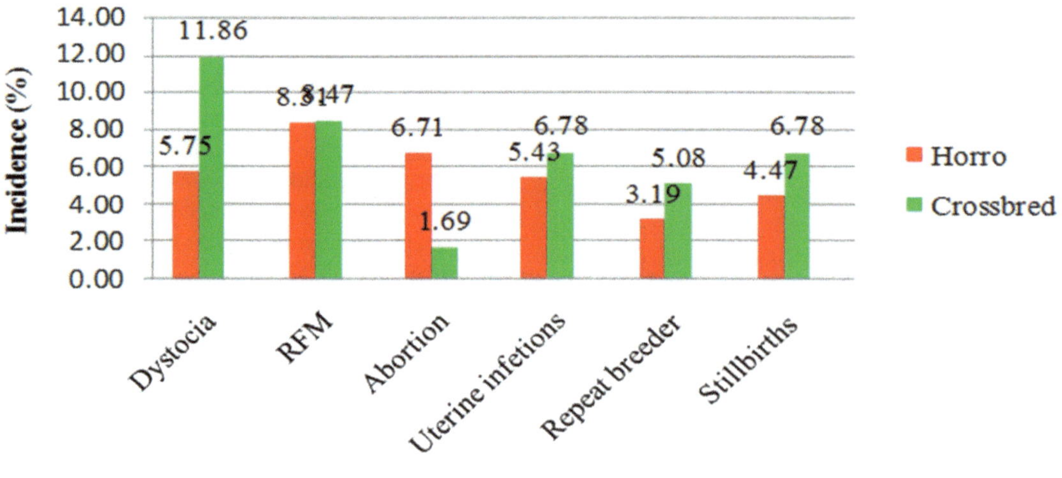

Figure 2. *Incidence of major clinical reproductive problems by breed of cows at Bako Agricultural research center, Western Oromia, Ethiopia.*

In this study, the overall incidence of abortion was found to be 5.9%, the incidence in local Horro and crossbred cows being 7.0% and 2.0%, respectively. Abortion incidence in relation to breed of study cows was also assessed and found to be statistically insignificant (p>0.05). In our study, most of the abortions occurred in the second and third trimester of pregnancy. On the other hand, the incidence of RFM in local and crossbred dairy cows was 8.31% and 8.47%, respectively, showing no effect of breed. Table 2 shows the relative frequency and incidence of RFM in cows when the data is explored further based on calf sex in both breeds of cows. Higher incidence of dystocia was observed in crossbred cows (11.86%) than in local cows (5.75%) though no statistically significant association was detected.

Table 2. *Relative frequency and proportion of retained fetal membranes (RFM) by breed and calf sex.*

Breed of dam	Calf sex	Total number of calvings	No. of cases	Incidence (%) of cases
Local Horro	Male	133	12	9.0
	Female	180	14	7.7
Crossbred	Male	34	2	5.8
	Female	25	3	12.0

The incidence and proportional morbidity rate of clinically observed major reproductive problems in the present study was given in the table below (Table 3).

Table 3. *The incidence and proportional morbidity rates (PMR) of major reproductive health problems of dairy cows at Bako between October 2008 and January 2010.*

Type of reproductive problems	No. of cases	Incidence (%)	PMR
RFM	31	8.3%	23.66
Dystocia	25	6.7%	19.08
Abortion	22	5.9%	16.79
Stillbirths	18	4.8%,	13.74
Endometritis	15	4.0%	11.45
Repeat breeder	13	3.5%	9.92
Pyometra	6	1.6%	4.58
Anestrous	1	0.3%	0.76

4. Discussions

In this study, the cumulative incidence of major reproductive problems of dairy cows was 35.2%. This means nearly one cow out of every three cows, regardless of various host related differences, encountered at least one of the described reproductive problems during the study period. This finding fairly agrees with previous reports from different regions of Ethiopia [10, 23, 24, 25, 26, 27]. However, much higher incidences were also reported from Ethiopia [28, 29]. On the other hand, our finding is higher than previous reports from Bedelle [30] and Asella [31] in Ethiopia. These variations could arise due to differences in management, breeds of the animals, and environmental factors. Differences in management systems and environmental conditions under which cattle are maintained could greatly affect the incidence of reproductive health problems [23, 32].

In the present study, no statistically detectable effect (p>0.05) of breed was shown on the cumulative incidence of major reproductive health problems evaluated. However, the incidence of the problem was higher in crossbred cows (40.7%) than in indigenous cows (34.2%). Consistent with our finding, other researchers [24, 33] did not detect the effect of breed on incidence of reproductive health problems in dairy cows in Ethiopia. Conversely, the lack of detectable effect of genotype on incidence of reproductive problems in our study is in disagreement with the previous reports from Ethiopia [4, 23, 25, 34]. Though our analysis could not detect significant effect of breed on occurrence of reproductive health problems, the higher incidence of the problems in crossbred cows could still suggest increased susceptibility of the animals to reproductive problems than local animals. The incidences of all the reproductive conditions assessed in this study were more common in crossbred cows than local cows. It is widely accepted that crossbred cows are less adaptive to tropical conditions such as high temperature, humidity and various diseases [4] which are typical characteristics of Bako and its surroundings. Though crossbred dairy cows require more intensive management, feeding and better health care than the indigenous zebu to attain better reproduction and production performances in the tropics [35], both the crossbred and local cows in the present study were managed under a similar management system.

The incidence of reproductive disorders among single parity and multiple parities were 38.5% and 33.8%, respectively and parity had no significant effect (p>0.05) on the incidence of the problems. This finding is in agreement with previous works in Ethiopia [24, 29] who did not detect the influence of parity on the incidence of reproductive problems in dairy cows. In contrast to this, other researchers [10, 23, 25] reported the effect of parity on occurrence of reproductive problems in dairy cows in Ethiopia. The effects of parity might be due to factors affecting reproduction in cows of greater parity. Aging cows and their reproductive systems probably involves more complex and permanent uterine changes than those cows with lower parities. Furthermore, an increase in parity not only brings reproductive problems but can also lead to serious locomotive, mammary and metabolic disorders [36]. The lack of influence of parity on incidence of reproductive health problems in our study could be due to, but not limited to, the much broader classification of parity category into primiparous (109, 29.3%) and pluriparous (263, 70.69%). The incidence of clinical reproductive problems were higher in cows that were bred by artificial insemination than those that were bred by natural service and those that gave birth to male calves relative to those that gave birth to female calves, though the differences were not significant (p>0.05). This could have been due to the larger calf sizes in both instances which predisposed the dams to developing the problems. Even though body condition score of the study animals did not influence the incidence of reproductive health problems in the present study, incidence was high in cows with poor body conditions (44.7%) than good (35.4%) ones. Other host related factors such as calf sex, age of dams and service type did not significantly influence (p>0.05) the incidence of reproductive problems in the present study.

The major types of reproductive health problems recorded in the present study were RFM, dystocia, abortions, uterine infections and stillbirths. In a similar fashion, several researchers [10, 23, 24, 25, 27, 28, 29, 33, 41] reported a closely similar results from different dairy farms in Ethiopia. In addition, a recent review paper [1] found that RFM, dystocia, abortion, stillbirth and twinning are the main reproductive and health problems affecting dairy cows worldwide.

The incidence of RFM in our study was 8.3%. Globally, the incidence varies from study to study but tends to be about 5-10% [1]. Our finding is in fair agreement with previous reports from Ethiopia [10, 25, 27, 30, 33] and elsewhere [37, 38, 39]. In contrast to our finding, higher incidences of RFM were reported from different farms in Ethiopia [23, 24, 28, 29, 40, 41]. In problem herds, the incidence may be much higher. The low incidence of RFM might be linked to the low incidence of abortion (5.9%), a known predisposing factor for RFM [42]. Other factors such as year of calving, season of calving, parity of dam, calf mortality, calving difficulty and fetal presentation have all been shown to affect the incidence of RFM [43].

In the present study, the incidence of dystocia of 6.7% is in agreement with previous reports [25, 28, 30, 33], but lower than the report of [44] from Ethiopia. Because definitions of dystocia vary in the literature, there is variation in the international incidence of calving difficulty. Internationally, reported incidence in dairy cattle of severe or considerable difficulty in calving varies from just below 2% to over 22%. However, assistance at calving (including lower degrees of difficulties) is much more prevalent, varying from 10% to over half of the calvings [19]. Higher incidence of dystocia was observed in crossbred cows (11.86%) than in local cows (5.75%) though no statistically detectable association ($p>0.05$) was found.

On the other hand, the present study revealed the occurrence of abortion in dairy cows to be 5.9%. This finding is slightly higher than the manageable limit, given the suggested target of 5% for dairy cattle [45]. Various researchers [10, 26, 28, 29, 44, 31] reported a closely similar findings from different areas of Ethiopia. Lower incidences of 1% and 2.6% were also reported from Jimma [24] and Hosanna [33] towns in Ethiopia. Conversely, widespread cases of abortion ranging from 12.5% to even 50% were also reported from both smallholder and large dairy farms in Ethiopia [27, 30, 34]. Most of the abortions encountered in the present study were late term which could have significant consequence on the effort to get replacement heifers and stock.

The incidence of repeat breeders in the present study was 3.5%. This finding is consistent with the report from Holetta town in Ethiopia [46], though both higher and lower incidences were also reported previously by different researchers from Ethiopia. Accordingly, higher incidence of repeat breeders were reported from different areas of Ethiopia [10, 26, 33, 44] and incidence as low as 0% was reported after regular follow up of pregnant dairy cows during peri-parturient period in Borena Zone of Ethiopia [27]. The difference in incidence of repeat breeders could partly be attributed to the difference in management of study animals. Majority of the higher incidences of repeat breeders reported above were based on dairy animals managed under extensive production in which cows in heat may not be properly followed and inseminated accordingly. In addition, lower incidence of repeat breeding in our study could be due to better follow-up of cows in heat for insemination and better technical efficiency of the inseminator. The incidence of stillbirths in this study of 4.8% was similar to other studies that had reported incidence ranging from 2.8% to 10% [1, 25, 28, 47, 48].

5. Conclusions

This study revealed the high incidence of major clinical reproductive problems in study animals. The most common type reproductive problems were retained fetal membrane, dystocia, abortion, uterine infections and stillbirths. This study revealed that nearly one cow out of every three cows encountered at least one type of clinical reproductive problems indicating the widespread occurrence of the problems among dairy cows kept on station at Bako Agricultural Research Center. However, considered plausible factors such as breed, parity number, body condition score (BCS), age of dams, calf sex and service type were had no significant influence on the occurrence of reproductive problems in the study farm indicating that some other factors are responsible for precipitating the conditions. It is, therefore, recommended that other factors that may precipitate the occurrence of the problems in the study animals should be identified and prevented to minimize the occurrence of these problems and associated losses not only to the center but also to the far demanding smallholder farmers in the area who hugely depend on the center for crossbred heifers.

Acknowledgements

The study was based on data collected from dairy cows at Bako Agricultural Research Center, the center to which the authors were affiliated. Thus, we, the authors would like to express our gratitude to the centre for allowing us to collect the data from the animals and the staff members of the dairy research team of the center who have been involved in data collection.

References

[1] Ghavi Hossein-Zadeh, N. (2013). Effects of main reproductive and health problems on the performance of dairy cows: a review. Span. J. Agric. Res. 11(3): 718-735.

[2] Bekana, M., Ekman, T. and Kindhal, H. (1994a). Ultrasonography of Bovine postpartum cows with retained fetal membranes. J. Vet. Med. A. 41: 653-662.

[3] Bekana, M., Jonsson, P., Kindhal, H. (1997). Bacterial isolates with retained fetal membranes and subsequent ovarian activity in cattle. Vet. Rec., 140: 232-234.

[4] Mukasa-Mugerwa, E., Azage, T., Tafese, M. and Teklu, Y. (1991).Reproductive efficiency of Bos indicus (Zebu) cows under artificial insemination. Anim. Reprod. Sci., 24: 63-72.

[5] Esslemont RJ, Kossaibati, MA. (1997). Culling in 50 dairy herds in England. Vet. Rec. 140: 36-39.

[6] Seegers, H., Beaudeau, F., Flourichon, C. and Bareille, N. (1998). Reasons for culling in French Holstein cows. Prev. Vet. Med. 36: 257-271.

[7] Stevenson, MA. and Lean, IJ. (1998). Descriptive epidemiological study on culling and deaths in eight dairy herds. Australian Vet. J. 76: 482-488.

[8] Asfaw, C., Gebreyohanes, G., Kebede, G., Kebede, K. and Tola, A. (2000). Reproductive performance and lactation yield of F1 (Bos indicus x Bos Taurus) animals at Bako. In: Proceedings of 7th Annual Conference of the Ethiopian Society of Animal Production (ESAP), held in Addis Ababa, Ethiopia, 26-27 May 1999: 386-396.

[9] Gebreyohannes, G. and Kebede, M. (2006). Herd life and lifetime calf crop production in relation to age at first calving in indigenous and crossbred cows at Bako, Ethiopia. Eth. J. Anim. Prod. 6(1): 55-65.

[10] Haftu, B. and Gashaw, A. (2009). Major Reproductive Health Problems of Dairy Cows in and around Bako, West Ethiopia. Eth. J. Anim. Prod. 9(1): 89-98.

[11] Kebede, M., Greyling, JPC., Schwalbach LMJ. and Duguma, G. (2006). Effect of season and supplementation on semen and testicular characteristics of Horro bulls in sub-humid environmental condition in Ethiopia. Eth. J. Anim. Prod. 6(1): 19-32.

[12] Fikru, A. (1988). Need for soil survey studies. pp. 15-20. In: Desta Beyene (ed.). Proceedings of soil science research review in Ethiopia. Institute of Agricultural Research (IAR), 11-14 February 1986, Addis Ababa, Ethiopia.

[13] Anon (1996). Omo-Gibe River Basin Integrated Development Master Plan Study. Final Report. Vol. VII. Land Resource Survey. B1. Federal Democratic Republic of Ethiopia. Ministry of Water Resources. Richard Woodroofe and Associates with Marcott, UK. 202.

[14] Sahlemedhin, S. and Ahmed, A. (1983). Phosphorus sorption characteristics of some Ethiopian soils. Eth. J. Agri. Sci. 5: 1-12.

[15] Gebreyohannes, G., Tegegne, A., Diedhiou, ML. and Hegde, BP. (2003). Reproduction efficiency of zebu and crossbred cows as measured by the inter-estrus and inter-service intervals at Bako. Proceedings of the 10th annual conference of the Ethiopian Society of Animal Production (ESAP) held in Addis Ababa, Ethiopia, August 21-23, Addis Ababa, Ethiopia.

[16] Alberro, M., and Hailemariam, S. (1982). The indigenous cattle of Ethiopia, Part I. World Anim. Rev. 41: 2-11.

[17] Ayana, T., Tafess, K., Mamo, G., Sisay, T. and Ameni, G. (2013). Isolation and molecular characterization of non-tuberculosis mycobacteria from skin positive reactors and pathological lesions of cattle at Bako, Western Ethiopia. Afr. J. Microbiol. Res. 7(20): 2190-2197.

[18] Peter, AT. (2000). Abortions in dairy cows: New insights and economic impact. Adv. Dairy Technol. 12: 233-244.

[19] Mee, JF. (2008a). Prevalence and risk factors for dystocia in dairy cattle: a review. Vet. J. 176(1): 93-101.

[20] Richard, W. (1993). Dairying. Tropical Agriculturalist, 1st ed. Macmillan Press London. 43 48.

[21] Kelton, DF., Lissemore, KD. and Martin, ER. (1998). Recommendations for recording and calculating the incidence of selected clinical diseases of dairy cattle. J. Dairy Sci. 81: 2502-2509.

[22] Clark, GM. (1982). Statistics and experimental design. A series of student text in contemporary biology. 2nd ed. Edward Arnold, London. 48-62.

[23] Gizaw, M., Bekana, M., Abayneh, T. (2007). Major reproductive health problems in smallholder dairy production in and around Nazareth town, Central Ethiopia. Vet. Online Int. J. Vet. Med. http://www.fourmilab.ch/rpkp/experiments/analysis.

[24] Gashaw, A., Worku, F. and Mulugeta, S. (2011). Assessment of smallholder dairy production and their reproductive health problems in Jimma Town, South-Western Ethiopia. Int. J. App. Res. 9: 80-86.

[25] Tesfaye, D. and Shamble, A. (2013). Reproductive health problems of cows under different management systems in Kombolcha, Northeast Ethiopia. Adv. Biolo. Res. 7 (3): 104-108, 2013.

[26] Esheti, G. and Moges, N. (2014). Major Reproductive Health Disorders in Cross Breed Dairy Cows in Ada'a District, East Shoa, Ethiopia. Global Veterinaria. 13 (4): 444-449.

[27] Benti, D. and Zewdie, W. (2014). Major reproductive health problems of indigenous Borena cows in Ethiopia. J. Adv. Vet. Anim. Res. 1(4): 182-188.

[28] Kassa, T. and Lema, M. (2005). Study on major reproductive problems of Zebu and Friesian x Zebu crossbred cows under small-scale dairy farms in Ada'a District, Oromia, Ethiopia. Eth. Vet. J. 9 (1): 109-122.

[29] Haile, A., Kassa, T., Mihret, M. and Asfaw, Y. (2010). Major reproductive disorders in cross breed dairy cow under smallholding in Addis Ababa milk shed. World J. Agri. Sci. 6(4): 412-418.

[30] Bitew, M. and Prased, S. (2011). Study on Major Reproductive Health Problems in Indigenous and Cross Breed Cows in and around Bedelle, South West Ethiopia. J. Anim. Vet. Adv. 10(6):723-727.

[31] Dinka, H. (2013). Major reproductive disorders of dairy cows in and around Asella town, Central Ethiopia. J. Vet. Med. Anim. Health. 5(4): 113-117.

[32] Mureda, E. and Mekuriaw, Z. (2008). Characteristics and constraints of crossbred dairy cattle production in lowland areas of Eastern Ethiopia. Live. Res. Rural Dev. 20(4).

[33] Haile, A., Tsegaye, Y. and Tesfaye, N. (2014). Assessment of Major Reproductive Disorders of Dairy Cattle in Urban and Per Urban Area of Hosanna, Southern Ethiopia. Anim. Vet. Sc. 2(5): 135-141.

[34] Tekelye, B., Kasali, OB. and Tsion, A. (1991). Reproductive problems in crossbred cattle in central Ethiopia. Anim. Reprod. Sci. 26: 41-49.

[35] Fielding and Matthewman (2004). Tropical cattle management In: Bovine medicine, diseases and husbandry of cattle. 2nd ed. (editors. Andrews AH, Blowey RW, Boyd H, and Eddy RG), Blackwell publishing company, Oxford, UK. 68-81.

[36] Hebert, AB., Bouchard, E., Dutremblay D. and Lefebure, R. (2011). Effects of reproductive disorder and parity on repeat breeder status and culling of dairy cows. Canad. J. Vet. Res. 75(2): 147-151.

[37] Erb, HW. and Martin, SW. (1980). Interrelationship between production and reproductive disease in Holstein cows. J. Diary. Sci. 63: 1911-1917.

[38] Gaines, JD. (1989). The role of record analysis in evaluating sub fertile dairy herds. Vet. Med. 84: 532-543.

[39] Correa, MT., Curtis, CR., Erb, H. N., Screlett, JM. and Smith, RD. (1990). An ecological risk factor for postpartum disorders of Holstein-Friesian cows form thirty-two New York farms. J. Dairy Sci. 73: 1515-1524.

[40] Mamo, T. (2004). Study on major postpartum reproductive problems of smallholder dairy cows in and around Debre Zeit. DVM Thesis, AAU, Ethiopia.

[41] Lemma, A. and Kebede, S. (2011). The effect of mating system and herd size on reproductive performance of dairy cows in market oriented urban dairy farms in and around Addis Ababa. Revue Méd. Vét. 162(11): 526-530.

[42] Arthur, GH., Noakes DE., Parkinson TJ. and England, GCW. (2001). Arthur's Veterinary Reproduction and Obstetrics. 8th ed. WB Saunders Ltd., Philadelphia. 864.

[43] Mee, JF. (1991). The incidence of retained fetal membranes on nine dairy research farms over a ten-year period (1978–1987). Irish Vet. J. 44: 48–52.

[44] Birhanu, A., Harlow, CR., Gidey, G., Tadesse, D., Desta, G., Gugssa, T., and Riley, S. (2015). Assessment of reproductive performance and problems in crossbred (Holstein Friesian X Zebu) dairy cattle in and around Mekelle, Tigray, Ethiopia. Anim. Vet. Sci. 3(3).

[45] Radostits, OM., Leslie, KE. and Fetrow, J. (1994). Maintenance of reproductive efficiency in dairy cattle. In Herd Health: Food Animal Production Medicine. 2nd ed. Philadelphia: W. B. Saunders Company, 141-158.

[46] Tigre, W. (2004). Major clinical reproductive health problems of dairy cows in and around Holleta. DVM thesis. Addis Ababa University, Debre Zeit, Ethiopia.

[47] Berglund, B., Steinbock, L. and Elvander, M. (2003). Causes of stillbirth and time of death in Swedish Holstein calves examined post mortem. Acta Vet. Scand.44(3): 111-120.

[48] Abuom, TO., Njenga, MJ., Wabacha, JK., Tsuma, VT. and Gitau, GK. (2012). Incidence and risk factors of periparturient conditions in smallholder dairy cattle herds Kikuyu Division of Kiambu District, Kenya. Eth. Vet. J. 16(2): 85-102.

Retrospective Study of Reproductive Diseases of Small Ruminants in Northern Barind Tract in Bangladesh

Md. Hemayatul Islam[1], Md. Jalal Uddin Sarder[1,*], Md. Siddiqur Rahman[3], Md. Ariful Haque[2], Md. Akhtarul Islam[1], Syed Sarwar Jahan[1], Rashida Khaton[1]

[1]Department of Animal Husbandry and Veterinary Science, University of Rajshahi, Bangladesh
[2]Institute of Biological Sciences, University of Rajshahi, Rajshahi-6205, Bangladesh
[3]Faculty of Veterinary science, Bangladesh Agricultural University, Mymensing, Bangladesh

Email address:
jalalnusa@yahoo.com (Md. J. U. Sarder)

Abstract: Context: The information of diseases prevalence give useful information on disease pattern and thus can be used in preventing diseases as well as formulating policies for future management to prevent diseases. Aim: This study is therefore aimed at determining the pattern of reproductive diseases encountered at the Barind tract in Bangladesh. Materials and Method: The primary data were collected by randomly selected location in each district of retrospective survey from the veterinary and vaccination camp of the study area. Records of 2667 clinical cases of small ruminants (2394 goats, 273 sheep) questionnaires report under this study, from July 2012 to June 2013 were analyzed to assess the importance of existing diseases. The computer program SPSS were analyzed the study and Chi-square and F test were used for significance test. Results: The small ruminants were significantly suffering from various diseases and disorders. The maximum 816 (30.6%) was affected by infectious diseases and lowest 18 (0.7%) was affected with poisonous diseases in small ruminants. The others diseases highest to lowest rate were 444 (16.6%), 354(13.3%), 345 (12.9%), 231 (8.7%), 162 (6.1%),102 (3.8%), 84 (3.1%),72 (2.7%) and 39 (1.5%) affected with gastrointestinal, respiratory, surgical, female reproductive disorder, deficiency syndrome, Integumentary involvement, diseases of sense organ, musculoskeletal system and disease of male sex organ respectively in small . The highest disease prevalence (89.8%) was observed in goat than in sheep (10.2%) and the total reproductive disease prevalence was 10.2%. The highest & lowest incidence rates of reproductive disorders in relation to sex were 32.5% & 1.9% in anoestrus and postitis. Similarly, the age had significant effect ($P<0.05$) and highest value were 20.4%, 7.9% & 4.5% observed in anoestrus of young, adult and old ages respectively. The season had significant effect and the overall disease prevalence was higher rainy season 40.4%, but the individual highest value observed in anoestrus 14.7% in winter season. Conclusion: The one tenth portion of disease prevalence got in reproductive related case, but most frequent reproductive diseases and disorder were in found in goat, female animal, young age, rainy season and particularly in anoestrus condition of small ruminants at northern Barind tract in Bangladesh.

Keywords: Reproductive Diseases, Prevalence, Age, Sex, Seasons

1. Introduction

The magnitude of contribution of the livestock sector to the GDP is 2.6 % in Bangladesh and 80% rural people rear indigenous animals. The present population of goat and, sheep are 22400000 and 2870000 respectively [1] (DLS, 2010). The Barind tract is situated in the Northern belt of Bangladesh. The area of Barind area in particular is known to tilt a farther 15M upwards in the west. On the other hand Barind Tract has a different geographic character than other parts of Bangladesh. Its soil formation is also different from others parts of Bangladesh. This northern part is 37 meter above sea level. People in this area used to cultivate rice once a year, but now produce various crops such as rice, white and pulses round the year. The other time of the year left that is suitable for grazing of animal especially small ruminants [2](Alice Mbugua 2011). Livestock sector provides full time employment to approximately 20% and part time employment to approximately 50% of the rural population of Bangladesh. It also generates an adequate amount of foreign currency every year by exporting hides and skin and their products. Besides, per capita income of Bangladesh is 750 US dollar and 49% of the total population of Bangladesh is malnourished. Per capita requirement of protein cannot be fulfilled by our protein sources. So, continuous protein deficiency causes various nutritional deficiency diseases followed by infectious diseases and reproductive disturbances. If the livestock sector develops, it will be able to fulfill the existing requirement of protein for the country. Disease is defined as inability to perform physiological functions at normal levels even though nutrition and other environmental requirements are provided at adequate levels [3] (Radositis *et al.,* 2007). Disease conditions always impair livestock production [4-5] (Akerejola *etal,* 1979; Lamorde, 1996). Apart from this, several other factors such as environment and nutrition, especially inadequate protein intake [6-7] (Kumidiake *et al.,* 1981; Smith and Somade, 1994) decrease reproductive performance. However, technological difficulties in these countries hinder extensive use of modern diagnostic techniques in disease surveillance [8] (Nwanta *et al.,* 2000). Diseases and climatic problems have been blamed as the main limitation to modern animal husbandry in tropical areas [9] (Loosli *et al.,* 1974). It is therefore important to understand not only the interactions between different diseases occurring in the same environment, but also the modulating influence of the climatic factors driving the seasonal variations usually observed [10](Onwuliri *et al* 1993). Such knowledge is essential in planning control strategies against reproductive diseases. Approximately 36% protein requirement is fulfilled by livestock sector. In the rural area of Plain land of Bangladesh livestock rearing such as beef fattening, goat rearing, buck rearing and sheep rearing are gradually increasing day by day. Small ruminants are allowed to roam throughout the seasons, thriving on indigenous browses growing in compound bushes and farm fallows with additional supplementation from kitchen wastes [11] (Okoli *et al.* 2003). The goat is called the "Poor man's cow" is the second important livestock in Bangladesh which plays an important role in the rural economy and earn substantial amount of foreign currency by exporting skin and others by products [12] (Kamaruddin, 2003). Each year goat production provides 127,000 MT meats, which accounts for 25% of total red meat in Bangladesh [13](FAO, 2007). Even in urban area goats and sheep are being raised under an intensive system of management by stall feeding with bran, fodder and tree leaves. So there is a lot of prospect to rear small ruminants in that area and Several reports have been written on livestock diseases in the country, but with very little attention to small ruminant's diseases especially reproductive diseases. These studies are usually emphasis to analysis the prevalence rate and evaluation of sex, age and seasonal influence on reproductive disease trends in small ruminants.

2. Materials and Methods

2.1. Sources of Information

The primary data were collected by randomly selected location in each district of retrospective survey from the veterinary and vaccination camp of the study area. The Health and Vaccination awareness camp was taken by primary questionnaire were filled up. The vaccination camps were in Nachal Upazilla Livestock office Chapainowabjong; Youth training centre, Noagoan; Moukhara High school field, Natore and Parila Primary School field, Paba, Rajshahi. The other data were collected from data record book of Veterinary Clinic and Artificial Insemination Center in the Department of Animal Husbandry and Veterinary Science, University of Rajshahi. Records of 2667 clinical cases of small ruminant (2394 goats, 273 sheep) questionnaires report under this study, from July 2012 to June 2013 were analyzed to assess the importance of existing diseases. The results were analyzed into eleven major diagnostic groups in small ruminants. The age of each animal was determined by asking the owner and by dentition. Diagnosis of these cases was made on the basis of signalment (age, sex and breed), clinical history and clinical examinations. To avoid overlapping of these diseases, certain adjustments were made so that each disease was counted under only one group. The data on the occurrence of clinical diseases and disorders were analyzed into eleven major diagnostic groups.

2.2. Data Processing

These groups were: (1) Gastro intestinal system involvement, (2) Respiratory system involvement (3) Musculoscletal system involvement, (4) Integumentary involvement, (5) Diseases of senses organ, (6) Infectious diseases (includes PPR, rabies, tetanus Naval ill, pregnancy toxemia, worm infestation and coccidiosis) (7) Deficiency and metabolic diseases, (8) Poisonous diseases, (9) Common Surgery, (10) Female reproductive diseases and (11) Male sex organ involvement. The age sex and seasonal influence on the occurrence of diseases were also analyzed. Accordingly, data were analyzed into three age groups: Kids/ lambs (below 12 months) adults (12 to 24 months) and older (more than 24 months) aged. Sex was male and female and. We considered three seasons as summer from March to May, Rainy from June to October and winter from November to February. The small ruminants' diseases of male and female reproductive involvement were selection for further revision. Data on clinical cases of reproductive abnormalities (in case of female) were abortion, anoestrus, cervicitis, dystocia, endometritis, pyometra, repeat breeding, retained placenta, still birth and vaginal or uterine prolapsed as well as in male it is orchitis, postitis, and urinary tract infection. Diagnoses at the health and vaccination campaign by the veterinarian were usually based on flock history, clinical sign and symptoms.

2.3. Statistical Analysis

Data were statistically analyzed by Statistical Package for

Social Science (SPSS) software 17.0 version [14]. Chi-square and F test was used to know the association between different groups in respective cases.

3. Results

The diseases and reproductive disorders observed in the different systems of small ruminants are shown in the Table 1-4. A total 2667 cases were presented to the study, and of these, 270(10.2%) were reproductive case. The percentage distribution of diseases according to species shows goat with the highest number of cases 2394 (89.8%), then sheep 273 (10.2%) (Table1). In the study it was found that small ruminant were significantly suffering from various diseases and disorders, where maximum 816 (30.6%) of small ruminants were affected by infectious diseases. The lowest number 18 (0.7%) small ruminants affected with poisonous diseases. The other number of diseases involve in small were highest to lowest rate 444 (16.6%), 354(13.3%), 345 (12.9%), 231 (8.7%), 162 (6.1%),102 (3.8%), 84 (3.1%),72 (2.7%) and 39 (1.5%) were in gastrointestinal, respiratory, surgical, female reproductive disorder, deficiency syndrome, Integumentary involvement, diseases of sense organ, musculoskeletal system and disease of male sex organ, respectively. The overall incidence rate of reproductive disorder was 10.2, where 8.7% in female and 1.5% in male sex involvement. The incidence rate (highest to lowest) of reproductive disorders involvement with relation to sex were 32.8%, 15.8%, 10.2%, 7.9%, 6.8%, 5.7%, 4.5% in anoestrus, abortion, dystocia , retained placenta, cervicities, mastitis and repeat breeding in case of female, but in male it was 5.7%, 5.3%, 2.6 and 1.9% in urinary tract infection, urolithiasis, postitis and orchitis, respectively (table 2). The study also revealed that the reproductive disorders of small ruminants were varied with aged. The incidence rate of cervicities, abortion, mastitis, retained placenta, anoestrus, repeat breeding, dystocia, urinary tract infection, postitis, urolithiasis and orchitis were 5.7%, 8.7%, 2.3%, 5.7%, 20.4%, 1.1%, 4.5%, 4.2%, 1.9%, 1.9% & 1.9% in young; 1.1%, 5.7%, 2.3%, 2.3%, 7.9%, 2.3%, 1.1%, 1.5%, 0%, 3.4% & 0.8% and in adult 0%, 1.5%, 1.1%, 2.3%, 4.5%, 1.1%, 2.3%, 0.8% ,0%, 0% & 0% in older respectively (table 3). The seasonal influence also diverse with the reproductive disorders of small in case of cervicities, abortion, mastitis, retained placenta, anoestrus, repeat breeding, dystocia, urinary tract infection, postitis, urolithiasis and orchitis were 1.1%, 3.4%, 3.4%, 1.1%, 9.1%, 0.0%, 2.3%, 2.3%, 0.8%, 1.9% & 1.9% in summer; 3.4%, 6.8%, 2.3%, 6.8%, 9.1%, 1.1%, 5.7%, 2.6%, 1.1%, 1.5% & 0.0% in rainy and 2.3%, 5.7%, 0%, 2.3%, 14.7%, 3.4%, 0%, 1.5%, 0%, 1.9% & 0.8% in winter respectively (table 4).

4. Discussion

The retrospective study provided preliminary information on the incidence and pattern of the reproductive disorder prevalent at the Northern Barind tract in Bangladesh. The frequency of reproductive disorder randomly distributed among the species. However, there were more cases affecting small (goat and sheep). This can be explained since small ruminants are in absolute terms, more numerous and it is relatively cheaper to rear small ruminants within the Barind area (Urban area) where they are simply allowed to roam freely and scavenge for food. The occurrence of diseases was predominate to be more in female than male [15] (Wazari *et al.*, 2006) due to the presence of higher number of female animals in the study area [16](Ali *et al* 2011) . This is consistent with the fact that females are kept for longer periods in the herd for breeding or milk supply than the males. Also, the peculiarity of the female's vulnerability could be a contributing factor and observed high frequency of anoestrus. The relationship between nutritional / management factors, poor feeding and present in infectious agent in the environment would be the second position of abortion. Twining poor feeding and management as a cause of dystocia [17-20](Arthur *et al.*, 1998; Dryendahl *et al.*, 1977; Bendixen *et al.*, 1987 & Islam *et al.*, 2013) may be associated with the relatively high incidence of dystocia and retained placenta observed in the study. Similarly the high incidence of urinary tract infection in male would be associated with service to any types of small ruminants, dry weather of the region and neglected of the infection.

Similarly the general frequency of the disease was randomly distributed throughout the year, but relatively more cases were encountered during the month of July to October (rainy season) followed by month of November to February (winter season) than the month of March to June (dry or summer season) which partially agree with Khair *et al.* [21] (2013) and disagree with Waziri *et al.*[15] (2006) The rainy season lies highest frequency may be due to the lack or scarcity of fodder and lack of grazing.

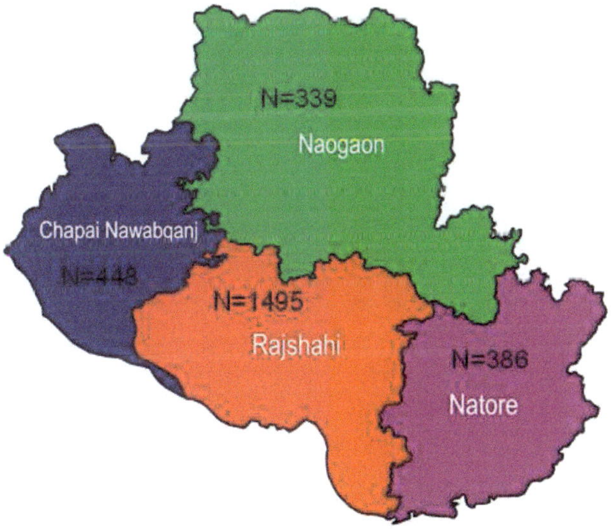

Figure 1. *Area of sample collection at Northern Barind Tract in Bangladesh.*

Table 1. Distribution of diseases of small ruminants.

Diseases	Small ruminants		Total
	Goat	Sheep	
Gastrointestinal	372 (13.9%)	72 (2.7%)	444 (16.6%)
Respiratory	327 (12.3%)	27 (1.0%)	354 (13.3%)
Musculoskeletal system	69 (2.6%)	3(0.1%)	72 (2.7%)
Female reproductive	183 (6.9%)	48(1.8%)	231 (8.7%)
Integumentary involvement	93 (3.5%)	9(0.3%)	102 (3.8%)
Disease of Sense organ	78 (2.9%)	6(0.2%)	84 (3.1%)
Infectious disease	750 (28.1%)	66(2.5%)	816 (30.6%)
Deficiency syndrome	153 (5.7%)	9(0.3%)	162 (6.1%)
Poison	12 (0.4%)	6 (0.2%)	18 (0.7%)
Male sex organ	39 (1.5%)	0 (0%)	39 (1.5%)
surgical	318 (11.9%)	27 (1.0%)	345 (12.9%)
Total	2394 (89.8%)	273 (10.2%)	2667 (100%)
F value	7.882	Significant	

Table 2. Distribution of reproductive diseases of small ruminants associated with sex.

Legend	Sex of small ruminants		Total
	Male	Female	
Cervicities	-	18 (6.8%)	18 (6.8%)
Abortion	-	42 (15.8%)	42 (15.8%)
Mastitis	-	15 (5.7%)	15 (5.7%)
Retained placenta	-	27 (10.2%)	27 (10.2%)
Anoestrus	-	87(32.8%)	87(32.8%)
Repeat breeding	-	12 (4.5%)	12 (4.5%)
Dystocia	-	21 (7.9%)	21 (7.9%)
Urinary tract Infection	15 (5.7%)	2(0.8%)	17 (6.4%)
Postitis	5 (1.9%)	-	5 (1.9%)
Urolithiasis	14 (5.3%)	-	14 (5.3%)
Orchitis	7 (2.6%)	-	7 (2.6%)
Total	41 (15.5%)	224 (84.5%)	265 (100%)
Chi-Square Test	Calculated value 251.506	Tabulated value 18.307	Significant P< 0.05

Table 3. Distribution of reproductive diseases of small ruminants associated with age.

Legend	Age of the small ruminants			Total
	Young 0<12 Months	Adult 12<24 Months	Old >24 Months	
Cervicities	15 (5.7%)	3 (1.1%)	0 (0%)	18 (6.8%)
Abortion	23 (8.7%)	15 (5.7%)	4 (1.5%)	42 (15.8%)
Mastitis	6 (2.3%)	6 (2.3%)	3 (1.1%)	15 (5.7%)
Retained placenta	15 (5.7%)	6 (2.3%)	6 (2.3%)	27 (10.2%)
Anoestrus	54 (20.4%)	21 (7.9%)	12 (4.5%)	87(32.8%)
Repeat breeding	3 (1.1%)	6 (2.3%)	3 (1.1%)	12 (4.5%)
Dystocia	12 (4.5%)	3 (1.1%)	6 (2.3%)	21 (7.9%)
Urinary tract Infection	11 (4.2%)	4 (1.5%)	02 (0.8%)	17(6.4%)
Postitis	5 (1.9%)	0 (0%)	0 (0%)	5 (1.9%)
Urolithiasis	5 (1.9%)	9 (3.4%)	0 (0%)	14 (5.3%)
Orchitis	5 (1.9%)	02 (0.8%)	0 (0%)	7 (2.6%)
Total	154 (58.1%)	75 (28.3%)	36(13.6%)	265 (100%)
Chi-Square Test	Calculated value 36.279	Tabulated value 31.410	Not Significance P>0.05	

Table 4. Distribution of reproductive diseases of small ruminants associated with Season.

Legend	Seasons of the Year			Total
	Summer (March to June)	Rainy (July to October)	Winter (November to February).	
Cervicities	3 (1.1%)	9 (3.4%)	6(2.3%)	18 (6.8%)
Abortion	9 (3.4%)	18 (6.8%)	15 (5.7%)	42 (15.8%)
Mastitis	9 (3.4%)	6 (2.3%)	0 (0%)	15 (5.7%)
Retained placenta	3 (1.1%)	18 (6.8%)	6 (2.3%)	27 (10.2%)
Anoestrus	24 (9.1%)	24 (9.1%)	39(14.7%)	87(32.8%)
Repeat breeding	0 (0.0%)	3 (1.1%)	9 (3.4%)	12 (4.5%)
Dystocia	6 (2.3%)	15 (5.7%)	0 (0%)	21 (7.9%)
Urinary tract Infection	6 (2.3%)	7 (2.6%)	4 (1.5%)	17(6.4%)
Postitis	2 (0.8%)	3 (1.1%)	0 (0%)	5 (1.9%)

Legend	Seasons of the Year			Total
	Summer (March to June)	Rainy (July to October)	Winter (November to February).	
Urolithiasis	5 (1.9%)	4 (1.5%)	5 (1.9%)	14 (5.3%)
Orchitis	5 (1.9%)	0 (0%)	2 (0.8%)	7 (2.6%)
Total	72 (27.2%)	107 (40.4%)	86(32.5%)	265 (100%)
Chi-Square Test	Calculated value 62.917	Tabulated value 31.410	Significant P<0.05	

Acknowledgements

We appreciate the assistance provided by farmer and the members of Bangladesh Livestock Society (BLS) to arrange the Veterinary Health and Vaccination Camp in data collection.

Authors' Contributions

Md. Hemayatul Islam designed the study, performed the data analysis and wrote the manuscript. Sarder MJU was supervised and contributed in development and pre-testing of the study questionnaire, data collection and reviewed the manuscript. The other authors read and approved the final manuscript.

References

[1] DLS (2010). Personal communication With Project Director, Animal Health Care, Management and Expansion Project, DLS, Dhaka.

[2] Alice Mbugua (2011) Research Report on Water Scarcity in Northern Bangladesh International volunteer, VSO and GBK staff, Parbatipur, Dinajpur: 1-25.

[3] Radostitis OM, Gay CC, Blood DC and Hinchcliff KW (2007) Veterinary Medicine. A Text book of the diseases of cattle, sheep, pig and horse, Ninth Edition, Bailliere Tindal, London, 1308.

[4] Akerejola OC, Schillhorn VT, Njoku CO (1979) Ovine and Caprine diseases in Nigeria. Bulletin of Animal Health and Production in Africa 27: 65 – 68.

[5] Lamorde AG (1996) The role of veterinarians on a developing economy. Nigerian Veterinary Journal (special edition) 1(1): 106 - 111.

[6] Kumidiaka J, Osori DIK., Ogwu D (1981) Incidence of genital abnormalities and physiological effect of genital pathology in indigenous cows. Nigerian Veterinary Journal 9: 52 - 54.

[7] Smith OS and Somade B (1994) Interaction between nutrition and reproduction in farm animals. IFS (International Foundation for science) Proceedings of a Regional Seminar on Animal Reproduction

[8] Nwanta JA, Hassan MI, and Alli-Balogun JK (2000) Epidemiology of PPR in northern states of Nigeria-An update. Proceedings25th Nigeria Society of Animal Production Annual Conference 19-23rd March 2000, Umudike, Nigeria.

[9] Maynard LA, and LOOSI JK (1969) Animal nutrition, 6th ed. McGraw-Hill Book Co., New York. 613pp.

[10] Onwuliri COE, Anosike JC, Nkem CN and Payne U K (1993) The ecology of animal parasitic nematodes in endemic areas of Jos, Nigeria. Applied Parasitology 34: 131-137

[11] Okoli IC, Ebere CS, Uchegbu MC, Udah CA, Ibeawuchi II (2003) A survey of the diversity of plants utilized for small ruminant feeding in south-eastern Nigeria. Agriculture Ecosystems & Environment 96 (1-3): 147-154.

[12] Kamaruddin KM (2003). Goat farming as a means of poverty alleviation. Proceeding of the BSVER symposium, Goats farming in Bangladesh; Problems and prospects. BAU. Bangladesh society for veterinary education research, BSVER Pub. No. 25 P- 26-34.

[13] FAO (2007). FAO production Year Book, Food and Agricultural organization of the USA, Rome, Italy. Vol 51.

[14] SPSS Inc. Released 2008. SPSS Statistics for Windows, Version 17.0. Chicago: SPSS Inc.

[15] Waziri MA, Adamu A and Bukar MM (2006) Analysis of Reproductive cases handeled at the state veterinary clinic Maidugure, Negeria. Negerian Veterinary Journal 27(2): 54-59.

[16] Ali MH, Bhuiyan MKJ and Alam MM (2011) Retrospective epidemiologic study of diseases in in Khagrachari hill tract District of Bangladesh. Bangladesh Veterinary Journal 11(1): 145-153.

[17] Arthur GH, Noakes DE, Pearson H, Parkinson TJ (1998) Veterinary Eproduction and Obstetrics, 7th Edition WB Saunders Co., Philadelphia: 185- 302.

[18] Dryendahl I., Mattson J and Peherson B (1977) Retained Placenta in cattle incidence, clinical data and effects on Postpartum release of fertility. Journal of the American Veterinary Medical Association 24: 529-541.

[19] Bendixen PH, Vilson B, and Ekesbo I (1987) Disease frequencies in dairy cows in Sweden. II. Retained Placenta. Preventative Veterinary Medicine 4:377-387.

[20] Islam MdH, Sarder MdJU, Jahan SS, Rahman M, Zahan M, Kader MdA and Mozaffor Hossain KM (2013) Retained placenta of dairy cows associated with managemental factors in Rajshahi, Bangladesh. Vet World 6(4):180-184, doi: 10.5455/vetworld.2013.180-184.

[21] Khairl MM, Alam1 AKMA, Rahman1 MT, Islam1 A, Azim and Chowdhury EH (2013) Incidence of reproductive and production diseases of cross-breed dairy cattle in Bangladesh. Bangl. J. Vet. Med. 11 (1): 31-36.

Permissions

All chapters in this book were first published in AVS, by Science Publishing Group; hereby published with permission under the Creative Commons Attribution License or equivalent. Every chapter published in this book has been scrutinized by our experts. Their significance has been extensively debated. The topics covered herein carry significant findings which will fuel the growth of the discipline. They may even be implemented as practical applications or may be referred to as a beginning point for another development.

The contributors of this book come from diverse backgrounds, making this book a truly international effort. This book will bring forth new frontiers with its revolutionizing research information and detailed analysis of the nascent developments around the world.

We would like to thank all the contributing authors for lending their expertise to make the book truly unique. They have played a crucial role in the development of this book. Without their invaluable contributions this book wouldn't have been possible. They have made vital efforts to compile up to date information on the varied aspects of this subject to make this book a valuable addition to the collection of many professionals and students.

This book was conceptualized with the vision of imparting up-to-date information and advanced data in this field. To ensure the same, a matchless editorial board was set up. Every individual on the board went through rigorous rounds of assessment to prove their worth. After which they invested a large part of their time researching and compiling the most relevant data for our readers.

The editorial board has been involved in producing this book since its inception. They have spent rigorous hours researching and exploring the diverse topics which have resulted in the successful publishing of this book. They have passed on their knowledge of decades through this book. To expedite this challenging task, the publisher supported the team at every step. A small team of assistant editors was also appointed to further simplify the editing procedure and attain best results for the readers.

Apart from the editorial board, the designing team has also invested a significant amount of their time in understanding the subject and creating the most relevant covers. They scrutinized every image to scout for the most suitable representation of the subject and create an appropriate cover for the book.

The publishing team has been an ardent support to the editorial, designing and production team. Their endless efforts to recruit the best for this project, has resulted in the accomplishment of this book. They are a veteran in the field of academics and their pool of knowledge is as vast as their experience in printing. Their expertise and guidance has proved useful at every step. Their uncompromising quality standards have made this book an exceptional effort. Their encouragement from time to time has been an inspiration for everyone.

The publisher and the editorial board hope that this book will prove to be a valuable piece of knowledge for researchers, students, practitioners and scholars across the globe.

List of Contributors

Vera Hossepian de Lima, Aline Costa Lucio, Leticia Zoccolario Oliveira and Luísa Cunha Carneiro
Department of Preventive Veterinary Medicine and Animal Reproduction, Estadual University of Sao Paulo, UNESP, Jaboticabal, Brazil

Mariney Flavia and Di-Tanno Ramalho
Research Center of Biotechnology, University of Sao Paulo, Sao Paulo, Brazil

Beatriz Costa Aguiar Alves and Carlos Alberto Moreira Filho
Department of Pediatrics, Medicine School of Estadual Universtiy of Sao Paulo, Sao Paulo, SP, Brazil

Hesham Elzorba, Hossney El Banna and Dina Derbala
Department of Pharmacology, Faculty of Veterinary Medicine, Cairo University, Giza, Egypt

Belkacem Behira
University of Es-senia, Faculty of Biology, Oran, Algeria

Bidjeh Kebkiba
Livestock Research Institute for Development (IRED), Ndjamena, Chad

Ban-Bo Bebanto Antipas
Faculty of Exact and Applied Sciences, University of Ndjamena, Ndjamena, Chad

Podkapaev Vladimir Michaelovich
Veterinary Academy in Moscow, KI Skriyabin, Moscow, Russia

Hanene Attia, Aymen Bali, Rabiaa M. Sghaier, Pablo A. Leon Martinez, Ghada Mkannez, Chiraz Atri, Khaled Chourabi, Fatma Z. Guerfali and Dhafer Laouini
Institut Pasteur de Tunis, LR11IP102, Laboratory of Transmission, Control and Immunobiology of Infections (LTCII), Tunis-Belvédère, Tunisia
Université Tunis El Manar, Tunis, Tunisia

Birhanu Hailu
Samara University, College of Veterinary Medicine, P.O.Box.132, Samara, Ethiopia

Berihu Gebrekidan, Solmon Raju, Alemselam Birhanu and Gebrhiwot Tadesse
Mekelle University, College of Veterinary Medicine, Mekelle, Ethiopia

Garba UM
Veterinary Clinic, Equitation Department, Nigerian Defence Academy, Kaduna, Nigeria
Sackey AKB
Department of Veterinary Medicine, Faculty of Veterinary Medicine, Ahmadu Bello University, Zaria, Nigeria

Lawal AI
Department of Veterinary Parasitology and Entomology, Faculty of Veterinary Medicine, Ahmadu Bello University, Zaria, Nigeria

Esievo KAN
Department of Veterinary Pathology, Faculty of Veterinary Medicine, Ahmadu Bello University, Zaria, Nigeria

Maryam Rassouli
Pathobiology Department, Shahmirzad School of Veterinary Medicine, Semnan University, Semnan, Iran
Pathobiology Department, Faculty of Veterinary Medicine, Semnan University, Semnan, Iran

Ghazaleh Aghazamani
Shahmirzad School of Veterinary Medicine, Semnan University, Semnan, Iran

Alemselam Birhanu Mekonnin, A. Forbes Howie, Christopher C. Harlow and Simon C. Riley
MRC Centre for Reproductive Health, The Queen's Medical Research Institute College of Medicine and Veterinary Medicine, University of Edinburgh, Edinburgh, United Kingdom

Berihu Gebrekidan, Gebregiorgis Ashebir, Goitom Gidey, Desalew Tadesse Tegegne and Gidena Desta
College of Veterinary Medicine, Mekelle University, Mekelle, Ethiopia

Tadesse Gugsa
Tigray Regional State Agriculture Bureau, Tigray, Mekelle, Ethiopia

Barde Israel Joshua, Kumbish Peterside Rinle, Chukwu Doris Isioma, Rimfa Amos Gambo, Akanbi Babatunde Olatunde, Moses Gyang Davou, Ahmed James Saidu and Okewole Philip Ademola
Department of Central Diagnostic Laboratory, National Veterinary Research Institute, Plateau State, Nigeria

Bale James Olaniyi Olabode, Oladele Sunday Blessing and Fatihu Mohammed Yakassai
Department of Veterinary Pathology, Ahmadu Bello University, Zaria, Kaduna State, Nigeria

Zulifqar Ali Laghari and Ayaz Ali Samo
Department of Physiology, University of Sindh, Jamshoro, Sindh, Pakistan

Baradi Waryani, Zameer Ali Palh, Khalid Hussain Lashari and Gulshan Ara Sahato
Department of Fresh Water Biology and fisheries, University of Sindh, Jamshoro, Sindh, Pakistan
Ghulam Murtaza Mastoi
Centre for Environmental Sciences, University of Sindh, Jamshoro, Sindh, Pakistan

Tahira Jabeen Ursani
Department of Zoology, University of Sindh, Jamshoro, Sindh, Pakistan

Rodríguez-Tobón Ahiezer
Postgraduate in Experimental Biology, Autonomous Metropolitan University-Iztapalapa, Iztapalapa, Mexico

León-Galván Miguel A.
Department of Biology, Autonomous Metropolitan University-Iztapalapa, Iztapalapa, Mexico

Arenas-Ríos Edith
Department of Biology of Reproduction, Autonomous Metropolitan University-Iztapalapa, Iztapalapa, Mexico

Bidjeh Kebkiba, Mahamat Fayiz Abakar, Assandi Oussiguere, Assane Kembe, Tchari Doungous and Keilar Aurelie
Department of Animal Health, Livestock Research Institute for Development, N'Djamena, Chad

Ban-bo Bebanto Antipas
Department of Faculty of Exact and Applied Sciences, University of N'Djamena, N'Djamena, Chad

Taïtouin Sounkreo
Epidemiology Unit, Directorate of Veterinary Services, N'Djamena, Chad

Stella Ifeanyi Smith, Muinah Adenike Fowora, Emmanuel Adedayo Omonigbehin and Margaret Iteun Ugo-Ijeh
Molecular Biology and Biotechnology division, Nigerian Institute of Medical Research Yaba, Lagos, Nigeria

Adedamilola Atiba, Tina Fingesi, Mary Ehi Adamu, Moses Bamidele and Peter Odeigah
Cell Biology and Genetics department, University of Lagos, Akoka, Lagos, Nigeria

Joseph Anejo-Okopi
Microbiology department, University of Jos/Jos University Teaching Hospital, AIDS Prevention Initiative in Nigeria department, Jos, Nigeria

Volkan Yilmaz
Department of Virology, Faculty of Veterinary Medicine, University of Kafkas, Kars, Turkey
Guash Abay
Abergelle Agricultural Research Center, Abyi-Adi, Ethiopia

Tilaye Demissie
Addis Ababa University, Addis Ababa, Ethiopia

Amene Fekadu
Hawassa University, Hawassa, Ethiopia

Teshale Teklue
Mekelle Agricultural Research Center, Mekelle, Ethiopia

Arenas-Ríos Edith and Rosado Adolfo
Department of Biology of Reproduction, Autonomous Metropolitan University-Iztapalapa, Iztapalapa, Mexico

Rodríguez-Tobón Ernesto
Masters in Biology of Reproduction, Autonomous Metropolitan University-Iztapalapa, Iztapalapa, Mexico

Rodríguez-Tobón Ahiezer
PhD in Experimental Biology, Autonomous Metropolitan University-Iztapalapa, Iztapalapa, Mexico

León-Galván Miguel Ángel
Department of Biology, Autonomous Metropolitan University-Iztapalapa, Iztapalapa, Mexico

Deny A. Iyai
Department of Animal Production, Faculty of Animal Sciences, Papua University, Jl, Gunung Salju, Amban, Manokwari, Papua Barat Province, Indonesia
Perumahan Dosen, Papua University, Jl, Tugu Jepang, Amban, Manokwari, Papua Barat, Indonesia

Desni T. R. Saragih and Frandz P. Rumbiak
Department of Animal Production, Faculty of Animal Sciences, Papua University, Jl, Gunung Salju, Amban, Manokwari, Papua Barat Province, Indonesia

Teshale Teklue
Mekelle Agricultural Research Center, Mekelle, Ethiopia

Temesgen Tesfay, Solomon Wayu and Tesfay Atsbha
Alamata Agricultural Research center, Alamata, Ethiopia

Tsigabu Nirayo
Axum Agricultural Research Center, Axum, Ethiopia

Birhanu Hailu
Samara University, College of Veterinary Medicine, Department of Veterinary Epidemiology and Preventive Medicine, Samara, Ethiopia

Alemselam Birhanu Mekonnin
MRC Centre for Reproductive Health, CMVM, University of Edinburgh, Edinburgh, UK
College of Veterinary Medicine, Mekelle University, Tigray, Mekelle, Ethiopia

Christopher R. Harlow and Simon C. Riley
MRC Centre for Reproductive Health, CMVM, University of Edinburgh, Edinburgh, UK

Goitom Gidey, Desalew Tadesse and Gidena Desta
College of Veterinary Medicine, Mekelle University, Tigray, Mekelle, Ethiopia

Tadesse Gugssa
Tigray Bureau of Agriculture and Rural Development, Tigray, Mekelle, Ethiopia

Issa Youssouf Adoum, Bada Algom Oumar, Adam Bakhit Mustapha and Ardjoun Khalil Djalal
National High Institute of Sciences and Techniques, Abeche (INSTA) Ex University Institute of Sciences and Techniques, Abeche, Chad

Mopate Logtene Youssouf
Livestock Research Institute for Development (LRID) Ex Zootechnical and Veterinary Research Laboratory, N'Djamena, Chad

Vounparet Zeuh
Livestock Polytechnic Institute of Moussoro, Moussoro, Chad

Ayssiwede Simplice Bosco and Missohou Ayao
Inter-State School of Sciences and Veterinary Medicine, service of Animal Husbandry Food Sciences (EISMV), Dakar-Fann, Sénégal

Martínez-Coronel Matías and Munguía-Pérez Alma Alicia
Department of Biology, Autonomous Metropolitan University-Iztapalapa, Iztapalapa, Mexico

Arenas-Ríos Edith
Department of Biology of Reproduction, Autonomous Metropolitan University-Iztapalapa, Iztapalapa, Mexico
Rasha S. Ahmed
Department of Anatomy, Faculty of Veterinary Medicine, University of Khartoum, Khartoum, Sudan

Holger Martens
Institut of Physiology, Faculty of Veterinary Medicine (WE02), Berlin, Germany

Christoph Muelling
Institut of Anatomy, Faculty of Veterinary Medicine, Leipzig, Germany

Asghar Arshi, Esmaeil Mahmoudi, Mohammad-Saeid Jami and Abbas Doosti
Biotechnology Research Center, Islamic Azad University, Shahrekord Branch, Shahrekord, Iran

Moshfe Abdolali and Cheraghzadeh Seyed Reza
Cellular and Molecular Research Center, Yasuj University of Medical Sciences, Yasuj, Iran

Rezaei Nasrabad Seyed Abbas, Zare Khafri Roohollah, Moein Masood and Parhizgari Najmeh
Student Research Committee, Yasuj of University of Medical Sciences, Yasuj, Iran

Arefkhah Nasir and Jamshidi Ali
Department of Parasitology and Mycology, Yasuj University of Medical Sciences, Yasuj, Iran

Ogunlade Jacob Taiwo
Department of Animal Production and Health Sciences, Faculty of Agricultural Sciences, Ekiti State University, Ado-Ekiti, Nigeria

León-Galván Miguel Angel, Cano Espinoza José Sulim, Guzman Ledesma Beatriz Samantha and Guevara-Chumacero Luis Manuel
Department of Biology, Autonomous Metropolitan University-Iztapalapa, Mexico

Rodríguez-Tobón Ahiezer
Postgraduate in Experimental Biology, Autonomous Metropolitan University-Iztapalapa, Mexico

Leyequien Abarca Lissette
Direction of the Sierra La Mojonera Flora and Fauna Protection Area, National Commission of Natural Protected Areas (CONANP), S.L.P. Mexico

El Banna H. A., M. Atef and Ghazal Nabil
Department of Pharmacology, Faculty of Veterinary Medicine, Cairo University, Giza, Egypt

Birhanu Hailu and Gezahign Alemayehu
Samara University, College of Veterinary Medicine, Department of Veterinary Epidemiology and Preventive Medicine, Samara, Ethiopia
Berihu Gebrekidan, Solmon Raju, Alemselam Birhanu and Gebrehiwot Tadesse
Mekelle University, College of Veterinary Medicine, Mekelle, Ethiopia

Mohamed E. Ahmed, Talha E. Abbas, Mojahid A. Abdlhag and Dafaalla E. Mukhtar
Department of Animal Production, Faculty of Agricultural Technology and Fish Science, University of ALneelain, Khartoum, Sudan

Saghir Ahmad and ZahidaTasawar
Institute of Pure and Applied Biology, Bahauddin Zakariya University, Multan, Pakistan

Lulzim Millaku and Jeton Orllati
Department of Biology, Mathematics & Natural Science Faculty, University of Prishtina, Prishtina, Kosovo

Resmije Imeri
Department of Biology, Agricultural & Veterinary Faculty, University of Prishtina, Prishtina, Kosovo

Artan Trebicka
Department of Biology, Natural Science Faculty, University of Tirana, Tirana, Albania

Ahmed Hassan
Department of Veterinary Pathology, Faculty of Agriculture, Iwate University, 3-18-8, Ueda, Morioka, 020-8550, Japan
Department of Poultry diseases, Faculty of Veterinary Medicine, Assiut University, Assiut, 71526, Egypt

Mostafa Shahata, Elrefaie Refaie and Ragab Ibrahim
Department of Poultry diseases, Faculty of Veterinary Medicine, Assiut University, Assiut, 71526, Egypt

Jun Sasaki and Masanubu Goryo
Department of Veterinary Pathology, Faculty of Agriculture, Iwate University, 3-18-8, Ueda, Morioka, 020-8550, Japan

Abdullah Varlik and Ibrahim Kalayci
Department of Geodesy and Photogrammetry, Faculty of Architecture and Engineering, Necmettin Erbakan University, Konya, Turkey

Sema Ozkadif
Department of Nursing, School of Health, Batman University, Batman, Turkey
Emrullah Eken
Department of Anatomy, Faculty of Veterinary Medicine, Selcuk University, Konya, Turkey

Birhanu Hailu, Gezahign Alemayehu and Nuru Seid
Samara University, College of Veterinary Medicine, Department of Veterinary Epidemiology and Preventive Medicine, Samara, Ethiopia

Abubakar Abdullahi Biu
Department of Veterinary Microbiology, Parasitology and Virology, Faculty of Veterinary Medicine, University of Maiduguri, Nigeria

Gwana Adamu Mohammed
Laboratory Unit, A.H.P Department, Mohamet Lawan College Agriculture, Maiduguri, Nigeria

Bukar-Kolo M. Yachilla
Department of Medicine, Faculty of Veterinary Medicine, Unimaid, Nigeria

Bako M. Modu and Umaru Buba Wakil
Department of Fisheries, Faculty of Agriculture, Unimaid, Nigeria

Abdullahi M. Mai
Department of Basic Science, Mohamet Lawan College of Agriculture, Maiduguri, Nigeria

Ali Abba Gana Benisheikh
Department of Basic Science, Mohamet Lawan College of Agriculture, Maiduguri, Nigeria
Biotechnology Centre, University of Maiduguri, Maiduguri, Nigeria

Adarju M. B.
Chad Basin Development Authority, Gambaru-Ngala Road, Maiduguri, Nigeria

Getahun Kebede Yadete
Ruminant Livestock Research, Debre Zeit Agricultural Research Center, Debre Zeit, Ethiopia

Gezahegn Alemayehu, Birhanu Hailu and Nuru Seid
College of Veterinary Medicine, Samara University, Samara, Ethiopia

Temesgen Ayana
Department of Veterinary Laboratory Technology, Ambo University, Ambo, Ethiopia

Tegegn Gudeta
Max Planck Institute for Developmental Biology, Tuebingen, Germany

Md. Hemayatul Islam, Md. Jalal Uddin Sarder, Md. Akhtarul Islam, Syed Sarwar Jahan and Rashida Khaton
Department of Animal Husbandry and Veterinary Science, University of Rajshahi, Bangladesh

Md. Siddiqur Rahman
Faculty of Veterinary science, Bangladesh Agricultural University, Mymensing, Bangladesh

Md. Ariful Haque
Institute of Biological Sciences, University of Rajshahi, Rajshahi-6205, Bangladesh

Index

R

S

T

V